Biotechnology Entrepreneurship

Biotechnology Entrepreneurship

Starting, Managing, and Leading Biotech Companies

Craig Shimasaki, PhD, MBA

President & CEO, Moleculera Labs and BioSource Consulting Group,
Oklahoma City, Oklahoma

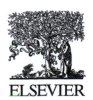

AMSTERDAM • BOSTON • HEIDELBERG • LONDON • NEW YORK • OXFORD • PARIS
SAN DIEGO • SAN FRANCISCO • SINGAPORE • SYDNEY • TOKYO

Academic Press is an imprint of Elsevier

Academic Press is an imprint of Elsevier
The Boulevard, Langford Lane, Kidlington, Oxford, OX5 1GB, UK
225 Wyman Street, Waltham, MA 02451, USA

Notices
Knowledge and best practice in this field are constantly changing. As new research and experience broaden our understanding, changes in research methods, professional practices, or medical treatment may become necessary.

Practitioners and researchers must always rely on their own experience and knowledge in evaluating and using any information, methods, compounds, or experiments described herein. In using such information or methods they should be mindful of their own safety and the safety of others, including parties for whom they have a professional responsibility.

To the fullest extent of the law, neither the Publisher nor the authors, contributors, or editors, assume any liability for any injury and/or damage to persons or property as a matter of products liability, negligence or otherwise, or from any use or operation of any methods, products, instructions, or ideas contained in the material herein.

British Library Cataloguing in Publication Data
A catalogue record for this book is available from the British Library

Library of Congress Cataloging in Publication Data
A catalog record for this book is available from the Library of Congress

ISBN: 978-0-12-404730-3

For information on all Academic Press publications
visit our website at store.elsevier.com

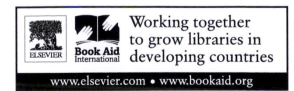

Working together
to grow libraries in
developing countries

www.elsevier.com • www.bookaid.org

To all the biotechnology entrepreneurs who have faced seemingly insurmountable odds and did not quit. Because of your vision and creativity you discovered resourceful ways to accomplish your goals, even at times using unconventional methods. Through your passion and persistence, many lives have been improved by your novel products that feed, fuel, and heal those in need. To all the biotechnology entrepreneurs who also pursued their goals with the same passion and vision as others, but who were never fortunate enough to see their creation reach the market—you too served a valuable purpose.

To each the biotechnology pioneers no longer with us who had the fortitude to blaze a trail that multitudes can now follow, we are grateful for your insight and vision that ushered in the biotechnology era. As the twelfth century author John of Salisbury said: "We are like dwarfs sitting on the shoulders of giants. We see more, and things that are more distant than they did, not because our sight is superior or because we are taller than they, but because they raise us up, and by their great stature add to ours."

To my mother and father who gave me opportunity and confidence; to my children Alyssa, Adam, and Lori, who inspire me to be a better father. Finally, to Verna, my loving wife of 36 years and my best friend, I am deeply grateful to you for being with me throughout our life journey together.

Contents

22. Your Business Plan and Presentation: Articulating Your Journey to Commercialization

Lowell W. Busenitz, PhD, MBA

Section VII
Biotechnology Product Development

23. Therapeutic Drug Development and Human Clinical Trials

Donald R. Kirsch, PhD

24. Development and Commercialization of *In Vitro* Diagnostics: Applications for Companion Diagnostics

John F. Beeler, PhD

25. Regulatory Approval and Compliances for Biotechnology Products

Norman W. Baylor, PhD

26. The Biomanufacturing of Biotechnology Products

*John Conner, MS, Don Wuchterl, Maria Lopez,
Bill Minshall, MS, Rabi Prusti, PhD, Dave Boclair,
Jay Peterson and Chris Allen, MS*

This is not just a book, but a compilation of experiences, advice, and lessons learned from biotechnology pioneers and leaders who have worked and served in this industry for many decades. There is an old saying "Learn from the mistakes of others because you will never live long enough to make them all yourself." We have all made a few of these ourselves, and experience is one of our greatest teachers. But without a recounting of lessons learned by others, we are destined to "relearn" these same lessons anew. What you are about to read are insights, guidance, and advice from veterans in this industry, sharing best practices in starting, managing, and leading biotechnology companies.

The biotechnology industry diligently pursues better, faster, and more effective methods of translating ideas into needed commercial products. Products are produced by companies, and companies are started and managed by entrepreneurial leaders. Therefore, it is vital to "produce" more effective entrepreneurial leaders and managers who are knowledgeable, better equipped, and have the acumen necessary to make wise decisions for building successful biotechnology companies. Seasoned entrepreneurial leaders are one of our scarcest resources and yet they are *the* most critical factor in predicting the future success of a company. Leaders and managers make decisions each day that affect the likelihood of success or failure for their organization and for the products they are developing. I believe that it is equally, if not more, important to develop knowledgeable and wise leaders who will shepherd the next generation of biotechnology companies.

The idea for this book came about primarily from two realizations. The first one was the recognition of my own inner frustrations while toiling through an inefficient, trial-and-error learning process as a serial entrepreneur of three biotechnology companies. I was fortunate to have started my career at Genentech in the early 1980s, and I witnessed first-hand the exciting opportunities and the unforeseen challenges of developing biotechnology products. However, even with that experience, I did not feel adequately prepared for the deluge of decisions that accompanied starting, managing, and leading a biotechnology company. As years went by, I recognized familiar overarching issues that arose at each successive company, and these issues were similar to those other entrepreneurs faced as they started and grew their companies.

The second realization came while listening to successful entrepreneurs and talented professionals who shared nuggets of wisdom and insight about their experiences and journey. Inspiration came while listening to fireside chats with Henri Termeer, former Chairman, CEO and President of Genzyme, who shared his experiences and gave us his insightful admonitions. More ideas came while hearing talks from seasoned industry professionals about how to strengthen intellectual property protection, pragmatic regulatory guidance, sensible market strategies, and practical fundraising advice. Then there was the realization that many of our early biotechnology pioneers were no longer with us. Sadly, there are relatively few books dedicated to teaching, training, and guiding new leaders and managers of biotechnology enterprises, and I found no written materials that comprehensively captured all of this knowledge.

My desire was to assemble a comprehensive work written by seasoned experts in the business of biotechnology, explaining the fundamental issues that students, practitioners, and future managers of biotechnology companies would need to know to be proficient in this industry. These writings are not only for them but also for the many professionals that support the biotechnology industry, government, and community leaders who are working to grow biotechnology clusters in their region, including individuals who want to be employed within this diverse industry.

In this book you will find a wealth of information and inspiration that provide the next generation of biotechnology entrepreneurs an improved chance of achieving success in this exciting, yet challenging industry. You will find this to be a guidebook to help entrepreneurial leaders, managers, practitioners, and industry supporters, gain "experience" through the lessons these individuals have learned. Within these covers you will hear first-hand accounts of early founders of biotechnology companies, confirming that starting and growing biotechnology companies is not a prescriptive endeavor. You will also hear from veteran entrepreneurs and industry professionals sharing insights about what they learned over many years in this industry. Topics such as: what is a biotechnology entrepreneur and what are the characteristics that make them successful; how to assess a technology product idea; growing biotechnology clusters in a region; licensing and protecting intellectual property strategies; what are the best sources of capital at different stages of development, angel capital, venture capital; product approval processes; reimbursement strategies; biotechnology partnerships; drug, diagnostics, and bioagriculture development processes; biomanufacturing; careers in the life science industry, and even bioethics.

The biotechnology industry and biotechnology entrepreneurship subject matter is vast and expanding with new knowledge and discoveries occurring almost daily and it is a formidable task to compile this subject matter. Yet it would be presumptuous to believe that this is an exhaustive treatment of all the information in this vast industry to everyone's satisfaction. However, this book aspires to be a major step toward compiling the essential parts and pieces necessary for biotechnology leaders, managers, and entrepreneurs to be informed of the key elements necessary to build and manage successful biotechnology companies.

Biotechnology companies are a melding of both science and business and, therefore, successful leaders are skilled risk managers of a scientific uncertainty business. However, one cannot manage the risks that they do not know. Our purpose and goal is to teach, train, and inspire current and future biotechnology entrepreneurs, leaders, and managers to be more successful in this rewarding and challenging industry. If we have accomplished that in any way, I will have considered this work a success.

I would greatly appreciate any feedback about this book and I solicit any suggestions on how we may improve its value to you. You may send any comments to me at cs@biosourceconsulting.com.

Craig Shimasaki, Ph.D, MBA
President & CEO
Moleculera Labs
BioSource Consulting Group
Oklahoma City, Oklahoma

Carl B. Feldbaum, JD

Among the fascinating aspects of biotechnology is the fact that this endeavor did not exist when the pioneers of the industry were growing up. Back in the day, it was not a career choice in high school or college—there were no courses you could take, no majors or minors you could elect to prepare you for what was to come. And I would be willing to bet that when asked what they wanted to be when they grew up, *no one* answered "a biotechnology entrepreneur."

With a scant background in biology, then short careers in law, national security affairs, and politics, I was "adopted" by the biotech village in 1993, when the Biotechnology Industry Organization (BIO) was first formed. Associating with those pioneer scientists, CEOs, and financial gurus has been the best part of my professional life. Put simply, their risk-taking behavior in uncharted territory, resilience, and dedication to helping others remain both inspirational and instructive.

When BIO was established 20 years ago, our infant industry was struggling to apply new molecular and genetic understanding to drug discovery, was running into financial and regulatory walls, and was attempting to adapt to proposals for comprehensive healthcare reform. Plus we encountered controversies over patents, cloning (remember Dolly?), NIH funding, GMOs, among others. Do these sound familiar?

Now, finally, we have this textbook, which serves as a roadmap and operating manual to guide the next generation of biotech entrepreneurs. The chapters that follow cover the waterfront—the whole constellation of issues you'll confront, the hardest nuts you'll have to crack. The authors of these chapters share their experience generously and forthrightly in a fashion that characterizes the best mentors of any industry, especially biotech.

Philosopher George Santayana's most famous reflection is often cited but too rarely heeded. Allow me to remind you that he said "Those who do not learn from history are condemned to repeat it." Trust me, it's worth learning from the biotech pioneers who have authored the chapters that follow. Having been there, done that, they can help you avoid many of the pitfalls that remain particular to this endeavor. They have made their mistakes, and for the most part have learned from them. What follows is high-value, even inspirational guidance.

Read on and go forth, but this will not be the end of the story. A confident prediction: biotechnology will transform the twenty-first century well beyond what chemistry and physics accomplished earlier. There is much further uncharted territory. Those are the chapters you will write.

Carl Feldbaum grew up in Philadelphia, graduated from Princeton University with a B.A. in Biology and a J.D. from the University of Pennsylvania Law School. He served as an Assistant District Attorney in his hometown, then as a prosecutor on the Watergate Special Prosecution Force in Washington, D.C. He later served as Inspector General for Defense Intelligence in the Pentagon, president of Palomar Corporation, a national security think tank, and as chief-of-staff to U.S. Senator Arlen Specter. In 1993 he helped found the Biotechnology Industry Organization and served as its president for 12 years until his "retirement" in 2005. In 2001 he was elected to the Biotechnology Hall of Fame. Carl now serves on several public and nonprofit biotech boards of directors.

Acknowledgements

I am immensely grateful to each of the many authors for their contribution to this book, and for being fervent supporters of the biotechnology industry. Each of them are successful in their own right and have selflessly authored their chapter in the midst of a demanding workload. They have graciously shared their knowledge, insights, and lessons they have learned during their professional careers in order to teach the next generation of biotechnology entrepreneurs.

I wish to thank Mr. Graham Nesbit, Acquisitions Editor of Elsevier, who recognized the value and need for such a book and who graciously accommodated the extended timeframe required to complete this comprehensive work.

Thanks to Ms. Cassie Van Der Laan and Ms. Debbie Clark for their tireless efforts and help in finalizing this manuscript and working out the necessary details to bring this work to print. Thanks to Dr. Mickey Young, neurologist and patent attorney, who graciously volunteered to review many of the chapters and who provided excellent feedback and comments.

A special thanks to my wife Verna who read and assisted in editing the seemingly endless revisions to many of the chapters in this book. Lastly, and without reservation, I acknowledge and give thanks to God, who makes all things that seem impossible—possible!

Chris Allen, MS Senior Manager Facilities and Engineering, Cytovance Biologics Inc., Oklahoma City, Oklahoma

Jack M. Anthony Founder and Principal, BioMentorz, Inc., Healdsburg, California

Norman W. Baylor, PhD President & CEO, Biologics Consulting Group, Inc., Alexandria, Virginia

John F. Beeler, PhD Director, Theranostics and Business Development bioMerieux, Cambridge, Massachusetts

Dave Boclair Manager Manufacturing Downstream Operations, Cytovance Biologics Inc., Oklahoma City, Oklahoma

Arthur A. Boni, PhD John R. Thorne Distinguished Career Professor of Entrepreneurship, Tepper School of Business at Carnegie Mellon University, Pittsburgh, Pennsylvania

Craig C. Bradley, JD Partner, Edwards Wildman Palmer LLP, Chicago, Illinois

G. Steven Burrill CEO, Burrill & Company, San Francisco, California

Lowell W. Busenitz, PhD, MBA Academic Director, Price College Center for Entrepreneurship, University of Oklahoma, Norman, Oklahoma

Robert J. Calcaterra, DSC President, St. Louis Arch Angels, St. Louis, Missouri

John Conner, MS Vice President Manufacturing Science and Technology, Cytovance Biologics, Inc., Oklahoma City, Oklahoma

Gerry J. Elman, MS, JD Elman Technology Law, P.C., Swarthmore, Pennsylvania

Steven M. Ferguson, CLP Deputy Director, Licensing & Entrepreneurship, Office of Technology Transfer, National Institutes of Health, Rockville, Maryland

Toby Freedman, PhD President, Synapsis Search Recruiting, Portolavalley, California

Susan Garfield, DrPH Senior Vice President, GfK Custom Research LLC, Wayland, Massachusetts

James C. Greenwood President & CEO, Biotechnology Industry Organization (BIO), Washington, D.C.

Neal Gutterson, PhD President & CEO, Mendel Biotechnology, Hayward, California

Phil Haworth, PhD, JD Principal, Biomentorz, Inc. Redwood City, California

Uma S. Kaundinya, PhD, CLP President & CEO, Aavishkar Innovations Inc., Bedford, Massachusetts

Donald R. Kirsch, PhD Chief Scientific Officer, Cambria Pharmaceuticals, Cambridge, Massachusetts

Joan E. Kureczka, MSEM Founder and Principal, Kureczka/Martin Associates and The Vivant Group, San Francisco, California

Lynn Johnson Langer, PhD, MBA Director, Enterprise and Regulatory Science Programs Center for Biotechnology Education, Johns Hopkins University, Rockville, Maryland

Maria Lopez Vice President Quality Systems, Cytovance Biologics Inc., Oklahoma City, Oklahoma

Lara V. Marks, D.Phil. (Oxon) Senior Research Fellow, Department of Social Science, Health and Medicine, King's College, London, England

Bill Minshall, MS Senior Vice President Regulatory Affairs, Cytovance Biologics Inc., Oklahoma City, Oklahoma

Jay Peterson Manager Manufacturing Upstream Operations, Cytovance Biologics Inc., Oklahoma City, Oklahoma

Rabi Prusti, PhD Executive Director Quality Control, Cytovance Biologics Inc., Oklahoma City, Oklahoma

Craig Shimasaki, PhD, MBA President & CEO, Moleculera Labs and BioSource Consulting Group, Oklahoma City, Oklahoma

Henri A. Termeer Former Chairman, CEO and President of Genzyme Corporation, Cambridge, Massachusetts

Gergana Todorova, PhD Assistant Professor, School of Business Administration, University of Miami, Coral Gables, Florida

Tom D. Walker CEO & President, TechColumbus, Inc., Columbus, Ohio

Robert E. Wanerman, JD, MPH Epstein Becker Green, P.C., Washington, D.C.

Laurie R. Weingart, PhD Carnegie Bosch Professor of Organizational Behavior and Theory, Tepper School of Business at Carnegie Mellon University, Pittsburgh, Pennsylvania

Gladys B. White, PhD Adjunct Professor of Liberal Studies, Georgetown University, Washington, D.C.

Don Wuchterl Senior Vice President Operations, Cytovance Biologics Inc., Oklahoma City, Oklahoma

Jay Z. Zhang, MS, JD Shuwen Biotech Co. Ltd., Deqing, Zhejiang Province, China and Momentous IP Ventures LLC, Salt Lake City, Utah

Biotechnology Entrepreneurship

Chapter 1

Unleashing the Promise of Biotechnology to Help Heal, Fuel, and Feed the World

James C. Greenwood

President and CEO, Biotechnology Industry Organization (BIO), Washington, D.C.

Biotechnology is a significant part of our lives, often in ways we may not realize. Biotechnology has enabled the creation of breakthrough products and technologies to combat disease, protect the environment, feed the hungry, produce fuels, and make other useful products. We can see biotechnology at work each day in our homes, workplaces, and everywhere in between. Biotechnology enables and improves the production of the food we eat, the clothes we wear, the consumer products we use, and the medicines we take.

Humans have used some form of biotechnology since the dawn of civilization. The biotech products of today might seem like miracles to our ancestors, but they are developed on a foundation of hard-won scientific knowledge discovered by countless generations of researchers and visionaries. As a biotech entrepreneur or investor, you will build on this foundation and be part of the most transformative industry of the twenty-first century. Your work will help save lives and improve the quality of life for potentially billions of people around the world.

The modern biotechnology industry emerged in the 1970s, based largely on a new recombinant DNA technique published in 1973 by Stanley Cohen of Stanford University and Herbert Boyer of the University of California. Recombinant DNA and subsequent discoveries have enhanced and accelerated our ability to develop practical biotechnology products to help us live longer and healthier lives, have a more abundant and sustainable food supply, use cleaner and more efficient processes for industrial manufacturing [1]. and reduce our greenhouse gas footprint. As of 2013, biotechnology is a more than $83 billion global industry. In 2012, the U.S. government released a *National Bioeconomy Blueprint* noting that bioscience industries are "a large and rapidly growing segment of the world economy that provides substantial public benefit." Nations around the world make large investments in the bioscience industry because they want the benefits of biotech innovation along with the good jobs and economic development that biotech brings.

The men and women of the biotechnology industry help heal, fuel, and feed the world. They also create immense economic value. This chapter will discuss a few of the many accomplishments of the biotechnology industry and some of the astounding breakthroughs on the horizon—new advances which you may play an important role in developing. It will also focus on the role that good public policy must play in supporting the biotechnology industry.

HEALTH BIOTECHNOLOGY: HELPING TO SAVE AND EXTEND LIVES

Biotechnology product developments are transforming the practice of medicine and providing new and better ways to detect, treat, and prevent disease. These products provide targeted treatments to minimize health risks and side-effects for individual patients. Biotechnology tools and techniques open new research avenues for discovering how healthy bodies work and what goes wrong when problems arise.

The first biotech drug for human use, human insulin produced by genetically modified bacteria, was approved by the U.S. Food and Drug Administration (FDA) in 1982. Today, the recombinant DNA technology that made production of human insulin and many other biologic medicines possible has been joined in the biotech tool kit by monoclonal antibodies, cellular therapy, gene therapy, RNA interference, stem cells, regenerative medicine, tissue engineering, new vaccine approaches, and other innovative technologies. (see Figure 1.1).

In the past decade, there have been approximately 300 new prescription medicines approved for use by the FDA [2]. There are more than 900 new biotech medicines in development for conditions including diabetes, blood disorders, Alzheimer's disease, autoimmune disorders, and many more. Biotechnology has revolutionized healthcare in many ways. Yet much more remains to be done in humanity's age-old battle against disease. Worldwide, more than 17 million

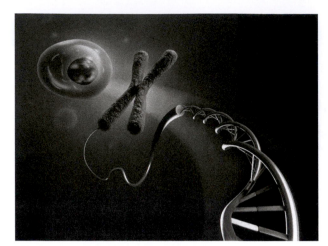

FIGURE 1.1 DNA is the genetic code for life

people die each year from cardiovascular disease [3]. More than seven million lives are lost to cancer [4]. More than a billion people, most of them in the developing world, are affected by deadly malaria, tuberculosis and sleeping sickness [5]. Approximately 300 million people suffer from one of the more than 7000 known rare diseases [6].

The promise of biotech is to reduce suffering and extend lives by developing better ways to detect, treat, and prevent diseases at a genetic or molecular level. This will give us all a better chance to enjoy longer, healthier, and more productive lives. Let's look at some of the ways biotech has made a difference and where we might find the next lifesaving breakthrough.

Saving Lives with Vaccines

Vaccines and immunizations represent the greatest successes of biotechnology in sheer number of lives saved. Most people in the developed world take it for granted that their child will not die struggling for breath inside an iron lung due to paralysis from polio. We have little worry that our kids will be permanently scarred from the ravages of smallpox or die from complications of measles or from whooping cough. Diseases that inspired fear and ended untold millions of lives for most of human history are now nearly forgotten. Vaccines make this peace of mind possible.

By the beginning of the twentieth century, vaccines existed for rabies, diphtheria, typhoid fever, and the plague. By the 1990s, smallpox and polio had been eradicated or nearly eradicated worldwide, preventing millions of deaths. Worldwide, 2.5 million child deaths are prevented each year by immunization. In this past decade alone, the biopharmaceutical industry has added to our arsenal new vaccines for shingles, pneumonia, human papilloma virus (which causes a common form of cervical cancer), and rotavirus (an infection fatal to many infants). Vaccine companies are now working to develop preventive vaccines against dangerous hospital infections such as group B streptococcus (GBS)

or *Staphylococcus aureus*; vaccines for neglected diseases such as dengue, malaria, and tuberculosis; and new pediatric vaccines. Research and investment in therapeutic vaccines has opened up new possibilities for treating hepatitis, many cancers, Alzheimer's, diabetes, and other conditions. Immunology and vaccine development continue to be a promising and vital field of health biotechnology (Figure 1.2).

Surviving Cancer Like Never Before

Biotechnology is helping us make substantial progress in the fight against cancer. For more and more patients, a cancer diagnosis is no longer the death sentence it once was. Due to new, more effective treatments and other medical advances, survival rates have increased significantly for many types of cancer. For example, childhood leukemia is now cured in 80 percent of cases, testicular cancer in more than 90 percent of cases, and Hodgkin's lymphoma in more than 90 percent of cases. Cancer nevertheless remains the third leading cause of worldwide deaths each year, with global rates expected to double by 2020 and triple by 2030, resulting in 17 million cancer deaths that year.

Biotechnology is helping us better understand the molecular and genetic basis of cancer. We can now develop targeted treatments that use gene-based tests to match patients with optimal drugs and drug dosages.

Oncology is approaching an era when cancer treatment will be determined more by the genetic signature of the tumor than by its location in the body. For example, one therapeutic cancer vaccine in development aims to stimulate the immune system to attack cancer cells common to lung, breast, prostate, and colorectal cancer cells while leaving healthy cells unharmed. There are now more than 350 new biopharmaceutical cancer medicines in development [7].

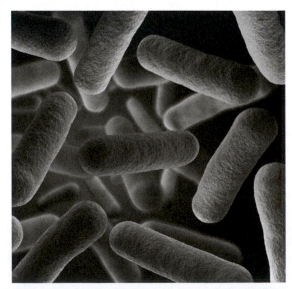

FIGURE 1.2 Vaccines are developed to combat infections from bacteria and other infectious organisms

Cancer treatment and prevention is another therapeutic area with high stakes and an urgent need for progress.

Improving Quality of Life

Even when biotechnology cannot yet offer a cure, biomedicines can greatly improve quality of life for patients with serious chronic illnesses. For example, innovative treatments are changing the outlook for multiple sclerosis (MS), an autoimmune disease that affects the brain and spinal cord. Due to nerve damage, MS patients can suffer severe symptoms in all parts of the body, including muscle loss, loss of bladder and bowel control, and vision loss. While a cure remains elusive, new biologic treatments have been shown to improve walking ability by 25 percent [8]. Similarly, a class of therapies called antiretrovirals has changed the prognosis for patients with HIV. Access to antiretroviral therapy has resulted in substantial declines in the number of people dying from AIDS-related reasons during the past decade. Mounting scientific evidence suggests that increased access to antiretroviral therapy is also contributing substantially to declines in the number of people acquiring HIV infection [9].

Other biologic medicines help some cancer patients avoid the debilitating side-effects of traditional chemotherapy, help certain cystic fibrosis patients breathe easier, and bring relief to many sufferers of rheumatoid arthritis and other immune disorders. Our ultimate goal is always to find cures and preventions for disease, but there is also great satisfaction in knowing that breakthroughs in biotechnology also help people with serious debilitating conditions move, breathe, and live a little easier.

Rare Diseases

If all of the people with rare diseases lived in one country, it would be the world's third most populous. A rare disease is one affecting fewer than 200,000 people. There are nearly 7000 such conditions. The vast majority of these conditions affect fewer than 6000 people each, but all of these rare diseases combined affect approximately 300 million people worldwide. Unfortunately, the healthcare needs of rare-disease patients are often unmet. The economics of developing a new drug for a small population are daunting and require strong public policy support, such as the incentives in the Orphan Drug Act, along with strong partnerships among biotech entrepreneurs, patient communities, healthcare providers, government, and others.

Today, fewer than 300 of the known rare diseases have FDA-approved therapies. Many of the existing treatments are biologic medicines and biotech companies currently have a record 460 medicines for rare disease in late-stage development [10].Treatment of rare diseases is a compelling opportunity for bioentrepreneurs who want to help meet the unique needs of this huge, yet often underserved, patient population.

Faster Detection, Better Accuracy, Greater Mobility

Biotech diagnostic tools have enhanced our ability to detect and diagnose conditions faster and with greater accuracy. There are more than 1200 biotech-based diagnostic tests in clinical use [11]. These range from faster and more accurate strep throat tests to tests that pinpoint-specific cancer cells to select treatment options. Genetic tests are available to detect approximately 2200 conditions, both common and rare, including tests for cancers, infectious diseases, and inherited genetic disorders [12]. Many require only a simple blood sample or mouth swab. Such tests can eliminate the need for costly and invasive exploratory surgeries. These tests analyze a patient's genetic material (DNA, RNA, chromosomes, and genes) as well as the molecular products of genes (biomarkers such as proteins, enzymes, or metabolites) that may indicate a disorder. Some newer molecular tests can also identify biomarkers indicating the presence of specific infectious agents, such as a virus, faster and more cost-effectively than can certain other existing alternatives (Figure 1.3).

Many biotech diagnostic tools are portable, allowing physicians to conduct tests, interpret results, and determine treatment during an office visit rather than having to wait for results to be developed in a potentially distant lab. These tools have improved access to healthcare in developing countries, many of which lack a sufficient healthcare delivery infrastructure.

Personalized Medicine

Advances in biotechnology also can help healthcare providers tailor treatments to the individual patient, guided by genetic information and biomarkers. This is an example

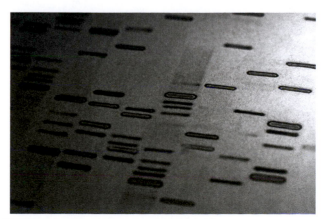

FIGURE 1.3   Genetic signatures and DNA ladders

of *personalized medicine*: leveraging information from an individual's genome and other unique biological characteristics to guide healthcare decisions, rather than treating every individual like the anonymous statistical average (Figure 1.4).

The cost of sequencing an individual's entire genome is rapidly falling, approaching the widely touted goal of sequencing an entire human genome for $1000 or less. As the cost declines, the possibility that full-genome sequencing will become a routine part of clinical care in the not too distant future increases. Current genetic tests can identify patients predisposed to developing various cancers, osteoporosis, emphysema, type II diabetes, and asthma. This information gives patients an opportunity to take early preventive steps by avoiding disease triggers such as poor diet, smoking, and other behavioral factors. This capability, combined with the diagnostic tools noted above, shows great promise for helping to prevent and treat chronic conditions and make overall healthcare more effective.

Genetic testing and molecular diagnostics also enable treatment regimens tailored to the individual patient. One study found hospitalization rates dropped 30 percent when genetic information was used to determine the best dosing for heart patients taking warfarin (the world's most-prescribed blood thinner) [13]. Another diagnostic test enables selection of the correct dosage of a powerful chemotherapy drug for pediatric leukemia. These tests have saved lives by preventing overdose fatalities. Other diagnostic tests look for specific biomarkers that indicate whether a patient is likely to benefit from a certain treatment. The transition to personalized medicine is expected to accelerate, enabling us to detect disease at an earlier stage when it can be treated more effectively. Personalized medicine can also reduce "trial and error" prescribing, emphasize proactive care, prevention and targeted

therapies, and shift the emphasis of medicine from reaction to prevention. By enabling these advances, biotech innovators help to reduce human suffering from disease, save lives, and revolutionize healthcare.

Looking Ahead

Biotechnology companies continue to develop promising new tools. Gene therapy, tissue engineering, and other advances are further transforming how we think about and treat disease, injuries, and disabilities. Scientists can now engineer replacement human organs for transplant using stem cells cultured from a patient's own body. Relatively simple organs like a bladder or trachea have been successfully used in surgery. Researchers are developing techniques to grow more complex organs, including hearts. The realm of the impossible gets smaller every day thanks to dedicated biotech scientists and entrepreneurs.

FOOD AND AGRICULTURAL BIOTECHNOLOGY: HELPING TO FEED THE WORLD

One of the challenges that biotech scientists and entrepreneurs are working to solve is how we address the needs of a growing world population. Today, there are more than 7 billion people living on our planet. However, by 2050, the global population is expected to reach 9 billion. That is many more mouths to feed. In fact, according to the United Nations Food and Agriculture Organization (UN-FAO), we will have to double world food production to do it. With most of the world's arable land already in production we'll need to make existing acreage much more productive. Biotechnology is helping us do so. The era of biotechnology-enhanced agriculture began in the 1990s with government approval for commercial deployment of biotech soybeans, corn, cotton, canola, and papaya. Because of their tremendous production advantages, biotech crops have become the most rapidly adopted technology in the history of agriculture and, in 2013, biotech crops were used by more than 17.3 million farmers on more than 420 million acres of farmland in 28 countries [14].

Biotech crops increase yields, thereby improving food security and enabling significant environmental, economic, and nutritional benefits. Animal biotechnology also contributes by increasing livestock production along with other benefits. A few examples of how agriculture biotechnology is helping to feed the world are found below.

Plant Biotechnology

Biotech tools enable plant breeders to select single genes that produce desired traits and move them from one plant

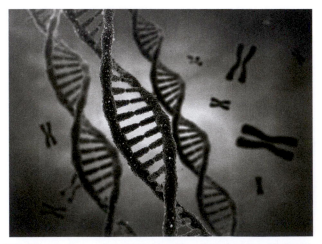

FIGURE 1.4 Personalized medicine utilizes the uniqueness of our genes

to another. These tools can also move genetic traits between plants and other organisms to achieve desired higher yields and other benefits (Figure 1.5).

- **Insect resistance:** Biotech crops with insect resistance (IR) traits reduce crop losses to insect pests. For instance, scientists have incorporated into corn, cotton, and other crops a gene from *bacillus thuringinesis* (Bt), a common soil bacterium that produces a protein that effectively paralyzes the larvae of the corn borer and the cotton bollworm—the most destructive pests to corn and cotton crops. This gives the crops a built-in defense against their most threatening insect enemies without the need to use spray-on pesticides.
- **Herbicide tolerance:** Herbicide-tolerant (HT) crops have genetic traits that make them tolerant of certain herbicides. This allows farmers to spray herbicide to destroy the weeds without damaging the crops. This method saves labor and fuel for motorized equipment and also promotes no-till farming, which can cut soil erosion by up to 90 percent. The most common herbicide-tolerant crops are cotton, corn, soybeans, and canola.
- **Resistance to environmental stresses:** Researchers are developing new products that have imported useful genes from other species to improve crop-plant tolerance for harsh conditions. Some of the products developed include plants with increased saline tolerance, drought tolerance, flood tolerance, and cold or heat tolerance. These traits will help farmers bring marginal lands into production and overcome some of the negative impacts of climate change.

Other Traits

Other engineered traits can help deliver benefits to farmers and society. For example, increasing the nitrogen-use efficiency of crops reduces the need for expensive nitrogen fertilizers and delayed-ripening (DR) technology will give farmers more flexibility in marketing their produce, reduce spoilage, and provide consumers with "fresh-from-the-garden" produce.

Biotechnology also can enable plants to produce healthier and more nutritious foods. Over time, these developments could help improve the nutrition of billions of people in the developing world by fortifying their staple crops with the nutrients that are typically missing from their diets. One example is "golden rice" enhanced with β-carotene to help fight Vitamin A deficiency, a leading cause of blindness in the developing world. Other innovations that have been undertaken enhance the iron content of some foods, which could help prevent anemia that affects 2 billion people worldwide due to insufficient iron in their diet. For some other food crops, biotechnology is used to express positive oil traits, such as Omega-3 fatty acids associated with improved cardiovascular health. Omega-3-enhanced soybean has been approved [15] and other enhanced-oil crops are in development. Scientists are also developing consumer-friendly improvements such as nonallergenic peanuts and improvements to the taste, texture, or the appearance of fruits and vegetables.

Stacked Traits

One of the most promising areas for the future of plant biotechnology is our expanding ability to "stack" traits, that is, to introduce more than one transgene into a crop to add multiple beneficial traits at once. The first commercial biotech crop with stacked traits was a cotton seed introduced in 1997 which had both insect resistance and herbicide tolerance traits. By 2011, 26 percent of all biotech crops planted had stacked traits [14].

Benefits of Plant Biotechnology

Biotech crops help farmers increase yields, which is essential if we are to feed the growing world population. Today more than 90 percent of corn, 90 percent of cotton, and 93 percent of soybeans grown in the United States are biotech crops [16]. Farmers have increased corn yield by more than 33 percent and soybean yield by 22 percent in the United States since the introduction of biotech crops. Through 2010, biotech crops have helped produce an additional 300 million tons of canola, cotton, corn, and soybean (Figure 1.6) [17].

Biotech crops also have significant environmental benefits. The adoption of HT crops has increased no-till agriculture by 69 percent [18], which reduces soil erosion and improves water quality. Through 2013, biotech crops have helped drive a 1.05 billion pound reduction in pesticide applications [17]. Reduced tilling and pesticide use also means less energy use and reduced greenhouse gas emissions. In 2011, biotech crops helped prevent the release of 23 billion kilograms of CO_2, the equivalent of taking almost 10.2 million cars off the road [17]. Biotech crops also

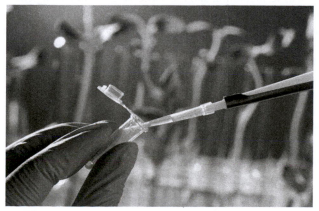

FIGURE 1.5   Genetic engineering for insect-resistant plants

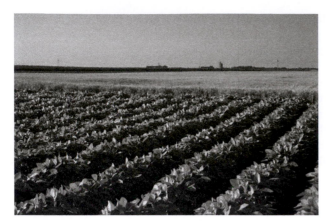

FIGURE 1.6 Biotechnology increases yields in soybeans

increase farmer incomes. In 2011, biotech crops created a net economic benefit of $19.8 billion at the farm level. More than half of these farm income gains went to farmers in developing countries [17]. Of the 17.3 million farmers growing biotech crops, more than 90 percent are small, resource-poor farmers from developing countries. The additional income generated by the use of biotech crops make a significant difference in their quality of life and ability to feed, care for, and educate their families.

In short, plant biotechnology helps feed the world, grow the agricultural economy, improve human health and nutrition [19] and make for a cleaner environment. Yet we are still in the early days of this technology, with many more potential benefits in store.

Animal Biotechnology

Rapidly rising global incomes and urbanization, along with population growth, is increasing the demand for meat and other animal products in many developing countries. Biotechnology contributes to meeting this rising demand by enabling healthier livestock populations and helping animal breeders better manage their herds for desired traits. Technologies such as embryo transfers, *in vitro* fertilization, cloning, and sex determination of embryos allow breeders to improve their herds. Biotech diagnostics, vaccines, and medicines help diagnose, treat, and prevent animal diseases in livestock. Other biotech products increase the digestibility of animal feed and improve animal nutrition, helping animals grow faster or, in the case of dairy cattle, produce more milk per unit of feed consumed.

Livestock can also be genetically engineered to use feed more efficiently and produce less manure. For example, the Enviropig™, which was previously under development, is a genetically engineered (GE) pig uniquely able to digest the phosphorus in cereal grain. This limits the amount of phosphorus in the pig manure, reducing pollution. Other developments are improving disease resistance in animals, such as birds that don't transmit the H1N1 (avian flu) virus

or cattle resistant to BSE (mad cow disease) and common infections such as mastitis. In aquaculture, scientists have developed a genetically engineered salmon that can reach its market weight in half the time of conventionally raised salmon.

Animal Biotech: Beyond Food

Animal biotech, along with plant biotechnology, offers a nearly limitless range of new applications for the next wave of scientists and entrepreneurs to develop. Scientists have engineered animals for many nonfood applications. These include:

- Xenotransplantation, using biotech animals as blood, organ, or tissue donors for human patients.
- Production of therapeutic agents, such as human antibody production in cattle, or the production of novel proteins, vaccines, drugs, and tissues.
- Models of human disease, like pigs that model heart disease or cystic fibrosis.
- In 2009, the FDA approved the first product from a genetically engineered animal. ATryn, an anticoagulant used for the prevention of blood clots in patients with a rare disease known as hereditary antithrombin (AT) deficiency, is made from GE goats [20].

INDUSTRIAL AND ENVIRONMENTAL BIOTECHNOLOGY: A BETTER WAY TO MAKE THINGS

Industrial biotechnology is one of the most promising new approaches to help meet the global challenges of preventing pollution, conserving energy and natural resources, and reducing manufacturing costs. The application of biotechnology to industrial processes is transforming how we produce existing products and helping to generate new products that were not even imagined a few years ago. Industrial biotechnology uses natural biological processes, such as fermentation and the harnessing of enzymes, yeasts, and microbes as microscopic manufacturing plants, to produce useful products. Among the products being made with industrial biotechnology are biodegradable plastics, renewable chemicals, energy-saving low-temperature detergents, pollution-eating bacteria, multivitamins, and biofuels. With the growing adoption of industrial biotech, we are in the early stages of an emerging biobased economy that meets some of the most important needs of our global civilization.

Working with Nature

Industrial biotechnology is grounded in biocatalysis and fermentation technology. Industrial biotech involves working with nature to maximize and optimize existing biochemical

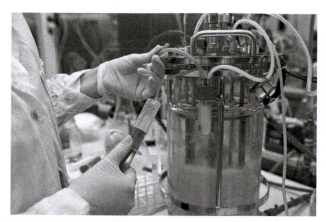

FIGURE 1.7   Lab-scale industrial biotechnology fermentation reactor

pathways that can be used in manufacturing. Researchers first seek enzyme-producing microorganisms in the natural environment and then search at the molecular level for the genes that produce enzymes with specific biocatalytic capabilities. Once isolated, such enzymes can be characterized for their ability to function in specific industrial processes and, if necessary, can be modified for greater efficiency. Typically these processes are carried out using a controlled environment, a bioreactor, in which microorganisms or cell lines are used to convert raw materials into the desired products, such as chemicals, pharmaceuticals, biobased materials, bioplastics, and biofuels (Figure 1.7).

Supporting Sustainability

Sustainability has become an important goal for society. For industry, sustainability means continuous innovation to make fundamental changes in resource consumption and product life-cycle management [21]. Companies are finding ways to reduce material inputs, save energy, minimize the generation of pollutants or waste in the manufacturing process, and either use renewable materials or produce recyclable or biodegradable products that minimize the end-of-life impact of products. Industrial biotechnology helps manufacturers accomplish these goals.

1. **Material inputs:** Many industrial products are petroleum-based. Petroleum is considered a nonrenewable resource that generates pollution, including greenhouse gases. Biotechnology enables manufacturers to reduce petroleum inputs by using biomass feedstocks. In most cases, this makes production cleaner and generates less waste.

2. **Saving energy:** Conventional manufacturing processes often require numerous energy-intensive steps, with many at high temperatures and high pressures. Industrial biotechnology can enable processing steps to be shortened or omitted altogether. This reduces energy requirements. For example, a biotech process for the bleaching

of pulp for paper production has been demonstrated to cut related energy uses by 40 percent. Biocatalysts, particularly enzyme-based processes, also operate at lower temperatures than conventional chemical processes, further conserving energy for some manufacturing operations.

3. **Reducing pollution:** Replacing traditional chemicals with biobased alternatives helps cut pollution at the source. As an example, biotechnology has revolutionized and simplified the production of vitamin B-2 (riboflavin), by reducing a traditional multistep chemical synthesis and purification process to a one-step fermentation process that reduces waste by 95 percent and leads to a 30 percent reduction of CO_2 [22].

4. **Biodegradable products:** A significant amount of plastic and other waste is not properly disposed of and often makes its way into the environment. Petroleum-based plastics don't break down well and may last for centuries. Industrial biotechnology has produced biodegradable plastic materials to replace many nondegradable petroleum-based plastics. One such bioplastic is polylactic acid (PLA), a biopolymer that uses corn or sugar beets as a feedstock. PLA is recyclable, biodegradable, and can be composted. It is used in fabrics, plastic films, food and beverage containers, textiles, coated papers and boards, and many other packaging applications.

Advanced Biofuels

Our present standard of living is largely built on fossil fuels. But our children's future depends on our ability to shift over time to renewable energy sources to reduce our reliance on fossil fuels and reduce greenhouse gas emissions. Global energy demand is projected to grow 56 percent between 2010 and 2040, [23] making this transition all the more urgent. Biotechnology is helping us move toward biobased, low-carbon or carbon-neutral fuels that are both renewable and better for our environment.

Conventional ethanol, typically produced from corn, accounts for most of the biofuel currently in use in the United States. Biotech innovation is helping to move us beyond the conventional biofuels to advanced biofuels like cellulosic ethanol, biobutanol, isobutanol, and other drop-in fuels. These are being developed so they can be made from next-generation feedstocks such as algae; crop residues like corn stalks, wheat straw and rice straw; wood waste; switchgrass, and other dedicated energy crops—even household trash. Advanced bioethanol made from such cellulosic feedstocks has the potential to reduce greenhouse gas emissions by as much as 128 percent, compared to reference gasoline [24]. This is possible because managed energy crops, such as switchgrass (Figure 1.8), are projected to become carbon sinks, since their root systems are generally undisturbed during harvest, which helps account for the estimated reductions of over 100 percent. The first several thousand commercial gallons of cellulosic biofuel in the U.S. were produced in 2012.

The key contribution of industrial biotechnology to the development of advanced biofuels is the identification of cellulases produced by microbes and fungi—and their production at industrial scales. Cellulases are enzymes that break down the cellulose found in plant cell walls into simple sugars that can serve as the raw materials for biofuels, as well as many of the biobased chemicals, plastics, and other materials discussed above.

Cellulose is the world's most common organic compound, estimated to make up half of all organic carbon on the planet. Biomass is therefore the most globally available and versatile renewable energy asset. There are enormous opportunities to tap this vast resource. Renewable fuels currently provide approximately 10 percent of U.S. on-road transportation fuel needs. A 2005 analysis by the Natural Resources Defense Council (NRDC) found that ethanol from cellulose could supply half of the U.S. transportation fuel needs by 2050.

The Biobased Economy

The big challenge for the industrial biotechnology sector is to develop a thriving biobased economy in which renewable agricultural feedstocks are converted to higher-value products such as biofuels, renewable chemicals, and biobased materials with biotech-enabled processes. As discussed above, industrial enzymes, microorganisms, and microbial systems are used today to produce chemical intermediates or in the manufacture of consumer products. The challenge ahead is to accelerate the growth of this biobased economy

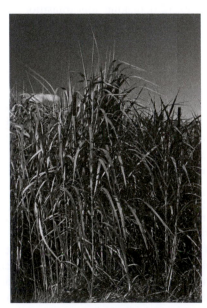

FIGURE 1.8   Switchgrass, a renewable bioenergy source

to revitalize traditional manufacturing, create new manufacturing opportunities, and generate high-quality jobs.

Industrial biotech products have a significant market footprint today which is expected to grow to as much as $547 billion by 2025 [25]. There is already a more than $2.9 billion global market for industrial enzymes [26]. By some estimates the global sustainable chemical industry could reach $1 trillion within a decade. Manufacturers use industrial biotechnology in industries such as food processing, pharmaceuticals, plastics, fuels, specialty chemicals, textiles and paper, and advanced materials manufacture. In 2013, there are more than 75 biorefineries active or under construction across North America for commercial production of advanced biofuels and chemicals from renewable biomass. Industrial biotechnology is bringing new, high paying, high quality jobs to communities and will underpin future economic growth across the world.

Synthetic Biology: A New Approach to Engineering Biology

Synthetic biology is a new evolution of biotech innovation that enables biotechnologists to go beyond manipulation of one or two genes and apply engineering techniques to make changes in entire genetic pathways. Some of the earliest researchers in synthetic biology came from the engineering field rather than the more traditional life science disciplines. These scientists can now "write" DNA code in a technique analogous to writing computer code. Synthetic biology provides astounding opportunities to the industrial biotech sphere—most notably an ability to custom engineer microbes, such as bacteria or yeast, to produce specific chemical compounds that the microbe never previously made.

Innovation for any industry is enhanced by increased speed, efficiency, performance, and cost-effectiveness within product development. Synthetic biology enables this type of innovation by allowing more complex, multistep fermentation of organic chemicals and longer gene synthesis. Synthetic biology describes a set of tools that will aid the continued evolution of biotechnology, including applied protein design, the standardization of genomic parts, and synthesis of full genomes [27]. Synthetic biology may speed development of biotech solutions for clean energy and chemical production.

Transforming Industries and the World

With a boost from synthetic biology and other advances, industrial biotechnology can transform all of the industries mentioned in this section, and many more. The momentum for industrial biotech is driven by global needs. For both the developing and developed world, industrial biotechnology presents enormous economic opportunities. By converting locally produced biomass and biological resources into value-added manufactured products and energy, people from all parts of the world have the opportunity to participate in this new, global, biobased economy.

THE PUBLIC POLICY ENVIRONMENT FOR BIOTECH INNOVATION

The best scientists and the smartest entrepreneurs cannot succeed without the right public policy environment. Public policy affects the ability of entrepreneurs to raise capital, protect intellectual property, carry out research and development, receive timely regulatory review and approval, and earn a sufficient return on their investment of time and capital in the development of new products. America's flourishing biotechnology industry is aided by smart and effective public policy that supports innovation and scientific advances. For this trend to continue, those interested in the field need to be active, engaged, and informed about how legislative decisions affect the industry. You should be familiar with the policies that support biotechnology and stay informed about the decisions of Congress, state legislators, and other policymakers that could help—or hinder—the success and growth of the biotechnology industry.

A number of landmark laws and foundational public policies enabled the growth of a robust biotechnology industry in the United States. They include:

1. **National Institutes of Health (NIH):** The NIH funds much of the basic medical research in the United States, spending about $31 billion annually in recent years. More than 50,000 competitive grants from the NIH support more than 325,000 researchers at more than 3000 universities, medical schools, and research institutions, in addition to research the NIH conducts at its own facilities. The NIH has invested hundreds of billions of dollars in public funding over 7 decades. This massive investment was a major factor in putting the United States at the forefront of biomedical innovation. NIH funding has helped scientists decipher the genetic code, sequence the human genome, and understand neurotransmitters and protein-folding, among many other fundamentals of biology.

2. **Bayh-Dole Act:** This law grants universities and nonprofit institutions exclusive rights to the intellectual property they produce through federally funded research. Since Bayh-Dole was adopted in 1980, more than 6000 U.S. companies have been founded to commercialize university research. NIH-funded research and technology transfer under Bayh-Dole spurred the rise of research universities as the hubs of biotechnology industry clusters.

3. **Food and Drug Administration (FDA):** Another advantage for the U.S. biotech industry is a favorable regulatory environment. New drugs and medical devices must receive FDA approval for safety and efficacy before entering the market. Globally, FDA approval is considered the "gold standard" of regulatory review—the most rigorous, predictable, and efficient system in the world. This has helped the United States attract the vast majority of global biomedical research and development.

4. **Hatch-Waxman Act:** This law strikes a balance between the public benefits of introducing low-cost generic drugs to the market with the need to maintain the incentives for investment in new biopharmaceutical innovation. Because of the lengthy product development, testing and review process, most drugs do not reach the market until a significant portion of their term-of-patent protection has already passed. Hatch-Waxman restores some of this effective patent life, while also creating a pathway for the eventual approval of generic drugs.

5. **Orphan Drug Act:** This law, passed in 1983, provides financial incentives to encourage companies to develop treatments for small patient populations. It provides developers with the exclusive right to market an orphan drug—a drug or biologic that treats a rare disease or condition—for that indication for 7 years from the date of FDA approval. According to the National Organization for Rare Disorders (NORD), more than 400 new drugs have been approved for treatment of orphan diseases since the signing of the Orphan Drug Act. In the 10 years preceding the approval of the Orphan Drug Act only 10 new therapies had been developed.

6. **Patent protection:** Because the majority of biotech companies are small businesses with no products on the market, they must rely on outside private investment, often raised from venture capital firms, to fund their research and development work. Biotechnology drug development is a lengthy and expensive process. Strong patents provide the needed incentives to attract the private funding from investors necessary to fund biomedical research.

7. **Drug reimbursement:** In general, the United States does not limit or restrict prescription drug prices, but allows the free market to work. With sound reimbursement policies in place, patients have greater and faster access to breakthrough therapies and medicines. Market-based drug pricing provides investors in new drug development with greater confidence they will be able to earn a sufficient return on their investment. Conversely, government price controls reduce incentives for investment in new drug development. As the largest purchaser of prescription drugs through Medicare, Medicaid, and other publicly-funded health programs, the United States government's pricing and reimbursement policies can have a huge effect on biomedical innovation.

These are only a few of many public policies that have helped the United States lead the world in the development of new biotech medicines. The right public policies are just as important for innovation in other sectors of the biotech industry. For the United States to remain the agriculture production leader of the world, we need sensible, science-based regulations and a predictable review and approval process for agricultural biotech products that is based on scientific evidence, and on the potential benefits to society and to the environment. Crops derived from modern biotechnology are among the most heavily regulated agricultural products. Currently, biotech crops and animals undergo intense regulatory scrutiny throughout the development process, which can take 10 to 15 years. Agricultural biotechnology is stringently regulated, and depending on the product, the regulators are some combination of the FDA, the U.S. Department of Agriculture (USDA), and the Environmental Protection Agency (EPA). Fair international trade policies and patent protection are also important to agricultural biotech, along with public funding for food and agricultural research.

Policies such as the Renewable Fuel Standard (which sets annual targets for the increased use of renewable fuels), tax credits, and other incentives have enabled the development of a biobased economy. These programs help companies attract the large investments needed to construct commercial-scale biorefineries by effectively guaranteeing a market for biorefinery products.

It is up to all of us in the biotech industry to educate the public about the value of biotechnology and to help policymakers understand the effects of their decisions on innovation. For instance, policymakers generally support developing new biologic treatments, but sometimes do not fully appreciate how expensive and high-risk biotech R&D really is—and thus how critical it is to have policies that maintain incentives for investors to back biotech innovation.

It is up to biotech innovators—those who understand the technology best—to share their experiences with friends, family, neighbors, and others. We should talk about our work and what we hope to accomplish for the world. It is up to us to educate people about the value of biotechnology and to present clear and accurate information about risks and benefits, so that public officials, and society as a whole, can make fully informed decisions. If we maintain and enhance public policies that support innovation, biotechnology will continue to fulfill its promise of offering powerful new solutions to some of the oldest human problems.

Promise for the Future

As President and CEO of the Biotechnology Industry Organization (BIO), I often have the opportunity to meet biotech entrepreneurs from across the United States and around the world. BIO represents more than 1100 innovative biotechnology companies and related organizations. Many of our members are small, emerging companies involved in the research and development of innovative healthcare, agricultural, industrial, and environmental biotechnology products. I am constantly amazed by the ingenuity of biotech researchers and by the almost infinite possibilities for using the science of life to improve the lives of everyone on our planet. The biotech breakthroughs discussed in this chapter barely scratch the surface of what the men and women of our industry have accomplished. Each day, biotech innovators build on the foundation of these past successes to develop new and better products to help heal, fuel, and feed the world. We are still in the early days of the biotech revolution, with an infinite amount to learn and boundless opportunities ahead. For you as an entrepreneur, the field of discovery is wide open.

REFERENCES

[1] Ahmann D, Dorgan JR. Bioengineering for Pollution Prevention through Development of Biobased Energy and Materials State of the Science Report. Washington, D.C: U.S: Environmental Protection Agency; 2007. EPA/600/R-07/028.

[2] Long G, Works J. Innovation in the Biopharmaceutical Pipeline: A Multidimensional View. Analysis Group with support from Pharmaceutical Research and Manufacturers of America; January 2013. http://www.analysisgroup.com/uploadedFiles/Publishing/Articles/2012_Innovation_in_the_Biopharmaceutical_Pipeline.pdf.

[3] World Health Organization (n.d.). "Major Causes of Death Fact Sheet." http://www.who.int/mediacentre/factsheets/fs310/en/index2.html.

[4] Globocan 2008. International Agency for Research on Cancer; 2010.

[5] World Intellectual Property Organization. (n.d.). "Neglected Tropical Diseases." http://www.wipo.int/wipo_magazine/en/2013/01/article_0004.html

[6] Global Genes Project estimates.

[7] PhRMA. Medicines in Development for Cancer. 2012. http://www.phrma.org/.

[8] Goodman AD, et al. Sustained-Release Oral Fampridine in Multiple Sclerosis: A Randomized, Double-Blind, Controlled Trial. The Lancet. February, 2009; 29, 373(9665):732–8. Available at http://www.thelancet.com/journals/lancet/article/PIIS0140-6736(09)60442-6/abstract.

[9] World Health Organization. Global HIV/AIDS Response, Progress Report. 2011. http://www.who.int/hiv/pub/progress_report2011/en/.

[10] PhRMA. Medicines in Development for Rare Diseases. 2011. http://www.phrma.org/research/rare-diseases.

[11] Allingham-Hawkins D. Successful Genetic Tests Are Predicated on Clinical Utility, Genetic Engineering and Biotechnology News 2008;28:14.

[12] Centers for Disease Control and Prevention. (n.d.). "Genomic Testing." http://www.cdc.gov/genomics/gtesting.

[13] Medco. Mayo Clinic Study Reveals Using a Simple Genetic Test Reduces Hospitalization Rates by Nearly a Third for Patients on Widely Prescribed Blood Thinner. Press Release. 16 March 2010. Available at http://www.prnewswire.com/news-releases/medco-mayo-clinic-study-reveals-using-a-simple-genetic-test-reduces-hospitalization-rates-by-nearly-a-third-for-patients-on-widely-prescribed-blood-thinner-87776257.html

[14] ISAAA. (n.d.). "Global Status of Commercialized Biotech/ GM Crops: 2012." *http://www.isaaa.org/resources/publications/ briefs/44/executivesummary/default.asp.*

[15] Monsanto. (n.d.). "Omega-3-Enhanced Soybean Oil." *http://www. monsanto.com/products/pages/how-omega-3-works.aspx.*

[16] USDA. (n.d). "Adoption of Genetically Engineered Crops in the U.S." http://www.ers.usda.gov/data-products/adoption-of-geneti- cally-engineered-crops-in-the-us.aspx.

[17] PG Economics. 2013. Press Release *http://www.pgeconomics.co.uk/ page/35/.*

[18] Conservation Technology Information Center. (n.d.). *http://www. ctic.org/BiotechSustainability.*

[19] ISAAA. (n.d.). "The Ideal Diet: Sufficient and Balanced." *http:// www.isaaa.org/resources/publications/pocketk/27/default.asp.*

[20] FDA. FDA Approves Orphan Drug ATryn to Treat Rare Clotting Disorder. 2009. http://www.fda.gov/NewsEvents/News- room/PressAnnouncements/2009/ucm109074.htm.

[21] Organisation for Economic Co-operation and Development. (1999(2)). "STI Review No. 25: Special Issue on Sustainable Development." Paris. p.68. *http://www.oecd-ilibrary.org/docserver/ download/9099251e.pdf.*

[22] Organisation for Economic Co-Operation and Development. "Indus- trial Biotechnology and Climate Change: Opportunities and Chal- lenges." Paris. 2011. *http://www.oecd.org/sti/biotech/49024032.pdf.*

[23] U.S. Energy Information Administration. International Energy Outlook 2013. Washington, D.C: DOE/EIA-0484. July 24, 2013. *http://www.eia.gov/forecasts/ieo/.*

[24] U.S. Environmental Protection Agency. Renewable Fuel Standard Program (RFS2) Regulatory Impact Analysis. February 2010, p.426. *http://www.epa.gov/otaq/renewablefuels/420r10006.pdf.*

[25] Department for Business Enterprise and Regulatory Reform. IB 2025: Maximising UK Opportunities from Industrial Biotechnology in a Low Carbon Economy. London: Industrial Biotechnology Innovation and Growth Team. May 2009 *http://www.industrialbiotech-europe. eu/wordpress/wp-content/uploads/2012/12/uk-get_file.pdf.*

[26] Erickson B, Nelson J, Winters P. Perspective on Opportunities in Industrial Biotechnology in Renewable Chemicals. Biotechnology Journal 2012 7(2):176–85.

[27] Erickson B, Singh R, Winters P. "Synthetic Biology: Regulating Industry Uses of New Biotechnologies. Science. 2, 2011;333(6047): 1254–6.

Chapter 2

A Biotechnology Entrepreneur's Story: Advice to Future Entrepreneurs

Henri A. Termeer

Former Chairman, CEO and President of Genzyme Corporation, Cambridge, Massachusetts

Henri A. Termeer served as the longest-tenured entrepreneurial CEO of any company in the biotechnology industry. His innovative approaches, achievements, and successes built Genzyme from a fledgling start-up to an international biopharmaceutical company with over $4.5 billion in revenue annually. Termeer is a compassionate, caring, and generous individual with a driving passion to find innovative ways of bringing new therapies for rare diseases to those who so desperately need them. Today, Genzyme remains the world's leading developer and manufacturer of orphan drugs. In February 2011, Genzyme was acquired by the Paris-based pharmaceutical company, Sanofi, for over $20 billion. That transaction was the second largest sale of a biotechnology company in history, following only Roche's acquisition of Genentech in 2009. This chapter is a brief overview of the entrepreneurial career path of Henri A. Termeer, and his advice to future biotechnology entrepreneurs.

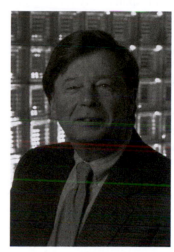

FIGURE 2.1 Henri A. Termeer.

There is an age-old question about whether entrepreneurs are "made" or "born." The theory is, if you are not born an entrepreneur, you cannot learn to become one. I am not certain about the correct answer to this frequently asked question; however, I believe that regardless of whether or not you are "born" an entrepreneur, you still must "learn" to be a good one if you want to be successful.

For me, while growing up, I had a natural interest in entrepreneurship and I seemed to gravitate toward entrepreneurial activities. I followed my natural interests with passion, and through this process I learned entrepreneurial skills in the areas I enjoyed. I grew up in the Netherlands and studied economics at the Erasmus University in Rotterdam. Even while I was studying economics, I was simultaneously involved in activities that allowed me to learn about the early commercialization process of companies. Throughout my formal education years, I continued to follow my interests, even when it meant leaving my home in Holland to study in England. From a very young age I always had a sense within myself that one day I would be an entrepreneur and be involved in starting a business on my own (Figure 2.1).

PATH TO ENTREPRENEURSHIP

My educational and early career years were characterized by following my passions and being involved in things that were exciting to me, especially entrepreneurial activities. Because of my interest in the commercialization process of companies, I decided to further my education and get an MBA, so I moved to Virginia to attend the Darden School of Business. While at Darden in the early 1970s, Baxter (then Baxter Travenol Laboratories) approached me with an offer for an exciting opportunity within their organization after my graduation in 1973. During their recruitment process, Baxter described themselves as a fast-growing healthcare company. At that time they were a small- to medium-sized company with about $200 to $300 million in revenue. Baxter told me they needed someone to become a General Manager in Europe who spoke European languages and understood the culture. This opportunity really interested me, coupled with the possibility that one day I could return to Europe to run one of their companies there.

After graduating, I joined Baxter, and it was at that time that I was first introduced to the medical world. Baxter was headquartered in Chicago, so I moved there from Virginia. After 3 years of training and grooming, I was sent to Europe as a General Manager to run Travenol GmbH in Germany. This was a great experience for me as I was just 29 years old, and yet I had full responsibility for all the operations and success of this company's products. Travenol was a premier company and had world-class clinical research and treatment programs for hemophilia. It was a wonderful learning experience as I had the freedom to develop and grow an organization in Germany, and I had the latitude to expand and manage the market for these products. In 1979, I returned to the U.S. where I was stationed in Los Angeles as the Executive Vice President of Baxter's new Biological Division, with responsibility for all global research and development, marketing, and regulatory affairs.

In the early 1980s Baxter was engaged in the beginning stages of the new biotechnology industry, and we were producing Factor VIII, blood clotting proteins, and other blood products. Our source of starting material was plasma, which we obtained by extraction from human blood. At that time we were just learning how to replace plasma extraction with newer biotechnology methods of production for our products. During this time, several early biotech companies such as Genentech, Genetics Institute, Genex, and Hybritech had already started, and I had the opportunity to negotiate deals on behalf of Baxter with these young biotechnology companies. Throughout these activities, I acquired valuable knowledge about the emerging world of biotechnology, which was still in its infancy. This was a very exciting time for me, and I had a strong sense that the possibilities were great for developing unique and novel products through biotechnology.

Interestingly, Baxter had also acquired a reputation as a company with great entrepreneurial instincts; where young people were given the chance to do something great. As a result, many Baxter alums were sought after and became instrumental in starting and growing many biotechnology companies, such as Genetics Institute, Hybritech, and Integrated Genetics. One reason for this concentration of biotech leaders from Baxter was that fledgling biotechnology companies desperately needed experienced management, and they looked for leaders in existing companies that had a good reputation. Harvard Business School published a book by Monica Higgins about the "Baxter Boys" [1] that chronicled the large number of biotechnology entrepreneurs that emerged from that company.

RISKS OF JOINING A BIOTECHNOLOGY COMPANY

In 1983, while at Baxter, I was approached by venture capitalists at Oak Ventures who invited me to become involved in the beginnings of Genzyme, a small biologics company they recently seeded with capital in Boston. After carefully considering the opportunity, I decided to make the move. I gave up what was a relatively comfortable role at Baxter, having worked there for 10 years, leaving a stable corporation for a new start-up in the emerging industry of biotechnology. Many others may have thought this move to be tenuous; however, I did not consider this move to be as big a risk as others might have. I had the distinct advantage in that Baxter produced human proteins, not through genetic engineering but through extraction of human plasma. Because of this experience, I was keenly aware of the medical significance of producing human proteins, and I also understood the risks and problems of acquiring them from human sources. Fortunately, protein-production risks had already been a part of my life for some time, so I felt very comfortable with my decision to move to a start-up company that would ultimately focus on orphan diseases. My thought process was that the first human protein product at Baxter, Factor VIII, was extracted from plasma and could have been thought of in some way as an orphan-type of disease also. When I compared all the product development and manufacturing risks we experienced at Baxter, such as the HIV and Hepatitis contamination risks, the risk of not finding enough plasma, the difficulties of storing plasma, and the product development and manufacturing risks, then moving to Genzyme did not seem to be an enormous leap to me.

There were also other reasons that convinced me to start from a clean slate at Genzyme. We had access to eight very enthusiastic full professors—seven from MIT and one from Harvard. We also decided to look for support from the top-tier group of venture capitalists to support our activities. Even though many others may have viewed this career move as risky, I was not tentative in my decision at all because I did not feel that the risks were enormous. In fact it was quite the opposite; I saw that an alternative way of producing human-derived proteins as very attractive, and to me, this was the "Holy Grail" kind-of-world.

GENZYME IN THE EARLY DAYS

Developing and growing a biotechnology company has never been easy, which was especially so in the early 1980s when there were no successful biotechnology business models to follow. When I started at Genzyme there was not much there, just a few very impressive scientists and the beginnings of a business infrastructure (Figure 2.2). However, we had the latitude and freedom to chart our own course and build something special. I reached out to other companies and became involved in discussions with biotechnology companies that were ahead of us, such as Genetics Institute, Hybritech, Genentech, and others; we were very impressed by their knowledge of biotechnology.

During the early days of Genzyme, we sold a few diagnostic enzymes, so we had a little bit of income, but in

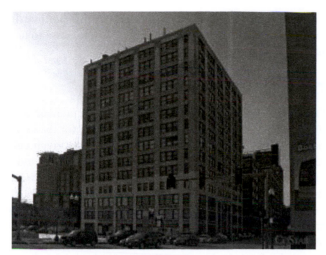

FIGURE 2.2   Early Genzyme office location. *75 Kneeland Street, Boston, MA (Source: LoopNet).*

reality we had no real sustainable capital. In addition, we had no real cash reserves to speak of, so I spent a disproportionate amount of my time in the early years raising money. I raised money any way I could. Because biotechnology was new, I even had to find new ways to raise money, along with creating cost-effective ways to get things done. During the first 2 years we raised just enough money to sustain ourselves for the following year, and we obtained two or three very small equity rounds. In the beginning, I thought I would go to pharmaceutical companies to secure our capital. Later, in doing this, I realized that this was a very costly route because pharmaceutical companies were not really interested in us as a company; they wanted to acquire our products and, of course, I wanted to keep our products for our company. Later we decided to raise money through selling equity. We tried many different routes to accomplish that, until we eventually went out with our IPO in 1986 and raised over $28 million. That capital reserve became the financial basis for us to accomplish all the rest of the activities at Genzyme.

THE IMPORTANCE OF UNDERSTANDING BUSINESS AND FINANCE

For a scientist without any financial experience or business background, starting a company can be very challenging. If you do not understand how financial systems operate, or you do not understand what the company financial goals are, or you do not understand what are reasonable terms to ask for during negotiations, you will feel extremely uncomfortable. In order to be successful, an entrepreneur must have confidence in both business and finance. Biotech entrepreneurs do not necessarily need to be accountants or financial analysts, but they do need to understand what is appropriate for a financial deal structure, including the best

approach for all aspects of accounting and financing of the company, understanding the impact on the company when giving up equity, the cost-of-capital, and the burn-rate risk to the company. Unfortunately, the consequences of raising capital and capital planning are often enormously underestimated, or even ignored, by young biotechnology companies and their entrepreneurs.

RAISING CAPITAL

The single most important value creator for a biotechnology company is sustainability. Not only do you need to conduct great science, you need to have a time continuum long enough to research the problem and complete the work so you can make it successful. The length of time you have to do this is ultimately determined by your financial strength. In order for biotechnology companies to raise capital they must give up something in return. It is critical to recognize what you are willing to give up because it may be very costly to the company. Obviously, the best asset a biotechnology company has is their first product that creates their equity value. Unfortunately, young biotechnology companies often give up their best asset in order to raise the capital they need. I believe a better approach is to use your second-best asset rather than giving up your most important asset. Another way of saying this in plain English is: Don't give up your "first-born." Or at the very least, if you must give it up, do it in such a way that the deal is so good for the company and shareholders that it cannot be refused. Young biotechnology companies are tempted to become short-sighted because they easily become focused on raising just enough money for the next day. On top of that, the asset they use to raise the money is the one that is the most advanced and the one with the greatest value to the company.

Young companies often presume they must relinquish their first product in order to raise capital, and then they can create a follow-on second product. However, what they do not appreciate is the enormous uncertainty and risks involved in creating a second product, not to mention the enormous amount of time and money required to accomplish that goal. Often companies end up being completely unsustainable because their first product has been "mortgaged" so to speak, and later they find themselves still in need of capital. It is important for the leader to recognize what it took for the first product to reach that stage of development and create its existing value. The flaw is that people presume they can easily develop a second successful product, which is an unrealistic assumption because you do not always know whether or not you can discover or accomplish that goal. Plus, most likely these steps often take 5, 10, or 15 years. I would venture to say that if you conducted a study on the thousands of companies that have had a relatively short life, often, almost all of them have some kind of collaboration early with a major company, and then they are unable to create a successful follow-on product. The truth is that the entrepreneur really does not know whether the company can create and successfully develop a second product. Unfortunately, this is how many companies get started and sadly their existence becomes limited.

There are, of course, different strategies of building a biotechnology company. Some entrepreneurs may just want to develop one product and find an exit for themselves. If your purpose and goal is to simply begin development for a short period of time and have an early exit then that is a different objective. However, if you want to build sustainability into your company and grow a strong business, do not give up your "first-born," give up your "second-born" instead. From the beginning at Genzyme, we intended to establish a sustainable business with revenues generated by our own products, and we sought to retain full rights to them. There are different beliefs on how to build a sustainable biotechnology company, but this is how we approached it at Genzyme.

MANAGING THE UNCERTAINTY OF BIOTECHNOLOGY

It is not uncommon for young leaders to look for and follow tried-and-true methods of success. However, building a biotechnology company and developing biotechnology products do not have straight-forward prescriptive paths. Every biotechnology company's path to success is in some way different from each other. I believe that any leader who does not recognize the enormous uncertainty of product development and the need to constantly learn and adapt, should not be in this business. In order to be successful in this industry, one must always be circumspect and never lose sight of the ultimate purpose and mission of the company, otherwise you may simply follow the path of least resistance. Successful entrepreneurs understand the principle of "hedging your bets." They plan for alternatives and think about "What would happen if this approach fails?" However, please do not take this as an endorsement for pessimism. You need to identify alternatives without losing the energy necessary to motivate your team and provide your idea or approach with the best possible opportunity for success. Managing the risks in the biotechnology industry is an important responsibility of the biotechnology entrepreneur. We know that the odds of picking successes are very small because even pharmaceutical companies with billions of dollars of R&D money cannot pick successes at a predicable rate. Big Pharma has a lot of experience, a lot of money, and yet they still often fail in their product development. They fail at trying to select what can be done better by thousands of smaller companies. Remember, you do not overcome this type of risk, you simply live with it and manage it. As an entrepreneur, you are destined to fail if you believe that biotechnology product development is *not* a risky business. Biotechnology is inherently a risky business; however, it is still enormously exciting and you can succeed at if you learn to adapt to and have well-thought-out alternative plans.

CORE VALUES

One of the most important things for an entrepreneur is to develop and establish a foundational purpose for the company. At Genzyme, we created a very purpose-driven culture which was to come up with important breakthroughs and develop and understand unique medical solutions; this purpose was larger than any single individual. When you work towards an important purpose, everyone gains a sense of urgency. Although this may seem strange, it is not about *me* just having some fun. It is about *us* making progress; it is about working together as a cohesive team and seeing needs in other areas of the company not necessarily assigned to you. The leader is key to spreading shared core values. If the leader does not possess good core values, he/she will not be emulated by employees. It is vital for the leader to create a culture of cooperation, shared values and responsibility, and the passion to meet unmet medical needs for patients.

INTEGRATING THE SCIENCE AND BUSINESS

I am a firm believer in having every stakeholder participate in examining what we did as a company, including the scientists, the business people, the receptionist, and even the person in the warehouse. This shared responsibility created a collective sense of purpose, because we were all aligned to one goal. I made sure that our scientists never had separation between what they were thinking and doing and what the business people were thinking and doing. We were an integrated company, and we kept it that way. As we grew in size, we naturally became quite diversified, but we still created ways for scientists and product development individuals to stay closely connected, even after our products reached the market. One cannot forget that there is always a certain amount of inherent natural tension created between the business and the science. But there is clearly less tension if you do not allow separation between these disciplines. Companies naturally grow in size and diversification; however, it is more problematic to allow separation between functions within companies. When employees feel engaged, it is more enjoyable for everyone within the company. When everyone feels connected, they experience an enormous sense of value being able to do something special for patients, especially when employees are involved throughout the entire project.

Early in the development of any project, when the product is making its way through the process to become a lead compound for a particular disease, we brought patients into the company. We exposed our scientists to the patient and the patient's environment and the patient advocacy organization, if one existed. Whenever there was an important meeting for that particular disease, we did not just have the marketing people sit in the room to discuss this, we included the scientists. Even after the product reached the clinic, we included the basic scientists and asked them to listen and make judgments about the progress; I encouraged our scientists to become involved in all these activities. As one can imagine, there were some scientists who preferred not to be involved in marketing discussions, and I accepted that. However, I would still invite scientists who were interested, to get close to the project and experience the entire process, because I understood the value of having collective interaction and participation from all disciplines. If an idea did not work or it just outright failed, it became a disappointment to the entire team. But they experienced this responsibility in a practical manner together as a team. If a project or idea did not work out, each team member learned something valuable and it allowed them to creatively think about alternative options to make it successful. Unless an individual is close to a project, it is very difficult for them to have the necessary motivation and understanding to attempt something new. Human nature is such that you do not learn much from an experience if you are not close to it. This is how I dealt with integrating the business and the science, for good or bad—there is no perfect formula.

THE VALUE OF A BUSINESS BACKGROUND AND EXPERIENCE

Building and growing a biotechnology company is a combination of business and science. Successful entrepreneurs understand the important aspects of each discipline. I came into this industry as a businessman and had gained many years of training at a very successful health sciences company. I had previously run several different large businesses at Baxter, including R&D, at the divisional or country level and at the sales and marketing and manufacturing level. By the time I started with Genzyme, my business background was fairly extensive and as a result, I was able to utilize my business experiences. Consequently, as the company grew I did not need to second guess my experiences and did not have a feeling that I would outgrow my ability to manage this business. I also made sure that the composition of the Board of Directors kept increasing in experience by bringing different people onto the board over time. Also, when we hired new employees, I made sure that people came with the right experience. We also did a lot of things that allowed people to continue their education. I knew we would experience growing pains, so we had regular meetings to try to identify how we could become a billion-dollar company and still be a company where all of us wanted to work. As we grew, we added

different business units, but we set up a system where we never really lost touch with people, and we allowed them to stay engaged with what the company as a whole was doing. We grew as new people came in, and a large company has a different feel than a smaller young one. However, our turnover was always very small—it had a very low turnover rate for a biotech company. We tried to be wise with regards to compensation, and we gave incentive compensation with options to everyone no matter what level they were in the company. Spanning almost 3 decades that I was there, Genzyme continued to retain an environment where people appreciated belonging; and up to the time I left, we had approximately 12,500 full-time employees. If you are the CEO of a start-up biotechnology company, your responsibility is to bring out good ideas from your team, inspire them, and provide the overarching vision that guides them to success.

One big flaw that can occur is when young entrepreneurs receive a lot of enthusiastic early financial and moral support from investors. As the company quickly develops, the support that was there in the beginning is no longer there later in the same way. Because of this, some entrepreneurs are surprised when suddenly they receive critical questions from these same investors, and the entrepreneur does not have answers. Entrepreneurs must expect hard questions because that is the only way an investor can stay in touch with the company and its progress. Successful entrepreneurs are not easily discouraged because they have broad shoulders and accept responsibility and feel in charge. If you do not feel in charge because strong investors seem to be the ones in charge, you need to ask yourself the question "can I overcome this issue?" If you become too irritated by having hard questions asked of you, you will not succeed. Always remember that the questions will never stop, especially when more development obstacles come. If this bothers you, you may not be the right person, or you may not be ready to lead a company.

DRIVEN FROM WITHIN

There is no formula for building a company and developing a biotechnology product, nor is it something you simply fill in the blanks to succeed. Every entrepreneur must have an internal navigation system and a high degree of self-motivation. I absolutely believe you cannot be successful without being driven from within yourself. You have to feel it. It requires total sensitivity 24/7. You live it. You think it. You must follow your instincts all the time because there are no universal predictable ways for success in this industry. Entrepreneurs must have these instincts and be connected with what is inside of them. If entrepreneurs need to wait for instruction from a board member as to what they can say, or be told what to do, they are in a problematic position. Investors and board members will want to tell you what to do because that is their business and it is their money. However, you should not wait for this to occur; you need to take your own cues, and you need to take the initiative before others begin telling you what to do. Yes, you can and should receive guidance from mentors and other entrepreneurs. You can, and should, bring other experienced people into your shop and share all the best advice and experience they have. Brainstorming can be very constructive; however, you must not sit back and wait for problems to occur before you do something. You should always take the initiative to actively lead your company from within. The entrepreneur must understand that he or she is the leader. You must take the initiative. It is a lonesome job in many ways because at the end of the day you cannot blame anyone else. Therefore, having self-confidence is important for entrepreneurs because their own instincts are critical to navigating through the challenges of building a company.

IN TOUCH WITH EVENTS OUTSIDE THE COMPANY

All entrepreneurs need to be able to work effectively with the world outside of the company's four walls. I believe this is *the* most decisive factor in facilitating your company's success. For instance, what do you need to do about reimbursement? What do you need to do about certain FDA regulations? What regulatory action needs to occur in order to get your product approved? What impact does the pricing for your product have? What is the impact of competition around the world? These are some of the things the CEO has to think about and have a feel for, even at the time of start-up. These outside issues must become a part of the entrepreneur's overall plan.

Biotech CEOs also need to be engaged with individuals outside of their company. Leaders need to become engaged in important meetings at the Biotechnology Industry Organization (BIO); they need to have colleagues they can talk to and exchange thoughts with. The entrepreneur needs to understand that these different elements of the outside world ultimately determine the economic success of the company. Recognize that the events which occur outside the company, impact the inside success. Successful entrepreneurs become part of that outside world on a continuous basis.

GOOD FORTUNE AND SUCCESS

Occasionally, good things happen to companies, such that when they look back at an event they can say "that was a fortunate break!" The entrepreneur must not forget that the opposite situation can also happen. Fortunate breaks occur when you create an environment that has ample opportunity and foresight to capture them. In other words, create a big umbrella. Companies that do not plan for contingencies or alternate events rarely have a chance to take advantage of fortunate breaks. It is probably true that in almost every instance of great success in companies, there were some fortunate series of events that catapulted them to success. Entrepreneurs need to know that they can increase their chances of "fortunate breaks" by incorporating foresight and planning for alternative events, and being prepared to take advantage of opportunities happening outside of their company.

CLOSING ADVICE

My advice to biotech entrepreneurs is "make a difference!" Work to create solutions for patients and help patients with physical limitations improve their life. We cannot afford *not* to come up with better treatments for diseases. As a society, this is where we should spend our best energy, use our best people, and focus our best efforts. Supporters of the biotechnology industry believe this is worth it. As a biotech entrepreneur, you can bring value and make a difference for these people. Look for a place to make a difference. Learn to do that which is important and operate by a different set of criteria than others.

I believe one of the greatest characteristics to becoming a successful entrepreneur is that you are not proud. Everything of great value required the help of other people. Don't limit yourself to your own resources. While you do this, live and operate with passion. Passion is what makes us who we are. Passion translates into a need to do something about a difficult situation. Successful entrepreneurs also have vision. Learn to see things that others do not. What you can visualize, you can carry forward. Ideas are simply an opportunity. Once you have the proof-of-concept you have a responsibility to take it forward. As you move things forward, learn to take calculated risks. The ability to pioneer something, and go places that no one else has ever been, is unique. Almost anyone can do things that are predictable. Remember, most initiatives will fail, but if you have the courage to take things forward and can identify alternatives, you can make your ultimate goal successful. I wish each of you the very best of success in your endeavors!

REFERENCE

[1] Higgins MC. How the Baxter Boys Built the Biotech Industry. Career Imprints: Creating Leaders Across An Industry. San Francisco Jossey-Bass: 2005.

Chapter 3

The Biotechnology Industry: An Engine of Innovation

G. Steven Burrill

CEO, Burrill & Company, San Francisco, California

In 1972, Stanford University Associate Professor of Medicine Stanley Cohen and University of California, San Francisco Professor of Bioechemistry Herbert Boyer famously met at a scientific conference in Hawaii and forged a collaboration over beer and sandwiches one night at a Honolulu deli. The two had been working on complimentary projects and combined their efforts to develop a method for isolating genes and DNA fragments and reproducing them. Boyer's lab had identified an enzyme that cut precise DNA fragments that coded for the production of specific proteins. Cohen had developed a method for inserting DNA fragments into bacteria cells. The process they developed for recombinant DNA essentially allowed a scientist to place DNA from higher organisms into bacteria or other cells and harness these cells as factories of desired proteins. Though the effort was initially undertaken as a way to produce materials for research, it was immediately recognized for its potential power in producing human therapeutics, such as insulin or antibiotics.

The fundamental work of Cohen and Boyer enabled the creation of the biotechnology industry (Figure 3.1). Though it was a second partnership that Boyer would forge that helped commercialize his invention and give rise to the industry. Robert Swanson, a venture capitalist who became convinced of the commercial potential of recombinant DNA, had been cold calling leading scientists in the field to see if they believed the technology was ready to be commercialized (Figure 3.2). While each agreed the technology had commercial potential, they told him it was at least a decade or two away. When he reached Boyer, not realizing the University of California, San Francisco (UCSF) scientist codeveloped the technique for recombinant DNA, and told him he wanted to start a company based on the technology, Boyer told Swanson he believed that the technology was ready to be commercialized, according to the historian Sally Smith Hughes in her book *Genentech: The Beginnings of Biotech*. Swanson convinced Boyer to meet with

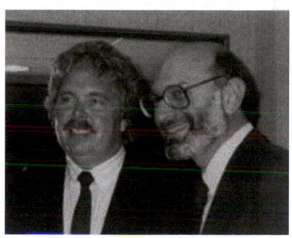

FIGURE 3.1 Stanley Cohen and Herb Boyer, inventors of the first genetic engineering tools.

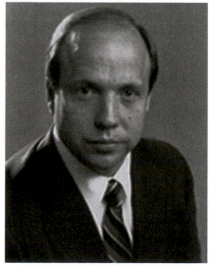

FIGURE 3.2 Robert Swanson, cofounder and first CEO of Genentech.

Biotechnology Entrepreneurship.

him and the two entered a partnership that would lead to the formation of Genentech in 1976. By the time the Swiss pharmaceutical giant Roche completed its acquisition of Genentech in 2009, the company was worth $100 billion, more than any pharmaceutical company at the time.

By 1979, Genentech had succeeded in producing the human protein somatostatin in *Escherichia coli* bacteria, an important proof-of-concept that a human protein could be produced this way. Next, the company set out to produce human insulin, a potentially lucrative market. At the time, insulin was primarily derived from the pancreas of cattle. But using bovine insulin carried a problem because some patients had immune responses to it that rendered it less effective. Being able to produce human insulin through the tools of biotechnology promised to deliver not only a safer and more effective product, but one that could be produced in whatever quantity was needed to meet demand. Once Genentech, working with scientists at the City of Hope, was able to demonstrate it was able to engineer bacteria to produce human insulin, it entered into a partnership agreement with the pharmaceutical company Eli Lilly, which at that time produced about 80 percent of the insulin for the U.S. market. Lilly provided an upfront payment of $500,000 to Genentech and milestone payments tied to the company meeting specific development milestones. Genentech would receive royalties of 6 percent on sales if the two companies were successful and brought the recombinant human insulin to market. The product, dubbed Humulin, won the U.S. Food and Drug Administration (FDA) approval to be marketed in 1982—the first genetically engineered product to win such approval (Figure 3.3).

The deal between Genentech and Lilly stood as an important model for the biotechnology industry that would be replicated again and again throughout its history. Genentech provided an important innovative product while Lilly provided capital and the expertise needed to develop the product, navigate it through the regulatory review process, and manufacture it. Though Genentech went on to develop a number of successful therapeutics that it manufactured and marketed, many small biotechs today have no desire to become fully integrated pharmaceutical companies. Instead, they see their strength in developing drugs to a proof-of-concept stage and believe they can do that more cost effectively than large pharmaceutical companies. Once they have clinical proof of a drug's potential, they seek to find a pharmaceutical partner willing to license the drug and take over development, regulatory approval, manufacturing, and marketing.

THE BIRTH OF AN INDUSTRY

In one sense, the world created in the wake of Cohen's and Boyer's invention was not new. Man has long harnessed biological processes for beneficial uses. Evidence suggests that for at least 6000 or 7000 years, fermentation was used in the ancient world to brew beer. And for thousands of years farmers have selected crops for desirable traits and, in the wake of Gregor Mendel's work in genetics, the agricultural sector cross-bred plants to bring about the characteristics they wanted (Figure 3.4). Biologics were also not new as healthcare products regulated by the U.S. FDA. Biological products, such as vaccines or blood-derived products, long predated the first recombinant biologics that reached the market. But the recombinant DNA technology ushered in a new era represented by an unparalleled ability to harness biological processes to make precise end-products, not only for therapeutic purposes, but also to engineer crops so they have specific

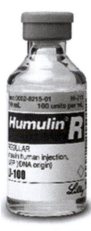

FIGURE 3.3 Recombinant human insulin: the first FDA-approved, genetically engineered product.

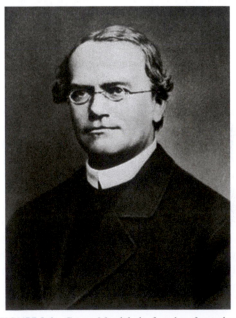

FIGURE 3.4 Gregor Mendel, the founder of genetics.

traits, such as resistance to drought or pesticides, as well as designing microbes to produce transportation fuels and chemicals used in industrial manufacturing.

Five years before the founding of Genentech, scientists Ron Cape and Peter Farley, as well as Nobel laureate Donald Glaser and investor Moshe Alafi, established Cetus in Berkeley in 1971. It also recruited Stanford's Cohen to its scientific advisory board. The company initially focused its efforts on finding microorganisms for industrial applications, but soon embraced recombinant technology and other new tools of the biotechnology industry. The company developed interleukin-2 which was used to treat certain cancers and viral infections and would eventually be marketed as Proleukin. The company also successfully cloned beta interferon which eventually became an important therapy for multiple sclerosis known as Betaseron. Its greatest contribution, though, was the development of polymerase chain reaction or PCR technology, a technique that allows someone to take minute fragments of DNA and amplify them into large quantities that can be used in a wide range of applications. Cetus employee Kary Mullis, who invented the process, won the Nobel Prize for his work (Figure 3.5).

In 1991, Cetus' next-door neighbor, Emeryville-based Chiron acquired the company. Chiron was also an early biotechnology pioneer. The company was founded by UCSF Biochemistry Department Chair William Rutter, with Ed Penhoet of the University of California, Berkeley and UCSF's Pablo Valenzuela. Chiron won success using the tools of biotechnology to develop vaccines and diagnostics.

In the San Diego region, Ivor Royston and Howard Birndorf formed Hybritech in 1978 with the plan to use monoclonal antibodies to advance research (Figure 3.6). The company, also backed by the venture capital firm of

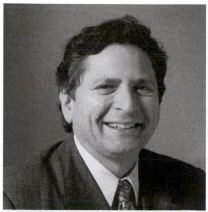
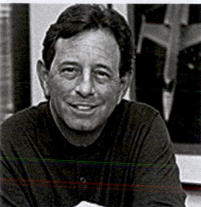

FIGURE 3.6   Ivor Royston and Howard Birndorf, founders of Hybritech.

Kleiner Perkins, though, quickly shifted its focus to using the technology to develop diagnostics. The company, San Diego's first, was acquired by Eli Lilly, which later sold it to Beckman Coulter. Hybritech's alums, however, have been a critical source of new company formation within the San Diego region. That same year across the country in Cambridge, Massachusetts, Harvard biochemist Walter Gilbert and MIT molecular biologist Phil Sharp, both who later separately went on to win Nobel Prizes, established Biogen. The company simultaneously established R&D headquarters in Geneva because of restrictions on the use of recombinant technology in Cambridge at the time. Within 2 years, the company discovered alpha interferon and beta interferon. The discoveries eventually led to the development of Avonex, which is used to treat multiple sclerosis.

Across the Charles River in Boston, entrepreneur Sheridan Snyder and Tufts University biochemist Henry Blair established Genzyme. Genzyme was developing products from engineered enzymes such as diagnostics, which provided it a faster path to revenue than most biotechs. Its defining strategy took shape when the company hired Henri Termeer in 1983 as president. Termeer, who had previously worked at Baxter, focused on enzyme replacement therapies for rare disease, a plan that allowed it to take advantage of the Orphan Drug Act, which provided a faster path to approval and other

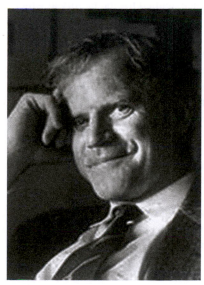

FIGURE 3.5   Kerry Mullis, inventor of PCR.

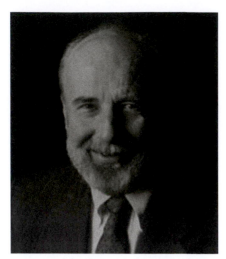

FIGURE 3.7   George Rathmann, founding CEO of Amgen.

incentives to companies developing therapies for diseases with patient populations of 200,000 or fewer. The company's first drug was developed to treat Gaucher's disease, a rare genetic lysomal storage disorder caused by a deficiency of a specific enzyme. The disorder is characterized by bruising, fatigue, anemia, low blood platelets, and enlargement of the liver and spleen. The drug, Ceredase, became available for these patients in 1989 and won full FDA approval in 1990. The pharmaceutical giant Sanofi bought Genzyme in 2011 for $20.1 billion and contingent value rights worth up to an additional $3.8 billion.

Around the time Genzyme was starting to make Ceredase available to patients, Amgen (short for Applied Molecular Genetics) won approval for the first of the blockbuster drugs it would produce. The FDA in 1989 approved the anemia drug erythropoietin alfa for patients with kidney disease. It's marketed as both Epogen and Procrit through its partnership with Johnson & Johnson. Amgen, in Thousand Oaks, California, was founded by venture capitalists Bill Bowes, who built a team of investors for the venture and recruited University of California, Los Angeles scientist Winston Salser to put a scientific advisory board together. Bowes recruited George Rathmann, who was a vice president of R&D for Abbott Laboratories, as CEO (Figure 3.7). Today, Amgen is the largest biotechnology company in the world with a $79 billion market cap, placing it above many Big Pharma companies, and revenue of $17.3 billion in 2012.

THE INDUSTRY TAKES ROOT

Though initially the earliest biotechnology companies sought to do everything from animal health to industrial applications of the technology, most of these companies quickly focused their development efforts on human therapeutics because of the high value of these products. The

early years of biotechnology have been dominated by companies seeking to use the technology to develop products for human health. The initial targets were for what was considered low-hanging fruit, such as human insulin and human growth hormone, where the therapeutic value was clearly understood and the molecules relatively easy to reproduce. However, while biotechnology was initially expected to allow drugmakers to develop products and bring them to market faster and more economically than their small molecule counterparts because they were expected to represent engineered versions of substances that naturally occurred in the body, in reality, particularly as new classes of biologics emerged, they faced similar development costs and the same long development and regulatory timeframes of traditional pharmaceuticals. As the technology emerged and the first companies seeking to commercialize biotechnology products were placing their stakes in the ground, there were high-profile debates over the safety and ethics of the new technology, questions about whether new laws were needed to restrict and control its use, fights over what could and could not be patented, and regulatory concerns about how to review and evaluate these new products. For the industry to take hold, there were several critical policy developments during the early years of the industry that set the stage for its subsequent growth and development.

Shortly after the development of recombinant DNA technology, scientists expressed concerns about unknown health hazards posed by the new technology. In response, the National Academy of Sciences called for a voluntary moratorium on recombinant DNA technology. Stanford University's Paul Berg, who later won the Nobel Prize for his pioneering work in recombinant DNA technology, assembled a conference for the National Academy of Sciences consisting of scientists, attorneys, and physicians in Pacific Grove, California that became known as The Asilomar Conference, named for the facility at which it was held. It explored whether any work needed to be prohibited and under what conditions experimentation in the field should be conducted. The 1975 conference established initial principles that called for containment efforts to match the risks of experiments. It also called for deferring experiments, such as cloning the DNA of deadly pathogens, because of the potential dangers it posed. But it also allowed the work to proceed.

In 1980, the U.S. Supreme Court put into place another critical piece for the young biotechnology. The case of *Diamond v. Chakrabarty* examined the question of whether genetically engineered organisms could be patented. Ananda Charkrabarty was working for General Electric when he developed a bacterium that would break down oil and could be used to clean oil spills. The U.S. Patent and Trademark Office rejected the applications saying living organisms could not be patented. A patent appeals court overturned that decision, saying the fact that something is living is irrelevant to the question of patentability. Sidney Diamond, the commissioner of the patent office, appealed the decision to the U.S. Supreme Court, which ruled in a 5 to 4 decision that the Chakrabarty's bacterium did not naturally occur in nature and was, in fact, the invention of a man and therefore capable of being patented.

That same year, the Patent and Trademark Law Amendments Act, commonly known as the Bayh-Dole Act, changed the rights surrounding intellectual property created through federally funded research. Until then, the government retained control of all patents resulting from federally funded research and licensed it out on a nonexclusive basis. The result was that most patents—some 95 percent of the 28,000 held by the government at the time of the Bayh-Dole Act—were never licensed, according to the Association of University Technology Managers. Without the protections of a patent or exclusive license, industry was generally unwilling to undertake the risk and expense of taking early-stage research and turning it into marketable products that benefitted the public and the economy. The new law established a policy for federally funded research that allowed universities, small businesses, and other recipients of research funding to retain the intellectual property they created with government-funded research and have the rights to license it. This allowed universities to become a critical source of biotechnology innovation that industry could then work to commercialize.

"The ties between biotechnology and university research have always been critical. Most biotech companies license technologies from nonprofit organizations. The continuation of this relationship—along with a strong, dependable patent system and flexible licensing practices—is essential to maintaining America's global leadership in biotech innovation," said Jim Greenwood, CEO of the trade association the Biotechnology Industry Organization in a 2012 report about the effects of the Bayh-Dole Act. "Federally-funded research and the incentives of Bayh-Dole lay the foundation for these successes, but turning basic discoveries into breakthrough medicines, cleaner energy, and enhanced crops takes years of hard work by entrepreneurial companies and investors willing to risk billions of dollars to fund that development."

THE INDUSTRY TODAY

Today, the biotechnology industry broadly represents more than an estimated 10,000 companies globally. By 2016, sales of biologics are expected to reach between $200 billion to $210 billion, up from $157 billion in 2011, according to IMS Health, a data service provider that tracks drug spending. In 2012 alone, life sciences companies globally raised nearly $90 billion in 2012, and potentially another $37 billion through partnering agreements. These companies include therapeutics, diagnostics, tools and technology companies, as well as companies working in agriculture,

and biofuels and renewable chemicals. As of the start of 2013, biopharmaceutical companies were using biological processes to develop more than 900 medicines and vaccines targeting more than 100 diseases, according to a report from the Pharmaceutical Research and Manufacturers of America or PhRMA. The trade group found more than a third of these drugs in the development pipeline—some 338 drugs—are targeting various cancers. Though the pipeline is full of more-established technologies, such as vaccines and monoclonal antibodies, it also reflects the growing importance of new biotechnologies and includes 69 cell therapies and 46 gene therapies.

But biotechnology's impact is not only being felt in healthcare. The trade group BIO says there are more than 13.3 million farmers around the world using agricultural biotech processes and biotech crops are grown on more than 2.3 billion acres of farmland worldwide. And in the industrial and fuel arena, companies are now moving from demonstration plants to building full-scale commercial production facilities.

Initially a clear delineation existed between pharmaceutical companies and biotechnology companies. Pharmaceutical companies traditionally developed and marketed small molecule drugs created through chemical synthesis whereas biotechnology companies produced large molecule therapeutics through recombinant technology. But the distinction between these sectors has blurred. Today, the world's largest pharmaceutical companies, mostly through licensing agreements and acquisitions, produce and market a large portion of the most successful biotechnology therapeutics available today. At the same time, these types of products have become important parts of the pipeline of these companies. In fact, seven of the ten forecasted best-selling drugs for 2016 are expected to be biologics, six of which are marketed by companies considered to be Big Pharma. At the same time, many so-called biotechs are today engaged in developing small molecule drugs, but are doing so with a deep understanding of the molecular mechanisms underlying the diseases they are meant to treat.

THE CHALLENGE OF DRUG DEVELOPMENT

Though much has changed since the early days of the biotechnology industry, some of the basic factors that shape the fundamental landscape in which therapeutic companies operate and give rise to the persistent challenges companies face in developing human therapeutics have only intensified. Drug development is a long, expensive, and highly regulated process. Not only has this reality remained constant, but during the history of the biotechnology industry development timelines have grown longer and costs have soared. Though estimates vary, on average it can take more than 10 years and $1.5 billion in capitalized costs to move a drug from discovery to the market.

In the United States, drugs are regulated by the U.S. FDA. Other countries have similar regulatory authorities. Before a drug can be sold on the market, it must go through a series of tests demonstrating it is safe and efficacious in order to win regulatory approval for marketing. These include preclinical tests in the lab and in animals before a drug can be tried in human subjects, a process that can take 3 to 6 years. Once a compound is selected for human clinical trials in the United States, a company must submit an Investigational New Drug application to the FDA documenting what is known about the molecule, its activity, and any known safety concerns, as well as plans for how the clinical trial will be conducted and what they will seek to demonstrate. During this process, researchers must determine such things as how a molecule would be delivered to a patient, what dosing would be used, and whether it could cause unintended effects. For every 250 drugs that enter preclinical testing, only five will ever make it to human clinical trials, according to the trade group Pharmaceutical Research and Manufacturers of America (PhRMA). If approved for human clinical testing, the molecule will be subjected to a series of progressively larger and more expensive human clinical trials to establish the safety, dosing, and efficacy of a particular drug to treat a specific disease. (See Figure 3.8.)

There are three stages to human clinical trials, known as phases. Early-stage or phase 1 clinical trials involve safety and dose testing, often in healthy subjects, to determine how much drug is needed to produce an effect in the body

and what level, if any, causes adverse reactions. These studies generally take about 6 months and involve up to 100 people. Mid-stage or phase 2 clinical trials can involve up to 500 people with the specific disease that the drug is intended to treat. The test subjects are generally divided into two groups with one group given the experimental drug and the other given a placebo. Safety and dosing are checked in these studies as well, but these tests are intended to provide a proof-of-concept and provide an indication that the drug offers benefits to someone with a given disease. Late-stage or phase 3 tests, depending on the disease, can involve as many as 5000 patients and go on for as many as 4 years.

If the clinical testing is successful, the drug developer submits a New Drug Application to the FDA—or a similar application to the regulatory authority in the country it hopes to market the drug. The application includes detailed data from the clinical trials. These submissions can be dense with information and include tens of thousands of pages of information. The FDA is expected to provide a response in most cases within 10 months of the filing. (See Figure 3.9.)

FALLING R&D PRODUCTIVITY

Drugmakers have faced a difficult period during the last several years as a number of trends have converged. The cost of drug development has soared, regulators have raised barriers for approval, governments have increased pricing pressures on drugs, and competition from generic drugs

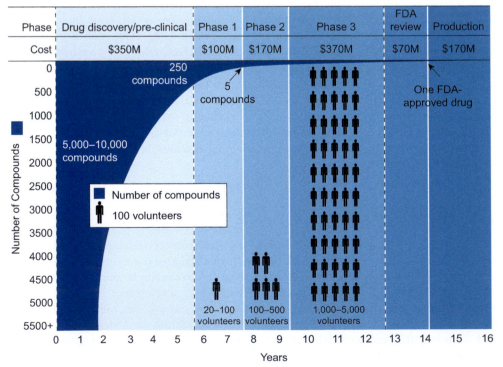

Source: U.S. Food and Drug Administration

FIGURE 3.8   Drug development process and attrition rates. *(From Burrill & Company 2013 Annual Report on the Life Sciences Industry.)*

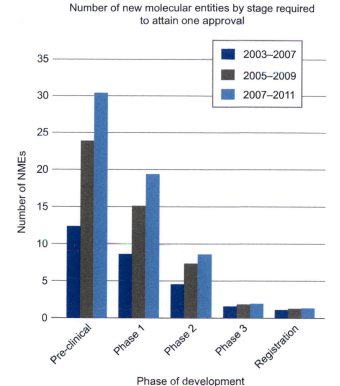

FIGURE 3.9   Declining number of new drugs reaching approval. *(From Burrill & Company 2013. Annual Report on the Life Sciences Industry.)*

has grown fierce and has rapidly eroded multibillion dollar franchises of the pharmaceutical industry's biggest revenue producers as patents on these drugs have expired. The sharp increase in the cost of drug development has failed to produce a concomitant rise in the output of new drugs and biologics. That, coupled with the prospect of billions of dollars in lost revenue to generic drugs as the biggest blockbusters lose patent protection, has forced the industry to reluctantly acknowledge that its existing business model is unsustainable. Though the so-called patent cliff has squeezed Big Pharma for several years, 2012 represented the steepest loss of revenue as drugs with annual sales in excess of $33 billion a year lost patent protection. The combination of poor R&D productivity, pricing pressures, and revenue loss has triggered broad efforts into new approaches to R&D that could provide more cost-effective methods and yield greater successes. (See Figure 3.10.)

Estimates of the cost of drug development vary widely. A December 2012 study from the independent U.K. research organization, the Office of Health Economics put the mean cost at $1.5 billion. The researchers based their numbers on 2011 dollars and new unpublished data from the period 1998 to 2002 gathered by CMRI (formerly the Center for Medicines Research) in confidential surveys. It said its findings are in line with other studies. Costs across therapeutic areas vary widely, with development costs for neurology, respiratory, and oncology the highest. At the low

end, drugs for HIV/AIDS and antiparasitics were among the least expensive to develop. Developing drugs for the most expensive indications can be twice the cost of developing drugs for the least expensive areas.

Out-of-pocket costs for drug development rose nearly sixfold from the 1970s to the 2000s, the researchers said. The rising costs, in part, are due to falling success rates for drugs in clinical development as drugmakers sought to tackle more intractable diseases, such as Alzheimer's and cancer. The study found that success rates fell to 1 in 10 in the 2000s compared to 1 in 5 during the 1980s. The increasing complexity of the science underlying drug development and rising regulatory barriers has slowed the process of bringing drugs through R&D to approval. In the 2000s, that time grew to 13.5 years from just 6 years in the 1970s. The report notes that the cost of capital has risen as well. In order to provide adequate returns to investors to attract the capital necessary to fund the risky process of drug development, drugmakers in the 2000s needed to provide an 11 percent return, up from 8 percent in the 1970s.

As pharmaceutical R&D productivity has worsened, biotechnology companies have become increasingly attractive as targets for acquisitions and licensing deals. These companies tend to produce products for unmet medical needs and for markets where there is limited or no competition. As such, these products can command higher prices and are generally less susceptible to competition from generic drugs, even though a world of so-called biosimilars—close copies of biologics that have gone off-patent— is on the cusp of taking hold.

THE CONSISTENT CHALLENGE

Though business models have evolved, one constant throughout the history of the biotechnology industry is that companies are in a near-constant state of fundraising. Drug development, as noted above, is a costly and time-consuming process, and with the prospect of revenues far off in the future for most biotech companies, they must find ways to raise the capital they need to fund development of their products.

There are many ways that biotechnology companies finance their business. The instruments available to a company will often depend on its stage of development, whether it is public or private, and whether it has product on the market or close to entering the marketplace. Among the many ways biotech companies raise money are listed below and more thoroughly described in Chapter 19: Sources of Capital and Investor Motivations.

- **Small Business Innovation Research Program (SBIR):** This program is intended to provide a source of funding to small businesses, such as biotechnology companies. The grants are awarded through a competitive

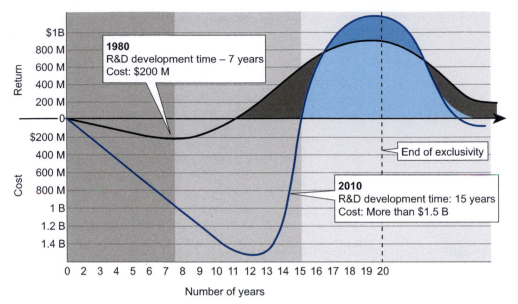

FIGURE 3.10   Time to recover R&D costs are being compressed. *(From Burrill & Company 2013 Annual Report on the Life Sciences Industry.)*

process and made through one of eleven federal agencies participating in the program, such as the U.S. Department of Health and Human Services and the U.S. Department of Defense. These grants are particularly attractive because they represent nondilutive capital. To qualify, a company must be at least 51 percent owned and controlled by one or more U.S. citizens and have no more than 500 employees.

- **Small Business Technology Transfer Program:** This is similar to the SBIR program except it focuses on forging public/private partnerships between small business and nonprofit research institutions.
- **Angel Capital:** This involves wealthy individuals who invest in high-risk, early-stage ventures. Angel investors within the biotech industry have grown increasingly sophisticated with former entrepreneurs and executives who have had success becoming investors. Through the formation of syndicates, Angel investors are playing increasingly important roles as venture capitalists have migrated away from early-stage investments in order to have shorter time horizons and more predictable exits from their investments.
- **Venture capital:** Venture capital has been the critical source of funding that gave rise to the biotech industry. These high-risk investors often take large ownership stakes in companies and provide not only essential capital to fund their growth, but also significant experience and relationships to guide the company and forge critical business alliances.
- **Strategic investors:** Strategic investors are corporations that invest in a company less for a financial return than a strategic reason. Within the biotech industry, this is usual in the form of a pharmaceutical company, often with its own venture capital arm investing alongside conventional venture capital firms. These investments can provide critical insight into new technologies and establish relationships that can later lead to licensing agreements.

- **Initial public offering (IPO):** Though still a viable financing option for biotechnology companies, public market investors have grown increasingly selective about investing in biotech companies, often insisting a company have marketed products or predictably will in the short-term. Although IPOs used to represent a way for a venture investor to gain liquidity from an investment, in recent years merger and acquisition (M&A) exits have become far more common as venture investors have often had to participate in IPOs as if they were another financing round for them.
- **Follow-on offering:** Once a company is public, additional offerings of stock are generally a much more cost-effective way to raise capital than other available sources.
- **Royalty financing:** A company with a marketed product or soon expected to have one can opt to raise money by selling the royalty stream to a specific drug in exchange for a lump-sum payment up front.

HOWDY PARTNER

Though the above examples are by no means the only financing alternatives, they represent many of the tools that biotech companies use to raise capital. One primary financing vehicle not included on the list above is licensing and partnering agreements. As with the very first product brought to market by the young industry, licensing and partnering agreements are a way that biotechnology companies can fund the development of a product, capitalize on the greater experience of a pharmaceutical company partner in navigating the regulatory arena, and tap into a well-established marketing, manufacturing, and distribution network.

Throughout the history of the biotechnology industry, partnering agreements have provided a critical source of funding to move drugs through clinical development and the approval process. Biotechnology companies have benefitted from the pharmaceutical industry's hunger to replenish its pipelines, particularly with the large amount of revenue being lost in recent years to patent expirations on top-selling drugs. These companies have grown increasingly reliant on biotechnology companies for innovative molecules as Big Pharma faced flagging productivity of their internal R&D engines. Though terms of collaborative agreements vary, they often involve an upfront payment to the biotechnology company, which generally hands off an experimental therapy once it has passed the proof-of-concept stage. Additional payments are usually tied to milestones along the development pathway and often include a royalty on sales.

Because these agreements can provide the potential for hundreds of millions of dollars in payments that never materialize because of clinical failures, the term "biobucks" has come to refer to the potential value of deals when they are announced. Despite the phantom nature of the total value of these deals, they are an essential mechanism for financing the development of innovative drugs. In fact, many companies are now formed with the sole purpose of developing drugs to proof-of-concept and then licensing them to a partner to complete development. This provides what many entrepreneurs and investors see as a lower risk and less capital-intensive strategy to realizing returns without building in the massive infrastructure needed to win regulatory approval, and to manufacture and market a drug. What's more, because companies can now contract outside companies and individuals to perform all the needed processes in moving a drug from discovery to market, a generation of so-called virtual companies have risen up to conduct drug development with relatively modest investment. These companies may license a drug from a university or a pharmaceutical company unwilling or unable to develop it and carry it to the proof-of-concept stage, at which point it can be partnered or sold.

THE END OF THE BLOCKBUSTER ERA

As the pharmaceutical industry undergoes a painful transition away from the blockbuster business model, biotechnology is leading it toward a new era of personalized medicine. The old model was based on hierarchical organizations with discovery and development conducted within the walls of the pharmaceutical company. The goal was to bring to market drugs for broad populations and heavily market them with a large salesforce. A "blockbuster drug" is considered to be one that has in excess of $1 billion in annual sales. The

world of Big Pharma had long been defined by the blockbuster business model.

Consider Parke-Davis Pharmaceuticals, which in 1986 made the decision to advance a compound that would be referred to as CI-981 into the clinic. It was not the company's lead compound in what was then a 4-year old program to develop a drug that could inhibit the liver enzyme HMG-CoA reductase, which is involved in the production of cholesterol. But when the development team was ready to advance the lead compound in the program into the clinic, the company learned that its competitor Sandoz already held patents on the molecule. As Jie Jack Li recounts in his book *The Triumph of the Heart,* Parke-Davis was late to the party in the emerging class of drugs known as statins. Merck would be first to market in 1987 with Mevacor. Three other statins—Merck's Zocor, Bristol-Myers-Squibb's Pravachol, and Sandoz' Lescol—were in late-stage clinical trials at the time Parke-Davis decided to enter the clinic. Those three other statins would make it to market well ahead of Parke-Davis' and there was debate within the company whether to even bother given the lead its competitors had. As *The Wall Street Journal* reported in a 2008 recounting of the history of the drug, animal studies suggested the Parke-Davis' drug was no better than its competitors. But Roger Newton, who codirected drug development at the company at the time, championed moving forward with it. "We'd spent a lot of years and blood, sweat and tears on this compound," he told *The Journal.* "Why would you spend all this money just to get to the edge of where you find out if it's viable?" By 1997 when the U.S. FDA approved CI-981, it had a new name: Lipitor (see Figure 3.11). Eventually, under the ownership of Pfizer, it would go on to become the top-selling drug in history reaching annual sales of $13.6 billion in 2006.

Around the same time Lipitor was heading to the clinic in 1986, a chance meeting between two researchers at the Denver airport would lead to another success story of a very different kind. It was there that Dennis Slamon, an oncologist at UCLA's Jonsson Cancer Center, met Genentech researcher Alex Ullrich. Their airport meeting, according to Robert Bazell in his book *HER-2: The Making of Herceptin,* would eventually lead to a scientific paper that suggested cancers that overexpress the protein HER-2 tend to spread quickly

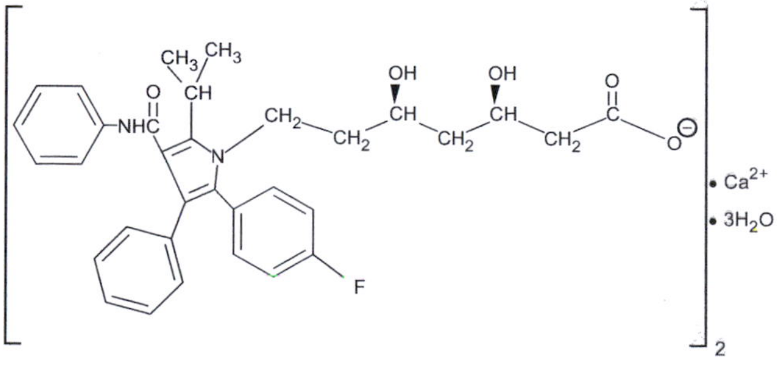

FIGURE 3.11   Lipitor chemical structure.

and metastasize. The two, though, ran into difficulty getting support for their work at Genentech. Bazell reports that by 1988, the company disbanded its oncology staff after its unsuccessful interferon-alfa trials and was no longer focusing on developing cancer therapies. That changed, however, when a senior vice president at the company learned his mother had been diagnosed with breast cancer and he pushed the project back on track. Their work led to a humanized monoclonal antibody, but as with Lipitor there were a number of obstacles along the way that made it an unlikely success story. Genentech's humanized monoclonal antibody was developed against a backdrop of spectacular industry failures around the technology, which can target a specific biological process involved in a disease. The drug faced great skepticism from within Genentech's ranks because no such drugs had yet been approved and many people questioned whether the technology would ever lead to an approved product.

Late in the development of the drug a big problem arose. With the company in the midst of a late-stage clinical trial, it became clear that the only hope of winning regulatory approval for what would become Herceptin, would require finding a partner to develop and commercialize a companion diagnostic similar to the home-brew assay the company was using in its clinical trials. The diagnostic test would enable doctors to determine whether a breast cancer patient was over-expressing the HER2 gene. Turned down by a Roche subsidiary that had no interest in developing a diagnostic for what it saw as too small a market, a team from Genentech found itself sitting over a meal of codfish in the dead of a Copenhagen winter negotiating a deal with representatives from a Danish company. Since then, Herceptin has helped transform the way biopharmaceutical companies think about drug development, companion diagnostics, and targeted therapies. Now a $5.5 billion-a-year product and growing, its success makes a persuasive case for personalized medicine.

Though Lipitor represented an impressive chemical engineering feat in how the molecule was synthesized, to a large extent it represents a business success story. While it benefitted from the eventual ability to demonstrate superiority to other statins that had beat it to market, it also enjoyed the massive investment over 10 years by its competitors to educate doctors about the value of the new class of drugs. It also benefitted from a strategic decision to aggressively price the new drug below the cost of the competing drugs already on the market. And, credit is due in part to an army of sales people—as many as 8000—who hammered away at doctors on the value and superiority of Lipitor during an age where drug reps still very much mattered and promotional budgets swelled. One 2007 study published in the *New England Journal of Medicine* found that by 2005, pharmaceutical spending on promotions rose to $29.9 billion in the United States, up from $11.4 billion in 1996. Pfizer spent $187.3 million to advertise Lipitor in 2007 alone.

THE TIMES THEY ARE A CHANGING

When Lipitor's patents expired at the end of 2011, it marked a symbolic end to the era of the one-size-fits-all blockbuster. It represented the way the industry long researched, developed, and marketed drugs, a model no longer in favor in the face of changing science, regulation, and healthcare economics. Today, it is unlikely that Parke Davis would have committed to the clinical development of Lipitor, the fifth drug in the category with no evidence at the time that it was any better than what was already on the market.

By contrast, Herceptin marked the birth of a new era of drug development and the shifting drivers of value in the industry. It not only represents an era where biology rather than chemistry is used to create drugs, but also one in which drug development is based upon understanding the molecular mechanism of disease, diagnostics that identify subpopulations of patients that will benefit from a specific therapy, and small, specialized sales forces that drive sales. The era of personalized medicine represented by Herceptin reflects a movement away from defining diseases by symptoms and locations within the body, toward understanding them through underlying genetic causes. Proponents of personalized medicine say it will increase the efficiency of drug development, cut wasteful spending on therapies that don't work for certain patients, and deliver more effective treatments to patients.

MAPPING THE HUMAN GENOME

Further fueling the advent of personalized medicine is a greater understanding of the human genome and the role it plays in wellness and disease. On June 26, 2000, President Bill Clinton stood at a press conference podium at the White House and announced that researchers at the Human Genome Project and a competing team from J. Craig Venter's Celera Genomics had completed a first draft of the human genome. The milestone fueled expectations about a new era for medicine. "With this profound new knowledge, humankind is on the verge of gaining immense, new power to heal," said Clinton. "It will revolutionize the diagnosis, prevention, and treatment of most, if not all, human diseases." Francis Collins, who at the time was the director of the Human Genome Project, said that the genetic diagnosis of disease would be accomplished within 10 years and new drugs based on that information would begin to emerge 5 years later. Within 20 years, Collins predicted, there would be a "complete transformation in therapeutic medicine." (See Figure 3.12.)

The complexity of disease biology, however, soon tempered the euphoria. Ten years after completing the rough draft of the human genome, the promised transformation, while hinted at, had yet to take place. "For biologists, the genome has yielded one insightful surprise after another,"

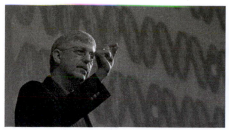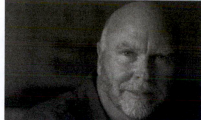

FIGURE 3.12 Francis Collins (left) and J. Craig Venter (right).

wrote Nicholas Wade in *The New York Times* on the tenth anniversary of the completion of the draft genome. "But the primary goal of the $3 billion Human Genome Project—to ferret out the genetic roots of common diseases like cancer and Alzheimer's and then generate treatments—remains largely elusive. Indeed, after 10 years of effort, geneticists are almost back to square one in knowing where to look for the roots of common disease." (See Figure 3.13.)

Venter, now chairman of the J. Craig Venter Institute, was blunter in his assessment when the German magazine *Der Spiegel* asked him in a July 2010 interview why it is taking so long for the information gleamed from the human genome to translate into benefits in medicine. "Because we have, in truth, learned nothing from the genome other than probabilities," he said. "How does a 1 or 3 percent increased risk for something translate into the clinic? It is useless information."

A transformation in medicine is underway, however, albeit a tad slower than many have expected. Though the mapping of the human genome hasn't yielded simple genetic explanations for diseases that have led to a medicine cabinet bursting with new drugs to cure them, a new understanding of the role genes play in disease has led to new therapeutics. In addition, there is a growing push among pharmaceutical companies to pair diagnostics to therapeutics. In part this represents an effort to accelerate drug development and cut costs of clinical trials by stratifying patient populations to increase the odds that a drug will be given to a patient who will benefit from it. At the same time, it reflects an effort to use therapeutics that are targeted to specific molecular mechanisms of disease to enhance the safety and efficacy of drugs and deliver on the promise of providing the right drug to the right patient in the right dose at the right time. Though the press reports marking the occasion of the tenth anniversary of the draft genome focused on the lack of drugs to grow out of new knowledge about genetics, it is changing the way drug research is being conducted. While there hasn't been a flood of new genomic-based drugs reaching the market, The *New York Times* noted that there is a mounting example of drugs that grow out of new knowledge about genetics ranging from targeted therapeutics for cancer that act on genetic abnormalities fueling a disease to recently approved therapeutics such as Amgen's osteoporosis drug Prolia and Human Genome Sciences lupus drug Benlysta. In fact, the newspaper noted that two-thirds of drugs being developed by Bristol-Myers Squibb have been touched in some way by genomics and one-third of Genentech's drugs in clinical trials and two-thirds of drugs in earlier development have been enabled by the genome project.

Still, as pharmaceutical executives told the newspaper, drug development remains a slow process and genomics is providing new drug targets, not drugs. "If on the first day we had discovered a new molecular target, it's still going to take 15 to 20 years to make the drug," Robert Ruffolo, Wyeth's former head of research and development told the *Times*. "Genomics did not speed up drug development. It gave us more rapid access to new molecular targets."

AN EVOLVING VISION

When people speak of personalized medicine they generally think about it in two ways. In simple terms, there is the notion of harnessing diagnostics and targeted therapeutics to attack the underlying molecular mechanism of a patient's individual disease. In this sense, personalized medicine is, as the saying goes, about delivering the right

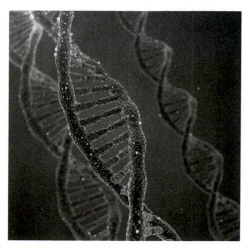

FIGURE 3.13 The Human Genome is comprised of over 3 billion DNA base pairs contained within 23 pairs of chromosomes.

drug, to the right patient, at the right dose, at the right time. It is here that personalized medicine has met with some of its most dramatic and earliest successes with early targeted therapies and companion diagnostics, such as Genentech's breast cancer drug Herceptin (Figure 3.14), which radically altered the therapeutic landscape for cancer therapies by identifying patients appropriate for the therapy through an understanding of the molecular mechanism underlying the form of the disease against which the drug would be effective. Herceptin works on what actually drives the growth and spread of the HER2 positive breast cancer, overexpression of the HER2 gene, rather than using less-discriminating toxins and hoping for the best. In this context, the term "personalized medicine" today is giving way to the newer term "precision medicine" as being more apt.

As pharmaceutical companies face increasing pressure from payers and regulators to establish the value of their products, they have come to embrace targeted therapies and companion diagnostics. In the old world, driven by a search for the next blockbuster drug, personalized medicine at first seemed like anathema. What drug company would go out of its way to marry a drug to a diagnostic that would guarantee eliminating a large number of potential customers, even if they would never benefit from using the drug? But as payers increasingly demand proof-of-value of new therapies and regulators seek greater certainty about the safety and efficacy of drugs, drug developers are focusing more on drugs that address unmet medical needs as a better route to clinical, regulatory, and economic success. They are also finding that the blockbuster era is not dead, only that the era of the one-size-fits-all blockbuster is coming to an end.

In 2012, newly approved personalized therapies included Vertex Pharmaceutical's Kalydeco for cystic fibrosis and Roche's Perjeta for the treatment of a certain form of breast cancer that has spread. The FDA in June 2012 approved Roche's Perjeta for HER2-positive metastatic breast cancer in combination with Herceptin and docetaxel chemotherapy. The approval was based on data from a late-stage clinical trial that showed previously untreated HER2-positive metastatic breast cancer patients who received the combination

of Perjeta, Herceptin and docetaxel chemotherapy lived a median of 6.1 months longer without their cancer getting worse compared to patients treated with Herceptin plus docetaxel chemotherapy. Progression-free survival in patients that received Perjeta in combination with the other therapies had a median of 18.5 months compared to 12.4 months for patients that received just Herceptin and docetaxel.

As with Herceptin, Perjeta is a personalized medicine that targets the HER2 receptor, a protein found in high quantities on the outside of cells in HER2-positive cancers. But Perjeta is believed to work in a way that is complementary to Herceptin, as the two medicines target different regions on the HER2 receptor. "Perjeta attacks HER2-positive tumors differently than Herceptin. Based on the way the two medicines work together, the combination plus chemotherapy can prolong the time before this aggressive cancer worsens compared to Herceptin and chemotherapy alone," said Hal Barron, chief medical officer and head of global product development for Roche's Genentech subsidiary.

In the case of Kalydeco, the FDA approved the drug for patients with a specific genetic mutation known as G551D, which drives the disease in roughly 4 percent of patients, or about 1200 people in the United States with cystic fibrosis (CF), a life-threatening disease that damages the lungs. It causes a cell-surface protein to function incorrectly, preventing a proper flow of sodium and fluid in and out of cells. Kalydeco works by restoring the function of that protein. "Kalydeco addresses the underlying cause of CF and the science behind the drug has opened exciting new doors to research and development that may eventually lead to additional therapies that will benefit more people living with CF," Robert Beall, president and CEO of the Cystic Fibrosis Foundation, said when the drug was approved. Cystic Fibrosis Foundation Therapeutics, the nonprofit drug discovery and development affiliate of the Cystic Fibrosis Foundation had long been in an R&D partnership with Vertex supporting the development of Kalydeco. Despite the small market for the drug, Vertex sales stand to be substantial. The drug carries an annual price tag of $294,000, according to Dow Jones Newswires.

CHANGING ECONOMICS

In fact, a 2012 study in *Drug Discovery Today* from Thomson Reuters and Pfizer makes a strong economic case for pharmaceutical companies to develop drugs for rare or orphan disease, diseases that afflict less than 200,000 people in the United States. The financial incentives put in place to encourage the development of drugs for rare diseases, such as the Orphan Drug Act of 1983, provide tax breaks, R&D offsets, R&D grants, waived FDA fees, accelerated approval, and extended periods of exclusivity. Orphan drugs also can generally command higher prices than drugs for nonorphan disease. As personalized medicine redefines diseases by their

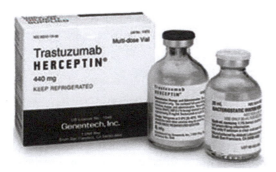

FIGURE 3.14   Herceptin, developed by Genentech.

underlying molecular mechanisms rather than their outward manifestations, it is breaking disease groups into smaller sub-populations, turning one-time broad diseases into subtypes of those diseases that by definition constitute rare disease.

"We're not just talking about the typical rare disease, what we are also talking about are the emerging subdiseases. You can take something like lung cancer; whereas before it might have been regarded as one cancer, typically pharma would try something to stick into lung cancer, now it's being talked of as 15 or 20 individual, small subdiseases," says Kiran Meekings, life sciences consultant at Thomson Reuters and lead author of the "Drug Discovery Today" study. "So if we look at crizotinib [Xalkori], approved last year, that is an orphan drug because it is targeting a very small population of a larger disease. This type of patient stratification or more personalized medicine approach is actually opening up new markets, which are smaller populations of larger diseases."

Pfizer's Xalkori was approved in 2011 to treat certain patients with late-stage, nonsmall cell lung cancers who express a mutated anaplastic lymphoma kinase, or ALK, gene. About 5 percent of patients with non small cell lung cancer, or about 9000 people a year with the disease, have the mutation. The drug costs $9600 a month or $115,000 for patients who use it for a year, according to *Forbes*. Xalkori was approved with a companion diagnostic test that will help determine if a patient has the abnormal ALK gene, a first-of-a-kind genetic test called the Vysis ALK Break Apart FISH Probe Kit. The companion diagnostics were approved ahead of the drug's 2011 approvals. "The trend in oncology research continues towards targeted therapies," said Alberto Gutierrez, director of the Office of In Vitro Diagnostic Device Evaluation and Safety in the FDA's Center for Devices and Radiological Health. "This test is an example of the important role companion diagnostics play in determining that the safest and most effective treatments are promptly delivered to patients living with serious and life-threatening diseases."

The Thomson Reuters study found that orphan drugs represent "an increasingly important component of the pharmaceutical market and have equal revenue-generating potential to non-orphan drugs." The authors said orphan drugs make up 22 percent of total drug sales, and the cumulative annual growth rate of the orphan drug market totaled 25.8 percent between 2001 and 2010. That compared to only 20.1 percent for the matched nonorphan control group. In fact, the study found that the mean annual economic value of orphan drugs, in 2010 terms, reached $637 million compared to $638 million for nonorphan drugs. While the present value of nonorphan drugs remained roughly constant between 2000 and 2010, the present value of orphan drugs nearly doubled during that period. "This analysis suggests that the impact of a smaller treatable patient pool is offset by the higher pricing of many orphan drugs, the increased market share, the

longer exclusivity period, and faster uptake rate that orphan drugs often garner as a result of the high unmet medical need in many of these diseases," the authors write.

A GREATER PROMISE

Beyond precision medicine, targeted therapeutics, and treatments tailored to individual patients, the greater promise of personalized medicine lies in radically transforming medicine away from treating symptoms of illness to not only addressing the underlying causes of disease, but also attacking disease at its earliest stages before it blossoms into a costly, chronic, or deadly threat. That's exactly what Stanford's Snyder was able to do with his own developing diabetes through his costly monitoring of the biological changes within his own body. Through improved diagnostics, new understanding of the human genome and biomarkers, and an array of new monitoring devices in the emerging world of digital health, healthcare is on the cusp of realizing the deeper vision of personalized medicine—or perhaps more accurately, personalized healthcare—defined by its focus on personal, predictive, and preventive care.

One of the primary drivers of that change is the rapidly falling cost of genome sequencing and the move of the genome from a costly and cumbersome research tool to a diagnostic tool with clincial utility. In 2012, the cost of sequencing was expected to fall below the $1000 mark, blowing away Moore's law (Figure 3.15). Though the Human Genome

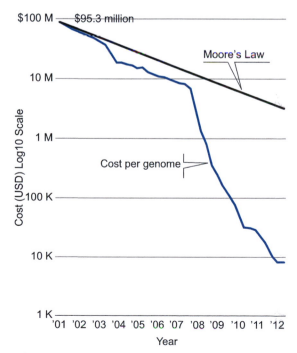

Sequencing cost per genome

FIGURE 3.15   Declining cost of sequencing a genome. (*From Burrill & Company. 2013 Annual Report on the Life Sciences Industry.*)

Project took 13 years and $3 billion dollars, the actual time and cost of sequencing the first human genome exclusive of other parts of the project has been estimated to have taken a year and cost about $500 million, according to officials at the National Human Genome Research Institute. In September 2012, Life Technologies began shipping its Ion Proton™ Sequencing System. The company said the chip-based system cost about a third of the genome scale sequencing systems that rely on light to read a genome and is small enough to fit on a desktop, saving researchers hundreds of thousands of dollars. The device can sequence exomes and transcriptomes in 2 to 4 hours. The company expects to release a second generation chip for the system around the end of the first quarter of 2013 that will be able to, in a few hours, sequence the human genome for $1000.

A World of Opportunity

Governments around the world are stepping in to advance life sciences in their countries to boost their economies and address the growing healthcare needs of their citizenry. In some emerging countries, such as Russia and China, the government is actively participating in funding startups and investing in new technologies that can be brought into their country, developed locally, and adapted to address unmet needs and add new fuel to their growing economies. In other countries, such as in Europe and the United Kingdom, regional organizations have formed investment funds to attract startups and strengthen their economies. While the developed world continues to be an important source of innovation and business opportunity, life sciences companies from startups to Big Pharma are taking advantage of global economic growth and healthcare initiatives both at home and abroad to capture value for their products and companies. These opportunities run the gamut from financial incentives and access to new markets to the chance to leverage the worth of an asset because of a regional medical practice or unmet medical need.

Sometimes a tax incentive intended to help startups develop novel products serves as the lure to locate research and development in a foreign country. Consider the case of AmpliPhi Biosciences, a semivirtual biotech based in the United States and the United Kingdom engaged in the development of phage-based drugs to treat infections. Bacteriophage, or phage, are naturally occurring viruses that attack and kill bacteria. If not properly contained, manufacturing phage could contaminate a facility that is also being used to manufacture other biologicals. So when AmpliPhi needed enough of its bacteriophage-based drug to run a late-stage trial to test it as a treatment of pseudomonas-based lung infections in patients with cystic fibrosis, it decided that it had to build its own manufacturing plant. AmpliPhi merged with Special Phage Services, an Australian company working on bacteriophage therapies to fight infections. After a global search for a contract manufacturing partner, the company decided it should build a plant at the lowest possible cost, but also be assured that it would operate under strict U.S. FDA standards for Current Good Manufacturing Practices. It decided that building in Australia would offer it the best opportunity. A major reason for selecting Australia was a relatively new R&D rebate program. The cash rebate from this program would end up covering a significant portion of AmpliPhi's R&D costs.

Australia's R&D Tax Incentive, implemented in July 2011 to boost innovation at a time when companies were struggling to access capital, offers a 45 percent refundable tax offset for R&D expenses in the form of annual cash rebates to companies that have less than $20 million in revenue and file tax returns in the country. AmpliPhi evaluated the option of partnering with a contract manufacturing organization or building a small facility, and decided to build and validate a facility outside Sydney. For a research-intensive biotech company without revenue, the tax credit was a welcome nondilutive source of funding for R&D activities.

INVESTING IN INNOVATION

As governments in emerging markets seek to move their countries from being centers of low-cost labor to centers of innovation and high-value jobs, they are becoming important sources of funding for early-stage life sciences companies in more-advanced economies. China, for example, has set ambitious targets to ramp up its innovation capability, and has targeted biotechnology as a strategic pillar for growth under its 12th Five-Year Plan. The plan aims to double biomedical R&D innovation funding from the previous Five-Year Plan to $300 billion and seeks to provide basic healthcare services to at least 90 percent of its 1.3 billion citizens by 2020.

PARTNERSHIPS OF CONVENIENCE

In some cases, early-stage biotechs are able to get partners in emerging markets to fund clinical development and still retain rights to those products outside of those markets. In other cases, they can help companies leverage an asset that they may be ill-prepared to commercialize in an emerging market and use market demands in those countries to accelerate the development and cut the cost and risk of bringing those products to market in developed countries.

Cleveland BioLabs' strategy is to create separate, independently funded entities to develop a broad pipeline of drug candidates and allow the company to move multiple drug candidates forward, with separate management teams focused on a smaller set of goals (Figure 3.16). While its treatment for radiation syndrome has shown positive results and is currently in pivotal trials, the company had

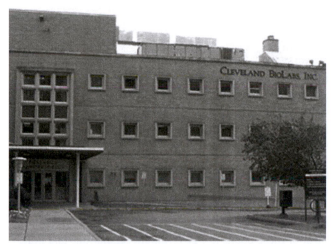

FIGURE 3.16 Cleveland BioLabs. *(Source: Site Selection Online, Upstate New York.)*

many other compounds in its pipeline for which it wanted to accelerate the development process. So it looked outside the United States to Eastern Europe and Asia, where it felt it could get its drugs to market sooner.

In 2010, Cleveland BioLabs found funding and partners in Russia for its anticancer therapies based on drug candidates of the curaxin family, forming the joint venture Incuron with Bioprocess Capital Ventures, a Russian government-backed venture fund that contributed $18 million. Cleveland BioLabs contributed two curaxins for oncology and orphan indications, taking a 75.8 percent stake in the Russia-based startup.

"This investment will enable us to support curaxin development through advanced human trials," said Cleveland BioLabs president and CEO Michael Fonstein, when the joint venture was launched. In April 2012, Incuron was given permission by Russian regulatory authorities to conduct early-stage human trials in Russia of an oral formulation of one of the compounds in patients with advanced solid tumors resistant or refractory to standard-care treatment.

Cleveland BioLabs partnered with Russian investors in a second joint venture in September 2011, this time with Rusnano, another Russian Federation-backed investment company. The venture, U.S.-based Panacela Labs, also majority-owned by Cleveland BioLabs, was formed to develop five preclinical drug candidates for cancer and infectious disease, giving Russia access to not only product candidates, but also global pharmaceutical expertise. Both ventures reflect ongoing efforts by the Russian government to strengthen its pharmaceutical industry which it sees as an important driver of economic growth.

Rusnano is investing up to $26 million over 4 years in Panacela, of which it paid $9 million upfront with future investments based upon the achievement of development milestones and the attraction of new investments to the

project. Cleveland BioLabs initially contributed $3 million to the joint venture and the preclinical candidates which were developed under the guidance of Andrei Gudkov, chief scientific officer of Cleveland BioLabs and a senior vice president at Roswell Park Cancer Institute.

The compounds are being developed and approved in Russia first. After the drugs are introduced into clinical practice there, Panacela intends to seek licensing and approval in other global markets, including the United States. In this way, Cleveland BioLabs can accelerate the development of its pipeline while Russia will get access to much-needed innovative drugs that it will be able to produce domestically.

In July 2012 Panacela Labs was awarded $4.6 million by the Ministry of Industry and Trade of the Russian Federation under the Russian Federation's "Pharma 2020" development initiative to support development of its xenomycin program. The initiative provides matching funds over a period of approximately 3 years. The money will be used to support preclinical and clinical studies of xenomycins as treatments for parasitic and fungal infections.

Russia's Pharma 2020 strategy aims to completely modernize the pharmaceutical industry in the country, mainly by transferring innovative technology from outside Russia to Russian companies. Partnerships with international companies, as well as investment projects of Big Pharma in Russia, are key elements of the strategy. The Russian government is committing about $6 billion through 2020 on the state level toward modernizing its domestic healthcare industry.

By leveraging the needs in emerging markets, companies such as Cleveland BioLabs can obtain access to nondilutive financing, reduce development risk, and develop multiple compounds at once. For emerging market countries, these deals provide a way to build their economies, decrease their dependence on drugs produced outside their borders, and increase the high-value technical skills of their workers as they address the health needs of their populations.

PROMOTING TECHNOLOGY TRANSFER

Emerging countries shifting their economies to high-value industries from a dependence on low-value commodities and manufacturing see biotechnology and other medical technologies as important drivers of economic growth and are investing heavily in education, infrastructure, and healthcare to develop homegrown industries to serve the needs of their people and fuel further growth of their economies. This provides an opportunity for companies to leverage an asset they may not be prepared to commercialize in an emerging market, and use the needs in those countries to accelerate the development and cut the cost and risk of bringing those products to market in developed countries.

Many nations are also leveraging their financial strengths to gain industry expertise. Russia is a leader in this trend. In order to diversify its economy from a dependence on natural resources toward more high-technology sectors, the Russian government in 2010 launched "Pharma 2020" as a national roadmap to develop the country's biomedical sector to meet the growing healthcare needs of its citizens. Then Prime Minister Vladimir Putin pledged about $12 billion over 10 years toward increasing the country's capacity to produce drugs and medical equipment, including the establishment of more than a dozen centers of innovation and the training of people to staff them. The goal is to increase domestic market share to 50 percent by 2020, from 20 percent in 2011. Eventually, the country hopes to become a major exporter of medicines—an ambitious goal at the time considering that few of the country's manufacturing facilities met international standards.

Russia is also seeking to build its biotechnology industry, which had been neglected for many years after the fall of the Soviet Union. "Twenty years ago we were one of the three or four biggest countries for biotech and now it is very little, which is awful," says Professor Konstantin Skryabin, head of the Department of Biotechnology at Lomonosov Moscow State University and venture partner with Burrill Russia. "So there was a definite need to push biotech as a priority in the country." Having biotech be a government priority will open up opportunities for other countries to participate, says Skryabin. "This is the motive of the initiative." As one of his last acts as prime minister, Putin formally signed the Russia "Bio2020" initiative in April 2012 to advance all areas of biotechnology in Russia. The plan includes an estimated $39 billion to be spent by 2020 in biomedical, bioagricultural, bioindustrial, aquaculture, forest biotech, environmental, and bioenergy projects.

Innovating is capital intensive, and governments realize that public funding is often not enough by itself. Because of that, they are taking steps to not only fund innovation directly, but also to encourage private investment. Russia sees technology transfer as a major component of its Pharma 2020 plan and several government-backed investment funds have been making significant bets in innovative Western life sciences companies that are willing to set up drug development and manufacturing facilities in Russia. Rusnano, for example, has made several investments in Western companies that include agreements to develop their compounds and commercialize them first in Russia.

Backed by $10 billion in government money, Rusnano entered into a $760 million equal partnership with U.S. venture capital firm Domain Associates in February 2012 to backup to 20 companies willing to develop their compounds in Russia. Most of the opportunities will be for late-stage products. By the end of 2012 they had invested $113 million in four Domain portfolio companies, three of which have transferred intellectual property rights to NovaMedica, a Moscow-based pharmaceutical company formed specifically to manufacture and distribute products from the partnership in Russia. On the Russian side, NovaMedica will

be eligible for special grants from the government that are provided to companies that engage in technology transfer of innovative products.

While drug sales in emerging markets are expected to grow by $157 billion over the next 5 years, reaching at least $345 billion by 2016, according to IMS Health, competition from local players will carve out a growing portion of that growth. Emerging markets differ in their demographics, governments, regulatory policies, economic structures, per capital income, and cultures—all things that must be taken into account when devising an emerging markets strategy.

As in developed countries, emerging markets governments face increased pressure to rein in healthcare costs. In most of these countries, government regulations and policy are designed to benefit local companies, and demand that foreign companies wishing to do business in their markets establish local subsidiaries and partner with local firms. Their regulatory bureaucracies can be difficult to navigate and businesses are often hampered by a lack of managerial expertise. Markets are often fragmented with many small players competing to get their products on government-essential drug lists.

Companies must also take into account that most of the population in emerging markets cannot afford to pay for high-priced drugs and many governments rely on drug price controls, so a return on investment is not assured. The potential market is huge however, and governments see the importance of investing in the life sciences to build innovation-based economies that can provide high-quality jobs. They see innovation as the way to transform their societies for the better, especially amid the austere economic conditions and global challenges facing the world today. The challenge for innovative companies is to understand and be able to take advantage of global opportunities when and where they arise. Those that succeed are poised to reap huge rewards for their efforts, both in monetary terms and in terms of improved human health and welfare.

NOT JUST ABOUT DRUGS

Environmental, energy, and food security risks posed by climate change and the rapid growth of economies and populations are driving nations to search for ways to move from a fossil fuel-based economy to a low-carbon economy—one that runs on renewable sources of energy and sustainable agricultural practices. Nations are turning to industrial biotechnology for sustainable solutions that could lead to energy security and mitigate global warming, while new agricultural biotechnologies hold promise for improving crops to both feed and fuel a growing world population that has surpassed 7 billion people and is expected to reach 9 billion by 2050.

Bioindustrial technologies are being developed to not only unlock the energy potential in plants, but also to turn industrial and municipal waste streams—currently discarded into the atmosphere or landfills—into feedstocks for the production of fuels and chemicals that are currently derived from petroleum. A new industry has been spurred, in part, by the establishment of the Renewable Fuel Standard, instituted by the Energy Independence and Security Act of 2007, which requires transportation fuels be blended with increasing amounts of biofuels. While biofuels today are primarily first-generation corn-based or sugar-based ethanol, new technologies are currently being scaled to manufacture next-generation bio-based fuels derived from biomass, algae, municipal wastes, and even carbon dioxide itself (Figure 3.17).

Many of these new technologies involve synthetic biology techniques to genetically engineer microbes, yeast, and algae to excrete the chemical or precursor molecule of value. On the biomass side of the equation, agricultural biotechs are developing crop varieties specifically suited for use as feedstocks for the biorenewables industry such as energy cane, sweet sorghum, and fast-growing grasses and other potential energy crops that can be grown in areas unsuitable for growing food crops.

EVERYTHING OLD IS NEW AGAIN

Biofuels are not new. The earliest engines were designed to run on biofuels—Henry Ford's Model T ran on hemp-derived ethanol. But as the large-scale exploration of crude oil took hold in the late 1930s and going forward, petroleum became the transportation fuel of choice. As oil prices have continued to rise, however, many governments have had to rethink the use of biofuels as a means of energy security. In the United States, the military has been one of the strongest proponents for the development of advanced biofuels. The

U.S. Navy, in particular, has a goal of getting 50 percent of its energy from low-carbon-emitting alternative sources by 2020, and has invested heavily to help develop bio-based diesel and aviation fuels. Even as the United States has reduced its dependence on foreign oil, for the military, using renewable fuels for transport and power is a matter of national security.

With fuel costs comprising more than a third of its average operating costs, the commercial aviation industry also wants sustainable renewable fuels in its mix both as a hedge against the rising price of fossil fuels and to reduce its carbon emissions. Globally, companies such as Dynamic Fuels, LanzaTech, Solazyme, Algae.Tec, Aemetis, Gevo, Amyris, and Neste, to name a few, are actively working to develop feedstocks and conversion technologies for the production of aviation biofuels. LanzaTech is partnered with Virgin Airlines, Solazyme has a supply agreement with Australia's Qantas Airlines, and Gevo has an agreement with United Airlines (Figure 3.18).

There also has been a strong drive among consumer goods, oil and chemical, and pulp and paper companies to access biorenewable technologies that can complement their existing products and at the same time reduce their carbon footprint. But in all these cases, bio-based products must meet the same performance standards as existing petroleum-based products and also be competitively priced.

THE CHALLENGE OF SCALE

Achieving commercial-scale production and cost-parity with fossil fuels takes an enormous amount of capital. While many of these companies have received significant backing from venture capitalists, strategic investment by the established oil, chemical, consumer goods, and agricultural industries has been imperative for the development of the biorenewables industry. Major global investors in this sector include the oil companies Shell, Total, and BP, chemical companies such as DuPont, BASF, Mitsui, Lanxess, M&G, and PTT, consumer goods companies such as Proctor & Gamble and Unilever, agribusinesses such as Monsanto, Syngenta, and Bunge, and waste handlers such as Waste Management, among many others. Partnerships with these strategic investors is the lifeline for many of these companies as they raise anywhere from $100 million to $300 million to build their first biorefineries, which started becoming operational in the second half of 2012.

Although many of these bioindustrial companies began with a strategy to make renewable fuels, many have turned their attention to producing renewable chemicals because they command lower volumes and higher prices. Although it was seen as ironic that Solazyme first marketed its customized algal oils in a line of cosmetics, it has been a trailblazer for success in a highly competitive industry. Other companies have followed Solazyme's lead to sell smaller

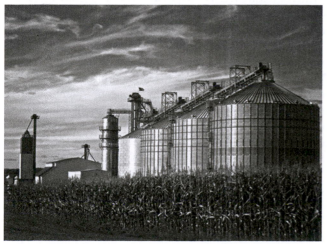

FIGURE 3.17 Corn as a renewable biofuel source.

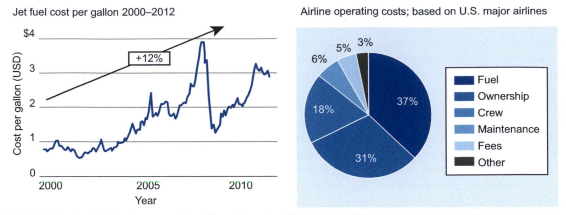

FIGURE 3.18   Jet fuel is the largest cost for airlines. *(From Burrill & Company 2013 Annual Report on the Life Sciences Industry.)*

volumes of their products into the consumer goods market as they develop their biofuels technology. Solazyme makes its renewable oils with genetically engineered algae grown in closed containers. Solazyme has secured contracts with the military and aviation industry to supply test amounts of aviation biofuels, and at the end of 2012 its algal-based biodiesel blend was offered in a successful pilot program at four gas stations in the San Francisco Bay Area.

IMPROVING YIELDS

Besides engineering crops for specific purposes such as a feedstock source for the production of bio-based fuels and chemicals, companies engaged in improving crops are taking advantage of a growing toolbox of biologic and genomic technologies to develop plants that can tolerate drought and other stressors, improve yield, and add nutritional value. While these technologies are still in the research phase, they may eventually find an easier route to market because they are outside the traditional definition genetic modification. Genetically modified crops, primarily corn, soybeans, and cotton are grown around the world and accounted for more than one third of the total seed market in 2011, with a market value of approximately $12 billion derived from seed sales and licensing revenue. Adoption rates are growing faster in developing countries, with Brazil, Argentina, China, and South Africa leading the rate of adoption.

Genetic modifications currently on the market include making crops herbicide-tolerant or pesticide-resistant. These transgenic modifications have been developed by a handful of big multinational agribusinesses: Monsanto, DuPont's Pioneer HiBred, Dow Agrosciences, Bayer Crop-Science, Syngenta, and BASF, which also make and market the agrochemicals used in conjunction with the crops.

While these agribusinesses control much of the crop-improvement market, they are looking at advanced breeding technologies that go beyond traditional genetic modification in order to develop superior hybrids without policy hurdles

faced by genetically modified crops in many parts of the world. Many of these new technologies work by modifying plant genes directly rather than by inserting foreign DNA as is the case in traditional genetic modification.

The agribusinesses are also looking outside their own research programs for innovation that can add to their toolkit. Monsanto and Syngenta, for example, have venture arms that invest in early-stage life sciences technology companies, especially those that support and complement their increased focus on the use of genomics, informatics, and biology directed at crop improvement. Both companies have made recent acquisitions in companies with RNA interference technology that can be applied to agriculture to develop topical or seed treatment products that can complement or replace agricultural chemical products.

The bio-based fuels and chemicals, or biorenewables, industry is young and agricultural technology has only recently embraced the power of genomics. For biorenewables, the industry needs to see some commercial successes at scales that can convince investors and the market that biorenewables can be a significant replacement for fossil fuels. As is the case with healthcare biotechs, companies that are nimble and flexible will be able to access capital and become acquisition targets.

Success will also depend on the aggregation and conversion of biomass from nonfood sources on a massive scale. This has not yet occurred and is still a future challenge. But energy and food prices are only going up, arable land is only getting scarcer, and demand on natural resources is only intensifying. In a finite world, biotechnologies that can move us to a low-carbon future will eventually gain in value, and deliver it to the benefit of mankind.

THE CHALLENGE TODAY

The reality for the pharmaceutical industry today is that sheer force of will and sales muscle will no longer drive multibillion successes for it. With the end of the one-size-fits-all blockbuster era, so too comes the end of the ability of drugmakers to shape markets for new drugs by deploying an army of sales people. That's evident not only in the shift of decision-making away from doctors to payers, but evident in the dramatic downsizing of pharmaceutical salesforces. In recognition of this fundamental change to the landscape, pharmaceutical companies are reaching out directly to payers to forge new partnerships and experiment with new types of payment models tied to the success of their products delivering real-world patient benefits.

Consider the biotechnology company Acorda Therapeutics, which in January 2010 won FDA approval for Ampyra, a drug that improves the ability of multiple sclerosis (MS) patients to walk. It was a major victory for the company after a long and challenging development path that resulted in a first-of-its-kind treatment, one that wasn't disease modifying, but improved function for MS patients. But once the FDA hurdle was cleared, the company faced new hurdles with payers. Like most small biotechs, Acorda had, until then, focused on the clinical and regulatory challenges it faced. Reimbursement had not been a major focus. The world that existed while the drug was being developed largely assumed that drugs that cleared regulatory hurdles wouldn't generally face issues on reimbursement.

But some payers wondered about the benefits of an MS drug that wasn't disease modifying. Ampyra is a potassium channel blocker that essentially restores the ability to conduct electrical signals to nerve fibers that have lost their protective myelin insulation. In retrospect, Ron Cohen, CEO of Acorda says, "If the company knew what it was going to encounter, it likely would have added elements to its clinical development program that would have been geared toward managed care acceptance, but might not necessarily have improved its chances of regulatory approval."

"This is not your grandfather's Buick anymore. If you grew up in biotech any time prior to the last five years, you need to reexamine your assumptions about the world of reimbursement. It has changed dramatically and it is continuing to change at really stunning speed," says Cohen, who says Acorda now engages payers in presentations of the company's early-stage pipeline in preparation for later discussion on clinical trial design once proof-of-concept is established. "If you are a developer, you need to understand it and if you don't have that expertise in-house, go get it, or hire it as a consultant at a minimum, because you need to do it."

Such discussions are not unusual for Big Pharma today, which has not only engaged with payers to get their input on clinical trial designs, but has also entered into research partnerships to address a variety of concerns and build a deeper dialogue with both insurers and pharmacy benefit managers. Payers now exert a greater influence on the market success or failure of a drug. AstraZeneca and Wellpoint announced a 4-year collaboration in 2011 to study the use

of already-marketed drugs. Sanofi and Medco, now part of Express Scripts, also in 2011 announced an agreement that gives Sanofi access to Medco's comparative data to help shape its drug-development strategy. And Pfizer that same year announced separate agreements with Humana and Medco. The Humana collaboration is focused on improving healthcare for seniors while the Medco collaboration focuses on identifying patient subgroups in which both experimental and marketed drugs would benefit.

In other cases, drugmakers and payers have entered into novel collaborations to share risks by linking the price paid for drugs to actual outcomes. A 2009 agreement between Merck and CIGNA described as "the first national outcome-based contract between a pharmaceutical company and a pharmacy benefit management company," provides payments to Merck that are based on how well its type 2 diabetes drugs Januvia and Janumet improve blood glucose levels in patients using the drugs. A separate agreement that same year between partners Procter & Gamble and Sanofi with the insurer Health Alliance calls for the drugmakers to cover the cost of treating patients covered by the insurer who use the osteoporosis drug Actonel and develop bone fractures.

Payers say what they want to understand is the value of new medications. Ideally, they say what they would like to see is clinical trials of new medications against standard of care to establish superiority, something they say pharmaceutical companies are reluctant to do because failure to demonstrate that could kill the market for a drug. "The value of the medication needs to be established. A lot of times a pharmaceutical firm will do some economic modeling for a drug and make some assertion that you can reduce other medical costs," says Edmund Pezalla, National Medical Director for Pharmacy Policy and Strategy for Aetna. He says this can include claims of medical cost offsets, such as a patient's use of a drug would help avoid having a stroke, other medical event, or the need to go to an emergency room. "But randomized clinical trials are not the best place to look for those medical costs offsets," he says.

In the absence of comparative effectiveness data, or data on offsets and actual use by patients that are better determined in real-world studies, there are things that payers would like to gather from clinical trials. These include understanding if there are subgroups of patients that benefit from a drug, not only through the use of biomarkers, but other measures such as medical histories or phenotypic data. They are also interested in measures of quality of life, such as whether the use of a drug improves the ability of someone to stay employed, do activities around the home, and remain productive.

"It's not just a matter of, 'here's a medicine and you can use it.' What we are trying to determine is, where does that medicine go?" says Pezalla. "Is it a medication that is for a niche population and that's how we should treat it; or is it a medication for a broader audience and it should be used after an existing generic; or is it a brand new sort of medication that really changes patient outcomes, really changes patient quality of life?"

THE MOMENT IS NOW

The pharmaceutical industry has for much of the past decade been bracing for the very moment in time it now finds itself. The patent cliff, long on the horizon, is now at its steepest point. The end of the one-size-fits-all blockbuster, a date marked not only by expiring patents, but emerging science, regulatory embarrassments, and payer frustration, has arrived as well. The day of reckoning for bloated and ineffective R&D operations has come also.

Then again, the new world the pharmaceutical industry has watched approach brings new opportunities as well. The shifting global economy has seen new demand and growth in emerging economies where spreading prosperity is giving rise to an emerging middle class. With longer life spans and changing lifestyles, prosperity is also bringing with it a growing incidence of chronic disease that will drive demand for treatments for cancer, heart disease, diabetes, and other conditions in markets such as China, Russia, Brazil and elsewhere.

The pharmaceutical industry has been involved in a variety of efforts to both create value by reducing costs, increasing efficiency, and improving the value of what it produces, while at the same time seeking ways to capture more value by focusing on drugs for unmet medical needs, rare diseases, and targeted therapies where value propositions are clear and pricing and competitive pressures are mitigated. A push to externalize research has accelerated. Pharmaceutical companies are forging deeper ties with academic institutions, disease advocacy groups, and independent research institutes. They are reaching further into the early-stage pipeline to partner on discovery-stage research with what for now are uncertain results. More than anything these activities reflect an acknowledgment that what has historically driven the industry is no longer producing adequate results and that it must find new ways to work. Consider Amgen's announcement in December 2012 that it would acquire the pioneering deCODE Genetics for $415 million. The Icelandic company has worked to identify links between genes and disease. Terry McGuire, general manager of Polaris Venture Partners and a deCODE backer, said in a blog post following the announcement of the deal that it may not fit analysts' expectations of drugmakers buying companies for promising mid-stage or late-stage drugs, but that there's a simple answer as to why Amgen did so. "There is a great need by large biotechs and pharma companies to show true and more predictable innovation," he wrote. "And Amgen's leaders know that the future of healthcare is laid on the foundation of producing truly innovative medicines and technologies."

But the challenges the industry face are multidimensional and its collaborations will need to extend beyond the traditional partners it has worked with to drive its pipeline, to build new relationships with patients, payers, providers, and nontraditional healthcare companies that will be essential to its future if it is to both create value for its customers and capture value for itself and its shareholders.

All of this remains good news for biotech companies that can distinguish their pipelines with drug candidates that can be seen to demonstrate value and provide products that can command premium pricing even at a time that pressure grows to use generics, impose price controls, and use other mechanisms to drive down the cost of drugs. Innovative biotherapeutics will not be immune from the same pressures that traditional small molecule drugs have faced, but they are better-positioned to withstand the assault that's ahead in a healthcare world that is rapidly transitioning to value-based models. A new world of biosimilars is emerging; payers and providers have already demonstrated that they are unwilling to pay for new therapies that are too pricey, and a growing number of countries are moving toward Germany's example in requiring some type of comparative effectiveness to justify pricing and use. That will make it harder for companies to pass off overpriced drugs or find substantial markets for ones that provide little or no improvement over existing therapies. But it will also bring a needed level of discipline to both investors and drug developers and will provide rich rewards for those who can produce true innovation.

For much of the history of the biotechnology industry, the practical question faced by therapeutics companies throughout the discovery and development process was, "Will we be able to get this approved?" The question of whether an experimental drug would produce adequate data to pass regulatory muster and what it would take to get there, was the practical question that executives and investors weighed. That has changed. Though companies are no less concerned about their experimental products proving to be safe and efficacious, the overriding question for executives and investors evaluating a potential product's worth has become, "Can I get paid for this?"

Healthcare is in the midst of an upheaval. As populations grow and age and chronic diseases affect a greater portion of the world's population, these intertwined trends are taking a greater toll on the financial wellbeing of healthcare systems. In response, governments around the globe are struggling with the seemingly contradictory goals improving the quality of care while simultaneously cutting costs. The pressures are driving reform efforts around the world and pulling healthcare systems away from fee-for-service to value-based care where instead of paying providers for procedures, they are paid for results.

For some, these pressures signal a move towards a dire future in which healthcare is rationed, cost is shifted to individuals, and new technologies are dismissed as nothing more than new opportunities for inflating costs and driving healthcare systems closer to the brink of bankruptcy. It is a world in which power is shifting to payers, and governments are wielding blunt instruments to cut costs such as price controls, formularies, and penalties for people who practice unhealthy behaviors. For drug and device makers, it represents new barriers to bringing innovative products to market. It is creating a bias against innovation. No longer will drugs and devices need only to demonstrate that they are safe and effective. Now, they will also need to establish they provide superior value to what's already available.

But the dilemma we face today presents new opportunities to address problems with healthcare that extend well beyond costs alone. We are in the midst of the most dramatic shift in healthcare in the history of humanity. That transformation is being driven by an unprecedented understanding of the molecular mechanisms of diseases as well as our emerging understanding of the human genome and the growing list of other omes, from the proteome to the microbiome. Scientists are uncovering how the molecules within the body interact with genes and how genes interact with diet and the environment to influence health and wellness.

Clinical practice is moving away from treating the symptoms of disease to treating the underlying molecular drivers of disease, and beyond that, to intervening before diseases manifest themselves. Although the earliest days of personalized medicine have been characterized by the advent of targeted therapeutics, the development of low-cost sequencing, and a deepening knowledge of the way genes interact with other aspects of their environment, the trial and error approach of matching a drug to a patient is giving way to a new era of precision medicine.

Accelerating the pace with which personalized medicine will take hold is the convergence of healthcare technologies with communication and information technologies that are giving rise to a new world of digital health. Smartphones are evolving into health guides, monitors, and an important new link between patient and providers (Figure 3.19). The family practitioner is giving way to accountable care organizations where the first point of contact may not be a doctor in private practice, but instead a nurse practitioner working out of a clinic located within a big box retailer or national drug store chain.

The evolving world is altering the way patients access healthcare and providers deliver it. But perhaps the greatest potential for digital health to alter healthcare practice lies in tying together disparate streams of data to guide and interpret the meaning of individual, real-time, biological changes to optimize health and wellness. The mapping of the human genome, rather than an end itself, represented only a start. The challenge is not only to integrate the genome with the other omes being cataloged, but to utilize the enormous computing power available today to overlay disparate datasets, such as insurance records, electronic health records, clinical data, real-time patient monitoring, pharmacy records, and more to decode what it tells us about health and wellness, what works and doesn't work, and which patients require intervention.

Though it is in healthcare where the biotechnology revolution is most visibly being played out, its effects touch on virtually all human endeavors including how we grow our food, fuel our machines, and produce our goods. The challenges faced in healthcare mirror the challenges faced in other segments as the pressure from growing populations and prosperity create demand for food, fuel, and industrial products where scarcity, financial costs, and societal costs have become growing concerns. Biotechnology holds the promise to provide answers to the growing problems we face.

A focus on value is not a bad thing. It should be embraced. It will help impose discipline in corporate decision-making and prioritize true innovation. Creating value alone, though, is not enough. Companies will need to figure out how to capture value as well, and that's something that will become a greater challenge in a world where there is increasing cost consciousness, and comparative effectiveness becomes a gatekeeper to the marketplace where patients are remade into healthcare consumers. Though it would be easy if value were an absolute, it is not. As with beauty, value is in the eye of the beholder—whether it is a payer weighing reimbursement for a product or a company weighing an acquisition, how that particular entity operates, its particular needs, and its alternatives will shape its view of the value of an asset.

VALUE IS TRANSIENT

When Human Genome Sciences received an unsolicited $7 billion bid from Amgen in 2010 to buy the company, it had its lead experimental drug, Benlysta, in late-stage clinical testing. The drug represented the first new therapy for lupus in 50 years. Two years later, the company had won approval for the drug and it was on the market, but when its partner GlaxoSmithKline made an unsolicited bid to acquire it, it

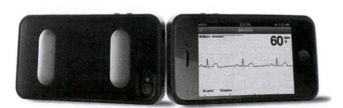

FIGURE 3.19 Digital health applications: AliveCor's heart monitor via iPhone. *(From AliveCor, LLC.)*

offered less than half what the company would have commanded just 2 years before. When Human Genome Sciences went looking for a white knight, neither Amgen nor anyone else was anywhere to be found.

VALUE IS GEOGRAPHIC DEPENDENT

What is the value of a five-bedroom, four-bathroom house? Well, according to the real estate information website Zillow, a 3210 square-foot lot on Margareta Street in Detroit sold in December 2012 for $55,001. Just 3 weeks earlier, a 2840 square-foot, five bedroom, four bathroom house on Austin Avenue in Los Altos, California sold for $2.5 million. There were likely many variables between the two homes, but chief among them was the location. Detroit is the United States' least-expensive housing market and Los Altos is its most expensive.

Differences in the location of a market can have a significant impact on the value of an asset. The cost of capital can also vary dramatically from market to market, allowing life sciences companies an opportunity to exploit geographic variations in value. One way this can be seen is in a number of deals involving countries that are seeking to build their own innovation-based biopharmaceutical industry (Figure 3.20). In these arrangements, the financial partner in the emerging country funds clinical development of the drug in exchange for rights to the drug in their home country. The innovator company can then use the data from those studies, which it owns outright, to seek approval for the drug in the rest of the world. These arrangements provide nondilutive financing, reduce development risks, and allow companies the ability to develop multiple products simultaneously.

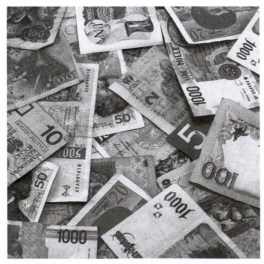

FIGURE 3.20   The value of a biotechnology company's asset and cost of capital varies with the market and the geographic region.

VALUE TO PAYERS IS NOT A CONSTANT

Life sciences companies must contend with growing cost-consciousness among payers, but what one payer views as an expense, another might view as an opportunity for savings, depending on the nature of the organization. Consider Kaiser Permanente, which ranked highest among 830 insurance plans in a Consumer Report survey at the end of 2011. *Time* magazine noted that Kaiser is both an insurer and provider. As such, it has a larger incentive to invest in preventive care, wellness classes, and free health education clinics. "Many other insurers and health systems avoid sinking money into such programs because patients switch insurers so frequently that such spending winds up benefiting another company," wrote *Time*. "But as the Consumer Reports' ratings show, Kaiser patient satisfaction is high and patient turnover low, so it makes more sense for the insurer to invest for the long haul."

By contrast, there is high turnover in most employer-sponsored insurance plans because employers frequently change health insurers in pursuit of lower costs. As a result, insurers have a disincentive to pay for preventive care. Researchers at Case Western Reserve University and Carnegie Mellon University looked at diabetes management and the lack of preventive care in a 2007 study and found the high rate at which Americans change health plans could be the cause. "It takes about a decade for insurers to recoup their investment in early diabetes treatment, and by then odds are that their customer has moved on to another health plan," wrote *Slate* magazine in discussing the study. "Alas, a lot of this turnover may be built in to the way Americans get health insurance. And it's the doing not of individual patients so much as their employers, who are always on the lookout to switch plans for lower-cost coverage" (Figure 3.21).

VALUE IS NOT A FUNCTION OF SALES AND EARNINGS

Multibillion dollar deals for life sciences companies that were years away from having products on the market are a reminder that these companies don't sell for a multiple of sales or earnings. Consider Gilead Sciences, which paid $11 billion to complete its acquisition of Pharmasset at the start of 2012. The bid, announced at the end of 2011, represented nearly a 90 percent premium over Pharmasset's closing price on the day before the announcement. Pharmasset's experimental hepatitis C drug, an oral therapy that promises to free patients from the use of interferon, which can cause flu-like side-effects, represented not only a potential best-in-class drug, but one that has a complimentary mechanism of action to a hepatitis C drug candidate already moving through Gilead's pipeline. That enhanced Pharmasset's potential value to Gilead since hepatitis C

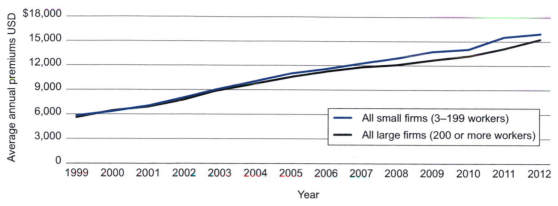

FIGURE 3.21   Average annual premiums for covered workers with family coverage from 1999 to 2012. *(From Burrill & Company 2013 Annual Report on the Life Sciences Industry.)*

therapies are expected to follow the path that Gilead so successfully forged with combination drugs for HIV/AIDS. Though Pharmasset's lead candidate had completed mid-stage testing, it is still undergoing late-stage clinical trials and is not expected to reach the market until 2014 at the earliest.

The Pharmasset acquisition changed the relative value of other hepatitis C drug developers as well. On the cusp of Gilead's purchase, its competitor Bristol-Myers Squibb purchased Inhibitex for $2.5 billion, a 163 percent premium over its close the day before the deal was announced. Inhibitex's lead drug candidate was in mid-stage testing, but things did not turn out well for Bristol-Myers. In August 2012, just 6 months after completing its acquisition, the drugmaker announced that it would discontinue development of the Inhibitex drug, leading *Motley Fool* to declare it "the most epic drug failure ever"—a reminder that value can be fleeting. Bristol-Myers said it would take a $1.8 billion charge related to the drug's failure.

THE CHALLENGE FOR LIFE SCIENCES COMPANIES

A world in which companies must evaluate their pipelines by asking whether a drug in development is something a payer would reimburse is a fundamentally different one than the world in which this industry has operated during the past. While companies today feel pressure to do more with less, improve their R&D productivity, and find ways to replace revenue lost to generic competition in the face of expiring patents, they also need to reconceive themselves in fundamental ways.

Biopharmaceutical companies that see themselves as being primarily in the business of developing and selling drugs will live in a world in which they will swim against stronger and stronger currents. Intense pricing pressure may lead to the industry producing more diamonds and less coal,

but in a world of value-based healthcare, it will be increasingly difficult for drugmakers to capture value through the products they create. Companies that are able to think differently about their assets, the value they can create through leveraging internal expertise, and novel approaches to serving the healthcare needs of patients, will find new ways to capture value outside of their products. Companies, from Web-based retailers such as Amazon with its cloud computing services to grocers such as Safeway capitalizing on loyalty card data mapping the buying habits of its customers, have found ways to do this.

The biotech industry continues to be one driven by vision, optimism, and enthusiasm for what can be, rather than necessarily what is. Such a world provides a perspective to see value differently. It is a world driven by innovation and focused on potential. As a result, it's also a perspective that is prone to rapid and sharp shifts as science, clinical data, policy, regulation, and competition alter the landscape with the suddenness of a temblor. The world in which these companies operate is changing. While there is much talk about value defining the new world of healthcare, governments and payers hold the power to determine price. The risk is that under the banner of value, governments and payers rely on the most expedient tools at their disposal to address costs without consideration of the value of a given therapy to a patient. We may be heading toward a world, to borrow from Oscar Wilde's "Lord Henry," where "people know the price of everything and the value of nothing." Innovation can bridge the gap between need and affordability. But for innovation to matter in this new world, it must create value for the customer, while providing adequate opportunity for industry to capture value along the way.

Our world faces many serious challenges, from feeding and fueling a growing population to addressing a worldwide epidemic of chronic diseases. As we look at the challenges before us, the biotechnology industry stands ready with solutions. We are at a time in the history of mankind that the secrets of the genome are being unlocked. Biotechnology is bringing about an era of personalized medicine where rather than treating symptoms of disease doctors will be able to address the underlying molecular mechanisms, or even intervene at the earliest stages to prevent illness. We have also begun to revolutionize industrial production by turning to biological processes to replace chemical ones. This industry has relied on the drive of entrepreneurs who have the imagination, vision, and fortitude to overcome the financial, scientific, and regulatory obstacles to change our world. The challenges have never been greater, but neither have the opportunities.

Chapter 4

What is Biotechnology Entrepreneurship?

Craig Shimasaki, PhD, MBA

President & CEO, Moleculera Labs and BioSource Consulting Group, Oklahoma City, Oklahoma

Biotechnology entrepreneurship is the sum of all the activities necessary to build an enterprise through the melding of both scientific and business disciplines. It is through these integrated activities that an enterprise creates, develops, and ultimately commercializes a biotechnology product. Some of the most amazing life-saving treatments and medical devices, advanced fuels, and efficient crops, have been created and developed through biotechnology enterprises. In this chapter, I will outline the unique aspects of entrepreneurship in the biotechnology industry contrasted with other industries, and then discuss the biotechnology entrepreneur's background and characteristics, and the forces that impact their decisions.

THE SIGNIFICANCE OF THE BIOTECHNOLOGY ENTREPRENEUR

All companies require a capable and skilled leader if they have any hope of becoming successful. However, without an entrepreneur there will be no company. Without a Rob Swanson and Herb Boyer, there would be no Genentech; without an Ivor Royston and Howard Birndorf there would have been no Hybritech (not to mention the numerous companies that their employees subsequently birthed in the San Diego area). Yes, diverse teams of people are essential to the success of any organization. However, without the leadership, vision, and the driving force of an entrepreneur, biotechnology products will never be brought into existence.

Biotechnology entrepreneurs are the backbone of the biotech industry and the source of its future innovation. Without them, there would be no biotechnology industry. Biotech entrepreneurs are leaders with vision and passion, driving them to pursue their goals with the belief that their product or service will ultimately impact the well-being of multitudes. Biotechnology entrepreneurs start companies for various reasons. Universally, they believe that their product or service can better diagnose, treat, cure, feed, or fuel millions of people. Most biotech entrepreneurs start companies with a heavy dose of altruism, and most often, this is the driving force that propels their work and efforts.

Without a doubt, biotechnology entrepreneurs believe financial rewards may await them. However, it is important to understand that these individuals are not *principally* driven by aspirations of financial prosperity. No doubt there are much easier and faster career paths for making a comfortable living. However, these individuals are motivated to prove that their discovery or invention can one day become a commercial product that is useful to the masses. This self-less motivation is an asset to the entrepreneur, especially when encountering challenging financial circumstances and still pressing forward without giving up or quitting. Unfortunately, this altruistic motivation can also become a detriment, particularly when sound financial and business decisions must be made. Biotechnology entrepreneurship can best be described as a journey down a challenging path to a satisfying and rewarding destination. The better-equipped entrepreneurs have a less-challenging journey than their counterparts. As we will discuss in more detail, most founders of biotechnology companies are typically scientists, physicians, engineers, or individuals with technical knowledge in a particular discipline.

THE INTEGRATION OF TWO DISTINCTLY DIFFERENT DISCIPLINES

Biotechnology entrepreneurship is based upon the integration of two distinctly different disciplines—science and business. Managing the complexities of this intertwined cross-discipline enterprise can take first-time entrepreneurs by surprise. Fist-time entrepreneurs in the scientific fields often start with the belief that completing scientific research is equivalent to success. Soon afterwards they learn there is a vast difference between completing a scientific project and building a successful company. When you include the need to make practical and strategic business decisions, which is not a typical skill set most scientists possess—leading a biotechnology company can be quite challenging.

The term *entrepreneur* as defined by *Merriam-Webster's Dictionary* is "one who organizes, manages, and assumes the risks of a business or enterprise." In other words, the entrepreneur is the owner and manager of the *business risks*. However, in a biotechnology enterprise, the entrepreneur is also the owner and manager of the *scientific risks*. This duplicity of roles requires an individual who understands both risks. This is because decisions made in one area impact the corresponding area, and scientific issues are often inextricably tied to business issues. For instance, your latest laboratory experiment may reveal an unforeseen requirement to modify your company's planned molecular target and therefore the team needs to modify the screening assays used to select the best target molecule. This, in turn, alters the original allotted time to reach your planned development milestone. Consequently, this change results in a requirement for more capital than originally anticipated in order to sustain the organization through this period. Without the necessary capital to continue development, a company will cease to exist. Creating successful biotechnology enterprises requires careful integration and management of *both* the business and the scientific issues, not to mention the myriad of other start-up issues an entrepreneur faces along the path of bringing a product to market. In this chapter, we will review several unique characteristics of biotechnology entrepreneurship and discuss the forces that influence the biotechnology leader's decisions.

BIOTECHNOLOGY ENTREPRENEURSHIP VERSUS GENERAL ENTREPRENEURSHIP

There are similarities between biotechnology entrepreneurship and general entrepreneurship activities. Both require a competitive idea, an experienced team to lead and manage the functions of the enterprise, capital to support the endeavor through to commercialization, and a dogged perseverance to overcome roadblocks encountered along the way. However, the differences between these two entrepreneurial paths are greater than their similarities. Biotechnology endeavors come with unique challenges other entrepreneurial endeavors do not face. These include, the need for enormous amounts of money to make incremental product development progress, longer development times, and stiffer regulatory approval requirements in order for products to be commercialized. Biotech products also have an inherent scientific uncertainty that often is not fully appreciated. Often, when developing these new products, the cause for the disease or condition which the product is targeting is not yet understood.

Time and Money Differences

Every entrepreneurial enterprise requires capital in order to develop a product and reach commercialization. However, biotechnology endeavors require orders-of-magnitude more capital and take much longer to develop than most other endeavors. Companies that develop Internet applications or consumer-oriented products may only require a few hundred thousand dollars in capital and a year or two in development before having a commercial product, whereas biotechnology enterprises require multiple millions of dollars and many years, possibly decades, before a product will reach the market. Because of the enormous capital required to produce a product in the biotechnology industry, maximizing your company's attractiveness to investors and industry partners is vital during the growth of your organization. No matter how great a product idea or technology concept may be, without continued and uninterrupted funding, it is nearly impossible for any biotechnology product to reach commercialization. Therefore, capital planning and the management's ability to raise capital are vital prerequisites for growth and development of a company in this industry. The biotech entrepreneur must have in their mind (and on paper) a good estimate of the total capital required to reach each value-enhancing milestone in order to remain attractive to subsequent investors. Funding gaps are not unusual for a development-stage company; however, it is incumbent upon the leader to be sure that these short-term and temporary funding gaps do not cause the demise of the company. In Chapter 9, "Understanding Biotechnology Sectors," we will discuss in more detail the cost estimates and timeframes for the development of different biotechnology products.

Regulatory Requirements

In addition to the cost and timeframe differences, the biotechnology industry is regulated by strict governmental requirements that must be met before any biotech product can be marketed. Regulatory agencies such as the Food and Drug Administration (FDA) in the U.S., the Medicines and Healthcare Products Regulatory Agency (MHRA) in the UK, and the European Medicines Agency (EMA) in Europe, to name a few, each require extensive preclinical and human clinical testing to prove that your biotechnology product is safe and effective before it can be commercialized. Just meeting these regulatory requirements may take several years and multiple millions of dollars. As technology and scientific methods advance and become more sophisticated, regulatory requirements also shift to keep pace with new discoveries uncovering the effects of biomedical and genetic products on human health. Since biotechnology products require numerous years of development, it would not be unusual to observe regulatory requirements modified or changed between the time your product development started and when your product is fully developed. Regulatory requirements differ for agricultural products, medical devices, laboratory tests, therapeutics, and biologics.

Understanding the specific regulatory requirements for your product approval is critical to raising capital and your commercialization success.

Biological Uncertainty Factor

One inherent factor within all biotechnology product development plans is "biological uncertainty". Each biotechnology product idea carries with it a finite amount of biological uncertainty, which is not fully known until the product is developed and finally tested in the laboratory, in the field, in animals or in humans. For medical devices and diagnostics, this biological uncertainty factor is not fully appreciated until the device or test is validated in a large-enough population of living beings, whether in animals or tested in large numbers of clinical specimens. For therapeutics and biologics, this biological uncertainty may erroneously be presumed to be minimized by having positive preclinical Phase 1 and Phase 2 testing results, only to discover that in Phase 3, the product is not effective in larger populations of people. For agricultural biotechnology products, this biological uncertainty can be hidden in the plant or animal species, through the unknown effect of a gene-trait, or its effect on the down-stream food chain or the eco-environment. This inherent biological uncertainty is a risk factor that must be managed in order to successfully bring any biotechnology product to market. It is impossible for an entrepreneurial team to eliminate this biological uncertainty; however, creative managers will find ways to adapt their product within the confines of these biologic uncertainties to ultimately produce a product that has great value to a target group of people.

ENTREPRENEURSHIP AND INTRAPRENEURSHIP

The vast majority of individuals reading this chapter may not intend to start a biotechnology company on their own. Even though you may not start a company, one thing is for certain—you will likely work for one. Much of what we discuss in this book is in reference to an "entrepreneur;" however, the entire content is directly applicable to *all* managers and leaders within any biotechnology organization. Each individual should learn what it means to operate as a biotechnology *intrepreneur* irrespective of their position within an organization. So what is an interpreneur? All companies have positions which carry broad responsibilities for a particular function, division, or department. The individuals who fill these positions, solve problems encountered within their department or function. An intrepreneur approaches problems and makes decisions as if they were solely responsible for the outcome; and they operate as if the consequences impact them personally. An

interpreneur works to complete not only the tasks and responsibilities assigned to them, but they also observe the functions around them to be sure they are being carried out properly, as they understand these can impact their own work and outcome. Great intrepreneurs know that their career advancement is determined in part by how they creatively solve problems and manage responsibilities their company entrusts to them. There are more career opportunities within the biotechnology industry than most individuals recognize. For those who want to learn more about the various career options available to individuals with biotechnology backgrounds, Chapter 31 entitled "Career Opportunities in the Life Science Industry" reviews the diversity of careers for new graduates or for current biotechnology professionals seeking to change job functions within this industry.

THE BIOTECHNOLOGY ENTREPRENEUR, MANAGER, OR LEADER

Leaders of entrepreneurial endeavors typically possess similar characteristics. Successful entrepreneurs also possess a variety of skill-sets and characteristics with the attempt to be identified. Many of these well-defined characteristics have been studied and taught in most business schools, whereas, I would like to list ten general entrepreneurial characteristics that I believe are essential to entrepreneurs in any industry. Although we will not take the time to elaborate on these general entrepreneurial characteristics, I would encourage you to reflect on the extent to which these operate within you. If you have uncertainty about any particular character trait, often by studying about them, you will find it is easier to emulate them and can find many good books devoted to them.

> **Essential Entrepreneurial Characteristics**
> 1. A driving passion for their work.
> 2. The ability to communicate their vision to others.
> 3. An innate ability to inspire others to follow.
> 4. Being unafraid to take carefully calculated risks.
> 5. Accepting responsibility and ownership for problems.
> 6. Humility and the desire to learn.
> 7. Viewing their environment through optimistic eyes.
> 8. Perseverance in the face of adversity.
> 9. The ability to multitask and manage critical activities simultaneously.
> 10. The ability to raise money and manage it well.

The biotechnology entrepreneur must also have an additional set of skills that I believe are crucial for success within the biotechnology industry. These additional skills are ones that help leaders reach great commercial outcomes. Unfortunately, these characteristics tend to be the ones that new leaders often struggle with the most. These essential characteristics are discussed below.

> **Essential Biotechnology Entrepreneurial Characteristics**
> 1. Awareness of the Unknown-Unknowns
> 2. Be a multidisciplined translator: the ability to speak and understand the language of business and science
> 3. Understand the purpose of negotiation
> 4. Having leadership wisdom
> 5. Possessing good core values
> 6. Having creativity and imagination

ESSENTIAL BIOTECHNOLOGY ENTREPRENEURIAL CHARACTERISTICS

Awareness of the Unknown-Unknowns

The term *unknown-unknowns* may sound like circular reasoning, but in reality it is a frequent peril in the development-stage of biotechnology companies. Its negative consequences have been painfully felt at some time or other in most all biotech enterprises. The biotechnology entrepreneur will encounter two types of unknowns. The first we call the *known-unknowns*. These are knowledge areas that you recognize as important, but you also realize that your understanding is limited in this particular area. All of us have experienced the sinking feeling of having limited knowledge in an unfamiliar area, whether it be accounting, finance, regulatory laws, human resources, or a particular area of chemistry, biology, or physics. Although you may wish you possessed a working knowledge in that particular area, you recognize it, and can hire consultants or solicit the advice of experts in that area. In other words, you are aware of what you don't know. The known-unknowns refer to having full recognition and awareness of limited information in an area that is critical to the company or future success, and you are also aware that you do not have enough knowledge to make rational decisions about how to proceed. There is safety in this awareness because entrepreneur leaders can then seek the advice of experts in these fields and proceed with caution.

Then there are the *unknown-unkowns*. This is when you do not possess knowledge about an area critical to the company, *and* you do not recognize your limitations, yet you proceed anyway. In other words, these are the things you do not know, that you do not know. For some familiar examples, think about Microsoft finding out after the launch of the new Windows 8 Operating System that a very large base of users don't like or understand how to use the interface? Was this something they did not know that they did not know? How about Coca-Cola and New Coke? After discontinuing the "Original Coke" recipe, they learned that most consumers did not like the New Coke. (Alternatively, some conspiritists believe this was a planned marketing ploy, meaning they believed Coca-Cola was smarter than most people thought). These are some examples of an organization thinking they understood something, but in reality they did not. The major difference between the unknown-unknowns for these large multinational companies and a start-up biotechnology company is that the former have large bank accounts and plentiful resources to recover from these mistakes, whereas the biotech company usually gets one chance at commercialization success. Missteps for a development-stage biotechnology company can cost millions of dollars and ultimately jeopardize their future existence. For large, well-established pharmaceutical companies, they can have multiple clinical trial failures and still survive another day to develop more products.

For Aviron, the biotechnology company that developed the FluMist influenza nasal vaccine in the late 1990s, the unknown-unknown was *not* utilizing the exact same manufacturing process for their commercial product which was tested in their Phase 3 clinical trials. It would appear that the company did not learn about this unknown-unknown until after submitting their Product License Application (PLA) to the Food and Drug Administration (FDA) in June 1998. This unknown-unknown required that the company confirm the clinical equivalence of their product manufactured by the new process, and compare it to the process for the product used in the Phase 3 clinical study. The result of this unknown-unknown was a delay in the FDA approval, additional capital consumed for more testing, additional clinical testing, and a drop in investor confidence. Fortunately for Aviron, they recovered and ultimately received FDA approval for their vaccine, and they were acquired in 2001 by MedImmune for $1.5 billion. Sadly, most unknown-unknowns in the biotechnology industry do not result in recovery and ultimate success such as this.

The unknown-unknowns are challenging to recognize because by definition you don't know what you don't know. A quote attributed to Socrates is "*The more I learn, the more I learn how little I know.*" One good way to avoid this pitfall is to always seek counsel and advice from experienced individuals in your field before embarking on what you are wanting to do. Often, because of the need to accomplish many things quickly, we move forward with a limited understanding of the issues, only to find out later there are unforeseen consequences. This can especially be true when planning and preparing for regulatory approvals and clearances for biotechnology and bio-agricultural products. Remember that regulations are constantly changing and without current regulatory knowledge and experience, it is extremely difficult to successfully satisfy the requirements for regulatory approval. Wise entrepreneurs surround themselves with many experienced and seasoned professionals they trust. These individuals may include other entrepreneurs, professionals in different fields, and experienced board members that bring expertise the entrepreneur does not possess. Also, don't be afraid to ask questions. Seek plenty of advice and guidance when planning, and before proceeding. Cultivate relationships with others who have led and managed successful companies (see Chapter 8 entitled "Building Human Relationship Networks"). When you are given advice, it is also worth noting that sometimes guidance can be, in reality, a personal preference rather than a strict requirement. Understand that everyone will have their own opinion and you don't have to follow the advice of all people. However, there is safety in the counsel of many wise individuals.

Before we leave this topic, it is important to understand the difference between *The Goal* and *A Method*. There are a myriad of issues a biotechnology entrepreneur must manage and navigate through when building a biotechnology company and developing a successful product. The goal rarely changes, whereas there are many methods to achieving your goal. Often, the advice from others is, in reality, their preferred method to reach your stated goal. Recognize that even your own belief about how (method) to reach your goal, is also an opinion. So listen to the advice of others as you may formulate an even better method that you did not previously consider. Remember, methods vary, but never lose sight of the goal.

Be a Multidisciplined Translator: The Ability to Speak and Understand the Language of Business and Science

All science- and technology-based companies experience a normal tension that rises at the interface of the technical and business/marketing functions. A good portion of this tension exists because of the absence of individuals who are multidisciplined translators of both the science and business goals of the organization. A development-stage biotechnology company usually starts with a small team of people, so it is imperative that someone within that team has the ability to communicate both the scientific and business goals of the company. A multidisciplined translator is someone who understands the business, financial, marketing, and corporate issues, but also understands the technical and scientific issues—and speaks both languages well enough for individuals in these respective fields to understand. Biotechnology companies are most often founded by someone with a technical background, such as a scientist, physician, or engineer. These individuals are very proficient and accomplished within their specific technical discipline. All too often, the business aspects, such as financing, marketing, and legal issues are not familiar to these individuals; or worse, they have no interest in learning or understanding them. Reticence to learning becomes problematic for a young organization. Even though the team may be accomplishing great work scientifically, its foundational business, market, and financial problems may eliminate the interest of potential investors or partners. For instance, if the technology is exciting and cutting-edge but there is no market need for such a product, there will be no investor interest. As such, the likelihood of raising large amounts of capital from sophisticated investors is small. In the opposite situation, where the founder is a businessperson and not a scientist, if they do not understand the scientific issues and limitations, they will operate in a pseudo-environment. They may believe that the technology can deliver a set of features and benefits, when in reality that may be impossible. In this case, the company may be promising future market benefits for a product that the science cannot deliver. Sadly, when prototype or clinical testing begins, there may be great disappointment, and most often, failure.

Scientists are trained to be analytical. They are adept at questioning theories and suppositions. They are great researchers because they are trained to be skeptical of information they don't understand until reproducible evidence is documented. Also, scientists naturally detect interpretation errors, and most scientists can quickly spot inconsistencies and problems within assumptions. These characteristics are ideal for making new discoveries, but they are ineffective communication tools when speaking to potential investors, businesspersons, and marketing people about your company's purpose and mission.

All entrepreneurs, whether a businessperson, scientist, or engineer, should speak to their counterparts in the vocabulary of the listener. At the very least, all entrepreneurs should communicate with the assumption that the listener has little or no prior understanding of the subject matter, including their specialized terminology. It is not a requirement that all entrepreneurs need to memorize a business and scientific lexicon. However, proficiency and skill is required in order to convey precise meaning so the listener understands what is communicated and not confused by the jargon. For instance, when a scientist is communicating to a businessperson or investor about the benefits of their technology, instead of going head-long into a discourse about "allelic-variation in single nucleotide polymorphisms and its haplotype chromosomal loci contribution to disease predisposition," you can just say "DNA modifications in genes increase a person's likelihood of getting a disease." The word "bacteria" works well for "*Bacteroides melaninogenicus.*" For the businessperson, their challenge is to translate the business concepts and define their terminology so it is understandable to the scientists and engineers. If a scientist asks the businessperson "how can we tell how much our company is worth," don't proceed to talk about "risk-adjusted discounts to future cash flows and future earnings," but rather explain concepts through analogies such as housing prices, where value is based upon what a willing buyer will pay at any point in time, then explain any other factors used for estimating value. To the degree that the technical individuals understand the business and marketing objectives, to that same degree these trained problem-solving individuals can help keep product development on track to meet business objectives and market expectations.

Learn to simplify all terminology common in your specialty, particularly when trying to communicate the value and significance of what you are doing to others. Use words that have meaning to the listener. Entrepreneurs should practice translating into the language of the listener and use analogies when describing complex scientific concepts or biological processes. Remember, verbal communication is simply a method of faithfully transferring thoughts and ideas to another individual. If the listener cannot comprehend what you are verbally communicating, they certainly will not know if your thoughts are worthy of consideration. Multidisciplined translators *think* about the issues encountered in other disciplines. Just as a proficient bilingual individual will tell you that they became fluent only when they began to *think* in that language. So it is with the biotechnology entrepreneur, they must think about the issues critical to both the science and the business. Scientists should practice thinking about the business issues, and businesspersons should spend time thinking about the issues in the science, and each should frequently ask questions of the other to be sure their understanding is consistent with fact. Businesspersons and scientists approach problems differently and each can benefit from the thoughts and solutions offered by each other. Also, learn to follow their thinking process rather than just accepting their end-result or conclusion. I have seen from personal experience that by sharing a scientific issue in a way that a nonscientist can understand, great ideas have been proposed, even though the listener was not knowledgeable of the technical issues. Don't be afraid to share issues with individuals whom you trust, even though they are skilled in other disciplines or other fields. They may surprise you with good ideas and solutions. At the very least you will have had practice simplifying the issues and concepts in a way that is understandable to others. You may even find that in doing this you solve your own problem by simplifying the issue. As we will discuss in the financing chapters, this is an essential skill when raising capital.

Understanding the Purpose of Negotiation

Frequently, the term *negotiation* conjures up an image of two parties sitting on opposite sides of a table emotionally arguing the terms of an agreement or price of an asset. The connotation is that of arm-twisting and demanding which are believed to be associated with these activities. The perception is that back-and-forth bantering is required until one party gets the upper-hand and pressures the other party to succumb to their demands. Negotiation in this sense does occur, but this image hopefully will not reflect the majority of negotiations the biotech entrepreneur will experience. It may be true that when you negotiate the value of your company with investors, it may sometimes resemble the above description; however, even then, it is best not to allow negotiations to deteriorate to a verbal wrestling match with the other party. The purpose of negotiation is to exchange something of value to one party for something different that

has value to another party. One aspect of negotiation important for entrepreneurs is that of:

- Balancing obligations made to different entities (investors, regulators, partners, customers).
- Balancing your limited time and resources.
- Securing *buy in* from those that hold or influence these resources.

Standard negotiation training seminars focus on techniques and the *dos* and *don'ts* of negotiation. However, negotiation is not just about technique, but rather understanding what is of importance to one party in order to exchange for something important to the other. Negotiation is about reaching agreeable compromise where each party receives enough value to come to agreement. Frequently, in negotiations one party states that *everything* is important to them and therefore there is limited compromise towards mutual agreement. In reality, every party has an order or hierarchy of importance for each of the terms or conditions in an agreement. The entrepreneur must learn to quickly find out what is of the highest value to the other party, and in exchange be sure to receive what is of the most value to them.

A better connotation for negotiation is the idea of a journey along an unfamiliar road navigating detours and roadblocks to ultimately arrive at your destination. Just as in this example, we sometimes say that we negotiated our way around these obstacles. So when we say we negotiated, we mean we figured out how to get past or go around obstacles in our path until we reached our goal. Great biotechnology entrepreneurs learn to be good negotiators in both of these senses, and they wisely negotiate as they traverse the obstacle-laden path of product development and commercialization.

Having Leadership Wisdom

As a society we are trained to value intellect and knowledge. Truly, without knowledge we make very few technological advances. However, there is an important difference between knowledge and wisdom. Wisdom is knowing when to apply a particular piece of knowledge in a particular situation at a particular time. We may know individuals who are full of knowledge because they can talk to you authoritatively on almost any subject. However, sometimes you may find that wisdom escapes these individuals. We can train ourselves to increase our wisdom just as we can train ourselves to gain knowledge. Often learning to increase in wisdom has to do with closing our mouths more often and listening carefully in order to understand the communicated thoughts and ideas of others. I did not say listen to the *words of others* because as we discussed above, verbal communication, or words, are just a surrogate for transmitting thoughts, ideas, concepts, and beliefs from one person to another. When we learn to readily grasp with fidelity the communicated thoughts, ideas, concepts, and beliefs of others, we can make better judgments and decisions about the best direction to take.

We all take action based upon what we believe. If we believe that there are severe consequences for missing a deadline, we usually alter our schedules and we then work longer and try to enlist resources to help meet that deadline. If we believe we can negotiate with the individual who gave us the deadline, we do not take the same actions, or at least not to the extent that we would have previously. These different actions are ultimately based upon what we believe. Unfortunately, often what we believe is not accurate, as in the case of the unknown-unknowns, where unforseen consequences lie ahead of us because we did not understand an issue. In situations like these, we falsely believe that the work we are doing is correct. Wisdom increases when we uncover truthful information we did not previously know, and it serves as a solid basis for our subsequent actions.

We all have a certain degree of expectation of wisdom from our leaders. We follow leaders because we believe they understand where they are going, we trust their judgment, and they inspire us by their vision and mission for the companies they lead. To become a more successful entrepreneur, you must increase your leadership wisdom because no one person can accomplish what a committed group of individuals can accomplish collectively. Cohesive and united entrepreneurial teams have accomplished some of the most amazing things that even larger, disorganized groups never achieve. Often the most significant difference between these two types of groups is that one of them has a leader with wisdom, and the team trusts the leader. There are many pitfalls to avoid for a development-stage biotechnology company. You will increase your likelihood of avoiding these pitfalls by increasing your leadership wisdom and by teaching your team to embody this same characteristic.

Possessing Good Core Values

Each one of us possesses a set of core values whether we recognize it or not. Core values are the sum total of the guiding principles upon which we operate and make decisions. Sometimes these core values are clearly defined, and other times these guiding principles are simply understood. The entrepreneurs that have built successful companies have been guided by strong core values. Foundational to a good leader is their core values. Any individual can be a leader, but having good core values determines the extent of their success and long-term value. It could be argued, based upon the strictest definition, that Fidel Castro was an effective *leader* because leadership is often defined as the ability to pull together resources, hold respect, spread a vision, and effectively execute a plan while inspiring others to follow. Few people think of Castro as a good leader simply because many of his actions were based on unethical core

values. Therefore the qualification of a good leader must be placed in the context of good core values. The leader's core values are the compass by which the organization will be directed. Be sure to examine your own core values and that of your leader because these are the principles and beliefs one reaches down into when individuals don't know what to do and are faced with difficult decisions. There are great books about leadership and core values that may be helpful for biotech entrepreneurs. I would recommend Jim Collins' book entitled *Good to Great* as a place to start [1]. Another easy book to read on core values is *Life's Greatest Lessons: 20 Things that Matter* written by Hal Urban. [2]

Having Creativity and Imagination

Creativity is not just an important characteristic for artists and musicians; it is essential for the success of every biotechnology entrepreneur. Creativity is not limited to artistic expression but rather is also necessary for arriving at great solutions that are not obvious from the circumstances. Albert Einstein once stated, "Imagination is more important than knowledge. For knowledge is limited to all we now know and understand…" Creativity and imagination allows one to see things others do not see in the midst of a difficult set of circumstances.

Creativity and imagination is what was used to establish each of the great architectural structures we see today. The Eiffel Tower was just a grand idea that existed in the mind of two engineers, Maurice Koechlin and Émile Nouguier, many years before the first steel girder was ever set in place. Even after the imagined structure was drawn on paper, Gustiv Eiffel and his two engineers encountered seemingly insurmountable challenges and were faced with many reasons to quit. There was great opposition to the building of the tower as criticism abounded, claiming it would cost too much, the design could not support its weight, and the land where it was to be erected was not solid (see Figure 4.1). However, through creativity and imagination, the founding team was able to overcome all these obstacles, including public opposition. As a result, the Eiffel Tower is appreciated and has become one of the most recognized structures in the world today. Never underestimate the value of creativity and imagination. Creative and imaginative entrepreneurs can accomplish great things when coupled with having leadership wisdom.

FOUR BACKGROUNDS OF BIOTECHNOLOGY ENTREPRENEURS

The typical biotechnology entrepreneur who starts an enterprise usually arises from one of the following four background types, although individuals from any background can start a biotechnology company—as long as they have the ideas, skills, and motivation. Unfortunately, the odds for

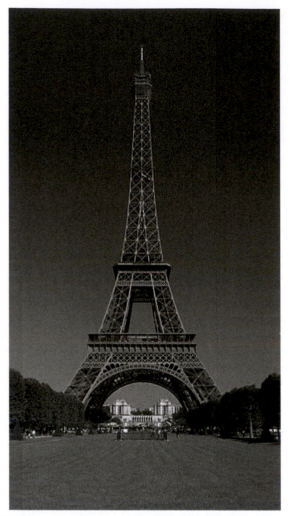

FIGURE 4.1   The Eiffel Tower: One of the most recognized architectural structures in the world. *(Source: Wikipedia)*

success are heavily weighed against anyone not from one of these categories. Each background comes with its own strengths and weaknesses. The four most common backgrounds of biotechnology entrepreneurs include:

1. The *scientist/physician/bioengineer* who comes from an academic institution (university, research foundation, nonprofit research institute).
2. The *scientist/physician/bioengineer* who comes from within the life science industry such as another biotechnology company.
3. The *business person*, such as a former executive in the life science, pharmaceutical, or venture capital industry, who is not a scientist/physician/bioengineer.
4. A *core group of individuals* that are spun off from another life science organization within the industry

Most biotech entrepreneurs and founders can be classified from one of these four categories and their backgrounds often influence the time required to raise capital. (See Figure 4.2.)

BEING THE ENTREPRENEUR FOR A SEASON

Because most early-stage biotechnology companies are founded by scientists, it is worthwhile to address the issue of how to be a biotechnology entrepreneur if you don't want to lead a company. If you are a professor at a university or research institution and you simply want the opportunity to see your research become a commercial biotechnology product, you do not necessarily need to leave your day-job and become a CEO. In fact, it may be ill-advised to become a CEO if you have no previous business experience. An academic scientist without prior business experience functioning as a CEO can be an impediment to a company raising money because investors bet on experienced people—not just technologies alone. Although there are examples of scientists leading successful biotech companies, unfortunately, stereotyping of scientists can and do occur. As a general rule, the more practical business experience you possess, the more confidence investors will have in your ability to successfully lead a company.

If you are an academic professor and want to remain in your position, you can still assist in starting and forming your new company and help develop the technology, and even participate in its value creation, without leaving your position. If you are considering leaving your academic position, you still don't have to run the entire organization unless that is your desire. There are several ways to participate in the entrepreneurial process without shouldering the full responsibility for the entire organization. There are valuable roles you can assume which still provide the opportunity to participate in the entrepreneurial process and better equip yourself for a subsequent entrepreneurial opportunity.

It is important to first decide your time commitment to the new entity. Are you interested in full-time participation or only part-time? Do you only want to participate in this new venture as a consultant on an *as-needed basis*? Would you like to start on an *as-needed* basis yet have the opportunity to later participate full-time? Identify your time commitment interest first because it will help in selecting your entrepreneurial options. If you are contemplating starting a biotechnology company but are not interested in leading the organization, here are some ways you can participate:

1. Take a position as *Chief Scientific Officer or Vice President of R&D*. Participate by leading the technology development but have someone else shoulder the business and financing responsibilities of the organization.
2. Participate as a *Scientific Advisory Board Member* and assist in the overall direction and in solving problems during the technology development.
3. Participate as *Scientific Consultant* and assist on an as-needed basis.

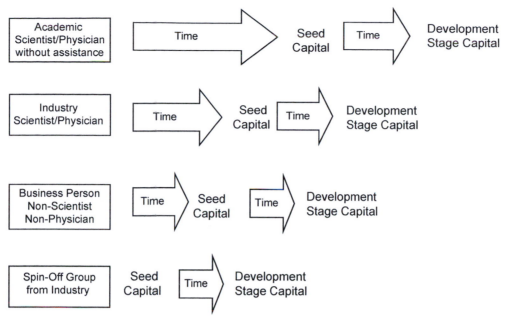

FIGURE 4.2   Different backgrounds of biotechnology entrepreneurs and relationship to time needed to raise capital. *(Adapted from Shimasaki, C. (2009). The Business of Bioscience: What Goes Into Making a Biotechnology Product. New York: Springer.)*

If you are a professor with minimal business experience, you may want to consider supportive roles in the new venture rather than taking responsibility for the entire organization. This way, you can learn by participating as a member of the team, rather than being solely responsible for the outcome of the company. By doing this, you will gain valuable experience which can be applied to your next opportunity. You can later lead with more confidence because you will then understand the start-up process and the many issues you may face. In the beginning, regardless of your long-term interest, you will be heavily involved in establishing the company, and must be willing to commit a large portion of your time during this phase. Afterward, you can then return to your academic research or medical practice while contributing in an alternate role as described above. As a founder of the company you will most likely be involved in securing seed funding for your new venture, which may come in the form of grants and/or seed capital funding from angel investors. During this time you must identify and recruit an experienced CEO or a former entrepreneur who can give you guidance on how to move the technology forward. Initially, the founding entrepreneur is the sole driving force behind the company. By participating in these supporting roles it will better prepare you for subsequent start-up options where you may want to assume the leadership role. It is essential to work with other experienced people because a good team is vital to business success. However, just because you are not leading the organization does not mean you cannot participate in shaping its future.

DRIVING FORCES BEHIND A BIOTECH ENTREPRENEUR'S DECISIONS

All entrepreneurs are presented with choices each day. The choices one makes can be analogous to a person deciding which path to travel along toward a desired location. Each decision, made over time, will advance you along a particular path that makes it easier or more difficult to arrive at your ultimate destination. For instance, if one lives in San Francisco and desires to travel to a final destination in New York City, there are literally hundreds of routes one can take to get there. Some paths may permit an individual to arrive faster and more economically than others, but as long as the traveler heads east and north, all travelers will eventually reach New York City. However, each time the traveler takes a south or westward step, that path will ultimately separate the individual further from their desired destination. Often there are obstacles along one's desired path, and these obstacles require creativity to navigate around, or to go over. Persistently applying the characteristics discussed above (creativity, imagination, wisdom, negotiation) will help the entrepreneur consistently move in the right direction. However, if you consistently yield yourself to follow the path of least resistance, you will never reach your goal. Each decision and choice an entrepreneur makes, plots a route toward a destination—intended or not. The take-home message is that biotechnology entrepreneurship is not forged by any single prescriptive path, even though there are facets of biotechnology that have strict requirements. The particular path you take, and the choices you make, may be different from that of another entrepreneur. However, the desired destination does

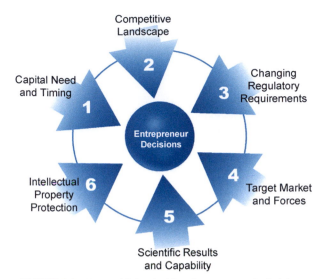

FIGURE 4.3   Forces driving the biotech entrepreneur's decisions.

not change. This analogy is another way of explaining the difference between a method and the goal. Different paths are the same as utilizing different methods but the goal always remains the same. All biotechnology entrepreneurs will have the best opportunity to arrive at their ultimate destination if they consistently find creative ways to navigate around and overcome obstacles within their path.

As illustrated in Figure 4.3, there are forces that affect the decisions a biotech entrepreneur makes. All decisions made during the growth of a company are knowingly or unknowingly impacted by each of these forces. I have included a few general comments to elaborate on these forces and give an example of how decisions in these areas can impact your company's future success.

Capital need and timing:
- How much capital do you need to make product development progress to increase your company value so you can then raise the next round of capital?
- How much capital is remaining and what time is left until the capital is exhausted?

Summary: *Decisions made on the when to raise, and the amount of capital you raise, will impact all the resources you have, and the time you are allotted to accomplish your goals.*

Competitive landscape:
- What is the strength of the existing competition and the likelihood of your future product remaining of competitive value?
- Are there existing substitutes being used comfortably and are there switching hurdles for these users?
- Can your product provide enough value to switch?

Summary: *The frequency and quality of competition, and the likelihood of new competitors, will impact the interest from investors and the latitude you have for the quality and types of features and benefits that are required for your product to be successful.*

Changing regulatory requirements:
- What are the current and future regulations that could affect your product approval; is there some precedent for your product or technology that make regulatory approval highly likely and less risky?
- Will you be able to provide enough supporting data to demonstrate safety and efficacy of your product or service to obtain regulatory approval?

Summary: *The decisions made on regulatory issues will impact the time it will take to reach commercialization or the likelihood of reaching commercialization.*

Target market and forces:
- Have you chosen the target market that has the greatest need for your product or service?
- Is there an educational or awareness requirement that can be managed easily so that those in this target market will readily adopt and utilize your product?

Summary: *Your decisions on selecting your target market for your product will impact the interest from investors and the likelihood of success once the product is commercialized.*

Scientific results and capability:
- Is there enough scientific evidence to support the likelihood that the future product would work and provide value to the target market selected?
- Do you possess, or can you retain, recruit, and hire, the key individuals that have the capability, and understand how to make the product perform in the manner required to provide significant value to your target market?

Summary: *Your decisions on the science and scientific personnel will impact the quality of the research and development, and ultimately the likelihood of reaching your product development goals.*

Intellectual property protection:
- Is there enough patent coverage to protect the product features you want in your product to warrant investor interest?
- Can you create broader intellectual property protection such that it would be increasingly difficult for others to provide an equivalent competitive product?

Summary: *Your decisions on the intellectual property protection strategy will impact your ability to attract investors and the sustainability of your product during commercialization.*

Each of these factors in some way have the ability to impact the other factors. For instance, decisions made in choosing your target market affect the likelihood of interest from investors, whereas your ability to attract funding impacts your ability to recruit and retain the best technical staff and resources. Product development decisions affect the likelihood of securing regulatory approval, whereas the ability to obtain regulatory approval impacts investor interest. Be aware of the effect of various decisions on other aspects of your company both now and in the future.

Number of years since starting	Year																
	1994	1995	1996	1997	1998	1999	2000	2001	2002	2003	2004	2005	2006	2007	2008	2009	2010
1	100.0	100.0	100.0	100.0	100.0	100.0	100.0	100.0	100.0	100.0	100.0	100.0	100.0	100.0	100.0	100.0	100.0
2	79.8	79.2	79.0	78.8	80.6	79.6	78.9	75.5	78.4	79.2	79.1	80.0	78.3	77.2	74.4	76.3	–
3	68.5	68.5	67.6	68.7	69.1	67.6	66.3	64.5	67.5	68.4	69.1	68.7	66.2	63.4	62.4	–	–
4	61.2	60.5	60.4	60.6	60.2	59.0	58.5	57.5	60.2	61.4	61.3	60.1	56.1	54.9	–	–	–
5	54.9	54.7	54.1	53.5	53.6	53.2	53.1	52.4	55.0	55.3	54.7	52.2	49.3	–	–	–	–
6	50.2	49.5	48.8	48.1	48.7	48.7	48.6	48.2	50.4	50.1	48.2	46.5	–	–	–	–	–
7	45.8	45.0	44.5	44.2	45.0	45.0	45.1	44.5	46.3	44.7	43.7	–	–	–	–	–	–
8	42.1	41.4	41.2	41.0	41.9	42.1	42.1	41.2	42.0	40.9	–	–	–	–	–	–	–
9	38.9	38.6	38.5	38.2	39.4	39.3	39.1	37.6	38.7	–	–	–	–	–	–	–	–
10	36.4	36.3	36.0	36.2	37.0	36.8	36.0	34.7	–	–	–	–	–	–	–	–	–
11	34.2	34.1	34.0	34.0	34.8	33.9	33.4	–	–	–	–	–	–	–	–	–	–
12	32.4	32.2	32.1	32.1	32.2	31.7	–	–	–	–	–	–	–	–	–	–	–
13	31.0	30.5	30.4	29.8	30.3	–	–	–	–	–	–	–	–	–	–	–	–
14	29.3	29.0	28.6	28.1	–	–	–	–	–	–	–	–	–	–	–	–	–
15	27.8	27.1	26.9	–	–	–	–	–	–	–	–	–	–	–	–	–	–
16	26.0	25.7	–	–	–	–	–	–	–	–	–	–	–	–	–	–	–
17	24.6	–	–	–	–	–	–	–	–	–	–	–	–	–	–	–	–

Note: Dashes indicate not applicable.

FIGURE 4.4   Percentage of failed companies across all industries based upon the number of years in business and the year started. (Source: *U.S. Bureau of Labor Statistics.*)

LEARNING FROM "FAILURE"

Sadly, there are many company failures within the biotechnology industry. These occur because of faulty product ideas, failed clinical trials, and choosing the wrong target market. The Small Business Administration (SBA) tells us that approximately 50 percent of companies in all industries fail within the first 5 years. Knowing the complexity of biological discoveries, the large capital requirements, and increasing federal regulations, it would not be surprising if the biotechnology industry has at least the same, if not a greater percentage of failures compared to other industries (see Figure 4.4).

Failure is true of any industry, not just biotechnology. However, the opportunity for success is what drives entrepreneurs and companies. The impact of biotechnology products on the life and well-being of our world is the motivation to seek more cures, better treatments, advanced fuels, improved crops, and safer foods. It is important for the biotech entrepreneur to understand there are failures, but not to presume that they are doomed to such a fate before they get started.

The correct definition of *failure* in this instance is *an unsuccessful company* or an *unsuccessful product*. However, failure sometimes incorrectly means more than that. All too often, failure is incorrectly intended to mean *a way of life*, or *an individual*. The biotechnology entrepreneur must remember that failure is just an *event* that occurred at a particular point in time. In reality, failure can be the most valuable learning experience and teaching resource for life—if the individual recognizes this difference. Thomas Edison understood the truth about what we call *failure*. His belief was evident when he replied to a question about his numerous unsuccessful attempts to find the perfect filament

for the light bulb by saying, "I never failed once, it just happened to be a 2000-step process." For the biotech entrepreneur, this is an important distinction to remember when building a business. There will be times you find yourself in unfamiliar situations that are extremely challenging and have grave consequences. You may even experience a failure or two along the way. For some, the natural human instinct is to draw back and retreat. Retreat shows up in various ways such as taking no more risks, avoiding most all decision-making, a lack of confidence, apathy, shirking responsibilities, and limited communication with your team. However, without the driving force of the entrepreneur there will be no life-saving products, no advancements in diagnostic technology, no treatments for rare diseases, no improvements in agricultural foods or crops, nor a host of other breakthroughs to benefit humankind.

SUMMARY

Biotechnology entrepreneurship is the study of the diverse activities essential to building a successful biotechnology company. The biotechnology entrepreneur is a company builder, a product developer, and a risk manager. They are the principal source of the motivation, vision, and forward momentum of the organization. Without them, the company would not exist. There are certain characteristics vital to all entrepreneurs and some that are essential to only those in the biotechnology industry. When an individual evaluates their weaknesses, then purposes to find help in the form of team members and mentors, they can avoid the unknown-unknowns. Biotech entrepreneurs daily face a myriad of challenges to their product and company success, and the entrepreneurial path can be likened to a journey toward a destination filled with roadblocks and detours along the way. There is no single prescriptive road that all entrepreneurs must take, but there are characteristics that will help you navigate around obstacles to your ultimate destination. Each decision an entrepreneur makes is influenced by the numerous forces described within this chapter. When risks are properly managed, and wise decisions are made, this endeavor will lead to some of the most rewarding life-long experiences of your career.

REFERENCES

[1] Collins J. Good to Great: Why Some Companies Make the Leap…and Others Don't, New York. New York: Collins Business; 2001.

[2] Urban H. Life's Greatest Lessons: 20 Things that Matter. 4th ed. New York: Fireside; 2003.

Five Essential Elements for Growing Biotechnology Clusters

Craig Shimasaki, PhD, MBA

President & CEO, Moleculera Labs and BioSource Consulting Group, Oklahoma City, Oklahoma

The first use of modern genetic engineering tools began in 1973 when Stanley Cohen and Herbert Boyer successfully excised a segment of frog DNA and transferred it into a bacterial plasmid to create a molecular factory for proteins. In 1976, 3 years after those humble beginnings, Genentech was founded with $500 each from Robert Swanson, at the time a young venture capitalist, and Herbert Boyer a University of California San Francisco Professor. *The biotechnology industry had begun.* In the ensuing 5 years, only a handful of companies followed, such as Cetus (which began in 1971 but not based on genetic engineering until after 1976), Biogen and Hybritech in 1978, Amgen in 1980, and Genzyme and Chiron in 1981. Less than 4 decades later, there are over 10,000 public and private biotechnology companies that collectively employ over 500,000 individuals worldwide. Today, the biotechnology industry continues to expand with cities, states, and local governments vying for the creation of biotechnology clusters in their region. Even though this industry is experiencing unprecedented growth, expansion is not occurring equally in all geographies, but is concentrated predominately in certain cluster locations. In this chapter, I describe Five Essential Elements that influence the growth and development of biotechnology clusters and stimulate the industry expansion over time within a particular locale.

The San Francisco Bay Area and the Boston/Cambridge area are recognized as the top biotechnology clusters worldwide. Many of the early biotechnology companies were started within these two geographic regions, and today they both are thriving biotechnology ecosystems, spawning new companies on a regular basis. It is estimated that approximately one-third of all U.S. biotech employees work in the Boston and San Francisco Bay areas where the concentration of biotechnology companies eclipse that of all other regions. Interestingly, these geographic regions have vastly different climates, almost opposite cultures, and distinctly different histories, yet both regions rapidly grew into thriving biotechnology hubs.

For the San Francisco Bay Area, one contributing factor that fueled their growth was the colocation of venture capital that previously funded the computer chip boom in the mid-1970s. Silicon Valley is proximal to San Francisco and is home to many entrepreneurial-minded leaders, with several academic institutions conducting ground-breaking research that fueled the birth of numerous biotechnology companies (Figure 5.1).

The Boston and Cambridge areas are also known for their top-ranked academic research institutions such as Harvard and MIT, but another key to Boston's transformation is its proximity to the large concentration of pharmaceutical companies (Figure 5.2). This colocation with a mature pharmaceutical industry gave ready access to an abundant resource of industry leaders and drug development team members for fledgling biotechnology companies.

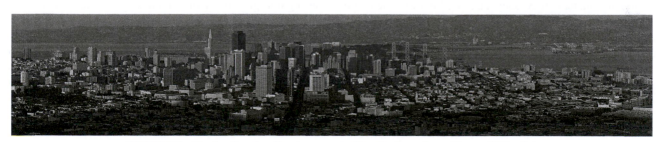

FIGURE 5.1 The San Francisco Bay Area, a major biotechnology cluster (*Source: Wikipedia*).

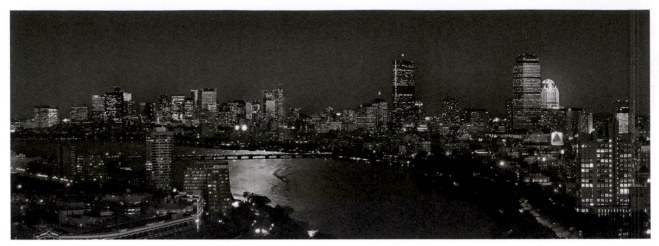

FIGURE 5.2   The Boston/Cambridge area, one of the top biotechnology clusters in the world *(Source: Wikipedia)*.

There are many other well-established and growing concentrations of biotech activity—literally all over the world. In a 2012 Life Science Cluster Report, Jones Lang LaSalle referenced the following as established clusters in the Americas: Greater Boston, San Diego, San Francisco Bay Area, Raleigh-Durham, Philadelphia, suburban Maryland/DC/Arlington, New Jersey/New York City, Los Angeles/Orange County, Minneapolis-St. Paul, and Seattle. They cite emerging biotechnology clusters in: Westchester/New Haven, Chicago, Denver, Cleveland/Columbus/Cincinnati, Salt Lake City, Dallas/Fort Worth, Southern Wisconsin, Central and South Florida, Indianapolis, Southern Michigan, and Atlanta, Canada, Brazil, Colombia, and Mexico. In the Europe, Middle East and Africa (EMEA) region, they cite established clusters in France, Germany, Netherlands, Switzerland, and the United Kingdom. They cite established biotechnology clusters in the Asia Pacific region as Japan, with emerging clusters in China, India, Indonesia, and Singapore [1]. Biotech clusters are growing in additional locations outside the United States, such as Medicon Valley which straddles the border of Sweden and Denmark and is home to over 100 biotechnology companies including large pharmaceutical companies such as AstraZeneca and Novo Nordisk. Switzerland's BioValley connects academia and companies of three nations in the Upper Rhine Valley, namely France, Germany and Switzerland. Australia has more than 400 biotechnology companies, predominately located in clusters in Sydney and Melbourne. There are more than 600 companies located in biotechnology clusters in Scotland, and in Oxford and London, biotechnology clusters are home to 163 and over 800 companies, respectively.

BIOTECHNOLOGY CLUSTERS ARE ACTIVELY DEVELOPING WORLD-WIDE

There is universal interest in developing biotechnology clusters in most all countries around the world. The providence of Ontario, Canada has a Biotechnology Cluster Innovation Program where the government is focused on funding and developing a competitive biotechnology cluster. Europe INNOVA was launched in 2006 as an initiative of the European Commission's Directorate General Enterprise and Industry which aspires to become the laboratory for the development and testing of new tools and instruments in support of innovation with the view to help enterprises innovate faster and better. They have brought together public and private support and providers such as innovation agencies, technology transfer offices, business incubators, financing intermediaries, cluster organizations, and others. Europe INNOVA also created NETBIOCLUE which stands for "NETworking activity for BIOtechnology CLUsters in Europe."

In 2006, the New York City Economic Development Corp., incorporated BioBAT (Figure 5.3), a nonprofit organization that is leading the biotech development at the Brooklyn Army Terminal and converting it into a massive new bioresearch and manufacturing facility. BioBAT, a 524,000-square-foot center for commercial bioscience is expected to create more than 1000 permanent jobs. The city invested $12 million in the project, and the state offered $48 million of funding. The Brooklyn Army Terminal is a 97-acre facility owned by the city and managed by the New York City Economic Development Corporation.

The Colorado Science and Technology Park at Fitzsimons is an example of what can be done to facilitate the organic growth of biotechnology in one's own state. A decommissioned Army medical center was closed down a decade ago in Denver, and 18 million square feet is being converted to house 30,000 new employees with many of the companies being spin-off technology companies from the University of Colorado Health Science Center (UCHSC). The state's investment of $4 billion will become an economic generator for Colorado and stimulate the development of many new biotechnology companies.

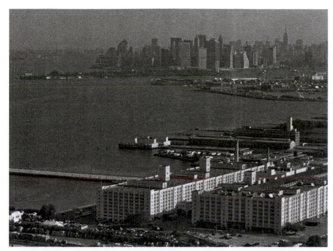

FIGURE 5.3   BioBAT at Brooklyn Army Terminal, a major biotechnology incubator in New York. (*Source: New York City Economic Development Corporation, NYCEDC*)

WHAT IS A BIOTECHNOLOGY CLUSTER

A biotechnology cluster is simply a very high concentration of organically grown biotechnology enterprises attached to a supportive ecosystem within a defined geographic region. Within this ecosystem each of the biotechnology companies are not typically interconnected to one another; however, they are all interconnected to their local bioscience providers and are sustained by the presence of the Five Essential Elements we will discuss below. Often, a biotechnology cluster will develop a subspecialty focus due to an inherent concentration of expertise and resources within that region. For instance, the greater Minneapolis, Minnesota region and surrounding areas are home to a high concentration of medical device companies, principally due to the historical presence of Medtronic, founded in 1949 with the development of the pacemaker, as well as 3M and Boston Scientific. High concentrations of therapeutic companies are located in the Boston area which was influenced by the large concentration of pharmaceutical companies clustered in New Jersey and the surrounding areas. A large number of agricultural biotechnology companies are clustered in Midwestern states of the U.S., principally due to the high concentration of agricultural research conducted at local universities and academic institutions.

WHAT ARE THE BENEFITS OF A BIOTECHNOLOGY CLUSTER?

In 2012, the U.S. government released the *National Bioeconomy Blueprint* noting that bioscience industries are "a large and rapidly growing segment of the world economy that provides substantial public benefit" [2]. The economic benefit and quality-of-life impact of a mature biotechnology cluster in its municipality and local government is significant. All regions support diverse economic development programs that are targeted to improve the quality of life and economic stability of their locale. Aside from the universal benefits of biotechnology products for health, agriculture, fuels, and energy, biotechnology clusters have much more to offer local regions and governments, with some of the benefits listed below:

1. **The biotechnology industry creates clean and high-technology jobs:** Regional municipalities and governments are searching for ways to attract and retain high-technology jobs which tend to be clean industries that generate fewer environmental issues. Based upon data from the U.S. Bureau of Labor statistics, the bioscience industry in the United States has led in job creation during the 2001 to 2010 period [3] when compared with other major knowledge-based industries critical for advancing high quality jobs (Figure 5.4). This was in spite of a nationwide decline in most all job categories. A primary reason for the resiliency of the bioscience industry is the diverse set of markets it serves. These markets span biomedical drugs, diagnostics and devices, agricultural products from animal health, to seeds and crop protection, and bio-based industrial products such as enzymes for industry chemical processes and bioremediation, biofuels, and bioplastics. The biotechnology industry has also fared much better than the overall economy through the recent U.S. recession and recovery.

2. **The biotechnology industry creates high paying jobs:** The average wages paid to bioscience industry workers reached $82,697 in 2010, more than $36,000 or 79 percent greater than the average paid in the overall national private sector [3]. Bioscience wage growth outpaced that of the private sector, increasing by 13.1 percent in inflation-adjusted terms since 2001 compared with a 4.4 percent pay raise among all other industries (Figure 5.5).

3. **New jobs and high paying jobs generate personal and sales taxes for local governments:** Because biotechnology employees tend to have significantly higher salaries than the national averages, these employees on average purchase more goods and services, generating more tax revenue to the local economy. All local governments need tax revenue to operate and support their infrastructure services for their community. As these amenities and services improve and increase, this in turn can attract other industries to the region with more job relocations.

4. **Biotechnology companies bring an innovative and skilled workforce:** Biotechnology companies require diversely skilled employees that are experienced in

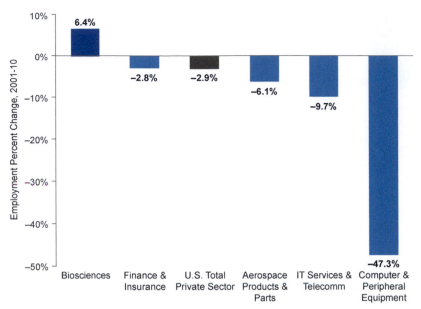

FIGURE 5.4   Job growth in bioscience compared to other knowledge-based industries, 2001 to 2010. (*Source: Battelle/BIO State Bioscience Industry Development 2012*)

various disciplines, including research and development, drug design, medical devices, mechanical and biomedical engineering, medical affairs, chemistry, molecular biology, regulatory affairs, clinical trials, and a host of other professional disciplines. Often industry professionals can contribute a portion of their time and

resources to the local economy by participating in various local support and philanthropic activities in their community.

5. **Biotechnology clusters attract collateral businesses and support services:** Biotechnology companies require a host of collateral support groups in order to be

U.S. Average Annual Wages per Employee, 2010		
Drugs & Pharmaceuticals	$	**99,486**
Finance & Insurance	$	84,516
Research, Testing, & Medical Laboratories	$	**84,065**
Total Biosciences	$	**82,697**
Bioscience-related Distribution	$	**80,049**
Professional, Scientific, & Technical Services	$	77,313
Information	$	74,382
Medical Devices & Equipment	$	**72,301**
Agricultural Feedstock & Chemicals	$	**70,869**
Manufacturing	$	57,511
Construction	$	49,588
U.S. Total Private Sector	$	**46,317**
Transportation & Warehousing	$	44,198
Real Estate & Rental & Leasing	$	43,779
Health Care & Social Assistance	$	43,732
Retail Trade	$	26,655

FIGURE 5.5   Average annual wages in the biosciences and other major industries, 2010. (*Source: Battelle/BIO State Bioscience Industry Development 2012*)

successful. These support services also tend to employ positions that are higher paying than the national average and they tend to be in clean industries. Some of the support services and professionals include corporate and patent attorneys, prototype development companies, accountants, public relations firms, medical service providers, clinical trial coordinators, medical consultants, and research technologists.

6. **Large talent pools bring cross-creativity and shortened development time:** As the critical mass of biotechnology company employees and their service providers increase in a locale, the speed for development of company technology and products tends to accelerate. This is principally due to the availability and quality of cross-creativity experts with the necessary experience to support these companies' product development needs. This increase in product development momentum is attractive to other companies that want access to those same resources and talent pools. Concurrent with industry growth comes greater expansion of support services and more professionals to support the industry—and the cycle continues.

THE FIVE ESSENTIAL ELEMENTS NECESSARY TO GROWING A BIOTECHNOLOGY CLUSTER

What key elements fueled the transformation of diverse locations such as Boston and San Francisco into two of the largest concentrations of biotechnology companies in the world? There are multiple factors that contribute to the growth and development of biotechnology cluster irrespective of location. However, some frequently described factors may indeed be contributing elements, but not all of them are essential. "Essential Elements" are those factors that when absent, or in limited quantity, directly prevents a biotechnology cluster from developing and expanding in any particular location. There are also "Nonessential Elements," which are contributors to the growth of a biotechnology cluster, but their absence or limitation does not prevent the industry's development in that location. Each Essential Element must be present in order to support the formation and expansion of a biotechnology cluster in that particular region. To the degree that any Essential Element is limited, to that same degree a region's biotechnology cluster growth will also be limited. The following Five Essential Elements are necessary to establish, stimulate, and encourage continued growth of the biotechnology industry within any geography.

Five Essential Elements

1. **Abundance of high quality, adequately funded academic research:** This Essential Element is basic academic research conducted at well-respected institutions, which is usually well-funded and always conducted by high-caliber researchers, scientists, physicians, or engineers. These researchers are well-published in top-tier peer-reviewed journals and are typically scientific and technology leaders in a particular field.

2. **Ready resource of seasoned and experienced biotechnology entrepreneurs:** This Essential Element is a supply of individuals who have the experience and expertise to shepherd fledgling companies through the difficult growth stages until commercialization or corporate partnership occurs. These individuals tend to be serial entrepreneurs who have started previous companies or served in key roles at previous biotechnology or life science organizations. Another experienced group consists of individuals with lengthy experience in senior positions at large multinational pharmaceutical, medical device, agricultural, or venture-funding corporations.

3. **Ready access to sources of at-risk, early and development-stage capital willing to fund start-up concepts:** This Essential Element consists of multiple funding sources, including angel investors, venture capital, or institutional capital located within, or proximal to, the local region. These are funding sources that actively invest in early- and development-stage life science enterprises. In addition, these sources can include local government-supported financing and granting programs directed to assist enterprises during the inception stages until significant value is realized.

4. **Adequate supply of technically skilled workforce experienced in the biotechnology industry:** This Essential Element is comprised of experienced scientists, technicians, and laboratory personnel that are well-trained in the particular techniques and methods required to advance the technology within that region. Such a workforce is necessary to support product development for these companies without them having to spend enormous amounts of time and resources for on-the-job training.

5. **Availability of dedicated wet-laboratory and specialized facilities at affordable rates:** This Essential Element is the supply of laboratory space and specialized facilities located in strategic areas that allow incubation of nascent companies time to prove their biological concepts or build working prototypes. These facilities should be state-of-the-art and must be offered at affordable rates to allow these early-stage companies to make value-enhancing progress in order to attract more investor capital.

"GROWING" BIOTECHNOLOGY CLUSTERS

A helpful analogy to understanding the process of growing a biotechnology cluster is the corollary to a farmer who wants to reap a harvest of a particular agricultural crop on his land. A farmer knows he cannot "make" crops grow. However, the farmer also understands he has the ability to greatly influence the likelihood of growth and the size of the harvest by ensuring that the essential elements are present when seed is planted. In this analogy, the "farmer" can be likened to the regional government or municipality and must include the joint efforts of both public and private sectors. The "agricultural crops" are fledgling biotechnology enterprises, whereas the "land" is simply the boundaries of the local geographic region in which the biotechnology cluster is desired. To carry this illustration further, if the farmer sows an abundance of fertile seed in nutrient-rich soil, provides an adequate supply of water and fertilizer, and removes destructive pests and weeds that inhibit growth, the seed will naturally flourish. Notably, if the farmer omits one of these elements or if an element is in short supply, such as water, it then becomes very difficult, if not impossible, to reap the desired harvest even though all other essential elements are in abundant supply. (See Figure 5.6.)

FIVE ESSENTIAL ELEMENTS TO GROWING A BIOTECHNOLOGY CLUSTER IN A REGION

Essential Element #1: Abundance of High Quality, Adequately Funded, Academic Research

This Essential Element of academic research must be plentiful, of high quality, and performed at local academic institutions by respected scientists, engineers, and physicians who are recognized as leaders in their field. Since the vast majority of all biotechnology products can trace their roots back to basic research originating at an academic institution, it is therefore necessary that within a region this element is abundantly present. An abundance of high-quality academic research is the "fertile seed," and without seed, there will be no crop harvested. The number of companies that can grow within that region will be proportional to the amount of high-quality research conducted within that region. If the seed is flawed in quality, or insufficient in quantity, a deficient or limited harvest will result. There is a direct correlation between the quality of a start-up company's products, and the quality of the underlying research that was licensed. Even though a company may still be formed from flawed research, the licensed technology will be a detractor to the company when trying to raise capital for its development. For the seed to be "fertile," both the research and the researcher at these academic institutions must be adequately funded, be leaders in their field, and have their results published in top-tier peer-reviewed scientific, medical, and related industry journals. Without the abundance of high-quality seed, there will be very few biotechnology companies birthed within these regions.

How is Quality Research Assessed?

The quality of the research can be assessed by the researcher's ability to secure sufficient grant funding to support their research. This is because research grants are typically awarded by peer review and prioritized by leaders in a related field and the most innovative and competitive research is typically funded. However, because of shrinking governmental budgets, _all_ innovative research is not funded adequately. Still, in spite of grant funding

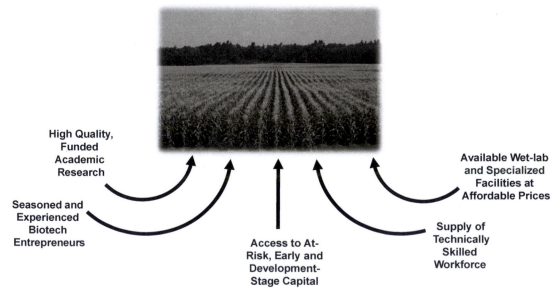

FIGURE 5.6   Essential elements that support biotech cluster growth.

limitations, these innovative and top-notch researchers are successful in attracting funding, and often from additional sources such as disease foundations, patient advocacy groups, and corporate donors. Another good measure of a region's likelihood of developing a biotechnology cluster, in general terms, is the amount of R&D spending within that region on a per capita basis. Figure 5.7 shows the relative R&D spending around the world on a country basis, but the same measure can be applied to any specific geographic region.

Choosing the Best Research Application

Even if great research abounds, there still must be an efficient process to identify and transfer great technology opportunities from academic institutions to commercial enterprises. Most all universities and academic institutions have a technology transfer office that is charged with this objective. Within these offices, it is not uncommon for institutions to accumulate "shelves" of intellectual property and patents that are without a commercial home. On average, the number of patents that remain unlicensed at a typical university may be as high as 60 to 75 percent of their intellectual property portfolio. In other words, the majority of ideas do not get licensed. I believe the reason that a large portion of these patents

remain on university shelves is not always due to non-innovative or poor quality science, but rather for three other reasons:

1. The product application that was chosen to demonstrate the underlying research is not of interest to potential licensees because it does not address a target market need that would support commercial success.
2. The institution does not have the necessary support personnel or the incentives to adequately identify the most strategic and best opportunities, and to actively solicit these to the most likely licensees.
3. The institution's academic researchers have limited interest, or minimal understanding of the steps necessary for translational development of their basic research, or they do not know how, or want to spin-out a company on their own.

Historically, solving these three issues were not objectives within the original charter of academic institutions. However, because of shrinking educational budgets and the need to find additional sources of revenue, technology commercialization can play a major role in finding new sources of revenue. Academic institutions can help improve this dilemma by placing emphasis on the expansion of basic research to encompass applied or translational focuses.

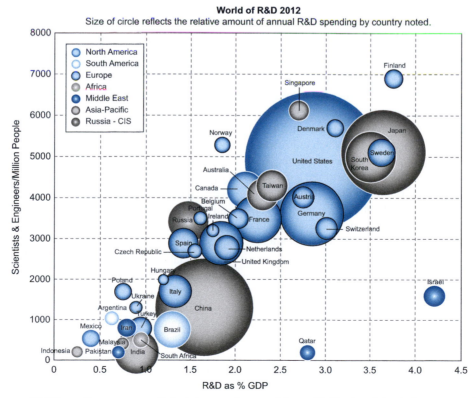

FIGURE 5.7 Summary of R&D spending on a per capita basis in countries around the world. The size of the circles represent the relative amount of the country's annual R&D spending. The position on the grid shows R&D spending as a percent of GDP and the number of scientists and engineers per million population. *(Source: 2013 Battelle/R&D Magazine Global R&D Funding Forecast)*

Many academic researchers have found that by taking their existing basic research and extending experimentation toward development of translational product concepts, they can build commercial value that attracts licensees to their technology. By incrementally advancing translational research, academic institutions may realize higher values for their licenses, or at least ensure that more of their portfolio is out-licensed for a future commercial applications.

For commercially-minded researchers who desire to see products developed from their work, they need to understand that successful biotechnology products all meet an important need for a paying customer. In other words, scientific technology must be viewed as a *solution* seeking the right *problem* to solve. Therefore, it is incumbent on the scientist or engineer to select the most important problem which has an audience who would gladly pay for that product or service. Technology application choices are conscious decisions that are at the discretion of the researcher. It is true that most all technology concepts have diverse applications. A researcher may select a particular application because they are more familiar with a seemingly obvious purpose, however, that may be a subpar market choice because there may be adequate products already serving that need. For instance, let's say a researcher discovers a molecule that inhibits a metabolic enzyme vital for growth of a streptococcal bacteria strain. The researcher's natural inclination may be to work on an application for the development of a new antibiotic to treat strep infections. However, unless that molecule works on drug-resistant strains of bacteria, there are already dozens of antibiotics that work effectively against strep—and inexpensively. This technology, although innovative, may never gain interest from future licensees or investors for future development. Alternatively, if that molecule could be found to inhibit other enzymes, (let's hypothesize that it would be a critical enzyme in the Alzheimer's disease pathway) if research was directed to modifying the molecule and inhibiting *that* enzyme, there certainly would be investor interest in that application! Therefore, one method in which universities and academic institutions may increase their licensing frequency is by reevaluating their technology portfolio and aligning the technology applications more closely with market needs. This activity requires the help of individuals with both technical and marketing knowledge to assist in the disclosures and patent application when professors and scientists initiate filings.

Awareness of Challenges with New Discoveries

Because biotechnology products are based upon a current understanding of science at the time of discovery, occasionally our current understanding is inadequate or insufficient to optimally develop an effective biotechnology product. In other words, the likelihood of success is not only the quality of the science, but also how much is understood about the condition or disease at the time. For instance, when the AIDS virus (HIV) was first reported in humans in 1983, it was unclear how this virus replicated within the body and how it evaded the human immune system. Many strategies for therapeutics and vaccines failed simply because of our limited knowledge of the infectious cycle of the HIV virus, and an unclear understanding of the human immune system. However, as scientists later discovered how the virus replicated and evaded the immune system, effective therapeutics were successfully developed by many biotech and pharmaceutical companies. If a researcher desires to see their technology become a therapeutic application, there must be adequate knowledge available about the mechanism of the disease or condition in order to support product development success. The better the understanding of the mechanism of a disease or condition, the more likely a therapeutic strategy will be successful when selecting a disease target.

Common Goals

Leaders of municipalities who want to build and cultivate a biotechnology cluster must garner support for this goal from their respective universities and academic institutions. Regions that want to accelerate their cluster development will do well by convincing government agencies to facilitate or incentivize university technology transfer offices to support spin-out companies within their locale. Assistance can also include creative programs to improve or increase the academic and translational research quality. One noteworthy program is Kentucky's "Bucks for Brains" where they are recruiting top talent to increase their research pool at local universities within their state. Bucks for Brains has enabled the University of Louisville to recruit and retain teams of research faculty from some of the best universities in the world.

Research at Academic Institutions Verses Commercialization at For-Profit Corporations

Although high-quality, adequately funded research is the fertile seed, a gap exists between the academic institutions that own them, and the commercial enterprises that develop and commercialize them. An academic institutions' original mission is that of gaining knowledge through basic research and teaching for the dissemination of knowledge. Whereas a commercial organizations' purpose for conducting research is that of creating products and services to meet a financially profitable market. Between these organizations and institutions (each having different purposes) a gap must be bridged in order to increase the flow of research into commercially viable and needed products for society. To the extent that both academic and commercial organizations make concerted efforts to bridge that gap, it is to that same extent that greater numbers of biotechnology companies will be birthed within that locale.

Essential Element #2: A Ready Resource of Seasoned and Experienced Biotechnology Entrepreneurs

Management experience and talent is one of the most significant factors in determining the success of start-up enterprises in every industry. For biotechnology companies, talented management is even more critical. Unfortunately, this Essential Element is in short supply almost everywhere, and this is one of the most critical rate-limiting Essential Elements in building biotechnology clusters. Financial investors, particularly venture capital firms, invest in talented teams and experienced leaders who have expertise and history within the biotechnology industry. These are individuals who can shepherd fledgling companies through the difficult growth stages in order to reach commercialization or partnering. Without an experienced biotechnology entrepreneur and a talented team, there will be no company. An important characteristic of these individuals (who are entrepreneurs by desire or by necessity) is the ability to translate both science and business issues, and to communicate effectively to both audiences. Some biotechnology entrepreneurs are former pharmaceutical and medical device executives with lengthy employment histories, or venture capital partners with past experience in leading start-up companies. Others are serial entrepreneurs that have started one or more biotechnology companies, or they may have served in senior roles at larger biotechnology companies. In the early days of the biotechnology industry there were no serial entrepreneurs to lead these nascent companies. Management talent was recruited from collateral industries. Interestingly, a high proportion of the early biotechnology leaders came from Baxter such as Ted Green, the first CEO of Hybritech and Henri Termeer, the former CEO of Genzyme [4].

In order to overcome the limited supply of these serial entrepreneurial leaders, many organizations within a region support an "Entrepreneur-in-Residence" program to recruit seasoned entrepreneurs who have started and exited previous biotechnology companies. The objective of such a program is that one seasoned entrepreneur leader can advise or manage multiple fledgling biotechnology companies until they gain enough intrinsic value to attract enough capital and can then hire a full-time CEO. Starting and growing a biotechnology company is not a straight-forward process. There are many obstacles that line the path of would-be entrepreneurs, and it takes seasoned individuals to successfully navigate these obstacles and reach success. As the biotechnology industry continues to mature and companies birth leaders who can become future entrepreneurs, this industry will be better equipped for rapid growth and expansion.

Successful and Unsuccessful Companies will Birth Other Companies

Just as harvested crops become seed for future crops, so do biotechnology companies give rise to seasoned entrepreneurs who start new biotechnology enterprises. Mature biotechnology companies will give rise to a fresh crop of biotechnology entrepreneurs who often start new companies in the same locale. An often repeated scenario is that one biotechnology company grows over time, then many of the early employees leave to start new ventures within the same region. A single mature biotechnology company can become the training grounds for a multitude of new entrepreneurs who often take experienced employees with them to accelerate the development of their new venture. This is principally how the San Diego biotechnology cluster was developed and expanded. In 1978, Ivor Royston, a Professor at UC San Diego, and his research assistant Howard Birndorf, started Hybritech with $300,000 in seed funding. Hybritech was focused on developing monoclonal antibody diagnostic tests and gained enough momentum to go public in 1981. The company grew, and in 1985 Eli Lilly purchased Hybritech for an estimated $500 million. Unfortunately, the formal corporate structure of Eli Lilly with its policies and procedures was imposed on the informal energetic entrepreneurial culture of Hybritech and it created culture clashes. Within a year of the Eli Lilly acquisition, most of Hybritech's key talent left the company and started new biotechnology enterprises in the San Diego area. More than 100 San Diego biotechnology companies can trace their roots back to Hybritech, such as Gensia, Gen-Probe and IDEC. Figure 5.8 lists a pedigree of some of these companies that trace their roots back to Hybritech. We see the same phenomena occur in other biotech clusters where the success and growth of one company breeds a large number of start-ups in the surrounding areas founded by former employees. Some serial founders also go on to be the financiers of new start-up biotechnology companies such as Ivor Royston, who became a Venture Capitalist and was an investor in many other companies in the San Diego area.

Essential Element #3: Access to Available Sources of At-Risk, Early-Stage and Development-Stage Capital Willing to Fund Start-Up Ideas

Without capital, even the best of ideas will not come to fruition. This Essential Element is usually one of the two major rate-limiting resources for the development of biotechnology clusters in any region. Capital is the fuel for development of biotechnology products and services. Capital limitations will hinder or delay product development progress and momentum, causing enthusiasm to

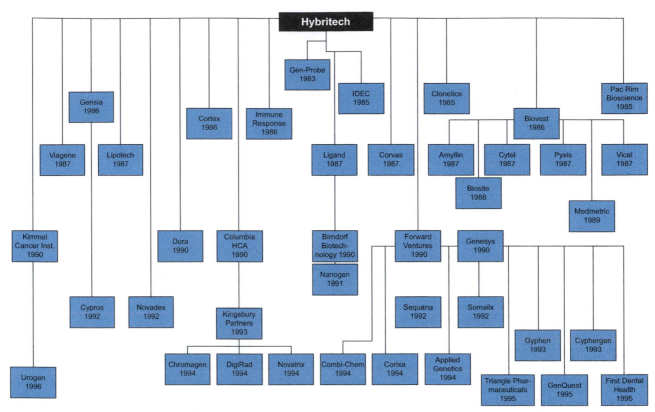

FIGURE 5.8 Companies founded by former Hybritech employees. *(Begatting Chart Courtesy: UC San Diego Extension and CONNECT)*

be lost if funding is delayed too long. Notwithstanding, many companies simply run out of capital before they can complete product development or they are unable to find investors soon enough before they are forced to downsize staffing. Occasionally, some funding issues have to do with poor planning on the leader's part by not understanding the length of time required to raise additional capital. However, seasoned entrepreneurs know that fundraising takes time. In other situations, the company may have missed an expected milestone and did not have enough capital to adjust or reposition their progress in time to find other interested investors. Apart from these situations, the major limitation for growth is the lack of early- and development-stage capital for companies within that region.

Early-Stage, Risk Capital Needed

It is a fact that capital is limited and there is not enough funds to support every start-up company having a good idea. However, it is also true that many "fundable" enterprises never obtain enough funding simply because of the lack of access to capital in their geographical region. Many investors, particularly early angel investors, invest in companies in their local region. A fledgling company needs access to "risk" capital, including angel investors, seed investors, and

venture capital to support their endeavors until significant valuation is realized. In order for a biotechnology cluster to develop, that region must have a continuum of investment capital resources for these companies to have the best chance of success.

Various regions have implemented funding programs to help fill this gap. Some programs are directed specifically toward life science or high-technology companies located within their geographic region. Different financing mechanisms have been created by local governments such as high-risk "loans" that are paid back (at a high premium) only if the company is successful, whereas if not, there is no further obligation. Other financing mechanisms include innovation grant awards that must be matched by private capital, thus incentivizing private investors to participate in the early-stage venture. Municipalities are also creating technology-commercialization centers to support their financing programs to add value with guidance, management, and board oversight for these young start-up companies. There are numerous ways that a regional government or municipality can support an early-stage biotechnology company's access to risk capital in their locale. The most important aspect is all of these sources must be readily accessible and directed toward early-stage financing of these innovative companies in order for a biotechnology cluster to be fostered.

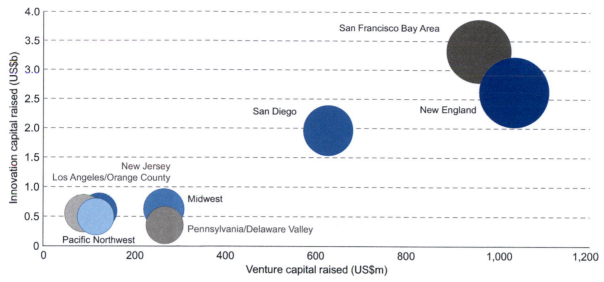

FIGURE 5.9 Capital raised by leading United States regions, 2012. As in 2011, the three leading regions for fundraising were the San Francisco Bay Area, New England, and San Diego. However, in 2011, New England had led the nation in both venture capital and innovation capital raised by a wide margin. In 2012, the gap closed, with the San Francisco Bay Area inching ahead in innovation capital while New England retained the lead in venture capital. The rest of the regions are clustered together. Bubble sizes show the relative numbers of financing per region. Innovative capital is the amount of equity capital raised by companies with revenues less than $500 million in U.S. dollars). *(From Ernst & Young, Beyond Borders, Biotechnology Industry Report 2013.)*

Needed Follow-On Capital During Development Stages

As discussed in Chapter 19 entitled "Sources of Capital and Investor Motivations," different investor groups have preferences for different stages of investment. Without a continuum of risk capital for companies within their locale, it is difficult to sustain a viable biotechnology hub. For instance, if a region has early-stage angel investors but little or no institutional investors or venture capital, companies may be started, but few will make it beyond the early stages of development. Without follow-on development-stage capital, what often happens is that the best organically funded companies relocate to other regions where access to capital is greater, or new funding is contingent on the company moving to the investor's locale.

Development-stage capital requires larger commitments of money than early-stage capital. Whereas early-stage capital for a biotechnology company can be as little as $100,000 to as much as $750,000, development stage capital may require $1 million to $3 million of capital for any one company. Often this amount of money is too large for angel investors and may be too small, and too early, for large venture capital firms. However, there are development-stage friendly venture capital firms that do invest at these stages, but they are not as plentiful. In order to fill this development-stage funding gap, some local government agencies have allocated a portion of funds toward development-stage companies, with private company matching requirements. Depending on the fund size, these local government agencies have become "super angels" and can

lead a funding round with a large group of individual angels matching.

Regions that have the greatest access to innovation capital (early-stage) and development-stage (venture-type) capital are the regions that experience the greatest growth in their biotechnology cluster development. Figure 5.9 shows regions in the United States with the most innovation capital and venture capital raised, whereas Figure 5.10 shows the same type of capital raised in other countries.

Essential Element #4: Adequate Supply of Technically-Skilled Workforce Experienced in the Biotechnology Field

Start-up and development-stage biotechnology companies require skilled and experienced teams of people to develop their products. This Essential Element is comprised of employees with specialized skill sets having the requisite expertise necessary to support development of the company technology. Expertise in a specialized technology is required because these individuals are the ones who must overcome technical problems during the development of a product. Fledgling biotechnology companies require these types of skilled team members, but cannot spend time with lengthy on-the-job training. Each team member added to the start-up company must contribute in ways that are not limited to someone having to train them. Each new member becomes the growing critical mass of expertise that must help advance the technology into a developed product. Because biotechnology can become

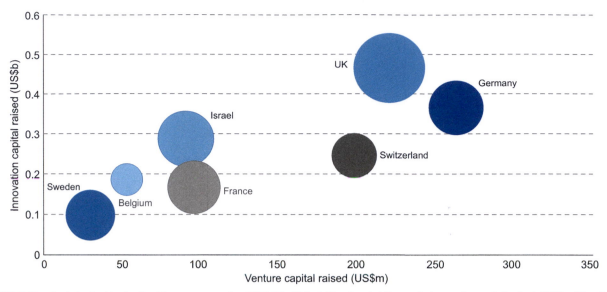

FIGURE 5.10   Capital raised by leading European countries, 2012. The United Kingdom led Europe in innovation capital raised ($467 million in U.S. dollars) as well as the number of financing rounds. However, Germany led Europe in the amount of venture capital raised ($263 million in U.S. dollars), in part because of two significant financings (CurVac and BRAIN) by family offices. Other leaders included Switzerland (third-highest amount of venture capital raised) and Israel (third-highest amount of venture capital raised). Bubble sizes show the relative number of financing per country. *(From Ernst & Young, Beyond Borders, Biotechnology Industry Report 2013.)*

so specialized in any particular sector, it is very difficult for a single region to have an experienced workforce that spans expertise in all sectors of the biotechnology industry. This is one reason why many biotechnology clusters naturally develop a sector focus due to the workforce expertise located within that region. This workforce specialization phenomena is evident in all industries, not just the biotechnology industry. For instance, auto manufacturing was originally clustered within the Detroit region of the United States, in part due to the high concentration of experienced autoworkers; whereas oil and gas clusters are strong in the Texas and Oklahoma regions. Having a supply of technically skilled workers is one reason that the existing biotechnology hubs of Boston and San Francisco continue to experience rapid formation of new biotech companies. Such industry specialty focus is attractive for recruiting other individuals with the same skills because they know that if necessary they can change jobs without ever changing zip codes.

Essential Element #5: Adequate and Dedicated Wet-Laboratory and Facilities at Affordable Rates

Adequate facilities are essential to fledgling biotechnology companies, allowing them to efficiently conduct research, and development and prototype testing. Biotechnology product development is highly specialized and requires specialized facilities and resources to service their product development needs. Inadequate facilities hinder product development and make a challenging product development

timeline even more challenging. Many regional municipalities and academic institutions are addressing the facility needs of start-up companies in creative ways. Most frequently this is accomplished through the creation of "incubators" which are often coupled with other resources. Incubators can assist young companies with the needed facilities and support to prove their scientific concepts or build working prototypes. The term *incubator* has been used to describe various types of facilities, but all incubators are not created equal. Some incubators provide subsidized rent along with support systems and personnel for a small fee. Other incubators are simply high-tech laboratory and office space at standard rates that are built and conveniently housed adjacent to an academic institution or university center. Ideally, an incubator program would be designed to support entrepreneurial companies by offering supportive resources and some assistance for nontechnical activities. In some cases these programs can be bundled to provide access to seed funding. Incubator programs are usually region-specific and have a mission to support local high-tech companies moving into their space for a period of time. Types of support can include nominal costs for access to common, but expensive, equipment or usage of resources such as animal facilities. These types of support programs help start-up companies accelerate product testing to reach a value-enhancing milestone that increases the likelihood of more significant funding.

Many universities have built their own dedicated life science incubator facilities to support university spin-offs, and give preference to serve their faculty or companies licensing their technology. In 1995, the University of Florida launched

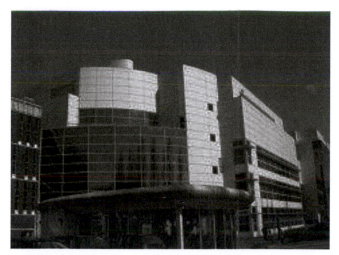

FIGURE 5.11 University of Manchester Innovation Center incubator building *(Source: The University of Manchester Innovation Center UMIC website).*

the Sid Martin Biotechnology Incubator with 40,000 square feet of labs, vivariums, greenhouses, fermentation facilities, and $1 million of shared scientific equipment and business-development services. In 2013 they were ranked the "World's Best University Biotechnology Incubator," based on an international study conducted by the Swedish-based research group, University Business Incubator (UBI). Other university-based incubator programs include the Harvard Innovation Lab, a 33,000 square-foot facility that includes all the schools stimulating a cross-pollination of ideas, including biotechnology. For about 10 years, the University of Manchester in the U.K. has incubated start-up life science companies in its University of Manchester Innovation Center (UMIC) (Figure 5.11) incubator building. Currently their state-of-the-art biotechnology R&D center includes over 85,000 square feet of bioscience incubator and related support facilities and include 16 turnkey laboratory suites with access to containment level 2 laboratories.

Irrespective of whether incubators are university or regional government-created and managed, biotech start-ups require these specialized facilities and support resources that these programs offer. For most regions, this Essential Element is one that can be remedied and should be a high priority, and not become a limiting factor. Building incubators and support systems for these fledgling companies does require a large one-time capital commitment, with supplemental capital to offset the building and maintenance expenses until the incubator is fully occupied and profitable or at minimum breakeven.

IMPORTANT CONSIDERATIONS

One important principle to recognize is that an abundance of one Essential Element does not compensate for the lack of another. Often there is a belief that a municipality

or local government can simply provide more of an existing resource to overcome their cluster growth limitations. However, this is not the case for the establishment of biotechnology clusters. For example, specialized facilities and laboratories are essential to support biotechnology throughout the lengthy development process. However, providing an over-abundance of state-of-the-art facilities, although they are needed, will not compensate for a lack of seasoned entrepreneurs with experience in starting and growing companies. All five of these Essential Elements must be present in sufficient quantities in order for a biotechnology cluster to take root and flourish.

Another important point to recognize is that there is a difference between "Convenience Elements" which are *good*, and "Essential Elements" which are *vital* to biotechnology cluster development. If a local government focuses a majority of its efforts on developing "nice-to-have" amenities, but does not first focus on missing or limited Essential Elements, biotechnology cluster formation or expansion will not occur. For instance, focusing first on accessible airport transportation in and out of the local region without first dealing with the hindrances and limitations for universities to out-license technology to local companies will have limited impact on cluster development. Some companies may indeed enjoy those additional conveniences, but by themselves these conveniences do not result in expansion of a biotechnology cluster if hindrances still remain to Essential Elements in that locale.

OTHER ENHANCERS OF BIOTECHNOLOGY CLUSTER DEVELOPMENT

There are various enhancers of cluster development but these are distinct from the Essential Elements. Some cluster enhancers include:

- Having a risk-taking culture.
- Having a collaborative spirit within the community.

"Enhancers" of biotechnology cluster development require something to enhance, so if the essential or "life giving" elements are not present, no enhancer will help with the development of a biotechnology cluster. Enhancers are certainly beneficial to the community and they help stimulate the attractiveness of that region, however, biotechnology clusters are unique in their requirements for establishing and flourishing. This, in fact, is what makes them more challenging to grow. Also, Enhancers are not easily imported, but rather are often innate characteristics inherent in the people living within a particular a geographic location. As a region experiences biotech industry expansion these enhancers may be self-generated or perpetuated concurrent with, or by, the growth of that cluster.

Risk-Taking Entrepreneurial Culture

Regions that have cultures of entrepreneurship and risk-taking are more successful than those without one. For any major work to be accomplished there must be a champion and a team of people that believe in the vision. The development of a biotechnology cluster is no different. It requires that many groups buy into this vision. A key enhancer that is either present or absent in the local region is an innovative and entrepreneurial culture. This is an attribute that is characterized by the people located in that region. Risk-taking cultures are those that are not afraid to apply capital toward valuable, risk-based projects. In the state of Oklahoma, the city of Tulsa was once known as the "Oil Capital of the World," and there were many risk-takers. This risk-taking culture was endemic throughout the majority of the state, and as a result, Oklahoma City has built a large Health Sciences Center with a major Life Science Research Park, having approximately one million square feet of class A wet-labs and office space. If a population of people will invest large sums of money to dig holes in the ground with hopes of striking oil, that risk-taking culture can certainly spill over into other industries within their region. Entrepreneurship is contagious.

Collegiality and Collaborative Spirit

In addition to a risk-taking culture, there must be an environment of collaboration within that region. Establishing and growing a new industry requires the support of organizations and teams of diverse individuals all cooperating together to achieve a common goal. Without a culture of collaboration, cross-discipline differences and conflicts can stall forward momentum and inhibit growth of a biotechnology cluster. If other industries within that region feel threatened by the focus or expansion of the biotechnology industry, there may be challenges to establishing a cluster. To avoid this, leaders should clearly and frequently communicate the collateral benefit to all stakeholders about the benefits of growing a biotechnology cluster within their region.

MAINTENANCE FACTORS VS. DRIVERS

Municipalities may be able to tout their climate as one of the best in the world. They may also be able to point out that their region has one of the lowest cost-of-living indexes in the United States. These can be likened to "maintenance factors" for growing biotechnology clusters because they are supportive and helpful, but they are not drivers of cluster development. If these maintenance factors were effectors rather than supportive, Boston's cold winter weather and high cost-of-living would drive away every biotechnology company there. In fact, biotechnology companies still flock to regions where the winter weather is bitter and the cost-of-living is astronomical, as long as the Five Essential Elements are in adequate supply in that region. Weather, cost-of-living, and transportation are truly supportive and helpful, but it is important to remember that they are not the drivers and effectors of biotechnology cluster development. That is not to say these maintenance factors do not need to be touted and even improved where humanly possible, but a region needs to be keenly focused on touting and enhancing each of the Five Essential Elements that truly drive the development of biotechnology clusters in any given region.

INHIBITORS OF BIOTECHNOLOGY CLUSTER GROWTH

Just as there are facilitators of biotechnology cluster development, there can be inhibitors of development also. These inhibitors can be qualitative or quantitative factors, people, or policies. Inhibitors of biotechnology cluster development may include such things as high taxes on a small business for incorporation in a particular region and corporate laws that apply equally to large corporations and small businesses without consideration. Inhibitors may also be other industries competing for the same government dollars or for special attention. It is important that the leaders of cluster development identify these inhibitors and work to remove or mitigate them while focusing on the missing or limited Essential Elements within their region.

THE ROLE OF GOVERNMENT IN DEVELOPING BIOTECHNOLOGY CLUSTERS

Government must play a role in the development of biotechnology industry clusters. Traditionally, the ways they have participated is in economic stimulation, financing, and incentives for companies and industries. Governments can stimulate private investments in biotechnology companies by providing investment tax credits for qualified investing in life science companies. Government can also provide research tax credits for research-based companies in incubators, which help reduce the capital required for the research and development of their products. Other government initiatives can include matching of private investments or the matching of federal grants, such as Small Business Innovation Research (SBIR) and Small Business Technology Transfer (STTR), for start-up biotechnology companies. Municipal and civic leaders can assist by starting or supporting industry trade associations such as their local Biotechnology Industry Organization (BIO). Federal governments can help by enacting supportive public policies that encourage biotechnology growth and expansion in all regions, such as the Bayh-Dole Act in the United States and the SBIR grant program. Because the federal government funds a portion of public university's budget, they should also include or allocate incentives for university technology transfer offices that facilitate the creation and start-up of new companies using university-developed technology. Governments can also support or contribute to the development of incubators associated with universities or geographic regions.

Many state governments have taken initiatives to create biotechnology clusters. Florida is an example of a state seeking to diversify its industry base by the wholesale development of a biotechnology hub within their state. They began a program of recruiting top-notch research institutions focused on life sciences and biotechnology. With a fund of $449 million they recruited the Scripps Research Institute and the Sanford-Burnham Medical Research Institute to expand to their state. With matching local government money they created a pool of $950 million for the development of a biotechnology hub. By April 2006, Florida moved into the top 10 ranking of biotechnology business centers as determined by Ernst & Young's Global Biotechnology Report. Although Florida has had success, government by itself will not be successful in initiating and stimulating biotechnology hub development

alone. Government must be a contributor and supporter of some of these Essential Elements but success requires that all stakeholders participate collectively.

WHERE TO START?

For regional governments, municipalities, and chambers of commerce that want to stimulate growth of a biotechnology cluster in their region, there are steps that can be taken to improve and increase the likelihood of that occurring. The first step is to objectively assess the quality and quantity of the Five Essential Elements within your local region. This should be performed by interviewing the existing biotechnology companies rather than determining this from talking only with governmental officials.

Figure 5.12 is a simple worksheet that will help initially rank your region against these five categories. Within each category, rank your region on a 1 to 5 scale, where 1 is minimal or poor quality, and 5 is outstanding quality and in abundance. The ranking scale should be in comparison to the best biotechnology clusters within your geographic providence or country, and not necessarily those within your state or neighboring municipality. Next, a gap analysis should be

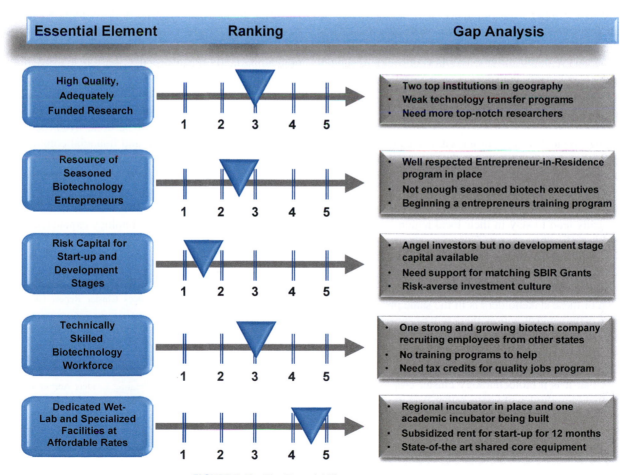

FIGURE 5.12 Five Essential Elements assessments.

conducted and the key shortcomings should be listed for each Essential Element. List the major roadblocks or inhibitors of each element rather than exhaustively listing all the contributing factors because communities can only focus on a few specific goals at a time. Be sure these are the real bottle-necks to the Essential Element because you do not want to address one issue, only to discover the real rate-limiting issue was not addressed. For any Essential Element that ranks a 3 or below, this should be a high priority and focus. Once the gaps and inhibitors are understood, develop a prioritized plan with creative solutions that is shared between government officials, civic and community leaders, and the private sector in order to address these limitations. Many regions are implementing creative programs to address their cluster development limitations, and these initiatives can be assessed and selected as to the likelihood of success in your region without having to implement them all yourself. Once specific solutions are identified for your region, create a timeline and assign responsibility to each stakeholder, with a time interval to report back with progress and improvements can be objectively measured. Recognize that your region's action plan will have different priorities and will likely focus on different limitations than another region. Do not adopt and utilize a plan that was created by another region without first assessing your unique hindrances and limitations to biotechnology cluster development. Your region's limitations to these Five Essential Elements can often be vastly different from another region's limitations, and your solutions should be directly tailored to your region's situation.

SUMMARY

Building a biotechnology cluster within a geography can be hugely successful for the local region and for diversification of the economy. Biotechnology jobs tend to be high-paying and highly skilled, and biotechnology tends to be a clean industry. Biotechnology companies that are established organically tend to stay in their local region because innovation is difficult to export. Governments, academic institutions, industry, and civic leaders must share a vision for innovation and have a commitment for risk-taking in order for a sustainable biotechnology cluster to come to fruition. If each of these stakeholders is in the same proverbial boat rowing in the same direction, there will be synergy. Growing a biotechnology cluster in a new or relatively new region should be thought of as a long-term growth plan and viewed in the same manner that a farmer does when growing crops, except that it is a biotechnology cluster crop and must be measured in multiples of years, rather than in seasons.

There are plenty of examples where regions are successfully growing and expanding their biotechnology cluster such as San Diego, Washington D.C., Seattle, and Raleigh-Durham for example. Outside of the United States there are good examples of biotechnology hubs emerging in Cambridge U.K., Berlin-Brandenberg, Munich, and others. The growth recipe for each of these regions is to ensure that all of the Five Essential Elements are present in quality and quantity. There is no "one" essential element that is more important than the others, and in order to grow a thriving biotechnology hub you need all five factors together in quality and quantity. There certainly are more than five elements that others may deem "essential" but in some way there may be iterations of these five. One thing is certain, that without these Five Essential Elements in abundant supply there will be limited regional growth of any biotechnology cluster. Recognize that biotechnology cluster development in new regions can take many years, possibly decades, so this is not necessarily a quick-fix program. However, by consistently focusing on targeted development of each of these elements, cluster development will eventually manifest and become self-perpetuating.

It is true that many early-stage biotechnology companies will fail, but business failure is normal in any industry. However, regions that succeed in developing a sustainable biotechnology cluster will reap dividends in their economy, in job creation, in diversification of an industry base, and more importantly, create products that can improve the quality of life for millions. It takes much time and a sustained effort to see significant cluster development in a region that previously has been unfamiliar with biotechnology. However, it can be done, and will be done by those with the fortitude, strategic leadership and financial commitment to do so. Like any endeavor, success follows leadership that understands how to guide a group of people toward a vision. Growing biotechnology clusters requires risk-taking and pioneering individuals. These individuals are the drivers and visionaries of future biotechnology expansion throughout the world.

REFERENCES

[1] Jones Lang LaSalle. Life Sciences Cluster Report Global; 2012. www.joneslanglasalle.com.
[2] Obama Administration. National Bioeconomy Blueprint; April 2012. page 1.
[3] Battelle/BIO. State Bioscience Industry Development Report; June 2012.
[4] Higgins M. Career Imprints: Creating Leaders Across an Industry. Harvard Business School, Jossey-Bass; 2005.

The Human Capital

Chapter 6

Characteristics of Successful Biotechnology Leaders

Lynn Johnson Langer, PhD, MBA

Director, Enterprise and Regulatory Science Programs Center for Biotechnology Education, Johns Hopkins University, Rockville, Maryland

Leaders of biotechnology companies face significantly different challenges and experience different life practices when compared with leaders of other businesses [1–3]. These differences include the manner in which biotechnology leaders have to continuously adapt and learn for their companies to be successful and the communication challenges that emanate from the different cultural worlds of scientists and business people—e.g., the different styles of social interaction and definitions of success. A more subtle, but perhaps even more compelling difference exists as well: Leaders of biotechnology organizations must balance the enormous financial pressures, the short-term development timeline concerns, and the urgency of saving human lives, against the need to carefully create and thoughtfully manage a company for long-term success. The biotechnology industry is unique in this regard. Because of the enormous cost of product development, there is very little middle ground in this industry where organizations can grow slowly and organically. At specific growth milestones, the organization must commit to success by investing in the infrastructure, staff, talent, and resources required to make it through development, clinical trials, regulatory approval, and into commercial production. Biotechnology product development can cost almost $1 billion for a single commercialized therapy.

Most biotechnology organizations are founded by scientists. Generally, scientist/founders' prior experience tends to come from the research laboratory. Leading a biotechnology organization is very different than leading or managing a research laboratory or even other types of business. Leading a research laboratory involves leading within an atmosphere with staff members similarly trained in scientific research where definitions of success are determined by peers rather than by the market and the uncertainty of approval and commercialization of drugs that lead to curing disease. Hence, the leadership demands of a research laboratory may not change over time, or at least not as rapidly as they do in a developing biotechnology company. The skills required of biotechnology

company leaders are also different from other nonbioscience businesses. Biotechnology companies must be market- and revenue-driven, the leaders are also expected to deal with complex and time-consuming regulatory factors and pressures, and with the ethics of testing on human subjects as they find cures for diseases where human lives are at stake. These differences between biotechnology companies and other organizations can frustrate a highly successful and respected scientist who has become accustomed to doing things his or her own way. These managers are often only accustomed to the style of leadership needed to run a successful laboratory.

There are businesspeople who start biotechnology companies who are not trained as scientists. These managers may not struggle with the same issues that scientist leaders do, however, nonscientist businesspeople will have different issues related to understanding the capabilities and limitations of the technology and its development time. This chapter briefly describes leadership pitfalls that scientists can find themselves in and discusses ways they can be overcome to lead to success. Business leaders in other industries must learn to adapt to changing organizational needs, but scientist/founders in the biotechnology industry must personally change in more dramatic and fundamental ways. The successful leader must evolve from a scientist, to a scientist leader, to a business leader. Hence, not only must the leader of a biotechnology company deal with the organizational chaos that frequently occurs in highly dynamic organizations, or what Peter Vaill [4] calls permanent whitewater, the successful biotechnology leader must also learn to change how he or she perceives the very nature of collegial relationships, how professional success is defined, and how the creative urge must be contained. Moreover, this continuous learning and adaptation must be carried out in a context in which the lead time to fully develop a product is much longer than in any other industry. This puts an additional strain on the leader because of the extraordinarily high risk of failure and the enormous financial costs involved. The scientist/founder, who may have seldom experienced personal or professional failure, finds him or herself in a situation where failure is common.

Because the scientist leaders often enter the industry with a strong and even primary desire to help humanity by finding cures for illnesses, as well as a desire to be financially successful, they are also motivated differently than other business leaders, including those in other science and technology-driven industries and in those companies with strong ethical concerns. A business leader's appropriate concern with how his or her company impacts the environment, acts in a socially responsible manner, or treats employees is very different than an immediate concern for human life and death. The combination of these different personal motivations and the scientist's ego make leading a biotechnology organization more complex than leading other organizations. This complexity is exacerbated by the highly regulated environment in which biotechnology organizations operate as well as the very nature of how these companies evolve and operate.

The biotechnology industry requires a controlled and sustained focus on preclinical testing and clinical trials over long periods of time. Traits that make many scientists successful in the lab may have the opposite effect when leading a biotechnology organization. Scientists' ability to be highly creative in a scientific endeavor may cause them to be too thorough, analytical, and creative when running a business. This can slow the process toward success. Leaders may be so accustomed to coming up with novel solutions in their research that they may not realize that business solutions may already exist. Such a focus on creativity can engender a level of ambiguity in an organization that must work in a highly regulated environment. In such an environment, the creative urges of the scientist often must be subsumed under the company's managerial needs for producing an approved drug that is marketable. This is not to say that scientist/founders' creativity is not useful in running their companies, but in some cases their creativity may prevent them from seeing solutions and providing the kind of sustained focus needed for success.

The underlying desire of many life scientists to help humanity, when starting a company means dealing with complex communication issues, stringent regulatory requirements, and often overwhelming financial considerations, makes leading a biotechnology company truly different from leading other organizations. To be successful in creating and leading biotechnology companies, the leader must continuously adapt and learn. Scientists may have an advantage here for by nature they tend to be curious and innately interested in learning. Because of the personal, financial, and organizational complexities of the biotechnology business only those few who are capable of continuous adaptation and learning are likely to be successful.

SUCCESS AND FAILURE

While no single leadership practice will guarantee success, one of the most important factors required is that the leader must be adaptable and able to lead effectively in a highly dynamic environment. Different styles of leadership are needed at different points in the company's evolution, often simultaneously. Leading a start-up, for example, requires a different approach than leading a company with hundreds or thousands of employees. Additionally, as the company grows, the leader needs to consistently articulate his or her vision. The leader also needs to be a strategic decision-maker and be flexible enough to allow the strategic vision to adjust to the culture and the environment. The leader needs to be able to communicate effectively and create an organization where communication flows efficiently at all levels. The leader also needs to recognize that clear cultural differences exist between functional groups and the leader must not give in to the common temptation among both scientists and business people to downplay the importance of these differences.

Organizational leaders need to empower their employees at all levels to make strategic decisions; but at the same time, the leader needs to know which decisions must be retained as his or her sole responsibility. The nature of leading biotechnology organizations requires leaders who are able to adapt their style and create learning organizations. There is no middle ground in this industry for slow, organic organizational growth and the leader must adapt quickly and use different styles of leadership almost simultaneously. Leaders of biotechnology organizations face enormous financial pressures and must balance these with the urgency of saving human lives. The biotechnology industry is unique in this regard.

Success or failure may result from the fact that most companies are founded by scientists who may have little experience or training in how to successfully create and lead a biotechnology company from start-up through commercialization. Classic examples of successful organizations started and run by scientist/founders include Genentech, Amgen, and Genzyme. The biotech industry is approaching 40 years old and there have been some blockbuster examples of success. These companies continuously adapted and grew from early start-up companies to multibillion dollar organizations. Yet because of the high entry barriers and high cost of biotech product development, many biotech start-ups fail. To bring a biopharmaceutical therapeutic product from the research bench to the consumer costs $1.3 billion [5]. Biotech leaders can ensure success by modifying their behavior and being open to change and adaptation. Over half of all biotechnology firms are founded by scientists, yet for every start-up biotech firm that succeeds, 15 to 20 fail and 8 out of 10 drugs fail in clinical trials [6–8]. Yet, there is much that can be done to improve the likelihood of success.

REQUIREMENTS FOR ACHIEVING SUCCESS: ORGANIZATIONAL

In the 1970s, Larry Greiner [9], argued that organizations go through five stages of growth that cause a significant change in leadership requirements and structure of the organization. These include a need for creative leaders from the outset of the company, to more directive leaders or when the company grows out of the early start-up phase. Greiner states that leaders need to learn to delegate, then coordinate and finally collaborate as companies grow large. However, Greiner's findings do not go far enough to describe the needs of the biotechnology organization and many of these traits are required in a more organic or constructivist way than a linear progression of requirements. Biotech companies evolve differently than other organizations due to the regulated nature of the biotechnology industry. They reach key crisis points that result in the requirement for major changes in leadership and structure. For example, early-stage biotechnology organizations with scientist/founders can initially be highly collaborative and entrepreneurial, but as the company grows, the decision-making styles and processes of communication must also change. This need for change is particularly true for biopharmaceutical organizations beginning clinical testing of their drug products in humans. As therapeutic-focused biotechnology organizations move into the clinical testing phase, the leader now needs to work within a more stringent United States Food and Drug Administration (USFDA)-regulated framework. Prior to human testing, the company is typically more research focused, and a collaborative style is expected and accepted. However, once a protocol for testing in humans has been established, changes can only be made with USFDA approval. Drug development companies require a decisive leader capable of delegating responsibility to expert senior executives in various, but interrelated, functional areas. At this point in the organization's development, decisions need to be made by the leader that cannot be easily changed due to the greater regulatory oversight.

The step to human clinical trials moves the biopharmaceutical company from a research orientation to a more operational, or product-development orientation. Regulatory bodies, such as the FDA and the European Medicines Agency (EMA) and the State Food and Drug Administration (SFDA) in China oversee and regulate all testing in humans and require substantial documentation. Maturing organizations need focused decision-making from their scientist/founders regarding testing in humans, but there also continues to be a need for collaborative leadership in other aspects of the organization. This is one of the paradoxes of leadership in biotechnology companies. Collaborative leadership continues to be critical in areas such as marketing, manufacturing, and the regulatory department as they work together to plan for the launch of a new product. This paradoxical challenge involves dealing with the complexity of simultaneously being both a directive and collaborative leader. Biotechnology organizations experience ever-changing leadership needs within the context of "permanent whitewater." [4] The essence of leaders who are learners and learning organizations is the ability to adapt and adjust as a complex and uncertain environment evolves. This evolution is not a linear process, but one that continuously circles back on itself while continuously moving forward.

Further, successful leaders recognize the requirement for different styles of leadership and decision-making within different functional areas of the organization. Researchers, for example, may prefer a collaborative style of decision-making whereas clinical and regulatory staff may prefer a more focused, decisive style. It is not unusual for scientists in general to have a highly collaborative management style because they are trained to collaborate and seek the opinion of others. This style of leadership may work well in the early stages of the organization. However, once a company advances its research to the product-development stage and begins preclinical and clinical trials, a new style of management is often needed. As the product moves from pure R&D to a regulatory environment that requires stringent oversight for testing in human subjects, the organization's managerial framework tends to become more rigid. For example, a Chief Medical Officer (CMO) at a biotechnology organization cannot accept changes in decisions related to clinical trials, or with commercialization of the product that may conflict or cause confusion with the regulatory requirements of getting a product through the critical USFDA approval process. Mid-stream shifts in business strategy, which may involve multiple organizational functions, can be tolerated early on, but not later when the drug begins to be tested in humans. For example, shifts in how, or to whom, the product may be marketed can no longer be easily dealt with as a collaborative decision once a product reaches a certain point. Such mid-stream changes are notoriously difficult to manage once a product moves out of R&D. Leaders of organizations with products in clinical trials need to trust and, in some circumstances, even defer to the opinion of the CMO or other experienced senior leaders. If the CEO is unable to trust or delegate some decisions to senior executives, a conflict may arise and company executives may become frustrated. This requirement does not mean that the CEO must give up all control but there must be staff in place that can be trusted to make the correct decision. There is a need for directive leadership by the CMO and collaborative leadership by the CEO. There is also the reality of the distribution and marketing systems, political and other realities, all of which require a fluid style of leadership by the CEO that enables him or her to be effective with the organization as a whole. Ultimately, when viewed from this perspective, the leadership is paradoxical. The leader must be simultaneously tough and directive, while at the same time being collaborative and compassionate, consistent and predictable, and adaptable and open to creativity and dissent.

Business leaders understand that scientists are frequently motivated by factors other than money, such as peer recognition, job satisfaction, environment, or scientific challenges. Scientists, on the other hand, need to understand that without a business focus, their discoveries may never be fully developed. Although each group may think they fully grasp these differences, their behavior and actions suggest they have not always understood how these differences can adversely affect an organization. Training is needed at all levels of the organization to help communicate across the cultural divides between science and business and to help ensure an increase in effective cross-departmental communication. Training should center on the fact that while both groups generally share similar goals for the organization, there is a need to view the company as a whole, with a systems view of the company. Without such a holistic systems perspective it will be difficult for the company to meet its goals and succeed.

While there are a number of requirements important for achieving success for newly emerging biotechnology organizations, these requirements center on the leader's ability to continuously learn and adapt to various organization growth stages and organization needs. Before a scientist even begins to establish a new organization it is very important for him or her to have a realistic understanding of the evolving requirements involved in starting and running a biotechnology company. A perception that the initial managerial, commercial, and scientific requirements will remain static may cause scientists to found organizations that will be at risk of failure as they grow beyond their initial stages. Because of the dynamic nature of this industry, scientist/founders need to learn how to suppress their ego and even be willing to give up complete control of the organization. As the company grows from its initial founding, it is very difficult for the scientist/founders to know all aspects of running a vital organization and they need to surround themselves with experienced people whose opinions they trust and to whom they can delegate responsibility. In addition, running a successful company will require scientist/founders to create an organization with high levels of communication and a culture of learning for all employees.

SIX FACTORS FOR SUCCESS

From researching successful biotechnology companies and their leaders, we find there are at least six factors that are strong indicators of success. The most important lesson is that these may be predictable practices that can be learned by leaders to increase the likelihood of success.

Be Adaptable

The dynamic nature of leading biotechnology organizations requires that leaders are able to continuously adapt their style and create learning organizations. The most crucial factor leading to success is that the leader must be adaptable to lead effectively in this highly dynamic environment.

This proves to be a paradox for many leaders who find that their style, while successful in some situations, may not be good for other situations.

Articulate Vision

Communication of the essence and culture of the organization will need to be carried out under the guiding principles created through the leadership of the scientist/founder. These principles need to be articulated and embedded within the culture so it will continue after the leader is gone. The company may not need to have an articulated mission statement to be successful, but a common understanding of the vision and goals of the organization is critical. Articulating the vision of the organization can be communicated directly by the leader when the company is small, but as it grows, other means of ensuring that employees at all levels understand the culture and mission of the company must be established. Slogans on the walls are only valuable if they reflect a genuine culture of what the company is in business for. If the business does not continually reinforce slogans with actions and tangible evidence of its vision, culture, and value, then it may come across as disingenuous.

The leader needs to consistently articulate his or her vision throughout the organization. Especially in changing times, everyone in the organization should have a solid idea of the vision. When the company is smaller, this can be done informally through discussion with employees; but as the company grows, the leader needs to take additional steps to ensure communication increases and in multiple ways. The leader needs to set an optimistic tone about the vision for the future and how the company can achieve this vision.

Strategic Decision-Maker

Often, scientist/founders have difficulty relinquishing control and trusting the judgment of others. If the leader can understand that the success of the organization depends on the leader's ability to make strategic decisions that almost necessarily require input from others who have had prior success then the leader may be more likely to accept advice from others. The leader needs to be flexible enough to allow the strategic vision to adjust to the culture and the environment. The leader needs to be seen as capable of decision-making, but also allow others in the organization to determine how individual goals will be met. They need to surround themselves with experts to help guide them in subject areas in which they themselves have limited experience. One way they can do this is through the use of an executive coach who has experience working with other leaders within the industry. Having a confidential coach with whom the leader may discuss concerns and fears may allow the

CONCLUSION

Based on observations of multiple organizations, interviews with their leaders and consultants, and from the literature, biotechnology companies require leaders who are able to continually learn and adapt to the continuous change of permanent organizational whitewater likely to be present as technology organizations mature and develop [4,16]. This ability to continuously learn and adapt is the single most important requirement to lead biotechnology companies to success. Without such a perspective, the leader and the organization will likely fail. To continuously learn, however, leaders must often suppress their own egos and relinquish control. Leaders also need to embody the story and the vision of the organization. Part of that vision should include creating a learning organization where all employees are encouraged and expected to continuously learn [4,17–19]. Such a learning organization should support and give confidence to employees so they will take on leadership roles within their own jobs [20].

In addition to being adaptable, a number of important attributes are required for establishing a learning organization that deals with the paradoxical nature of successful biotechnology companies. First, the leader should be a visionary manager who is able to consistently articulate his or her vision throughout the organization. Second, the leader needs to be a strategic decision-maker and be flexible enough to allow the strategic vision to adjust to the culture and the environment. Third, the leader needs to be able to communicate effectively and create an organization where communication flows efficiently at all levels. Such communication can be extremely difficult in fast-growing organizations where effective communication is needed across cultural, geographic, or functional boundaries. Fourth, the leader needs to recognize that clear cultural differences exist between functional groups. The leader must not give in to the common temptation among both scientists and business people to downplay the importance of these differences. Within the organization, cultural differences need to be respected, whether they are between people from different countries or people with different functional backgrounds, such as science and business. Finally, organizational leaders need to empower their employees at all levels to make strategic decisions; but at the same time, the leader needs to know which decisions must be retained as his or her sole responsibility.

REFERENCES

[1] Langer L.J. How Scientist/Founders Lead Successful Biopharmaceutical Organizations: A Study of Three Companies. Ph.D. Dissertation; 2008.

[2] Langer L.J. Leadership Strategies for Biotechnology Organizations: A Literature Review. In: Grant T. Savage, Myron Fottler, editors. Biennial Review of Health Care Management: Meso Perspectives. Advances in Health Care Management. vol. 8. Emerald Group Publishing Limited: 2009.

[3] Langer L.J. Moving Beyond the Start-Up Phase. Life Science Leader, Jameson Publishing; March, 2011. Vol. 3, Number 3. p. 60.

[4] Vaill P.B. Learning as a way of being. San Francisco: Jossey-Boss; 1996.

[5] Tufts E-News. (n.d.). The ballooning pricetag. Retrieved February 5, 2012, from http://csdd.tufts.edu/news/complete_story/pr_outlook_2011.

[6] Federal Reserve Bank of Dallas. A conversation with Nancy Chang: taking the pulse of biotech. pp. 8–9. Retrieved June 6, 2007, from http://www.dallasfed.org/assets/documents/research/swe/2007/swe0702e.pdf. http://www.dallasfed.org/research/swe/2007/swe0702e.pdf; March/April, 2007.

[7] Stanford, Graduate School of Business. (n.d.). Biotech innovators and investors assess challenges, opportunities. Retrieved, June 6, 2007, from http://www.gsb.stanford.edu/NEWS/headlines/biotechnology.shtml.

[8] Zhang J, Patel N. The dynamics of California's biotechnology industry. Retrieved, May 29, 2007, from http://www.ppic.org/content/pubs/report/R_405JZR.pdf; 2005.

[9] Greiner L. Evolution and revolution as organizations grow. Harv Bus Rev 1998, May–June:55-66.

[10] Amgen Investors facts. Retrieved February 3, 2014, from http://investors.amgen.com/phoenix.zhtml?c=61656&p=irol-newsArticle&ID=1894412&highlight=.

[11] Contract Pharma. Top 10 Biopharma report, 2007, July/August. pp. 94–109.

[12] Herper M, Langreth R. Forbes. Amgen's Latest Mess. Retrieved August 2, 2007, from http://www.forbes.com/2007/02/16/amgen-cancer-pharmacuticals-biz_cx_mh_0216amgen.html; 2007.

[13] Fortune 100 best companies to work 2007; Retrieved, August 2, 2007, from http://money.cnn.com/magazines/fortune/bestcompanies/2007/full_list; 2007.

[14] Arnaout R.A. Amgen's CEO discusses company's secrets of success. The Tech Online Edition, Vol. 6, p. Issue 116. Retrieved August 8, 2007, from http://www-tech.mit.edu/V116/N6/amgen.6n.html; 1996.

[15] Grupp R.W, Gaines-Ross L. Reputation management in the biotechnology industry. J Commercial Biotechnol 2002;9(1):17-26.

[16] Heifetz R.A. Leadership without easy answers. Cambridge. MA: Belknap Press of Harvard University Press; 1994.

[17] Bennis, W.G., & Nanus, B. (1997). Leaders: Strategies for taking charge (2nd ed.). New York: Harper Business.

[18] Gardner, H. (1995). Leading minds: An anatomy of leadership. New York: Basic Books.

[19] Senge, P. (1990). The fifth discipline. New York: Doubleday.

[20] Wergin J, editor. Leadership in place: How academic professionals can find their leadership voice. Bolton, MA: Anker; 2007.

Chapter 7

Building, Managing, and Motivating Great Teams

Arthur A. Boni, PhD*, Laurie R. Weingart, PhD** and Gergana Todorova, PhD***

*John R. Thorne Distinguished Career Professor of Entrepreneurship, Tepper School of Business at Carnegie Mellon University, Pittsburgh, Pennsylvania, **Carnegie Bosch Professor of Organizational Behavior and Theory, Tepper School of Business at Carnegie Mellon University, Pittsburgh, Pennsylvania, ***Assistant Professor, School of Business Administration, University of Miami, Coral Gables, Florida

This chapter focuses on the essentials of building and growing effective, collaborative, team-based organizations that are capable of creating both disruptive and sustained innovations in biotechnology. Entrepreneurs and innovators, who found, build, and grow knowledge-based organizations that are technologically driven, must be market focused. Although the technology is very important and may in fact define the company, it is the caliber and experience of the team that will determine whether or not the company is successful. Therefore, it is critical for the entrepreneur to focus on developing collaborative teams with diverse skill sets and areas of expertise. The content herein is specifically addressed to biotechnology organizations, but is also pertinent to most technology-driven businesses. Entrepreneurs pursuing opportunities in the biotechnology and biomedical fields are faced with special constraints that must be addressed by the teams and their firms. These organizations are characterized by long industry life cycles (or time to market). They are also highly capital and risk-intensive, are regulated by a set of complex and changing government systems, and are constrained in their profitability by reimbursement from third parties. These issues compound and confound the entrepreneurial challenges of any start-up. As with any start-up organization the founding team is challenged to reduce risk—technology, market, team, and business model. We advocate building interdisciplinary, collaborative teams that can manage and balance the science with the business issues while including the capacity to interact effectively with partners, investors, and a multitude of service providers to complete and validate their business models. Equally important are two issues that are related to any knowledge-based, human-intensive business.

The first issue of importance is building and growing an entrepreneurial culture. The second and closely related issue is incorporating mechanisms to motivate the highly creative talent at the core of the enterprise. We present a framework for motivation that includes *ownership*, defined to include both *equity participation* for potential capital gain, and also "*psychological ownership*" of the direction and future of the organization itself. The culture created and nurtured by the founders and early employees (and their investors) evolves organically and guides the company through the challenges that occur across the company life cycle: e.g., technology development, regulatory issues, financing intellectual property challenges, and the entrance and exodus of key personnel as the organization grows through its life cycle, etc.

In this chapter we identify and discuss the principles and best practices for building entrepreneurial companies from two perspectives: (1) "experiential learning" gathered over years of working with and observing early-stage and growth-stage entrepreneurial organizations and (2) "academic learning" that is focused on the principles of building effective teams based on selected academic or scholarly literature and studies. Our perspective thus blends real-world lessons filtered through and framed by a more scholarly approach based on case literature and research-based studies.

The "theory and practice" of building a biotechnology company is presented with emphasis on the entire company life cycle—start-up, development stage, clinical stage, growth, and exit. We begin with a description of the entrepreneurial process and note the importance of high-performing teams in building and growing the organization. We then stress that an effective organization incorporates as a foundation, building and growing a culture that encourages and rewards collaborative interdisciplinary teams for their contributions to the success of the venture. The principles outlined are applicable to "fully integrated emerging and mature companies" as well as to those organizations that employ "open-innovation" business models which are businesses that rely on partnering for sourcing and developing new products and services. The chapter outlines, from an academic and experiential perspective, those fundamental issues that must be addressed when building teams: *tasks to be performed, people/skills required, norms, and processes.* We also include a "lessons learned" summary based on interviews and experiences with numerous early-stage teams and their investors. This summary incorporates principles that guide team formation, management, and motivation. In particular, how do you find, hire, and motivate teams that are effective (or not) in the biopharmaceutical industry?

ENTREPRENEURIAL PROCESS FUNDAMENTALS RELATED TO TEAMS

Building an entrepreneurial team for a biotechnology company incorporates a daunting set of challenges and tasks. As with any such endeavor the *entrepreneurial process* focuses on the following three separate, but related parts (as described by Timmons and Spinelli) [1] (Figure 7.1):

1. Identifying the *opportunity* and developing a strategy capable of creating sustained and differentiated competitive advantage.
2. Acquiring the *resources* needed to develop the opportunity, thereby developing, creating, and capturing value in the marketplace, e.g., financing, partnerships for market access (channels) and customer relations, etc.
3. Building the *team* needed to exploit the opportunity. In science-based companies, teams must include people with expertise in science/technology and business plus other related "tasks," e.g., product development, laboratory and clinical testing, intellectual property development, etc.

In addition, and most importantly, *leadership* is needed to continually balance the opportunity with the resources and the team needed to exploit it. Leadership is also required to evolve the entrepreneurial process, continuously and seamlessly as the organization engages in the innovation process—inspiration, ideation, and implementation—and evolves through the company life-cycle stages of start-up, development, clinical testing, and market introduction/growth. Another essential

part of leadership is to create the appropriate culture consistent with the vision and mantra, and to maintain that culture through growth and "turbulence" expected during company development; e.g., both internal and external factors must be managed.

An important component of a strong leadership team is the presence, guidance, and mentoring provided by external parties such as advisors and the board of directors. As noted, it is essential that the founders and their advisors create a vision and mantra that establishes the culture and strives to grow and maintain that culture. All organizations grow and adapt as continuing challenges are faced, handled, and new ones arise (some expectedly and some not). The competitive landscape, the financing environment, the regulatory environment, the human motivations, and ambitions are but a few of the variables that must be dealt with effectively and in a timely manner.

It is well established that entrepreneurs create new jobs and advanced innovation. As biotechnology entrepreneurs initiate new ventures or undertakings, a key task is to form the start-up organization needed to create significant, differentiable and sustainable value through technology. The team is also charged with development of the business model to deliver the innovation (and value) to the marketplace, and return shared value (in the form of wealth and return-on-investment) for the innovators, entrepreneurs, investors and partners. The founding entrepreneurial team is the de facto organization in these new ventures since by definition the organization is created by the founders, their advisors/directors, and in many cases by the investors to commercialize the particular innovation. Many would argue that the team design, composition, and expertise in new ventures are perhaps the most important determinants of the ultimate success of a new venture. The entrepreneurial team must be developed with the ability to function as a successful organization in the entrepreneurial context of a high-risk competitive environment, dealing with complex incentive and financial structures.

Additional team building challenges for entrepreneurs and innovators are emerging as a result of pressures in the pharmaceutical space (diminishing product pipelines, regulatory failures, and a lack of capital availability). Therefore, in today's economy there is a recognition that the start-up team would be well served to utilize "open-innovation" approaches to leverage expertise, to gain the needed skills to commercialize complex technologies, all the while preserving capital to ensure good returns on investment for all constituencies. An important corollary here is that it is also important to ensure that rewards are apportioned to those who create value and who assume risk; i.e., entrepreneurs and investors as well as partners. We hypothesize that entrepreneurs are more highly motivated by ownership that includes both psychological factors (such as the ability to influence the direction of "their firms") as well as financial factors via equity ownership.

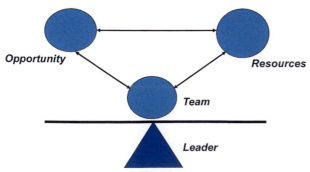

FIGURE 7.1 The entrepreneurial process model. (*Adapted from Timmons and Spinelli, 2007.*)

Given these challenges to innovate, the industry is beginning to see a trend toward creation of more "virtual companies" (another version of "open-innovation") whereby a *small but highly experienced core team leverages the expertise and resources of an extended network of partners, collaborators, and resources.* Successful firms are increasingly reliant on open-innovation which involves interactions with outside agents such as investors, partners, customers, experts to obtain ideas, technologies, expertise, access to market channels, etc. As such, entrepreneurial firms may be nested or embedded within multiple external networks with different structures and flows of capital (human and financial) and services. Research on teams and innovation uses the term "boundary-spanning activities" to denote the interactions of team members with external agents including all activities of team members related to the flows of resources between the team and external agents. We illustrate some of these principles in a mini case study later in the chapter.

Highlighting the importance of collaboration, a recent Kauffman Foundation study surveyed firms in the first 4 years of their operations from 2004 through 2007 [2]. The authors reported that 25 percent of competitive advantage is attributed to collaboration with another firm and 8 percent of competitive advantage was due to collaboration with a government laboratory or with universities respectively. We would expect these numbers to be even higher in biotechnology (and in other industries with long, capital intensive commercialization pathways). While the Kaufmann study [2] and other works discuss the trend towards development and adoption of open-innovation business models, the literature does not discuss in any detail the motivation of entrepreneurial teams/firms to leverage and share expertise and capital returns within these networked models of innovation. The open-innovation framework [3,4] suggests that technology companies adopt a networked approach to high-performance innovation sustainably and efficiently—that is, companies

exchange ideas, information, and technologies and bring to market new products through alliances and other forms of interfirm collaborations. These distributed, or networked organizations are expected to add to the complexity of the team challenges involved. (See Figures 7.2 and 7.3).

We have taken a team design perspective in our search for a better understanding of the interactions of entrepreneurial firms at both the firm level, and extending to include interactions with external agents (i.e., boundary spanning activities in networks). In particular, in ongoing work we have been attempting to quantify the effect of ownership structures on these interactions. As prior research on entrepreneurship suggests, young entrepreneurial firms highlight the importance of the entrepreneurial team as a means to bring innovations to market. Therefore, in our research we have sought to better understand the motivational nature of teams and collaborations to better understand the internal and external predictors of success of entrepreneurial firms.

In this chapter we introduce two recent undertakings as examples to illustrate evolving alternative structures for open innovation with an emphasis on capital efficiency and improved innovation outcomes. This is offered to provide insight into new organizational structures and the impact of such emerging structures on the extended teams that must be implemented to create a more adaptive approach to innovation in the biopharmaceutical field.

The Importance of Building and Maintaining an Entrepreneurial Culture

The onset of a company formation starts with the vision of the founders and the articulation of the culture that they want to build into the "DNA" of the start-up organization. The goal is to build and then sustain that vision and culture as the company grows through its life cycle. While each company is different in regard to its culture and mission, the challenge faced by the founders can be reduced to the following ingredients

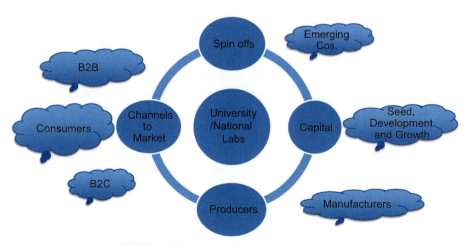

FIGURE 7.2   The science-based innovation ecosystem

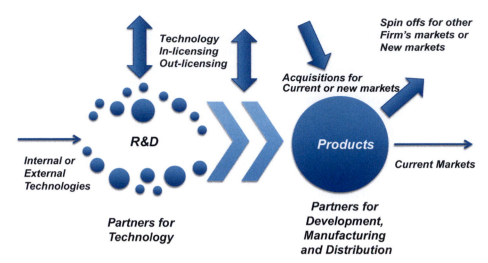

FIGURE 7.3   An open-innovation network for sustained and disruptive innovation. *(Adapted from Chesbrough et al., 2006 [4].)*

articulated by Boni [5] in a review of the book written by the second CEO of Amgen, Gordon Binder [6] entitled *Science Lessons—What The Business of Biotech Taught Me About Management* who had the opportunity (and challenge) of following the legendary George Rathmann:

- Build a talented and balanced management team in a culture that incorporates an interdisciplinary, team-based, collaborative approach with leadership throughout.
- Encourage and reward performance.
- Organize around autonomy and innovation.
- Tolerate risk and learn from failure.

All of us can learn a few lessons from Amgen, which is arguably one of the most successful biotechnology companies in the relatively short history of the industry. We suggest that in building a management team, there are some best practices that have proven to be successful over the years. First and foremost is the challenge and principal objective to *build an entrepreneurial culture* that incorporates the necessary values and ingredients to capture and grow market share and which utilize the principles of sustained or disruptive innovation including business model innovations. Herein, we focus on the "secret sauce of innovation" which is the *human capital and processes* needed to create and deliver innovations to the market and capture value for the organization sustainably.

The following additional cultural traits are required for successful organizations:

- A focus first on the needs of the market, which comes from being close to the customer or user
- Implementation of a reward system that values contribution and success and incorporates both psychological ownership of the outcome and equity ownership
- Embraces an open-innovation model to take advantage of ideas and collaborations beyond the "borders" of the company itself

The second challenge is to *imbue in this culture the following values* as identified in a recent *Harvard Business Review* article by Steven Prokesh [7], entitled "How GE Teaches Teams to Lead". (See Figure 7.4.)

- Challenge and involvement
- Freedom
- Trust and openness
- Time for ideas
- Playfulness and humor
- Conflict (creative tension but not destructive)
- Idea support
- Debate
- Risk taking

These common principles form the basis for building a managerial team and creative culture needed to innovate. A paraphrase from Phil Jackson, the most winning professional sports coach in history is appropriate here: "The strength of the team is each individual member—the strength of each member is the team."

We cite a book written by Wayne McVicker [8] entitled *Starting Something: An Entrepreneur's Tale of Control, Confrontation and Corporate Culture* to illustrate some other essential lessons learned in building and growing an entrepreneurial culture. While this is an example of a "dotcom" company, NeoForma was one of the first e-commerce companies in the healthcare space and the lessons are applicable to biotechnology companies or to any other technology-driven, but market focused (or customer centric) company. The book describes an insider's perspective that provides both the "dark and bright sides" of corporate culture. In the final chapter entitled "Afterthoughts," McVicker includes 12 things (which we paraphrase below) to keep in mind when starting (and growing) something—most of which deal with corporate culture. McVicker

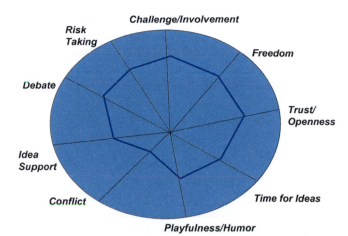

FIGURE 7.4 Attributes of an Effective Organization. (*Adapted from GE [7]*.)

advises aspiring entrepreneurs to focus on the team and the culture!

1. Be who you are—otherwise your company's culture will suffer, as will you.
2. Hire for culture first, experience second—if someone feels wrong, they are.
3. Communicate empowerment—don't waste the potential of any employee.
4. Learn to release without letting go—enable but monitor progress.
5. Balance is not always found in the middle—communicate decisions clearly, even if you need to change your position.
6. Do one thing well and then do it better—focus.
7. Regularly wear your customer's clothes—don't forget that's why you're in business.
8. The unsatisfied customer is the most important customer—that's where the opportunity lies.
9. Never let your competitors drive your business decisions—stay focused and listen to your customers.
10. Never let your investors drive your business decisions—keep the long-term view.
11. Listen to all advice but trust what you know—ideas that require customers to change behavior often take 10 or more years to implement.
12. Enjoy yourself—it is fun to create something new and useful.

SUMMARY OF "LESSONS LEARNED" (THE EXPERIENTIAL PERSPECTIVE)

Prior to providing an academic perspective on the fundamentals of building, growing, and motivating high-performance teams, we provide in this section a "practitioner-originated" summary of issues regarding building and growing teams in start-up, developing, and growth-stage biotech companies.

In this regard, one of us (Boni) is the founder and national co-chair of an Entrepreneurship Boot Camp (from 2005) hosted and logistically managed by the international Biotechnology Industry Organization (BIO) at its annual meetings. One session deals with a moderated interview of a company chief executive officer (CEO), chief technical officer (CTO)/chief scientific officer (CSO), and one of their BOD members/investors. Different companies are incorporated into each Boot Camp, so the following represents a summary of the "hot topics" that are consistently discussed each year.

Each panel is charged by the moderator with discussing a number of key issues and exchanging views on how they are handled "in the real world" during the start-up and development stages of the organization. Most organizations represented are still at the development/clinical level or just entering the market growth stage. The audience has an opportunity to ask questions and to engage in discussion with each other and with the panelists and Moderator. Over the years the following four topics and a brief summary of recommendations gather the most questions and discussion:

1 Virtual Start-Ups versus "Bricks and Mortar"

Acquiring capital is very difficult if not impossible until a considerable amount of risk (technology, intellectual property [IP], clinical, and team) is reduced. However, progress must be made to interest investors. Therefore, founders most often need to acquire nonequity resources (government, economic development, and selling of services) or funding from individual angels to raise limited seed capital. It is also beneficial to do so to increase market capital and reduce dilution. So reducing the amount of capital needed is recommended by leveraging resources; e.g., use of academic facilities, outsourcing product development, and clinical work to others. It is recommended not to invest in facilities except for the bare minimum; instead, invest in key people who may or may not join the company full time and have the founders fill multiple functions on the management team. "Cash is king" so use it wisely. Eventually you will need some facilities so consider locating in an incubator or leveraging common space with existing organizations in a research park. Invest in "hard assets" only when this is justifiable after evolving down the commercialization path.

2 The First Hires and Building Boards

Start with a small core team that originally consists of the founders (two or three) and a few part-time consultants—noted above. Identify key advisors and directors who can provide you with good advice and credibility and pay them with equity (it's worth the dilution). Find an attorney that will work on a contingent basis (not always possible) and consult with them on creative and legal ways to handle compensation, stock, and corporate partnering issues. However, make sure that a vesting (time-based) schedule is used for stock options. Alternately, issue restricted stock. Consider what happens to the stock if key people leave. If it is gone with the departing person it will dilute those who remain since the person has to be replaced. Pay the core team less-than-competitive salaries until funds are raised—the early-stage employees will make up for their reduced compensation with their stock grants. Hire for the essential tasks that need to get done but make sure the fit is good (see below). Use mentors to help you and to locate advisory board members and directors. Initially you should have no more than three to five science/business advisory board members (nonfiduciary positions) and three board members (with at least one outside, credible, and experienced person). Advisors and directors surrounding and supporting (and mentoring) the core team will facilitate progress with commercialization and will lead to downstream success with fundraising and partnering.

Hiring progression/priority will generally proceed in the following order of priority:

1. Business, scientific/technical, and market/business development leadership team.
2. Clinical/medical, regulatory, and intellectual property (IP) expertise (can be outsourced with inside leadership via a key employee at the appropriate time).
3. Personnel to contribute to the scientific and business agenda associated with commercialization according to the organizational priorities (generally product development and customer/user development).
4. Financial management (once significant funds are raised, especially A-round financing).

Keep in mind that as new team members join they must buy into the culture that has been created by the founders. So these first members are key and will build and preserve the corporate culture. We highlight that "fit," shared values, relevant experience, and ability to execute are all important considerations.

A subset of this discussion always revolves around the issue of "splitting the equity pie" and dilution. We could write an entire article on this topic; suffice it to say that the initial equity should be split among the founders and early hires (if any) based on what they have contributed to the company formation, what they will contribute going forward, and the level of risk each person takes. We encourage the founders to engage a good lawyer to help with this because it is always a contentious issue as to who contributed what and who will do so going forward. Most prominent among the contentious issues is the debate about the

weighting of science versus business in equity participation. Make sure that the founders get rewarded for their founding contributions (value is attributed to both technology and business acumen), and make sure that those who take the risk and actually join the company are rewarded for that as well. Small equity pools are then created for advisors/directors and for stock options for employees to be hired prior to the next funding tranche—typically 15 to 20 percent of the total for all parties. The pool will then be replenished prior to the next equity raise (investors will most often insist that the dilution will be taken by the insiders and not the investors). Many entrepreneurs worry excessively about dilution. For those who have been through this many times however, there is a realization that creating value that builds the capitalization of the company is the key outcome to be pursued, and taking outside money is essential to value creation and risk reduction, i.e., a "small piece of a large pie" is better than the alternative. Getting to the end game is the objective!

3 Balancing Science and Commercialization

In biotechnology and biomedical companies there is always the need to continually advance the science (to prove principle, build the platform, and the IP portfolio). However, progress down the commercialization pathway is necessary to generate the funding that will be needed to attract subsequent team members. Therefore, priorities and a sense of urgency to advance the technology and business have to be established early on at the founder and board level and managed carefully by the CEO and CTO or CSO of the company. Many organizations maintain close ties to a university where scientific advances can be handled (but be careful of IP and conflict of interest issues). Commercialization involves clinical demonstration in parallel with product development, which is difficult in a regulated environment. Once funding is raised make sure to allocate a small portion to advance the science and also consider some government augmentation (via the Small Business Innovation Research [SBIR] program) to achieve those objectives. While SBIR funding is nondilutive, sometimes the timing is not consistent with commercialization priorities.

4 Managing Through Transitions

Along the commercialization pathway, company leadership and the board will need to deal with the evolution of the team as people join the team and leave the team—either voluntarily or involuntarily. Sometimes founders take "lesser roles" as new leadership is required to move forward through the clinic and into the marketplace, or to raise venture capital and/or partnership funding. We have not found the perfect formula for dealing with these issues. One thing that can be counted on is that it will happen in virtually every company. In order to manage this process the right people must be on the board or on the advisory group to assist with the people issues—the addition or subtraction as well as the team remaining. Nothing can destroy team chemistry faster than a mismanaged transition. The best advice is to handle the situation quickly and professionally with good communication to all of the constituencies of the company appropriate to the specific situation. It is rare that a founder who becomes the CEO of a biotechnology start-up can survive through to the acquisition or the initial public offering (IPO).

In Conclusion

In conclusion, we present one current and timely thought that is becoming increasingly important for building and funding biotechnology companies. As these organizations are built, consider using more capital-efficient business models. Capital efficiency (achieving more, faster, and for less expenditure) can be achieved via various methods; e.g., outsourcing, partnering, use of agile methods borrowed from software development, etc. Capital-efficient, agile development is essential for biotechnology and biomedical companies where it is important to reduce technical, market, and team risks prior to bringing in the extensive amounts of capital required. As noted, the formation of win-win partnerships, while maintaining the ability to share significantly in the value that has been created by the team is recommended. For example, iterative (through repeated cycles) product and market development can lead to lower capital expenditures and faster time-to-market (even though the regulatory authorities tends to slow down the cycle time—this is not as much of an issue for other technology companies where lean and agile methods are being employed). There is much discussion in the field of biotechnology about the use of leveraged capabilities and assets including the building of "virtual companies" using management teams that have prior experience with bringing products to market and/or by partnering with outside organizations. Also consider creating value and reducing risk via a proof-of-principle demonstration in a clinical setting (even if offshore) prior to raising large amounts of capital. An extensive discussion on this topic is beyond the scope of this chapter, however suffice it to say that virtual companies can be created to leverage expertise by using open-innovation principles to partner for technology, market access, product development and clinical testing, manufacturing, and even management teams. Why build capacity that already exists? Sharing value might be a better option. The challenge is to build a core team that is equipped with the processes and networks to access and effectively manage these relationships. However, keep in mind that it will be necessary to have expertise on the extended team to manage the partnered or outsourced tasks. This will require the existence of talent that has experience with product development, clinical testing, etc. The subject of building teams in open-innovation environments is a topic of current work and research.

Keep in mind that the overall objective in building a team is to address one key component of risk reduction for the organization—demonstration of the ability to execute. The team addresses market risk, regulatory risk, IP risk, and risk associated with reimbursement. Other sections of the Boot Camp deal with the reduction of technical risk and are not addressed explicitly herein except how they are addressed by having the right people on the team at the right time.

KEY QUESTIONS TO ASK WHEN BUILDING THE TEAM—THE ACADEMIC PERSPECTIVE

Building a team is comprised of three phases summarized by Thompson, [9] each of which must be revisited as the organization and the team transitions from start-up to the development and commercialization stage, and then proceeds to market launch, growth, and maturity (Figure 7.5).

Phase One: Consists of *task analysis*. Specifically, what is the work that needs to be performed and what is its focus, how much authority and autonomy does the team have to manage its own work, what is the degree of interdependence among the team members, and are the team members interests aligned or competitive?

Phase Two: Consists of the *people required* to perform the tasks to achieve at least the next milestone or two. How many people are needed, what technical, task management, and interpersonal skills are required, and what diversity is optimal for the team?

Phase Three: Consists of *processes and procedures required* to achieve success. What are the explicit or spoken norms, what are the implicit norms, which norms are conducive for performance, how are ineffective norms revised, and how much structure is required? We would argue that a team contract be employed to provide a framework for the explicit and implicit norms of behavior expected with the team.

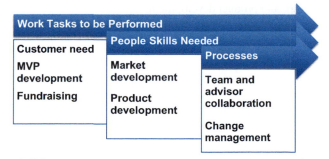

FIGURE 7.5 Three phases of building an effective team. (*Adapted from GE [7].*)

Underlying these tasks, people and processes is the entrepreneurial culture that is desired. That is, those organizational characteristics and norms noted above plus the "expected entrepreneurial style of the people engaged," e.g., willingness to assume "some" risk, thriving on chaos, not controlling, positive, passionate, perseverant, and motivated to make an impact, or perhaps even to change the world.

Building a Biotechnology Organization

Most early-stage biotechnology companies, as with most technology companies, start with two or three founders. The founders bring their passion, vision, and mantra for a new company, along with the needed expertise, skill sets, and networks to provide leadership for the two key and critical dimensions: (1) *technology advancement*, and (2) *business/market development*. In effect, upon founding, the *task analysis* and *people required* phases occur simultaneously and the founders form the kernel of a viable start-up. The focus on developing and advancing the technology and the market in parallel is the "essential task, or job to be done," and the founders are the key people who perform those tasks, which are organization specific. This initial founding team (and their advisors added as needed) then evolves through Phases One and Two of the Thompson "model" in parallel where team members are acquired to evolve the technology and the market/industry dimensions while advancing the commercialization process and developing the business model. It is understood that they must also acquire the needed financial resources to move forward. In most biotechnology start-ups, where both technology leadership and business leadership are essential, decisions are most often made informally and by consensus with input and perspective from both dimensions. But over time, these roles evolve into a more formal structure, with decisions by the CEO and the CTO or CSO. In most technology-enabled organizations (including biotechnology) the task analysis indicates that leadership is required to:

- Provide vision, strategic direction, fundraising, team building, and overall leadership.
- Lead scientific advancement, technology commercialization, and product development.
- Lead business development and partnering.

Additionally for biotechnology companies specifically, it will be necessary to add the capacity to deal with the following activities:

- Regulatory compliance and clinical demonstration.
- Intellectual Property (IP) development.
- Reimbursement.

Early on, these tasks can be accomplished by the members of the founding team and/or by part-time talent. These people expand from the kernel to comprise the core of the start-up and development-stage team that most often has several individuals, with perhaps two C-level positions designated to handle both *inside and outside functions*— these include simultaneous development of the product while working in parallel to more thoroughly understand and address customer/user need and the external environment. Acquiring people assets in biotechnology/tech companies is as important as acquiring financial assets, but one is required to accomplish the other—while advancing the opportunity and proposed solution. In effect an additional key task is developing the organization—most often consuming a significant part of the CEO's time allocation, along with acquiring funding! A quote here is appropriate to consider when building and growing biotechnology companies which are knowledge-based organizations. "Your most precious possession is not your financial assets. Your most precious possession is the people you have working there, and what they carry around in their heads, and their ability to work together" —attributed to Robert Reich, former Secretary of Labor in the Clinton administration and now a professor at the University of California, Berkeley.

The team that comprises an early-stage organization is not complete without developing its "periphery" —team members who serve in a more advisory function and contribute to the organization on an as-needed basis. It is critical for early-stage organizations to develop a set of directors/advisors that bring specialized expertise, connections, and access to networks for funding, partnering, hiring, etc. Most important is the need to institute a formalized, but small board of directors (BOD) of at least three people, including independent director(s), perhaps growing to five as equity investments occur. The BOD is responsible for fiduciary control, provides overview of strategic direction and operations, and also ensures that corrective actions based on internal and external changes and issues are addressed in a timely manner. Note that an advisory board is also important in that it performs different functions from a board of directors. Whereas the BOD will have fiduciary responsibility, other boards can be formed that are advisory only—most often providing specialized knowledge and guidance such as science/technology, clinical development, etc. These bridges between the internal organization and the external environment also provide credibility and validation of the opportunity being pursued via the reputation of the people engaged with the organization. These directors and advisors are most often compensated via equity using industry norms as guidelines for a directors and advisors stock option pool.

Therefore, the leadership team consists of both the core members (i.e., the people on the ground) who have committed and are willing to take a risk to join the company, as well as the peripheral members, the BOD/advisory board. This extended team is expected to provide expertise, networks, perspective, and discipline as follows:

- Access to people, capital, partners, and markets/customers.
- Access to counsel and expertise for IP, regulatory, reimbursement, clinical trials, and corporate agreements.
- Advice, experienced perspective, and mentoring.
- Adherence to a plan and fiduciary responsibility.

As noted above, the characteristics of this extended team include the knowledge, skills, and expertise, coupled with the requisite interpersonal skills (diversity, collaborative, and communicative), and who have a shared value system (a common purpose and vision, trust, and a sense of humor). In addition, since in many technology-based organizations one is dealing with large egos, it is advisable to be able to "check your egos at the door."

Finding and Hiring Good People

Finding and hiring good team members is the most important challenge faced by any company let alone a start-up or early-stage organization! Especially at the earliest stages of any organization the CEO and other founders must be personally engaged in the hiring process since the "organizational DNA" or culture is imprinted starting with the hiring process. Selecting the right people "with the right DNA" is important to building the desired cultural norms—both spoken and unspoken. All start-ups should strive to hire only "A players" since excellence is essential to company success. Don't just hire to get the job done—make sure that the person "fits" and can also do the current task or job as well as grow with the organization. Hiring is expensive and time consuming, so hire right. A bad fit can be bad for the organization and replacing someone is also problematic and expensive. But if replacement is necessary, do it quickly and professionally, otherwise the "bad fit" will affect the organization itself.

Diversity is good since there are many skill sets required to build a successful company and diverse perspectives and experience sets provide more enlightened and innovative solutions. In a biotechnology or biomedical company diversity includes various scientific backgrounds, business development/industry knowledge, and expertise ranging from IP to regulatory to reimbursement. Additionally one must deal with perspectives gathered in small companies and in larger, more mature organizations, e.g., pharmaceutical or large medical device companies. All of these key elements of the extended management team need to be integrated into the entrepreneurial and innovative culture being built. We advise embracing diversity, but not leaving the synergies to chance as the team is built up over the life cycle of the company. It is important to build mechanisms and processes to manage diversity not only internally, but also across the boundaries of the firm as networked innovation and partnering emerge as a norm in the biotechnology/biopharmaceutical industry. This open-innovation business model is becoming increasingly important as industry convergence continues, blurring the boundaries between pharmaceutical and the biotechnology organizations. The team, culture and vision sharing are as important as skill sets so that there is trust, liking, and respect (unspoken norms) across the team and organization. Most successful organizations build this mentality into the hiring process and walk away from talented people if the cultural fit is not there.

It is important to understand and deal with factors that motivate entrepreneurs, and to address them individually with team members as the team is built and expanded. Boni has discussed entrepreneurial characteristics that are pertinent to biotechnology companies in his review of Binder's book [5].

What Makes Teams Work, or Not? The Academic Perspective

To discuss what works and what does not, we need to deal with three key factors: (1) The structure of the team, which includes roles and routines; (2) Behavioral integration—managing the diversity; and (3) Team norms—goals and shared values, team motivation, and processes for coordinating, communicating, managing conflict, making decisions, running meetings, and enforcing norms.

Larson and LaFasto [10] list the following necessary conditions for effective teamwork:

- A clear, shared and elevating goal.
- A results-driven structure, that includes:
  - Clear roles and accountabilities.
  - An effective communication system.
  - Monitoring of individual performance and providing feedback.
  - Fact-based judgments.
- Competent team members (technical and interpersonal).
- Unified commitment.
- Collaborative climate.
- Standards of excellence.
- External support and recognition.
- Principled leadership.

We refer the reader who is further interested in building effective teams to several good *Harvard Business Review* articles by Billington [11] and Katzenbach and Smith [12]. While these articles are not targeted specifically at knowledge-based biotechnology companies, the authors address the issue of what makes the difference between teams that perform and those that don't. These are universal lessons. To be effective, a team must go beyond just being a group or a collective of individuals. The team is defined as "a small number of people with complementary skills (competence) who are committed to a common purpose, set of performance goals, and an approach for which they hold themselves mutually accountable." The Billington article points out that mutual accountability differentiates a team from a group. In a team, if the team fails (or the company), all fail together. If the team succeeds all are rewarded in proportion to their contributions. Another way to keep motivation high, something that is important in any start-up organization, is for the leadership team (and its board) to establish and maintain a sense of urgency. Kotter [13] identifies the sense of urgency as the first and essential step in his 8-step process for leading change identified in extensive case studies. From a practical perspective we advise that the team consider spending a lot of time together outside the workplace and inside (which is inevitable in a start-up environment).

Mini-Case Analyses of Emerging Open-Innovation Organizational Structures in Biotechnology

The material in this section is included to specifically emphasize the challenges faced by teams in "nontraditional" organizational forms. Historically most biotechnology companies (and their pharmaceutical counterparts) have been built and developed as "vertically integrated organizations" —most if not all functions of the organization accomplished internally with teams contained in the organization. However, it is important to recognize that a new paradigm is emerging with the recognition of open collaboration/innovation, and the introduction of virtual companies and networked organizations. This evolution to what has been referred to as "the Pharma 3.0 model" is driven by the need to improve the efficiency of the biopharmaceutical innovation process through engagement of a broader set of ideas, technologies, resources, and capabilities. Collaboration across organizational and geographical boundaries is expected to provide a more capital-efficient, shorter-development, and approval cycle with a higher success rate. However, no benefits are achieved without challenges. In this case the complexity of creating high-performance collaborative, cross-boundary teams adds a new dimension to the challenge.

Therefore, in this section we discuss several new and promising models for bringing complex, high-risk, long development-cycle products to commercialization in biopharma. The mini-case section closes with a short summary of selected issues dealing with building teams to lead and grow these new organizations. We also note that at the time of this writing we are at the dawn of this new approach to innovation, so whether or not these forms will be effective as a solution to the "biopharma innovators dilemma" is yet to be proven or demonstrated.

Inherent in these emerging organizational models is the ability to identify and source opportunities by assembling diverse and disparate resources that permit the identification and exploitation of promising disruptive technologies that address significant market need while validating the need, efficacy, and safety in close collaboration with corporate partners, e. g., extant pharmaceutical organizations. As such, the markets-first approach to commercialization proceeds in parallel with developing and validating key parts of the business model, including the partnership, channels to market, and customer interaction components.

Team development in these new organizational forms also proceeds via a multistep process. However, now the leadership team is comprised of:

- Industry leaders who are very experienced in commercialization and have thorough understanding of both the technology and the business aspects.
- Individuals who are well-networked in the industry and financial communities (and perhaps the academic community).
- Those who really understand the market need and most probably includes pharmaceutical partners

These leadership teams can then build, acquire, and mentor multiple founding scientific teams who would then pursue specific commercialization opportunities with ideas, technologies, and capabilities acquired from the overall network (including clinical testing and manufacturing). The coupled management leadership team and scientific team(s) can then be linked to partner corporations (e.g., pharmaceutical companies) and early stage investors—both well known to the leadership management team.

There are several promising emerging organizations using such an approach, but we highlight herein only two for brevity. The first organization highlighted, Enlight BioSciences [14] illustrates some essential features dealing with innovation in a networked environment. The second organization highlighted in this mini-case is summarized in some recent undertakings led by David U'Prichard and others from Druid BioVentures [15] and then BioMotiv LLC [16]. Taken together they illustrate partnering across the entire value chain of biopharma and incorporate disparate sources of participants ranging from technology sourcing to commercialization expertise to efficient channels to the market.

Enlight BioSciences, a Boston-based company, was founded by PureTech Ventures, a life science venture capital firm, and a team of industry leaders and academic luminaries in 2007 [14]. Enlight and PureTech provided the team leadership and early-stage financing to identify new technologies to meet identified market need. They then developed the scientific leadership team to form a dedicated new company(s) to commercialize the opportunities. The areas of focus which they identified included: imaging, safety/toxicology, predictive models, chemistry/biochemistry, synthesis/ production, biomarkers, formulation/delivery, and biologic platforms. Investment funding was provided by PureTech and a series of pharma partners that included Abbot, Johnson and Johnson, Eli Lilly and Co., Merck, Novartis, and Pfizer. This investment and leadership group provided initial funding of $78 million plus in-kind expertise to Endra Holdings, LLC, which then in turn invested in Endra, Inc. as the commercialization entity. Endra, Inc. was one of a series of companies that were expected to emerge to pursue specific commercialization opportunities in the suite of the eight areas of interest identified by the Enlight BioSciences team and their partners.

For the start-up company Endra Inc., the venture creation model consisted of: a "seasoned management team" assigned from Enlight, coupled with a team of founding scientists who had been recruited from a laboratory (e. g., a university or government lab) as part of the founding team. Considering this specific case, we highlighted the challenges of team interactions, motivations at several, coupled levels, and "boundary-spanning activities" involving the management team from Enlight, PureTech Ventures, their partners and advisory boards, the science team from the start-up (i.e., the boundary-spanning activities), and teams from the supporting network of investors and corporate partners. A very complex undertaking indeed. All of the team dynamics were present here, but as noted, was complicated by the various interests of the participating parties and their respective corporate cultures.

Other so called "virtual organizational models" have been discussed and pursued in recent years. David U'Prichard, former Chair of Global R&D at SmithKline Beecham (now GlaxoSmithKline) and ICI/Zeneca has pioneered two recent undertakings [15,16]. The need for these organizations are driven by several trends: (1) the lack of capital for pharmaceutical innovation in the "valley of death" (between early-stage development and clinical validation), hence the need for capital efficiency; and, (2) shrinking of the "pharma pipeline." There has been a shift from a fully integrated company model (FIPCO) in which the sponsor "owns" the entire drug development process from synthesis to marketing, toward a networked model of innovation, referred to as a FIPNet (or fully integrated pharmaceutical network). FIPNet's engage all of the major stakeholders involved in the drug-development process, blending the core competencies of each to leverage capabilities, enhance efficiency, and boost output.

Dr. U'Pritchard and his partners at Red Abbey Venture Partners and NeuroVenture Capital attempted to create a model (Druid BioVentures) where the plan was to acquire early-stage drugs, develop them (under the leadership of a very experienced drug-development team in a virtual company), and then license the drugs to a pharmaceutical company when the "valley of death" was traversed successfully—value added and risk reduced. After several years and the failure to close a round of venture capital financing, the need to identify and pursue other opportunities led to the next iteration of this model. The Harrington Project is a $250 million national initiative to accelerate breakthrough discoveries into medicines. A national consortium of academic medical centers (the Harrington Discovery Institute and an Innovation Center) translates promising discoveries into BioMotive, which is a national bio-accelerator to promote commercialization and entrepreneurship in medicine. BioMotive is a for-profit entity that is an "evergreen" holding company that invests in and manages a portfolio of early projects, each structured as a virtual, single-asset development corporation. A full-time staff in Cleveland, Ohio is complemented by a larger group of very senior pharmaceutical consultants in greater Philadelphia and in Oxford, UK. BioMotive "sources" the best opportunities from around the country, leveraging nonprofit assets, utilizes a team of experienced and connected advisors, and accelerates development to exit via partnership with pharmaceutical companies (at the late discovery stage through Phase Ib). They anticipate significant and sustained financial returns from developing a portfolio of programs. Dr. U'Prichard is the CSO and Chairman of BioMotive, Baiju Shah (former President and CEO of Bio Enterprise in Cleveland) is CEO and they have assembled a very impressive team of consultants and advisors. The intent of the Harrington Project (BioMotive) is to accelerate breakthrough discoveries into medicines.

To summarize, in both mini-cases, we note boundary-spanning flows of knowledge, ideas, and financial resources across teams nested in networks. How does this complexity affect the processes and performance in entrepreneurial teams that exist at multiple levels of the entire organizational network and is distributed geographically and organizationally? In these more complex organizational structures it is important to understand the factors that enhance or inhibit these boundary-spanning flows with a focus on motivation. In particular, how does the role of employee ownership (psychological and financial) affect performance? It is our hypothesis that ownership structure and motivation in entrepreneurial firms afffects the distribution of risk and reward across networks and value chains. Interest alignment that determines the competitive advantage [17] is particularly complex in highly novel, multiagent, and uncertain contexts such as these.

AN APPROACH TO UNDERSTAND FACTORS THAT MOTIVATE TEAMS

There are a variety of team-related motivational factors that lead to increased innovation throughput and capital efficiency in entrepreneurial firms. These factors help bring innovations to market. Our particular goal is to better-define the role of team motivation through employee ownership, both psychological and financial. We have focused first on the entrepreneurial team itself (how the firm optimizes its performance). The approach outlined below incorporates a design that may be extended to deal with the more complex issue of how the performance is optimized in the supporting

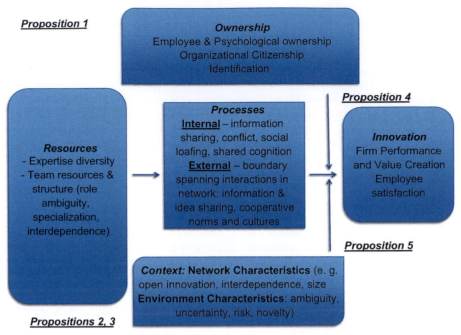

FIGURE 7.6 Framework for motivation of entrepreneurial teams incorporating employee ownership.

network. We have noted in this chapter that networked teams clearly incorporate new dimensions of building, motivating, and growing entrepreneurial teams.

Framework for an Entrepreneurial Team Motivation Model

In this section we present a model that attempts to frame the issues involved in motivating team members and partners. Our basic assumption is that the young entrepreneurial firm can be modeled as an entrepreneurial team because of its small size and the high interdependence of activities within the firm. As this work proceeds to incorporate later-stage companies and collaborative networks, we would consider the nodes in the open-innovation network to be entrepreneurial team-based organizations and/or firms working in concert to pursue innovation. (Figure 7.6)

To gain new insights about motivation in entrepreneurial teams, we investigated whether employee ownership in terms of financial ownership was reflected in psychological ownership, citizenship behaviors (defined as voluntary contributions to the firm), and identification with the firm. Based on the literature cited later in this chapter and using the IPMO (Input, Process, Moderators, Output) framework for the study of teamwork, we developed hypotheses about employee ownership (both financial and psychological) and its effects on team interactions and team performance.

We hypothesized that the choice of ownership structure plays a pivotal role in team motivation. Employee ownership was expected to promote value-creating dynamics of interactions of entrepreneurial firm/team members both

with inside and outside stakeholders. The ownership structure can strengthen or weaken the boundaries between entrepreneurial teams and the networks of stakeholders. The strong boundaries between an entrepreneurial team and its external stakeholders can both benefit and harm the activities of entrepreneurs. The strong boundaries can motivate knowledge sharing within the team through stronger identification with the team and psychological ownership. However, they can also discourage knowledge sharing between the team and external stakeholders because of in-group biases and intellectual property ownership risks and ambiguities.

To test whether team motivation via employee ownership (both financial and psychological) enhances team interactions with both internal and external stakeholders and improves outcomes in entrepreneurial firms/teams, we conducted a preliminary quantitative research study summarized below. We tested the following hypotheses about the role of motivation via employee ownership:

Hypothesis 1: Employee ownership (financial) leads to high *psychological ownership*, more citizenship behaviors, and higher identification with the firm.
Hypothesis 2: Employee ownership (both financial and psychological) enhances the *internal processes* of information and idea sharing, and divergent task conflict in the firm/team.
Hypothesis 3: Employee ownership (both financial and psychological) enhances *boundary-spanning (external) interactions (flows* of knowledge, ideas, and financial resources) between the firm/team nested in open innovation networks and the key external agents.

Hypothesis 4 (which is yet to be tested): Employee ownership (both financial and psychological) enhances innovation *outcomes* in entrepreneurial teams nested in open-innovation networks.

These hypotheses were tested using a quasi-experimental approach and two-group comparison. Group one was composed of start-up company teams initiated by Carnegie Mellon University graduate students and group two was composed of a parallel cohort of graduate students performing entrepreneurial projects sponsored by external companies [18,19]. The first group represented entrepreneurial firms with high employee ownership (financial), while the second group represented entrepreneurial firms with low employee ownership (financial). We did statistical analyses on the two groups to compare their motivation through employee ownership, their organizational citizenship behaviors, internal team processes, boundary-spanning (external) interactions in the network of open-innovation, and team longevity and innovation outcomes. Our preliminary findings are summarized briefly below:

> **Finding 1:** In support of hypothesis 1, we found that psychological ownership was significantly higher for the teams with high employee ownership (financial) than for the teams with low employee ownership (financial). Employee ownership (financial) also increased the voluntary contributions of team members (higher citizenship behaviors) and the identification with the team.
>
> > **Lesson learned 1:** Employee ownership (financial) improves team motivation. It increases psychological ownership, voluntary contributions of team members (i.e., citizenship behaviors), and identification with the team.
>
> **Finding 2:** In support of hypotheses 2 and 3, we found that the higher level of employee ownership (both financial and psychological) led to enhanced team interactions. In teams with a higher level of employee ownership, there was higher internal idea sharing, higher external idea sharing, and higher creative conflict.
>
> > **Lesson learned 2:** Both financial and psychological employee ownership improves innovation—enhancing team processes such as idea sharing (both internal and external) and creative conflict.
>
> **Finding 3:** In support of hypothesis 4, we found that higher psychological ownership was related to higher satisfaction (both with the team and with the project). We also noted that team satisfaction is important because it predicts the willingness of the team members to stay with the team and thus enhances its longevity. Psychological ownership also had a positive effect on value-added in terms of "usability" of innovation project outcome— whether the innovation outcome fills a need, has utility, and has a favorable timescale of return.

> > **Lesson learned 3:** Psychological ownership represents an important motivating factor in teams because it improves team satisfaction and "usability" of innovations. Since employee ownership (financial) increases psychological ownership as per finding 1, both financial and psychological employee ownership represent essential motivating factors in entrepreneurial teams. In the future we plan to examine how the open-innovation network characteristics influence the importance of ownership in enhancing innovation in extended networks.

SUMMARY AND CONCLUSIONS

In this chapter we have covered the topic of building and growing collaborative, interdisciplinary teams that identify and commercialize promising biotechnology innovations and grow successful companies. We have tried to illustrate one significant conclusion: the importance of the team in generating a successful outcome cannot be overemphasized. Without an effective team most companies will not achieve their potential, or will fail. We have also highlighted the necessity of building and sustaining an entrepreneurial culture as a means to differentiate and sustain successful organizations. The authors also stress that leadership must recognize and reward team (and partner) contributions to company value creation, and to incorporate mechanisms and processes to encourage employees to "own" and identify with their organization. We then illustrate the principles underlying building and growing high-performance teams as encountered in both traditional and emerging organizational structures. We point out that new organizational forms including collaborative, networked partnerships present human resource management challenges regarding (extended) team development, management, and performance.

AN ABRIDGED OVERVIEW OF TEAM PERFORMANCE LITERATURE

We provide this concluding section as "further food for thought" for practitioners and academics interested in understanding the current literature in relation to team building and performance. We also suggest areas that require further thought and elucidation for those who are more "research oriented" and are seeking new opportunities for research.

We have integrated prior research in three areas that have been disconnected previously and that have influenced the development of our Model for High-performance, Motivated Teams. These three areas are: (1) innovation networks; (2) team motivation, boundary spanning, and internal processes; and, (3) research on shared ownership.

We expanded and further developed the input-process-output model of strategic entrepreneurship [20], who developed a theory that explains and predicts value creation in entrepreneurial firms. They elaborate on how the inputs affect the outputs, e.g., value creation, and argue that understanding the inputs is not sufficient. The processes that transfer the inputs into new value, termed "resource orchestration processes," often determine whether an entrepreneurial firm will be successful in its value creation efforts [20]. Focusing on these processes, we have investigated specific internal and external processes that are at the core of "resource orchestration." Furthermore, we extended the model to elaborate on important characteristics of the context in which the entrepreneurial teams operate. We considered the open-innovation network model to identify the contextual factors that drive value creation, and conceptualized the entrepreneurial organization as a team to enrich the understanding of how an entrepreneurial organization creates value.

Although much academic research has focused on the structure of innovation networks and on the processes in innovation teams, there is little theoretical or empirical work on the effects of external innovation networks and boundary-spanning resource flows on the processes and performance of entrepreneurial teams especially in start-up companies. The entrepreneurial teams nested within open-innovation networks represent an interesting and unique setting because they are exposed to more ambiguity and uncertainty than innovation teams nested within mature and established organizations.

A recent meta-analysis of team level predictors of innovation shows that *team process variables* have the strongest effect on product innovation [21]. These results provide evidence that motivation (vision/goals and task orientation) and external communication displayed the strongest positive relationship to innovation and creativity. External communication, in particular, had a strong positive effect on product innovation.

Teams develop distinct strategies in their interactions with external agents: some specialize in particular activities, some remain isolated from the external environment, and others engage in multiple external activities. These points are illustrated in a seminal research paper by Ancona and Caldwell [22], which provides evidence that different boundary-spanning activities require different internal processes and have different effects on performance. Recently, Ancona and Bresman [23] argue that the external activities of teams gain in importance and also investigate the idea flow between a team and its external agents. Zott and Amit [24] investigate business models of entrepreneurial firms in terms of boundary-spanning interactions and their effects on the performance of entrepreneurial firms.

In a recent review of research on boundary-spanning activities, Joshi et al. [25] conclude that the important predictors of boundary-spanning activities are team composition, the contextual characteristics, i.e., uncertainty, and the task-based factors such as task interdependence and the team-development stage.

The shift towards external alliances for new product development in the pharmaceutical industry was discussed more than a decade ago by Whittaker and Bower [26]. Organizational models such as those outlined briefly in this chapter, increases the importance of boundary-spanning activities as different firms in the networked organization carry out more and more activities efficiently in the value chain. Recent theories on innovation networks suggest that network research is largely focused on structure and outcome, but does not examine the crucial processes that take place between a firm and its network partners. Dhanaraj and Parkhe [27] suggest that a firm must actively manage its interactions with external agents in the network through managing knowledge flows, innovation, network stability, and appropriability (an economic term regarding the environmental factors that govern an innovator's ability to capture profits generated by an innovation).

Recent research on the knowledge exchange between firms suggests that commitment-based human resource practices represent an important managerial tool for fostering boundary-spanning activities [28]. One of the commitment-based human resource practices is the compensation practice such as employee ownership that focuses employee motivation on *group and organizational performance indicators.* Employee ownership may also be related to psychological ownership, which has been shown to enhance citizenship behaviors and firm performance; c.f., van Dyne and Pierce [29]. Employee ownership represents an important motivational tool in organizations [30]. Research shows that the economic and social employee-organization relationship influences psychological ownership, which in turn influences performance [31].

Shore and Singh [32] identify the need to study how employees perceive employee ownership and whether their ownership perception is an important factor that affects the performance outcomes of employee-ownership practices. Furthermore, Gong and Chang [33] establish a positive relationship between HR practices such as pay contingent on performance, participation in decision-making, and employment security, which are all related to shared capitalism, and organizational citizenship.

A recent study on employee ownership and firm performance shows that the alignment of internal processes and goals represents an important factor for success in life science industries [32]. We extend the research to consider in-depth the effects of employee ownership on teamwork in entrepreneurial organizations. We argue that contextual factors may explain when the relationship between employee ownership and performance is more positive. It is clear that both the internal and the external processes will provide a better understanding of how and why employee ownership can enhance innovation in early-stage firms nested in open-innovation networks.

ACKNOWLEDGEMENT

The article previously published by Boni, A.A, and L.R. Weingart. (2012). "Building Teams in Entrepreneurial Companies." *Journal of Commercial Biotechnology*. 18(2). http://dx.doi.org/10.5912/jcb507 is incorporated into this chapter as modified by the authors with approval of the publisher of the *Journal of Commercial Biotechnology*.

The authors acknowledge that framework for motivation of entrepreneurial teams incorporating employee ownership was supported by the Foundation for Enterprise Development (FED), La Jolla, California. We appreciate the input and support of Mary Ann Beyster, CEO. Dr. Boni also acknowledges the leadership and team-building lessons learned as part of the leadership team led by Dr. J. Robert Beyster, founder and Chairman of FED and of Science Applications International Corporation (SAIC). During a decade of high growth at SAIC, spanning early stage to the largest U.S., employee-owned technology company was a great learning experience on building and working with geographically dispersed high-performance teams.

REFERENCES

[1] Timmons JA, Spinelli S. New Venture Creation, Entrepreneurship for the 21st Century. 7th ed. ; 2007. McGraw Hill Irwin.

[2] Robb A, Ballou J, DesRoches D, Potter F, Zhao Z, Reedy EJ. An overview of the Kauffman firm survey: Results from the 2004–2007 data. Published on Kauffman Foundation of Entrepreneurship webpage; 2009. *www.kauffman.org*.

[3] Chesbrough H. Open Innovation: The New Imperative for Creating and Profiting from Technology. Cambridge, MA.: Harvard University Press; 2003.

[4] Chesbrough H, Vanhaverbeke W, West J, editors. Open Innovation: Researching a New Paradigm. Cambridge, MA: Harvard University Press; 2006.

[5] Boni AA. "Science Lessons: What Biotech Taught Me About Management." A Book Review of Gordon Binder and Philip Bashe. J Commercial Biotechnol 2009;15(1):86–91.

[6] Binder G, Bashe P. Science Lessons—What The Business of Biotech Taught Me About Management. Harvard Business Press; 2008.

[7] Prokesh S. "How GE Teaches Teams to Lead Change,". Harvard Business Review 2009. Reprint R0901J.

[8] McVicker WW. *Starting Something –An Entrepreneur's Tale of Control, Confrontation, and Corporate Culture*. Los Altos, CA: Ravel Media, LLC; 2005.

[9] Thompson L. Making the Team. A Guide for Managers. 4th ed. Prentice Hall; 2011.

[10] Larson CE, LaFasto FMJ. Teamwork: What Must Go Right, What Can Go Wrong. Newberry Park, CA: Sage; 1989.

[11] Billington J. The Three Essentials of an Effective Team. Harvard Business Review Reprint; 1997. U9701A.

[12] Katzenbach JR, Smith DK. The Discipline of Teams,. Harv Bus Rev 2005. Reprint R0507P.

[13] Kotter JP. Leading Change. Boston, MA: Harvard Business Press; 1996.

[14] Ernst & Young. (2010). "Beyond Borders, Global Biotechnology," published by Ernst & Young, edited by Giovannetti, G.T. and J. Gautam.

[15] U'Prichard DC. Private communication from BIO Entrepreneurship Bootcamp organized by Boni and Steve Sammut; 2013. Held in Chicago, Illinois.

[16] U'Prichard DC. New Paradigms in Drug R&D: A Personal Perspective. J Commercial Biotechnol April 2012;18(No. 2).

[17] Gottshalg O, Zollo M. "Interest Alignment and Competitive Advantage. Acad Manage Rev 2007;32:418–38.

[18] Boni AA, Weingart LR, Evenson S. Innovation in an Academic Setting: Designing and Leading a Business Through Market-Focused, Interdisciplinary Teams. Acad Manage Learn Educ 2009;8:407–17.

[19] Boni AA, Emerson ST. An Integrated Model of University Technology Commercialization and Entrepreneurship Education. Adv Study Entrepreneurship, Innov Economic Growth 2005;16:241–74.

[20] Hitt MA, Ireland RD, Sirmon DG, Trahms CA. "Strategic Entrepreneurship: Creating Value for Individuals, Organizations, and Society. Acad Manage Perspect 2011;25:57–76.

[21] Hulsheger UR, Anderson N, Salgado JF. Team-Level Predictors of Innovation at Work: A Comprehensive Meta-Analysis Spanning Three Decades of Research. J Appl Psychol 2009. September 2009, 5, pp. 1128–45.

[22] Ancona DG, Caldwell DF. Bridging the Boundary: External Activity and Performance in Organizational Teams. Adm Sci Q 1992;37:634–65.

[23] Ancona DG, Bresman H. Begging, Borrowing, and Building on Ideas from the Outside to Create Pulsed Innovation Inside Teams. In: Thompson L, Choi HS, editors. Creativity and Innovation in Organizational Teams. Mahwah, NJ: Lawrence Erlbaum, Associates; 2006. pp. 183–99.

[24] Zott C, Amit R. Business Model Design and the Performance of Entrepreneurial Firms. Organ Sci 2007;18:181–99.

[25] Joshi A, Pandi N, Guohong H. "Bracketing Team Boundary Spanning: An Examination of Task-Based, Team-Level, and Contextual Antecedents. J Organ Behav 2009;30:731–59.

[26] Whittaker E, Bower DJ. A Shift to External Alliances for Product Development in the Pharmaceutical Industry. R&D Manag 1994;24:249–59.

[27] Dhanaraj C, Parkhe A. Orchestrating Innovation Networks. Acad Manage Rev 2006;31:659–70.

[28] Collins CJ, Smith KG. Knowledge Exchange and Combination: The Role of Human Resource Practices in the Performance of High-Technology Firms. Acad Manage J 2006;49:544–60.

[29] Van Dyne L, Pierce JL. Psychological Ownership and Feelings of Possession: Three Field Studies Predicting Employee Attitudes and Organizational Citizenship Behavior. J Organ Behav 2004;35:439–59.

[30] Rousseau DM, Shperling Z. "Pieces of Action: Ownership and the Changing Employment Relationship. Acad Manage Review 2003;28:553–70.

[31] Aryee S, Sun LY, Zhou Q. Employee Organization Relationship, Psychological Ownership and Contextual Performance: A social Exchange Perspective. In:Academy of Management Proceeding, vol. 2009, No 1, pp. 1–6. Academy of Management.

[32] Shore L, Singh G. Uses and Impact of Shared Capitalism: Final Report. San Diego: Paper presented at the 2009 Foundation for Enterprise Development Symposium; 2009.

[33] Gong Y, Chang S, Cheung SY. High performance work system and Collective OCB: A Collective Social Exchange Perspective. Hum Res Manage J 2010;20(2):119–37.

Chapter 8

Building Human Relationship Networks

Tom D. Walker

CEO & President, TechColumbus, Inc., Columbus, Ohio

Human relationships are just as important to companies as they are to individuals. This chapter is about building and utilizing human relationships to advance and accelerate the creation and development of a start-up biotechnology company. While there are many aspects of entrepreneurship that are unique to biotechnology businesses, when it comes to purposeful and enduring business relationships, entrepreneurs in biotech are in the same lab space as other entrepreneurs. Relationship building takes time, focus, and, in order to be used to its best advantage, is an element of the business plan from day one.

The first thing a biotechnology entrepreneur needs to do when it comes to relationships is develop a *networking mindset*. By networking mindset, I mean that the entrepreneur holds the deep belief that purposeful relationships with a variety of people through formal and informal structures over time can help CEOs and chief technology officers create, grow, and operate the business.

A networking mindset is based on these beliefs:

- I need help; without it my company can't succeed.
- My resources are limited.
- I don't, can't, and won't ever know everything I need to know about building a company. I don't even know what I don't know.
- There are many people nearby who have traveled the path before me. They do know what I don't know. Many are happy and eager to help.
- The way I reach these people is through relationships that provide benefits to all parties involved.

Purposeful networking leads to mentoring. Effective mentoring leads to advising. Successful advising leads to productive investor and board of directors relationships. Effective investors and board of directors relationships lead to profitable exits.

Throughout my career, I and the companies I've led have benefited from the networked relationships that we've built over time. In this chapter, you will read first-hand the practical advice provided by three outstanding early-stage investors who mentor and serve on boards: William

Botts, serial entrepreneur and investor; John O. Huston, founder/manager of Ohio TechAngel Funds and Angel Capital Association Chairman Emeritus, and Bill Payne, serial entrepreneur and founder of four angel groups. I've been involved in entrepreneurship and early-stage investing for more than 20 years and I continue to seek wisdom and advice from individuals with more and different experiences. I encourage you to start building that habit now. As Bill Botts says, *"There is a great pool of talent available for entrepreneurs to use as sounding boards, particularly when the company is small and early stage. Go ahead and dream big, but get some help. Don't diminish the vision and the dream, but to keep it going, get some help to implement and stay focused on your mission."*

All entrepreneurs have personal relationships which may or may not provide ancillary business benefits. Among the personal relationships you already have, there may be some individuals who can offer you connections and business advice. However, in this chapter, we are talking about an additional frame for relationships—*purposeful relationships*, those that the entrepreneur develops expressly with the business in mind. Some of these business relationships may evolve into close personal relationships, but the primary reason for these relationships is to create informal and formal human connections that can help grow a company.

PURPOSEFUL NETWORKING IS A WAY TO EXPAND LIMITED RESOURCES

The "What," "Why," and "How" of Purposeful Networking

The term *networks* describes the myriad of interconnected human relationships that exist between people. The basic fact of all human networks is that any two people who feel connected have something in common. They might both know the same person. They might be from the same industry, live in the same neighborhood or have graduated from the same university. They may both be CPAs, patent-holders, attorneys, or parents of an autistic child. They may share a need, goal, problem, or a solution. They may be looking to raise money, invest money, train, or be trained.

The "why" of networking is simple. Human networks are a way for an entrepreneur to increase resources and fill in the gaps in his or her own experience and capabilities. There is nothing wrong or underhanded about building relationships to enhance your business. It makes sound business sense to augment the natural "geekiness" of a bioscience team with the expertise to build key business relationships. Seeking the coaching and advice of others will help you better manage the business as well as expand the company's reach into the marketplace so that it is easier to make productive contact with potential business partners, investors, and aquisitors.

The process of purposeful networking is especially critical in biotech because in the beginning stages of a biotech company, resources are always limited and achieving milestones is very, very difficult. From the proof-of-concept through subsequent seed stages, especially when the science is in the early development stage, the resources that the innovator garners—usually through grants or awards—are appropriately put toward development of the technology. It continues to be that way for some time. Not only is there limited funding, the employee roster is very thin. Often it's just the innovator/founder (that would be one person, not two). That person understands the science; knows his or her way around research lab and academia, and is often a relentless expert at experimentation, but likely doesn't know much about starting a business—and doesn't have the funding to hire the missing expertise. Initially, the innovator—now turned entrepreneur—has to find ways to augment his or her scientific expertise by increasing his or her understanding of how business works.

The "how" of building a network happens formally and informally. With a networking mindset, you can recognize opportunities for purposeful networking every day. The goal is to build networks that are sticky. A good way to do that is to begin with human connections that are already there. Successful scientists and innovators know how to network. Most have collaborated with other scientists and have built up networks for those types of relationships very well. An entrepreneur founding a company can put those same techniques to work building business relationships. Do not be afraid to sit down with business people to brainstorm challenges or ask for advice. That's the single best way to build networking relationships.

It's always a risk to generalize, but in the interest of making this chapter as beneficial as possible, I want to address those innovators who find it challenging to connect, or who plain don't like talking with nonscientific folk. In a few words, get over it. If you are going to succeed at starting a company, you must engage with people in finance, marketing, and, sales. If you can't develop the ability to engage with these folks who often are very different in temperament, process, and mindset from scientists, then find

another entrepreneur to start your company and you can take the role as chief technology officer.

The model for networking is straightforward. Start by talking with other entrepreneurs. They will be the easiest to reach. They've been where you are and have done what you are trying to do. They know how hard it is, and as a group are very willing to help the next entrepreneur. It's easier to build relationships with individuals who are in close proximity. Get to know people in your own geography to build relationships that are within arms' reach. These will form the foundation of your network. Building a human network is a lot like building a house; if you have strong foundation, you can do a lot to that structure over the years. Networks are like that. Build them in layers.

Prebuilt, Organized Support Networks: Build on Connections That Are Already There

With the emphasis on new company start-ups as a driver of economic growth, most regions have organizations that support new company formations. Plot a roadmap of these and figure out how your company can benefit from the available programs and services. There are all sorts of ready-built entities and networking points: Chambers of Commerce, universities, incubators, and organizations responsible specifically for small business or broader economic development. Identify these organizations. The more you get comfortable reaching into these groups that are established for networking, the faster you will be able to build the unique foundation of human connections that your company needs.

Many regions these days have some level of specific focus on entrepreneurship. Often that's an economic development organization at least partially funded by the state. It's fairly common for those entities to have people on their teams that bring networks of other people to bear in a very public or private fashion. If you aren't naturally inclined to network, these intermediaries make it easier for you. They have structured settings, receptions, and meeting formats to help you connect with people. Once you build relationships, you utilize them like you would any business service.

Some parts of the country even have robust entrepreneurial centers with websites that list the types of advisors that entrepreneurs can access once they become part of that center. For example, TechColumbus is an entrepreneurial-development organization that would be considered one of these intermediaries. One of the things we bring to our region is a robust, pre-assembled network of professionals that are experts-in-residence, to help entrepreneurs with networking in the early formation phases of the companies.

Entrepreneurial centers are a good starting point; however, an entrepreneur needs to be clear about what he or she needs from the center. Many entrepreneur centers serve diverse industries and broad markets and take a shotgun approach. They also serve a range of entrepreneurs and innovators. It's your task to study the organization and decide what is useful for you and your company in your situation and what you can skip.

Begin by setting up a meeting with the head of the center—the president or the director. A 15 or 20 minute meeting will do. Be prepared to offer a synopsis of who you are and what you are trying to accomplish. Describe your business—briefly—and then express interest in how the center can help. The president or director of the place will likely steer you to someone else on the staff for the details or programs and the like, but it's a good practice to make this initial contact with whoever is in charge.

Once you engage with the center, don't kill yourself by going to every meeting or event. Determine how much time to spend in attending networking events versus building relationships one-on-one. It's often a matter of attending the next happy hour reception (easier) versus identifying and getting to know individuals who can help you address gaps in your knowledge and expertise (requires more forethought and planning). Be targeted. Participate in the right things; don't participate in everything. Participate in activities that impact you and your company at the stage of your business that you are in. If you are preproof-of-concept, you don't need to focus on term sheets yet. This isn't to say that you won't build relationships with an eye to future needs, but you have to be smart about how you use your time. By participating in these organizations you are receiving, but you are also giving back. You are getting to know people in the community. You are becoming part of other people's networks. You are building expertise and relationships that may lead to you being a mentor or an advisor concurrent with your existing role or a role sometime in the future. You may have just the expertise that another person needs.

Investors Can Be Sources of Mentoring and Advice Long Before They Are Sources of Capital

Make an effort to know angels and venture capitalists—not as sources of capital, although eventually they may become that for you, but as experts and mentors. Likely, no person understands more about the biotechnology landscape than angels and venture capitalists who invest there. The time to start is when the company is at the concept stage, i.e., when you are proving your business idea and developing your first business plan. Keep in mind that you are building relationships with individuals to help you gain access to the sources of equity capital that your business will need 18 to 36 months down the road. Entrepreneurs will be surprised at the willingness of many investors to share what they know with attentive and hard-working innovators. Investors, especially those who invest in medical devices or biotechnology, are always interested in scientific developments. A bioscience entrepreneur

may have perspectives and contacts with other scientists or institutions that can help make preinvestment relationships with angels and venture capitalists a mutually beneficial two-way street.

It's never too early to begin thinking about investor terms and an exit strategy—even if those events are likely 3 to 5 years away. Exiting a biotechnology business is complicated and specialized. An angel who makes it a practice to invest in this industry can help you understand things from an investor's perspective. There are angel groups across the country that specialize in biotech deals. You will find many groups listed on the website of the Angel Capital Association (ACA) *www.angelcapitalassociation.org.* This site and the site of the Angel Resource Institute (ARI) *www. angelresourceinstitute.org* also provide extensive resources for entrepreneurs.

Sooner or later, every biotechnology business that survives will need to raise significant capital. If you have been wisely building connections to the individuals who are in this targeted and narrow field of investing, you will have a leg up on the capital-raising process. You will have contacts, you will understand the perspective of potential investors and you will know how to talk with them. You will understand the vocabulary and common investment terms, and you will be better equipped to approach the capital-raising process with a CEO mentality when your company reaches that stage.

As a serial investor, Bill Botts is careful not to get mixed up as either an investor or a board member with an entrepreneur who won't open up his or her mind and listen to advice from outsiders with experience. *"If they are so self-centered and cocky that they won't listen to anybody, it's not worth risking my money, time, and effort. I've been involved with angel groups for years. In the due diligence phase when we are considering the management team, one of the key factors is will the person listen, i.e., is he or she mentorable? They don't have to take all the advice, but as an investor, I want to know that they are going to be receptive, take it in, and consider it. Otherwise, I will just walk away."*

Engage Your Contacts and Associates at University and Research Institutions to Widen Your Network

Innovators typically have deeply rooted associations in the academic and research communities. These are natural networks for biotechnology entrepreneurs. University technology transfer offices (TTOs), as an example, exist to help their researchers transfer technologies to the commercial market. Recently, we've seen several examples of these departments strengthening their own networks by linking with alumni networks. The alumni connection can be an interesting path to find key strategy partnerships, investors, potential populations for clinical trials, or even future acquirers. Most research universities also have good business schools. More and more of these schools have entrepreneurship programs that extend across disciplines in a focused attempt to bring the lesson of entrepreneurship directly into the course of study for science and engineering disciplines. Most entrepreneurship programs involve internships and company case studies.

There are all sorts of opportunities for researches to network with those entrepreneur programs, from engaging an intern, to mentoring student teams in business plan competitions. I've witnessed several examples where the ideas for a potential biotech start-up served as the company model for a business competition, and the marketing plans and research that were developed for the competition were actually used in the business. We have a medical device company here where the researcher developed the idea and then worked with a student team who won their business plan competition and this gave the company more resources to launch.

Small Business Innovation Research and Small Business Technology Transfer Programs Are Vital Sources of Funding for Prototyping and Commercialization

The importance of the federal government's Small Business Innovation Research (SBIR) and Small Business Technology Transfer (STTR) programs to the landscape of biotechnology start-ups cannot be overstated. Competing for these awards (which range from $150,000 to millions of dollars) is arduous, but they can mean survival to biotechnology seed-stage companies. Biotechnology businesses can't get through seed stage on private equity. Some of the best and most successful biotechnology companies we have worked with participate in the SBIR/STTR process early and often. With at least 17 federal agencies offering this funding, the rules are varied and complex. The thing to remember about the federal government is that technologies cross agency needs. An innovative approach to treating a disease might be of interest to the National Institutes of Health (NIH) as well as to the Department of Defense (DoD).

Winning approval is both science and art. When it comes to SBIR/STTR, there are multiple constituencies with which to build person-to-person relationships. Most regional and state economic development entities have some level of understanding about SBIR/STTR programs and proposal writing. Sometimes there is state funding for entrepreneurial assistance. This is another area where regional incubators and economic development organizations typically have contacts and expertise. Talk to them. There are consultants who understand how to improve a company's odds of winning grant funding. An entrepreneur can reach out to contacts within the agencies themselves.

Federal procurement regulations allow you talk to people on the funding side. Their interests and needs are public information. Asking federal program managers to talk about what they are looking for gives the innovator an opportunity to talk about the company's technology.

Associations and Industry Groups Are a Source of Connections and Leadership Opportunities

Industry and trade associations are a great way to stay connected at a national or even international level with other people and companies in biotechnology and related fields. At the lowest level of involvement, associations will provide website and event and meeting access for entrepreneurs. Beyond that, the utility is a function of how active and comprehensive the association's reach and services are. Industry associations can be an avenue to find and forge strategic partnerships—from technical to marketing and distribution—and to seek out referrals for service providers (legal, accounting, marketing, and public relations). Associations are sometimes a source of operating metrics, providing ways to measure your company against others in your field. Serving on a committee or accepting more of a leadership role provides visibility and public relations (PR) opportunities for the entrepreneur and the company. If the group has a newsletter, you can volunteer to write an expert article. The tradeoff between a more active or passive role is one of time management.

Media Relationships: Members of the Media Can Be Your Friends

A start-up company doesn't have the budget to pay for advertising or PR, but there are other ways to attract attention that don't require a large budget. Local media are also looking for local stories about innovation. Figure out the local publications in your region and state—newspapers, business press, newsletters, and blogs from universities and economic development organizations. Volunteer to write or contribute to an article. Offer your experience as an expert source. Reports are always looking for experts to quote. Sometimes newspapers run innovator awards. Look for those opportunities to get your name and your company name and story out early.

Community Leaders Are Always Looking for the Next Crop of Leaders-to-Be

In every community, there are people out there already doing the spadework—gathering together those in the region that want to be part of an entrepreneurial ecosystem. In that group, there will be individuals—often highly successful entrepreneurs themselves—who want to give back to fulfill a part of their own personal needs and goals, and who, in so doing, will also receive a benefit from the entrepreneurs they support and mentor. When you do connect with community leaders in meaningful productive ways, it can help in every other area of building relationships.

Networks Are Fluid and Change Over Time

The best human networks are dynamic. They change with different types of talent and different associations as the company gains traction and grows. There will be a small number of people that you'll remain in steady contact with over time, and you will be in less frequent contact with most others; however, you don't want to lose track of the valuable contacts you've made.

It's important to set up a system to capture the names and contact information of the people you meet. Obviously you need an electronic address book that you protect and backup. Invest time in creating a top-notch profile on LinkedIn. The whole idea of networking is to build up your own personal directory of people who can help your business grow. Out of that, the entrepreneur with a fundable business will have the best chance of finding the right kind of resources and funding he or she needs.

HUMAN NETWORKS LEAD TO MENTORING

Entrepreneurs Need Mentoring First, Capital Comes Later

Thinking back over all the entrepreneurs I assisted in the last 20 years, most have one thing in common. They come in the door looking for money. It's the rare person who has said, "I need this kind of business mentoring." Instead, people say, "I'm looking for capital." Human relationships are third, fourth, or tenth on the list. Most entrepreneurs—especially those in biotechnology—have it backwards. The first thing you need is mentoring, not money. It is very difficult to start a company. Until they are knee-deep in alligators, most entrepreneurs don't realize how hard it actually is. A lot of it you have to learn for yourself, but there's also a lot that you can learn from entrepreneurs who have gone through this before and from experts in fields other than yours.

Bill Payne who teaches best practices to angel investors and entrepreneurs says, *"Mentors provide advice and counsel based on our experience. We expect entrepreneurs to listen to our advice, to be coachable, but not to act on every piece of advice. We provide the entrepreneur with information to make their own decisions about the direction of the company. It's the entrepreneur's company. It's going to be successful based on what he or she does, not necessarily on what we mentors say."*

Mentoring is the meaty part of the human resource network. With mentors, you are building around your personal expertise the core disciplines that are going to

help immediately at the proof-of-concept stage and then carry through as the company progresses along the entrepreneurial path, tackling the milestones that will lead to your goals. *"Mentors guide, not control,"* Bill Payne says. *"We are good listeners. We expect entrepreneurs to be good listeners as well. We have to listen through issues and make sure we have a full understanding of what the entrepreneur is facing. Effective mentors ask a lot of questions to provide entrepreneurs with a set of options to review before the entrepreneurs make a decision."*

The first step is to overcome any reluctance to ask for help. Don't be afraid to sit down with someone and ask for advice. That's how you can build off of what others have built for you. The second step is to map your networking plan, considering the critical milestones that must be achieved at your point on the entrepreneurial path. The more targeted you are on the type of mentoring you need, the greater success you will have at building a strong network to serve you over time. Angels like Bill Payne have a kind of give-back motivation for mentoring. *"We enjoy working with entrepreneurs. We were probably mentored ourselves at some early stage in business or at some other phase of our life. We enjoy sharing in the success of start-up companies,"* he says.

Say you are in the concept stage, still proving feasibility. Wouldn't it be cool to talk to the founder of a company who has been in your shoes? Someone who has done the exact same thing that you are trying to do—someone who has all kinds of life and business experience to help you grow and accelerate your company. That's the kind of thing targeted mentoring can do. However mentors aren't foolproof. They know a lot, but not everything. *"We mentors have to be ready to say 'I don't know.' It's okay, more than okay, even necessary that we say we don't know how to proceed in a certain situation rather than let the ego kick in and cause us to give a strong opinion when we may not have addressed the particular issue in the past,"* Bill Payne says.

What Mentoring does a Bioscience Entrepreneur Need?

- **Technology experts:** This is the easy one. Scientists usually have their technology networks built out fairly well—sometimes to the extent that they extend far beyond a local region, even to being global. Most innovators are good at this. They understand these relationships—how to build them and how valuable they are. The next step is to build on that robust scientific network. How you built that network of technical cohorts can be your personal template for augmenting those incredibly talented people with others who have different expertise.

- **CEO perspective:** Starting out, most bioscience entrepreneurs lack the CEO perspective—particularly if their formal training has always been in the sciences and they haven't been to business school. Reach out to other people who have founded start-ups, especially those who have started more than one company. It's as important to talk to entrepreneurs who have failed as well as those who have achieved success.

- **Company formation:** You need someone to talk with about early-stage company formation in bioscience from a legal perspective. Should you organize as a C-corp. or an LLC? What are the advantages and disadvantages to each? What kinds of capital can a bioscience entrepreneur raise and at what stage. Seek out individuals with an understanding of the continuum of capital—from federal grants to angel investment to VC funding. You aren't looking to raise capital at this point, just to understand how the decisions you make early on can affect investors' willingness to invest at a later stage. "I'm not trying to raise capital; I'm trying to learn" can open lots of doors.

- **Exit strategy:** It may sound like strange advice to suggest that a bioscience entrepreneur who is thinking about starting a company also think about "ending" it, but that's what you must do. Because of the enormous investment required to bring medical innovations to the marketplace, successful bioscience start-ups are almost always acquired, so you want to anticipate that from the start. Biotechnology business models are well understood in the marketplace; however, there are also lots of subtleties. There may be angel investors in your region who specialize in bioscience. Ask them how they help their portfolio companies plan exit strategies. Ask them how you can learn the ropes.

- **Legal advice:** Good legal advice is never free and seldom cheap. This is one area where you need to budget early. Buy a few hours of time from an attorney who specializes in advanced technology start-ups. If the person has experience with biotechnology businesses all the better, but this isn't a requirement. Sometimes attorneys have special rates for start-up companies. Ask around for referrals. Economic development organizations can be a good source of information about people who work with early stage businesses.

  Recognize that a biotechnology company will need different legal skills at different stages of development and that not all attorneys are created equal at every stage. I've always believed in building a diverse network of legal talent, especially for companies in the biotechnology industry. At a minimum, in addition to corporate counsel, you will need expertise in intellectual property (domestic and international) and in licensing.

  There is generally an attorney in every family. This is the attorney you should *not* use for legal advice. You can use family-member attorneys as business advisors and mentors, for referrals, or to point you in the right direction, but resist asking them for legal counsel.

- **Business development and marketing:** This is the Achilles heel for many innovators. Most have little experience in marketing and zero experience in sales. Yet these functions are the lifeblood of any successful company. Don't fall into the trap of thinking that the founder/innovator's job is only the science. While the company may literally be years away from business development and marketing, thinking about potential customers and markets, the problems they have that need solving, and about what the competition is doing or might do in the future—all these considerations help define the most appropriate commercialization path and help the innovator develop a mindset of application as well as research.

- **Tactical financial:** The single biggest problem that entrepreneurs face is running out of cash. Tactical financial mentoring can help you figure out how to make the money you have stretch as far as possible. For this, talk to entrepreneurs who have weathered the gap between proof-of-concept and Series A investment. Find out how they did it. From Skyping instead of traveling, to sharing office space, to stretching out the life of laptops and servers, talking to those who have done it will yield lots of useful ideas.

- **Strategic financial:** Every new business requires a capital strategy and plan. As a starting point, turn to the organizations in your region with services to support entrepreneurs. You will learn the vocabulary of capital markets and the sources and stages of capital that match the milestones in the entrepreneur's path. Work through your mentors, professors, and other contacts to meet angel investors—not to pitch your company, but to learn about the mindset of angels who invest in biotech.

- **SBIR/STTR awards:** There are companies in every state who have been successful with SBIR/STTRs. Seek them out. There are national consultants who are experts at developing SBIR/STTR proposals. Even if the company won't reach the grant-writing stage for months, we recommend seeking referrals and then talking to one or two of these specialists—even if you have to pay for their time. They can help you plan and structure your trials and reports to best match the information that agencies will require. The results of the trials will be the results, but agencies are very specific about the information they require and the formatting of that information. Compliance is usually straightforward—as long as the entrepreneur understands the requirements before trials start.

- **Regulatory:** Getting drugs and diagnostics to market requires an understanding of the legal and regulatory environment. University technology transfer offices, research institutions, and individual innovators are all excellent sources of mentoring on how to manage the FDA process. It's important to speak to experts *before* you structure experiments and studies to ensure that the methods you employ and the way you structure the reporting of outcomes is synchronous with the requirements of the regulatory bodies you aim to convince.

Informal human networks can help you build the business in early stages, and you don't have to give up equity. At the proof-of-concept and seed stages, as the company progresses along the entrepreneurial path and you become engaged in the community, meet people, and interact with some of them as mentors, you might be ready for a more formal structure. Multiple heads are always better than one. The entrepreneur's goal: close and trusted working relationships that help the company achieve the milestones of the entrepreneur's path.

BOARDS OF ADVISORS AND DIRECTORS CAN HELP ACCELERATE COMPANY SUCCESS

Building an Advisory Board to Help Your Company Early On

A board of advisors is a group of at least three, but not more than five people, who you know and trust. Advisors participate at the invitation of the entrepreneur. They are there to provide insight, to offer suggestions, and to serve as a sounding board when you want to talk a problem or opportunity through. Advisory boards, unlike boards of directors, do not carry legal or fiduciary responsibilities.

When it's time to start forming an advisory board, ask yourself this question: How do I supplement the skills and talents of my current team with volunteers who have expertise, interest, and are willing to prioritize advising my company for some period of time? Think in terms of the actual functional areas that you need to build around you to make you a more successful entrepreneur.

I've always found that entrepreneurs who seek advice *before* they begin asking people to serve as advisors build better boards. John Huston advises, *"As you build advisory and board relationships, have people with relevant experience, have people who can ask the questions that you haven't heard of or thought of, and bucketize so there is no question around the table who is primarily responsible for providing each essential business skill."*

There are no hard and fast rules for setting up an advisory board, but here are some guidelines that contribute to a more successful experience for entrepreneur and advisors.

- Decide what kind of help you need from your advisory board. Look for talent, not bulk. If your strong suit is technology, then focus on marketing, finance, or other disciplines where you have little or no experience. Expertise in regulatory considerations is always a plus. John Huston says, *"Look first for someone who has failed—someone who sat on the board of a company that ceased operating. That's very important because half these start-up*

ventures expire. If a director has had success, make sure it was productive success. There were people who made tens of millions but can't replicate it because it was during the .com time, and they never learned that it was their timing more than their brilliance." It may work well for a bioscience venture to begin with a clinical advisory board of one or two experts and then move into adding business expertise over time. One caution: it is natural and more comfortable for scientists and researchers to interact with other scientists and researchers. The purpose of advisors is to supplement the knowledge you already have. Don't lose sight of this important principle.

- Have a timeline, but don't be in too much of a hurry to fill out your advisory board. Many successful advisory teams are created one member at a time. A slower approach gives the entrepreneur time to work with members as they come and to figure out where the gaps in expertise lie.
- When you talk to people about being advisors to your company, be clear about what you expect. Be straightforward about the importance you place on the board. Ask respectfully, *but ask*, if the individual will have the time and interest to participate at the level you anticipate. Ensure that there are no conflicts of interest. Bill Payne says, *"When mentors step up to the plate, they agree to make the entrepreneur a priority, maybe not the highest, but still a high priority. When the entrepreneur is looking for help, the mentor will make herself available as a relative high priority, depending on the urgency of the situation,"*
- Choose people who will be able to work together, but resist building a team of people who are too like-minded. Seek a mix of strategic and tactical talent.
- It's logical to draw on your pool of mentors as well as professors or academic advisors. These individuals contribute in two possible ways. You may want to ask them to be advisors or you may ask them to suggest others who have the time, interest, and skills that match your needs.
- A bioscience company will benefit from having a recognized authority on the advisory team. A well-known name in the industry adds instant credibility and can open many doors.
- Friends and family members have their place in entrepreneurial ventures, but that place is not on the advisory board. The same is true for employees.

Following a few straightforward operating practices with your advisory board will produce more efficient and effective results as well as help you prepare for working with a formal board of directors if and when that comes about.

- When asking for help from an advisor, be clear about what you need. If you just want to brainstorm a problem or talk to think, frame the discussion that way. Your advisors are busy people. Help them help you by being specific as you can. Bill Payne says, *"When entrepreneurs face a fork in the road, they often want mentors to just tell them which road to take. But that is not how mentors help entrepreneurs. Providing entrepreneurs with options from the mentor's personal experience that will help the entrepreneur make the decisions can be an important learning experience."*

- Meet with the advisory board as a whole every quarter or so. These meetings can be face-to-face, via Skype, or even on a conference call.
- Have an agenda and stick to it. Update the group on company progress, but make the primary focus a time to discuss opportunities or issues to receive the benefit of the board's collective thought. It's your agenda.
- Summarize meeting discussions with advisory board notes. Include action items and owners. Promptly (within the same week) email the notes to board members. Create a follow-up process. Keep a retention file of these notes.
- Provide periodic email communications to keep the advisory board updated on company progress, key milestones, and challenges. Take the appropriate steps to ensure the confidentiality of these communications.
- Consider appropriate compensation for your advisory board. It's tough to pay board advisors when you lack the money to hire employees. There are degrees of compensation that evolve as your company and board evolves, including structured and common methods of providing options for board members that vest over time. Certainly many advisors want to give back, but if you want to ensure priority and focus, compensation is one tool.
- The company always pays for any expenses the board incurs. That's part of the reason in the beginning to choose people who are local. Creating and working with a board of advisors is a great way to learn some things about how to work with a formal board.

The Right Board of Directors Can Help You and Your Company Succeed

Once the corporation has raised external capital, the shareholder documents will require the company to have a board of directors. Everything the entrepreneur has learned from building and working with a board of advisors is applicable to working with a board of directors. That doesn't mean that the entrepreneur has learned everything there is to learn—for example, boards of directors have legal responsibilities—but the board of advisors experience gives a biotechnology entrepreneur a great head start of working with a formal board.

Considerations for Selecting Your Board of Directors

Ohio TechAngels tell their directors that they have three things to do for the young start-up company: (1) coach, mentor, and, if necessary, fire and replace the CEO; (2) never let the company run out of cash, and (3) sell the company.

"Everything else helps or hinders these overarching goals," John Huston says.

When you secure your first round of equity funding, your investors will require one or two board seats. If you are the founder/CEO you will take a third. You have the opportunity to exert significant influence over the selection process for the remaining members of your board. When choosing advisors and directors, focus on those who have relevant experience.

"One of the huge myths in this business is that people who have vast experience on public boards are qualified to sit on private company boards. Nothing could be further from the truth," John Huston says. *"How many times do you really think that those companies talk about survival? Rarely would the meeting of a large public company Board start by anyone saying, 'We have $133,412 in the bank, and our burn rate is $43,000 so unless something changes we will be on fumes in 4 months.' Our start-up directors discuss 'Months to Fumes' at each meeting. Another myth is that because start-ups are so much smaller enterprises, directors' challenges are less daunting than those facing large company boards. That's no more true than thinking that a baby is just a small adult. A baby isn't a small adult: Babies are frightfully fragile with a set of survival needs. We need directors who know how to nurture babies."*

Here are some guidelines that can help you make the board of directors experience a good one for your company and for you personally.

- Go to your mentors who are CEOs. Ask them how they built their board. What criteria should you be thinking about? Use the Internet to gain information and perspective. There is quite a bit of high-quality, easily searchable material on this topic.
- Before you seek additional board members, ensure that the financial and strategic expectations and objectives of the investors (via their representatives on your board), founder, CEO, and any other company officers are fully aligned and communicated.
- Pay particular attention to the exit strategy and also to investors' feelings about the experience and attributes of an operating CEO. In many biotechnology businesses we've worked with, investors recognized that a business-oriented CEO teamed with a founder/chief technology officer, makes a more-effective management team than one person wearing two or three hats. Understand this reality. Bill Botts says, *"I've seen numerous high technology companies where the founder and technical guru is the Chief Technology Officer while the CEO is the business person. I've seen CTOs who fought to build their technology and have created incredible know-how and patent portfolios, but knew they didn't have, or want, the ability to run a company. Sometimes they knew this because they've failed a couple of times. Really smart technology entrepreneurs might ask, why should*

I learn a whole different field, when there's a world full of people that already know how to do those things?"

- Be proactive with board selection. Create and prioritize a list of candidates. Discuss these with your investors. Be prepared to talk about the skills you need and why you think these candidates could help the company achieve critical milestones.

Now is the time that the mentoring and advisory relationships you have built so diligently really come into play. Use these human resources to help you figure out what type of expertise you need. What talent, experience, and contacts will complement you and the investor members? Do you need marketing, financial, engineering, or regulatory expertise?

Do you know people you want to ask to join the board, or do you want to use your relationships as a source of recommendations and referrals to people you don't yet know? You may choose to keep your advisory board intact, especially if their expertise is more on the scientific side, or you may choose one of these individuals as a member of your formal board.

- Investors may also require board observer seats. The corporate attorney may also be an observer.
- Who your board members know can be as important as what they know. Would you benefit from having a board member who knows the industry, perhaps one who has contacts with the companies that could be players in your exit strategy?
- Be wary of egos—especially your own. The folks you will be considering for your board will be confident achievers in their fields. You want people who are able to work collaboratively and who will listen to different perspectives—people who can state their opinions and who also can modify their points-of-view when presented with alternative facts and opinions. Boards are most effective when the members are able to collaborate and work as a team to help the company achieve the key milestones of the business plan. As Bill Botts says, *"I tell entrepreneurs, You don't have to accept everything your advisors tell you, but you better integrate it all into your thought processes to see if there's merit. This applies to technical issues, and especially to business issues. If you've built a decent board, they are going to know a lot more about many things than do you. Tap that resource!"*
- Remain coachable. Collectively, your board knows more than you know. They have the power and authority to change your duties and responsibilities. Bill Botts says, *"Sure entrepreneurs who don't seek outside help also succeed, but, many times, they have a lot more trouble than those who are willing to get help along the way. If an entrepreneur won't listen, but is successfully executing, you can say 'terrific job,' but when he starts stumbling, he is frequently out and everyone loses."*

If your board is required to be a five- to seven-member team there will be two to four open seats. (Keep an odd number of seats on your board, and no more than the number required to fill in order to supply the expertise you need.)

The Role and Responsibilities of Boards of Directors Are Specific and Prescribed by Law

Boards of directors' legal responsibilities are very specific. You can and must learn the details of the fiduciary *duties of care and loyalty* from your corporate counsel. Be aware that boards of directors are bound to protect and grow the corporation, act in the corporation's best interest, and never engage in conflict of interest or use information obtained as a director for personal gain.

The board is in place to serve the company. The help that a company needs from the board varies from point-to-point on the entrepreneurial path. It's important to match the effort to the timing of milestones to be achieved. As the company evolves, the definition of the roles of the board, and for that matter the CEO, will also evolve. Boards are not authorized to sign contracts on behalf of the corporation, but they do elect the corporate officers (this includes you) who then have the responsibility for day-to-day operations of the company. This means that once you have a formal board, that board has the power to hire and fire the CEO. It is useful in the beginning to document the roles and responsibilities of the CEO and the board. Define which CEO decisions (including dollar limits) require board approval. Define term limits for board members and how the chairperson of the board will be chosen.

Board Meetings—Set a Consistent Calendar and Format and Follow It

Monthly board meetings are common for companies in seed to early-growth stages. The CEO has the responsibility to set the tone and tempo of the meetings. Talk to your advisory board, other entrepreneurs, mentors, and board members to find out what they have seen to be effective. In-person meetings are the best if at all possible. Convening online may save time and money, but board relationships aren't the place to cut corners. There is so much for the entrepreneur and the business to gain from getting board members together for a period of time to focus entirely on the company.

Invest the appropriate time and focus to preparing for board meetings. The CEO and the board chair should work together to develop meeting agendas. Discuss every topic with every board member ahead of time. Not only will you avoid surprises—which everyone will appreciate—you will also receive valuable feedback that may suggest ways to improve what you are doing or the way you are doing it before the meeting takes place. Don't assume that board members will remember all the details from meeting-to-meeting. Provide updates. Send out board meeting materials at least two days ahead of the meeting. Include detailed financial information. Boards know how to read financial statements and can do that offline. Limit yourself to one financial chart in the board presentation. Use most of the meeting to talk about challenges and opportunities.

Standardize the format of your communications—board books, financial reports, capitalization table, and requests for grants of equity. As the company develops past the seed stage and adds employees or rewards contributors already on board, you will be requesting equity grants. Create a standard format that includes the capitalization table whether it has changed or not. A set procedure and a consistent report format facilitate compensation discussions and cause the awarding of grants to proceed more smoothly and efficiently.

Include your senior managers in board meetings. This gives the board and your management team an opportunity to get to know each other. You can have a closed executive session to talk about personnel, compensation, or other confidential matters. Bill Botts' philosophy has always been to construct boards with all outside directors plus the CEO. *"Boards that are made up of inside executives result in board meetings being more like staff meetings, with the same old ideas and fixes by the same staff members,"* Botts says. *"I always make board meetings open to the executive team. They participate just like they are on the board, except they don't have a vote. I have staff meetings every week as well. Frankly, I don't need a board that's another staff meeting. I need board meetings where my team can react with outside experts to get other views and advice. Management teams tend to become ingrown and don't always have the benefit of outsiders who have taken different approaches to solving similar problems."*

Board minutes are important. They provide a continuous record of the company and can be used in legal proceedings. Get advice from your corporate counsel, investors, and board members who have served on other boards as to the level of detail.

Compensation Usually Takes the Form of Options that Vest Over Time

The company will pay all directors' expenses. To have an engaged and enthusiastic board, the company needs to compensate them. Since cash is so limited, in seed and early stages, a common practice is to award directors with corporate options (typically 0.25 to 1 percent of outstanding shares) that vest in 3 to 5 years. Angels and venture capitalists who serve as a requirement of the investment do not receive additional compensation. Clearly define how the options vest. Ensure that the charter of the company defines the limits of the directors' liability. The company must also provide directors and officers (D&O) liability insurance to protect the participants' assets.

PERSONAL TRAITS AND CHARACTERISTICS
All Effective Relationships Are Built on Trust and Mutual Respect

In the entrepreneurial world there is an extra something in the mix—the excitement that comes with invention, discovery, and building a whole business around the innovation of a new idea.

Relationship building comes naturally to many entrepreneurs. For others, it is a learned skill. Either way, certain attitudes and behaviors foster relationships that can be as valuable to a company as assets on a balance sheet. Other traits can derail the best-intended connections between human beings.

- Operate with complete integrity. Follow the intent as well as the letter of the law. Match your words and deeds.
- Respect others, from the small to the large. Do what you say you will do. Be timely for meetings and with any other follow-up. Keep confidences.
- Remain coachable. Don't wait until you need to ask for help. Listen, especially when your first instinct is to disagree. Be willing to change your mind, say you were wrong, or stand your ground.
- Reciprocate. Give back to the relationship—in appreciation and expertise. There will always be entrepreneurs coming along behind you. Do for them what others did for you.
- Collaboration is the secret sauce of mutually beneficial relationships. Learn to work with others. Give credit where credit is due.

CONCLUSION

Purposeful and productive business relationships are assets that don't appear on the balance sheet. Formal and informal networks can help the entrepreneur grow the company. Even if the venture doesn't succeed, well-founded, purposeful business relationships endure.

The innovator's mantra of relationships are:

1. I can't build a successful company without help.
2. Commercialization and science are two entirely different disciplines.
3. The things that make me good at one thing, may cause me to be less effective at the other.
4. There are many people with all kinds of experience and skill who are eagerly available to help entrepreneurs.
5. It's my job to find mentors and advisors, meet them, and then demonstrate that I and my company are worthy of their attention and assistance.
6. I can't count on the scientific method when it comes to building relationships with other human beings. I must learn new techniques.

7. I will be eagerly coachable and listen to what mentors and advisors have to say, recognizing that while I may be an expert in my field, great science is only the first step in great company formation.

Building and nurturing purposeful, diverse relationships is a critical success factor for becoming a successful entrepreneur. The benefits are enormous—from coaching and mentoring that money can't buy, to ensuring friendships that evolve and endure far beyond capital rounds, product launches, and profitable exits.

Anyone who has an interest in problem solving, a thirst for learning, and a passion for his or her business can become a builder of meaningful relationships. I know because I've seen dozens and dozens of scientists and researchers do it successfully year after year.

The Technology

Chapter 9

Understanding Biotechnology Product Sectors

Craig Shimasaki, PhD, MBA

President & CEO, Moleculera Labs and BioSource Consulting Group, Oklahoma City, Oklahoma

When we speak about the "biotechnology industry" it is in broad reference to a diverse group of treatments, biologics, diagnostics, medical devices, clinical laboratory tests, instruments, agricultural, industrial, and biofuel applications. The biotechnology industry encompasses many diverse sectors which are ever-expanding as new scientific and technical discoveries are uncovered and new applications are found. The goal of biotechnology is to produce unique products and processes that improve life, health, and well-being of individuals and society as a whole. On the surface, the biotechnology industry may appear to be complex because of the seemingly endless and diverse array of products that biotechnology is capable of producing. However, it is surprising how each sector utilizes many similar tools and methods to create these diverse products.

The purpose of this chapter is to introduce you to the major sectors of the biotechnology industry and equip you with a better understanding of each of these segments. Each product sector has unique aspects, including specialized technical and regulatory hurdles. Regardless of what particular sector you may be working in, having a basic understanding of all sectors will help relate the work of your organization to the broader biotechnology industry as a whole. Understanding other biotech sectors can also spark new ideas for novel product development within your own sector and provide solutions to problems encountered during product development. Often, the convergence of these sectors produce products that are more efficient and more effective than those that could be created by any single technology sector alone. For example, the category of Combination Device/Therapeutics resulted from the introduction of vascular stents (metal scaffolds which are medical devices) which were later improved though the addition of anticoagulant drug coatings (therapeutics) resulting in more efficacious drug-eluting stents which have now replaced the original stents used for coronary artery narrowing.

New sectors within the biotechnology industry will no doubt continue to emerge. For instance, just 20 years ago

there were no such things as "biochips" or "microarrays," whereas today, most research laboratories and pharmaceutical companies routinely employ instrumentation that utilizes microarrays and microchips in their research and development (R&D). Possessing a working knowledge of each of these sectors is invaluable to biotech entrepreneurs, managers, and biotech executives. This overview will provide a framework to aid you in later study of other product sectors that may be of interest to you. Should you find a particular biotechnology sector of interest, you are encouraged to seek the many additional resources to expand your detailed working knowledge of these sectors.

BIOTECHNOLOGY PRODUCT AND TECHNOLOGY SECTORS

Biotechnology sectors can be classified by their *technology* or their *product* category. For instance, "genomics" and "proteomics" are indeed "sectors" of biotechnology but these classifications are based upon the *technology* that they employ, rather than the resulting *product* that is produced from the technology (Figure 9.1). It is important to recognize that any individual *technology* is capable of producing many different biotechnology products each belonging to different *product sectors*. For instance, the use of *genomic technology* can result in a *diagnostic test* by measuring mRNA transcripts. Alternatively, genomic technology can result in a *therapeutic* by utilizing antisense DNA to block or inhibit a disease process. *Genomic technology* can also result in a *research instrument* by utilizing gene-based microarray analysis. Although *genomic technology* can result in a diagnostic, therapeutic, and research instrument product, as described, each has vastly different development pathways, different costs, and different development timeframes. Since our focus is on biotechnology product commercialization, in this chapter we will discuss *product sectors* rather than *technology sectors*. As we review these sectors, remember that any particular technology can cross multiple product

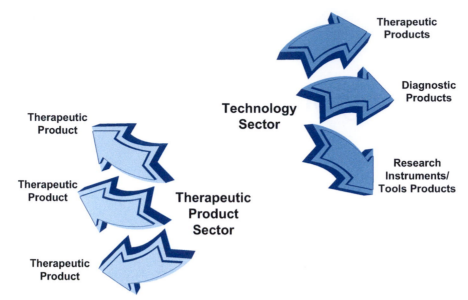

FIGURE 9.1　Technology sectors versus product sectors. Any one technology is capable of producing multiple products in different sectors, whereas one product sector focuses on multiple products within the same sector.

sectors, but the manner in which it is applied to a problem and the solution solved will determine the product category in which it resides. When reviewing the product sector list below you may also recognize the absence of nanotechnology as a product sector. Nanotechnology has significant promise yet it is also a technology that can be applied to a variety of product sectors from therapeutics to medical devices to diagnostics. Its applicability is so broad that nanotechnology can also be utilized within nonbiotechnology applications such as in the paint and electronics industry to name a few. Without reservation, the categorization of biotechnology by *technology* has merit, especially for researchers, but in the context of this chapter, we will be focusing on *product* sectors and their commercialization aspects.

Biotechnology Product Sectors

In this chapter, I want to share with you ten of the most common biotechnology product sectors. No doubt there may be more and there are certainly other ways to subdivide these sectors. However, this categorization will provide a suitable framework for understanding the characteristics and features that comprise each of these sectors, including the differences in costs, development timeframe and market applications for each of these categories. Within each product sector we will discuss the function of products within this sector, pertinent characteristics of each product sector, product examples, and briefly describe how these products are regulated.

1. Therapeutics
2. Biologics and vaccines
3. *In vitro* diagnostics and personalized medicine
4. Medical devices

5. Combination device/therapeutics
6. Digital health IT applications
7. Research instruments and tools
8. Biocrops
9. Biofuels
10. Industrial biotechnology

PRODUCT DEVELOPMENT COSTS VARY BY SECTOR

Before we discuss the individual biotechnology product sectors, it is helpful to understand the general range of costs required to complete development and reach commercialization for each of these product sectors. There is no getting around the fact that *all* biotechnology product development is expensive and requires large amounts of capital to bring a product to commercialization. Many biotechnology companies have started with a great technology concept and novel product idea, but for lack of funds at a critical time period these noble product applications have vanished. One of the many reasons for this shortfall can be attributed to poor financial planning and a lack of familiarity with the overall development costs and the need for continual fundraising. No one should undertake an endeavor, particularly a biotechnology enterprise, without first counting the financial costs, or at least *understanding* these costs before starting. A reference from scripture reads: "*Suppose one of you wants to build a tower. Will he not first sit down and estimate the cost to see if he has enough money to complete it?*"[a] Starting, growing, and leading a biotechnology company is no different. At the outset of starting an enterprise it is critical that

---

a. Gospel of Luke chapter 14, verse 28, (NIV)

TABLE 9.1 Biotechnology Product Development Cost Estimates

Product Sector Categories	Development Cost Estimates
Therapeutics	$250 million to $1.5 billion
Biologics and vaccines	$250 million to $1.5 billion
In vitro diagnostics and personalized medicine	$5 to $100 million
Medical devices	$15 to $100 million
Combination device/ therapeutics	$75 to $250 million
Digital health IT applications	$250,000 to $15 million
Research instruments and tools	$5 to $75 million
BioAgriculture	$75 to $200 million
Biofuels	$50 to $150 million
Industrial biotechnology	$15 to $75 million

the leader recognize and appreciate all the costs of product development, testing, and regulatory approval within any of these sectors. Careful planning and timing for fundraising that is tied to meeting key milestones along with proper fiscal management, can provide the greatest opportunity for a good product idea to reach commercialization. Few industries face the enormous expense, lengthy development time, and challenging regulatory hurdles inherent within the biotechnology product-development process. However, in contrast, few industries carry the medical impact that biotechnology has on the health and well-being of millions of lives. The reader will benefit by understanding the range of costs and the typical commercialization timeframes attributed to each of these product sectors.

Table 9.1 lists range estimates of the various development costs for each of these product sectors. These ranges take into account the costs for research, development, clinical testing, regulatory, and approval costs prior to commercialization. Within some product sectors the cost ranges are extremely broad simply because of the diverse types of products that can be produced within that particular category. For instance, within the *in vitro* diagnostic and personalized medicine category there is a wide cost range of $5 to $100 million. This is because follow-on diagnostics using existing platform technologies require less development costs than a new diagnostic testing category using a relatively new technology platform. For instance, a hypothetical new diagnostic test for the detection of Lyme disease based upon several newly identified proteins utilizing existing point-of-care lateral-flow technology may be able to complete development and reach commercialization at the lower end of the cost range. Whereas

a complex genetic test that uses RNA expression analysis to predict the likelihood of cancer recurrence for the prediction of breast cancer may require development costs at the upper end of the category. A general rule is that an improvement in an existing diagnostic test (one that is faster or more sensitive) than a test already on the market would most likely be at the lower end of the sector cost range, whereas totally new platforms and/or new diagnostic categories (tests not previously available) will typically be at the higher end of the cost range. For all products, the overall costs for development increases in proportion to the amount of laboratory, animal, and human clinical data that must be collected in order to demonstrate safety and clinical efficacy of a product. In addition, each of these sector development costs are impacted by the technology utilized, the target market, and the complexity of the product.

For therapeutics, biologics, and vaccines, the upper-end product development cost of $1.5 billion takes into account the estimated number of research failures encountered when advancing one successful product to commercialization. In actuality, any one single therapeutic or biologic product-development program may have development costs at the lower end of the range; however no one can predict which one will be successful. Therefore most large pharmaceutical companies use upper-end estimates that include the typical failure rates incurred along the way.[b] In the sector of BioAgriculture, product development costs can vary depending on the type of product and the number and types of genetic traits incorporated into a product, including the amount of field testing required to prove safety.

Although I have listed general range estimates for development costs within each of these product sectors, it is essential to determine more precise cost estimates for your particular product when creating and establishing a product development plan and business plan. Precise product development cost estimates will help you assess the number and size of financing rounds required in order for your product to reach various development milestones and, ultimately, commercialization. Understanding the process required to arrive at accurate product development cost estimates will help ensure you don't run short of capital and it will also assure investors that you understand the capital requirements for bringing your product to the market. When calculating product development costs be sure to build within your estimates an allowance for unexpected events and contingency plans. Rarely, if ever, do product development plans proceed as anticipated. More often than not, unforeseen roadblocks, delays, and development challenges arise which extend the originally estimated timeframe, which translates into additional costs. When estimating product development costs, consider adding a contingency factor of 15 to 25

---

b. 2013 PhRMA's Pharmaceutical Industry Profile: http://www.phrma.org/sites/default/files/pdf/PhRMA%20Profile%202013.pdf

percent of the costs for certain development phases that are unpredictable. Alternatively, determine your own contingency estimates based upon your particular product sector, the technology utilized, the target market, and the number and types of features your product must possess in order to be successful. Your goal is to arrive at the best and most reliable cost estimate of the entire development process from concept through to commercialization.

PRODUCT DEVELOPMENT TIMEFRAME VARIES FOR BIOTECHNOLOGY SECTORS

Just as the development costs vary, so do the product development timeframes. Each product sector requires varying amounts of time for R&D, prototype testing or animal testing, human clinical or field testing, and regulatory approval. It is equally important to determine an accurate timeframe required for your product to move from concept through each stage of product development and ultimately into the market.

Suffice it to say that all biotechnology product sectors (with the exception of digital health IT applications) require numerous years to move a product from concept through development, testing, regulatory approval, and into the marketplace. Table 9.2 lists a range of development timeframes for products within each of these sectors. Because of the expansion and mass adoption of digital and information technology (IT), many digital health IT applications have emerged which can potentially reach the market within 1 to 3 years of product concept, whereas therapeutics and biologics may require 12 to 15 years to reach commercialization. The product development timeframes listed encompass the time spent on research, development, prototype and clinical testing, regulatory, and approval processes.

Just as with sector costs, development timeframes vary between product sectors and within a sector depending on the particular product. For the biotech entrepreneur or company leader, it is important to outline a timetable throughout each of the various development stages for your particular product. Mapping a development timeframe for your particular product is essential because reaching certain product development milestones provide value-enhancing events for the company. In addition, as discussed in Chapter 19 entitled "Sources of Capital and Investor Motivations," there are certain company stages that investors prefer to invest in and these are tied directly to product development milestones. For instance, value-enhancing events for therapeutic and biologic companies include most all product-development milestones.

Examples of Value-enhancing Milestones for Therapeutics and Biologics

1. Completion of basic and translational research.
2. Completion of development and *in vitro* testing.
3. Completion of lead/process optimization.
4. Completion of preclinical testing in animals.
5. Filing of an Investigational New Drug (IND) applications with the FDA.
6. Initiation or completion of each stage of clinical testing (Phase 1, 2, and 3).
7. Filing of a New Drug Application (NDA) with the FDA.
8. Regulatory review and product approval.
9. Scale-up and manufacturing.
10. Marketing and growth.

For medical devices and diagnostics there are different value-enhancing milestones.

Examples of Value-enhancing Milestones for Medical Devices and Diagnostics

1. Completion of basic and translational research.
2. Completion of the proof-of-concept phase.
3. Completion of prototype development.
4. Completion of clinical validation.
5. Filing of a 510(k) or a PMA with the FDA.
6. Completion of a regulatory review and approval or marketing clearance.
7. Scale-up and manufacturing.
8. Marketing and expansion.

Each product sector has its own unique value-enhancing milestones. A company should recognize and outline each value-enhancing milestone that confers significant product development progress and increases interest and confidence in the company and its future. By outlining and achieving these milestones a company can progressively increase its value and continue to attract greater funding interest for the company throughout subsequent development stages of the product.

TABLE 9.2 Product Sector Timeframe Estimates

Product Sector Categories	Timeframe Estimates
Therapeutics	12 to 15 years
Biologics and vaccines	12 to 15 years
In vitro diagnostics and personalized medicine	3 to 7 years
Medical devices	3 to 5 years
Combination device/therapeutics	5 to 10 years
Digital health IT applications	1 to 3 years
Research instruments and tools	3 to 7 years
Biocrops	7 to 16 years
Biofuels	5 to 10 years
Industrial biotechnology	2 to 4 years

CREATING VALUE

Regardless of the product sector, the goal of all start-up or early-stage biotechnology companies is to create value within the product being developed and within the company. Imperceptibly, throughout the entire product development process, value is created. Value is not created all at once, nor is it created proportional to the time or money invested. Value is created incrementally every time a product development milestone is successfully reached. Completing certain product development milestones confer more value than others and, with each successful milestone reached, risk is simultaneously reduced—value increases as risk is reduced (See Figure 9.2). Steady progress through product development in a financially efficient manner creates a situation where more investors will want to participate in your endeavor. Understanding the concept of value creation is important for entrepreneurs because investors and future partners have expectations about product development progress, costs, and milestones. Everything the company does should be viewed in a way that it does not detract, but rather increases the value of the product and the company and decreases the risk, thereby increasing the likelihood of raising additional capital. By properly estimating development costs and timeframes, and reaching value-enhancing milestones along the way, value is attributed to the company and it makes the task of raising capital for subsequent financing rounds easier, because without continuous sources of capital no product will reach the market.

OVERVIEW OF PRODUCT SECTORS

Therapeutics

Therapeutics generally refer to any drug or medicine that is used to treat a disease or condition with the intent of curing or lessening its severity. The FDA does not list a definition of a "therapeutic" but does list a definition for a "drug" as *"A substance recognized by an official pharmacopoeia or formulary; a substance intended for use in the diagnosis, cure, mitigation, treatment, or prevention of disease; a substance (other than food) intended to affect the structure or any function of the body; a substance intended for use as a component of a medicine but not a device or a component, part or accessory of a device."* The word "therapeutic" as defined by *Merriam-Webster* states *"relating to the treatment of disease or disorders by remedial agents or methods"*

Overview **of the various sectors and subcategories:**
1. **Therapeutics**
   a. Small molecules
   b. Peptides and nucleic acids
2. **Biologics and vaccines**
   a. Oligonucleotides and antisense
   b. Proteins
   c. Monoclonal antibodies
   d. Stem cells
3. **Diagnostics**
   a. *In vitro* diagnostics
   b. Molecular diagnostic
   c. Predictive and prognostic diagnostics
   d. Companion diagnostics
   e. Personalized medicine
   f. Clinical laboratory services—CLIA laboratory
4. **Medical devices**
5. **Combination device/therapeutic products**
6. **Research tools and reagents**
   a. Sequencers
   b. Microarrays
7. **Digital health and healthcare delivery IT**
8. **BioAgriculture**
9. **BioFuels**
10. **Industrial biotechnology**

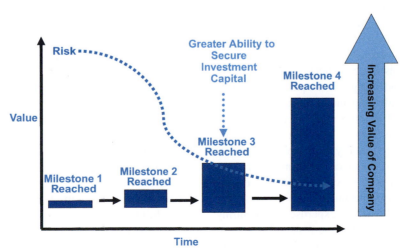

FIGURE 9.2 Value increases and risk reduces with each milestone reached.

or by others as *"…pertaining to the treating or curing of a disease."* The terms "drug" and "therapeutic" are often used synonymously in various contexts, and for this sector category we will consider them the same. For the general public who first learns about the biotechnology industry, they most often associate this industry with therapeutic treatments for different diseases or conditions, such as AIDS, Alzheimer's, or cancer. Indeed, therapeutics comprise a very large portion of the development activity within the biotechnology industry and this segment consumes the largest portion of the capital raised. However, therapeutic companies make up a limited portion of the total number of biotechnology companies within the industry and they represent only a portion of the multitude of products produced by biotechnology.

Prior to the emergence of the biotechnology industry, therapeutics were developed and commercialized by the large pharmaceutical companies around the world such as Merck, Schering, Hoffmann-La Roche, and Burroughs Wellcome to name a few. Many of these companies originally started as chemical manufacturers, apothecaries, and pharmacies. Merck, in Germany, originated as a pharmacy located in Darmstadt in 1668 and was possibly the first company to move in the direction of pharmaceutical manufacturing. The main focus of the pharmaceutical industry has primarily been on the discovery and development of *"small molecule"* therapeutics which are chemical compounds that can be studied in isolated assays and synthetically produced by chemists (see Chapter 23 entitled "Therapeutic Drug Development and Human Clinical Trials"). Many successful small molecule chemical entities were developed and produced by these pharmaceutical companies such as acetylsalicylic acid (ASA) or aspirin. The pharmaceutical industry steadily grew as more small molecule drugs were successfully developed and commercialized such as analgesics (pain), antipyretics (fever reducers), barbiturates (acting on the central nervous system), and others.

These pharmaceutical companies experienced many successes and great demand for their products, which created the growth and expansion of these multinational mega companies. However, over time, the number of novel small molecule drug opportunities became less abundant as evidenced by the declining successes in finding and commercializing small molecule therapeutics. This issue, coupled with increasing drug-development costs, and changes in the patent exclusivity period laws, pharmaceutical companies sought methods and opportunities to create and develop more successful therapeutic products. Once biotechnology tools and recombinant DNA techniques emerged in the early 1970s, pharmaceutical companies saw the value of biologics. After many of these biotechnology products proved successful, pharmaceutical companies began acquiring biotechnology companies as a means of augmenting their biological expertise and acquiring access to biotechnology products. More and more pharmaceutical companies slowly began transitioning to the development of biologics and the acquisition of biotechnology companies.

Further dissolving the distinction between pharmaceutical and biotechnology companies, we now have emerging a category of companies referred to as "biotherapeutics companies." Major biotechnology company acquisitions continue to occur such as in 2008 when Cambridge, Massachusetts-based Millennium Pharmaceuticals was acquired by Japanese Takeda Pharmaceutical for $8.8 billion. In 2009 Swiss-based Roche purchased the remaining shares of South San Francisco-based Genentech for $46.8 billion completing its full acquisition since it first acquired a 56 percent majority ownership in 1990. And in 2011, the French pharmaceutical giant Sanofi-Aventis acquired Boston-based Genzyme for $20.1 billion. It is important to recognize that in one sense, the term "therapeutics" does include "biologics," because biologics are also used for treating diseases and conditions. However, the reader should know there are product development and regulatory distinctions between "therapeutics" and "biologics." We will discuss biologics in the next section but for now will elaborate on the differences and examine these two categories as clearly distinct entities. However, as time goes on there appears to be less of a distinction between traditional therapeutics and biologics.

The vast majority of what is described as traditional therapeutics can be categorized as:

- Small organic molecules
- Peptides and nucleic acids

Small molecules are chemical entities that are usually chemically synthesized, administered orally, and absorbed through the intestines into the bloodstream. The overall product development goal for a therapeutic is to produce a pill or capsule that contains the chemical entity which can be conveniently administered by mouth and quickly produce the desired effect within the body. As previously mentioned, small molecules, such as peptides and nucleic acids can also be utilized as diagnostics and as reagents in clinical tests, whereas therapeutics utilize these types of molecules for the purpose of treating a disease or condition.

Mechanisms of Action for Therapeutics

Common mechanisms of action for many therapeutics are to block or interfere with a chemical reaction within the body, block a receptor, or to block or inhibit a process in an undesirable microorganism. These interferences and blockages can be targeted against critical enzymes that are involved in a disease process, or receptors on cells which trigger downstream events such as a transcription of RNA and translation of proteins. By interfering or blocking a specific biological or chemical process in the body or in a microorganism, therapeutics can "treat" a wide variety of diseases or conditions. To the degree that the therapeutic is specific enough and can target a single process or a single receptor, to that same degree a therapeutics' "side-effects" are minimized. However, within the body many similar reactions occur simultaneously, and similar receptors can be found in various cells and organs throughout the body. As a result, most all therapeutics have "side-effects" which can range from minimal to very significant. The proper prescribing of a therapeutic is typically based upon an analysis of the risk/benefit to the patient by the physician. If the potential benefit of the therapeutic outweighs the risks of side-effects or potential consequences, then the clinician will prescribe the treatment. In certain therapeutics, side-effects can be extremely severe or even life-threatening such as the case of chemotherapeutic drugs used in the treatment of certain types of cancers. However, in some cases, the physician may determine that the risk of no treatment may be worse than the risk of treatment side-effects.

Therapeutics are created that can also target or interfere with biological processes that are not found in our own body, but rather in microorganisms that attack our body. For instance, antibiotics belong to a class of anti-infectives (which also include antivirals and antifungals), which are small molecules designed to inhibit a specific biologic process in the growth cycle in bacteria. Some of the processes that antibiotics target include inhibiting the synthesis of the bacteria's cell-walls or the synthesis of its protein, thus slowing down or stopping their reproduction. Antibiotics are developed with the intent of inhibiting or blocking bacteria-specific biological processes, and since bacteria possesses unique enzymes and proteins that differ from those in the human body, most of these drugs tend to be quite effective and usually elicit minimal side-effects. However, because bacteria possess the ability to transfer genes to other bacteria and confer antibiotic resistance, this reduces the effectiveness of antibiotics over time and creates drug-resistant strains of bacteria. As a result, biotechnology can play an important role in identifying and creating antibiotics that may encounter minimal resistance from bacteria.

Therapeutic Categories

The number of therapeutic categories is large and growing as new biological mechanisms are discovered and new conditions emerge. The following list outlines 50 different therapeutic categories established by the U.S. Pharmacopeia and listed on the FDA website [1]:

- Analgesics
- Anesthetics
- Antibacterials
- Anticonvulsants
- Antidementia agents
- Antidepressants
- Antidotes, deterrents, and toxicologic agents
- Antiemetics
- Antifungals
- Antigout agents

- Anti-inflammatory agents
- Antimigraine agents
- Antimyasthenic agents
- Antimycobacterials
- Antineoplastics
- Antiparasitics
- Antiparkinson agents
- Antipsychotics
- Antispasticity agents
- Antivirals
- Anxiolytics
- Bipolar agents
- Blood glucose regulators
- Blood products/modifiers/volume expanders
- Cardiovascular agents
- Central nervous system agents
- Dental and oral agents
- Dermatological agents
- Enzyme replacements/modifiers
- Gastrointestinal agents
- Genitourinary agents
- Hormonal agents, stimulant/replacement/modifying (adrenal)
- Hormonal agents, stimulant/replacement/modifying (pituitary)
- Hormonal agents, stimulant/replacement/modifying (prostaglandins)
- Hormonal agents, stimulant/replacement/modifying (sex hormones/modifyers)
- Hormonal agents, stimulant/replacement/modifying (thyroid)
- Hormonal agents, suppressant (adrenal)
- Hormonal agents, suppressant (parathyroid)
- Hormonal agents, suppressant (pituitary)
- Hormonal agents, suppressant (sex hormones/modifiers)
- Hormonal agents, suppressant (thyroid)
- Immunological agents
- Inflammatory bowel disease agents
- Metabolic bone disease agents
- Ophthalmic agents
- Otic agents
- Respiratory tract agents
- Sedatives/hypnotics
- Skeletal muscle relaxants
- Therapeutic nutrients/minerals/electrolytes

Other Characteristics of Therapeutics

Most therapeutic drugs have three or more names assigned to them. These names include the *brand name* or *trade name* which is given by the company, such as "Lipitor" by Pfizer. There is also a *generic name* "atorvastatin calcium," and a (usually long) *chemical name*

"[R-(R*,R*)]-2-(4-fluorophenyl)-β,δ-dihydroxy-5-(1-methylethyl)-3-phenyl-4 [(phenylamino)carbonyl]-1Hpyr-role-1-heptanoic acid, calcium salt (2:1) trihydrate."

Regulation of Therapeutics

Therapeutics (and biologics) are some of the most stringently regulated sectors in any industry. Due in large part to the potential for unwanted side-effects, the regulatory approval route for therapeutics, including the requirements for safety and efficacy in animal and clinical testing, is very strenuous and lengthy, often taking 10 to 15 years for a therapeutic product to reach the market. Whether the approval is in the United States under the FDA or in other countries through their own regulatory agencies, the therapeutic and biologic sectors have become the most costly segments in time and money to develop. Estimates for the cost of the development of a new therapeutic drug has been calculated to be about $1.3 billion [2].

Therapeutic Products in Development

There is a vast number of therapeutic drugs under development and in clinical studies. In a 2013 report [3] the Analysis Group identified 5400 drug products in clinical development for cancer to cardiovascular disease and diabetes to neurology to name just a few areas. They reported that a high percentage of new molecular entities (NME)-focused development activities were *potentially first-in-class*—in other words, drugs that work by a unique pharmacological class distinct from those of any other marketed products. The pharmaceutical and biotechnology industries are continuously identifying new drug targets and new methods for treating some of the most chronic and debilitating conditions. (See Figure 9.3.)

Biologics and Vaccines

Biologics can also be thought of as "therapeutics" in the sense that they are utilized to treat a disease or condition. The official FDA definition of "biological products" or "biologics" is any virus, therapeutic serum, toxin, antitoxin, or analogous product applicable to the prevention, treatment, or cure of diseases or injuries of man. The European Union regulations defines "biological medicinal products" as a protein or nucleic acid-based pharmaceutical substance used for therapeutic or *in vivo* diagnostic purposes, which is produced by means other than direct extraction from a native (nonengineered) biological source. Biologics differ from the above-mentioned therapeutic small molecule drugs in several characteristics. One of the most important characteristics of a biologic is that they are large complex molecules which require complex processes to manufacture and produce. (See Figure 9.4.) Whereas small molecule therapeutic drugs are often stable in most environments and can be chemically synthesized and administered orally. Biologics are usually fragile, and most often administered by injection into the bloodstream for treatment, as most biologics would be digested or

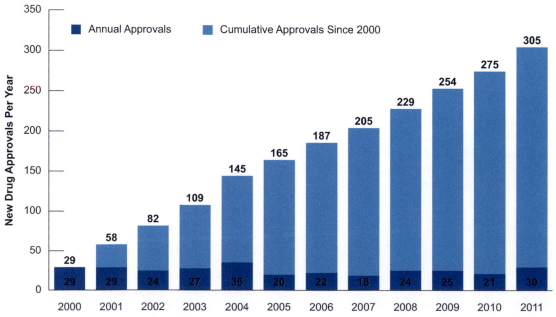

FIGURE 9.3 Annual and cumulative new drug approvals since 2000. Note: new drug approvals include new molecular entities and biologic license applications (BLAs). *(Reprinted by permission from Macmillan Publishers Ltd: Mullard, A. "2011 FDA drug approvals",Nat Rev Drug Discov 2012 Feb 1;11(2):91-94.*

broken down if administered orally. Rarely can a biologic be chemically synthesized because of their complexity and size (with the exception of oligonucleotides and antisense DNA), and are often produced by a process that utilizes a protein expression system in a mammalian or insect cell line or in a bacteria. Biologics also rely on complex "posttranslational modifications" that are carried out by these living expression systems. Posttranslational modifications include different glycosylation patterns within these proteins which affect the activity (potency) of the protein, its three-dimensional structure (protein folding pattern), and rate of clearance from the body (elimination and half-life). Biologics are very complex and difficult to fully characterize, and for this reason they often are characterized by their manufacturing processes. The manufacturing processes of biologics are complex, and slight changes in temperature during processing or other factors can impact the final product and affect how it works in patients. As a result, regulatory agencies require that changes in the manufacturing process or facility may require additional clinical studies to demonstrate safety, purity, and potency (see Chapter 26 entitled "The Biomanufacturing of Biotechnology Products").

Biologic categories include:

- Proteins, enzymes, and growth factors.
- Monoclonal antibodies.
- Blood components such as blood factors, stem cells, or proteins.
- Oligonucleotides and antisense DNA.

It is important to remember that many of these same biologic entities can also be utilized in certain processes to identify disease conditions (diagnostics). For instance, monoclonal antibodies, coupled or used with detection and signaling molecules are commonly used to identify or capture molecular markers within the body or in a specimen. In this section we differentiate the usage of these biologic products as treatments, whereas in the diagnostic section we will elaborate on the usage of monoclonal antibodies for diagnostics purposes.

Mechanisms of Action for Biologics

Most biologics are replacements or substitutes of actual human proteins that are either missing or at low levels within the body of the individual being treated. Genetic engineering tools have given us the ability to "cut" and "paste" various genes that code for human proteins, and transfer them into the genome of bacteria, insect, or mammalian cells and grow them in culture so that they can express (produce) the desired human protein. Because most biologics are replicas of actual human proteins, their function is identical to the natural purpose of the original protein in the human body.

Examples of Biologic Products

Monoclonal Antibodies

Monoclonal antibodies are biologics that have shown increasing promise as candidates for treatments of diverse diseases because of their ability to bind specifically to almost any target molecule. Antibodies (Abs) are immune system proteins that recognize and bind to foreign substances, usually with very high affinity. "*Monoclonal*" antibodies (mAbs) refer to the fact that only a "single" antibody clone is being produced, as opposed to "polyclonal" where "multiple clones" or different antibodies with different specificities are being produced. In 1975, Köhler and Milstein [4] discovered a method to produce mouse monoclonal antibodies directed against any specific target. This provided the ability to engineer a mouse monoclonal antibody directed against a desired target. For this monumental work and discovery these scientists won the Nobel Prize in 1984. With the further advent of additional biotechnology tools we can now genetically engineer and produce completely *humanized monoclonal antibodies* that are directed against desired targets and

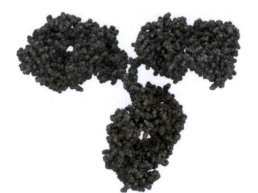
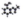

FIGURE 9.4 Biologic versus a small molecule drug. (Left) Biologic: molecular structure of a monoclonal antibody approximately 150,000 molecular weight. (Right) Small molecule drug: aspirin molecular structure approximately 180 molecular weight. (approximate - not drawn to scale)

thus eliminate the potential for rejection by the human immune system of an antibody from a mouse species. As of 2013, a total of 33 mAbs were approved by the FDA as biologics for a variety of therapeutic targets. Because mAbs are specific enough to allow targeting of unhealthy cells without harm to healthy cells, they have been particularly important in fighting cancer, and more recently, have shown great promise for autoimmune diseases such as rheumatoid arthritis. Two successful monoclonal antibody biologics include Herceptin® produced by Genentech/Roche, which is a humanized mAb used in the treatment of certain types of breast cancer, and Remicade® manufactured by Centocor/Janssen, which is a human mAb that binds and neutralizes TNF-alpha, an inflammatory cytokine overproduced in rheumatoid arthritis.

Human Monoclonal Antibody Products in Development

Other important human mAbs are in clinical testing with great promise. A mAb has been designed to block the protein cytokine messenger interlukin-13 (IL-13) that communicates between cells and triggers inflammation in the airways which is a key mechanism of asthma, a condition suffered by over 25 million Americans, including 7.1 million children.[c] Another mAb in development is targeted to interleukin-17 (IL-17), a cytokine involved in the inflammation process of psoriasis. Another mAb, which is FDA approved for cancer treatment, targets the epidermal growth factor (EGFR) linked to the growth of many types of cancer. Originally, this mAb was FDA approved for the treatment of certain metastatic colorectal cancers, but additional clinical studies have found that the absence of certain gene mutations could predict a patient's response to this treatment. About 65 percent of patients without this gene mutation are likely to benefit from this treatment.

Vaccines as Biologics

Vaccines have been utilized as early as 1796 when Edward Jenner discovered that by injecting cowpox into an individual, he could create immunity to smallpox, the devastating viral disease that is now considered to be eradicated. Later, in 1885, Louis Pasteur successfully developed the first rabies vaccine. Since then vaccines have been developed against diphtheria, tetanus, anthrax, cholera, plague, typhoid, and tuberculosis. The premise is that small amounts of attenuated infectious agents injected into the body can stimulate the natural immune system to develop immunity to these organisms and prevent future disease. Through biotechnology, vaccines are now being developed for HIV and even used as therapies for the treatment of cancer.

c. American Lung Association.

Therapeutic Vaccines

Therapeutic vaccines utilize a patient's own immune system to fight an existing disease rather than immunizing for protection against future disease. In 2010 the U.S. FDA approved the first therapeutic vaccine, Provenge®, manufactured by the Dendron Corporation, a novel method for treating prostate cancer. The treatment involves taking a patient's own white blood cells and using a drug that trains them to more actively attack cancer cells. The patient's white blood cells are collected and certain immune cells are isolated. The cells are then incubated with a protein often found on prostate tumors combined with an immune system booster. The treated cells are then infused back into the patient three times over the course of a month. Provenge® is intended for men whose prostate cancer has spread throughout the body and it is personalized for each patient.

A virus-based therapeutic vaccine for the treatment of melanoma is also in clinical development. This product is a genetically modified virus that replicates only in tumor cells and expresses an immune-stimulating protein that causes the death of cancer cells and stimulates the immune system to destroy other cancer cells. This therapeutic vaccine trains the immune system to recognize and eliminate the cancer cells while not harming normal cells.

Stem Cell Therapy

Stem cells are unique from other cells within the body. Stem cells are undifferentiated and have the potential to become any other specialized cell within the body, and does so based upon various signals internal and external to the cell. Stem cells also act as a repair system for the body to replenish body tissues as cell turnover occurs. They have the capacity to divide for long periods of time and they retain their ability to make all cell types within the body. All stem cells—regardless of their source—have three general properties: they are capable of dividing and renewing themselves for long periods; they are unspecialized; and they can give rise to specialized cell types.

There are two origins of stem cells:

1. **Embryonic stem cells** (ES) are isolated from tissues of a developing human fetus during the blastocyst phase of embryological development.
2. **Adult stem cells** or **somatic stem cells**, are isolated from tissues of the adult body. Bone marrow is the most common source and is rich with stem cells that can be used to treat certain blood diseases and cancers.

The stem cell controversy is the ethical debate primarily concerning the creation, treatment, and destruction of human embryos incident to research involving embryonic stem cells. An important point is that not all stem cell research involves the creation, use, or destruction of human embryos as there are adult stem cells, amniotic stem cells, and induced-pluripotent stem cells which do not involve human embryos and are providing discoveries and answers for human health treatments. Stem cell research is rapidly advancing and may soon result in treatments for Parkinson's disease, diabetes, cerebral palsy, heart disease, and many other chronic conditions.

In 2006, Professor Shinya Yamanaka's team at Kyoto University demonstrated that it is possible to reprogram a mature adult cell to take on the properties of an embryonic stem cell. These cells are termed induced pluripotent (not fixed and capable of developing into other cell types) stem cells, or iPS cells, which provide an unlimited source of pluripotent stem cells for adult tissues and have no associated ethical issues. This potential, together with the possibility of deriving stem cells from any individual, has tremendous therapeutic applications from drug screening to regenerative medicine. (See Figure 9.5.)

Gene Therapy

Gene therapy is the insertion of genes into an individual's cells and tissues to treat or prevent disease instead of using drugs or surgery. In gene therapy, DNA is packaged into a "vector," which is used to get the DNA inside cells within the body. Once inside, the DNA becomes expressed by the cell resulting in the production of a therapeutic protein, which in turn treats the patient's disease. One gene therapy employs an adeno-associated virus (AAV) as a vector to deliver to the gene neurturin which has been found to restore cells damaged in Parkinson's patients and protect them from further degeneration. The first FDA-approved gene therapy experiment

in the United States occurred in 1990 for the treatment of ADA-SCID, Adenosine Deaminase deficiency, an inherited disorder that damages the immune system and causes severe combined immunodeficiency (SCID). Individuals with SCID lack immune protection from bacteria, viruses, and fungi. Subsequently, over 1700 clinical trials have been conducted using a number of techniques for gene therapy. (See Figure 9.6.)

Although gene therapy technology is still in its infancy and has experienced some failures, it has also been used with some success. Different forms of gene therapy include:

- Replacing a mutated gene that causes disease with a healthy copy of the gene.
- Inactivating, or "knocking out," a mutated gene that is functioning improperly.
- Introducing a new gene into the body to help fight a particular disease.
- Introducing a DNA-encoding therapeutic protein drug (rather than a natural human gene) to provide treatment.

Currently, gene therapy is only being tested for the treatment of diseases that have no other cures. Gene therapy holds promise for a number of diseases including inherited disorders, certain types of cancer, and certain viral infections. Gene therapy still has risks and more clinical trials are underway to be sure that it will be safe and effective.

RNA Interference

RNA interference (RNAi) is a process in which RNAi molecules are used to inhibit gene expression. Specific RNAi sequences are introduced into the cell which binds to and destroys its mRNA target. RNAi molecules can either increase or decrease a gene's activity, for example by preventing an mRNA from producing a protein or by blocking an expression inhibitor. Potentially any disease-causing

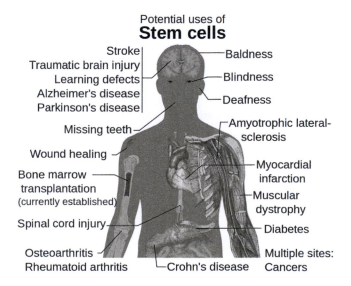

FIGURE 9.5 Potential uses of stem cells. (*Source: Wikipedia.*)

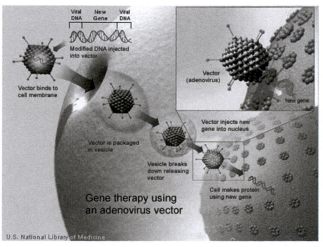

FIGURE 9.6 Example of viral-vector-based gene therapy. (*Source: U.S. National Library of Medicine.*)

gene, cell type, or tissue can be targeted with RNAi. The first major RNA therapeutic was approved by the FDA in 2013 designed to lower cholesterol for patients with a rare condition that leads to very high cholesterol levels in their blood. The RNAi drug named mipomersen (Kynamro) was developed by Isis Pharmaceuticals under a 2008 partnership with Genzyme, now a part of the French Pharmaceutical company, Sanofi.

As of 2013 there were over 50 companies and partners developing over 75 RNA interference drugs. One RNAi therapeutic in development targets Duchenne muscular dystrophy (DMD), a recessive X-linked form of muscular dystrophy, afflicting 1 in 3500 newborn boys and is the most severe form of muscular dystrophy in childhood. Early clinical trials of the drug have demonstrated improved expression of the dystrophin protein which is associated with skeletal muscle cells and is absent in Duchenne muscular dystrophy. RNA interference may provide novel therapies for patients, especially those with genetic disorders.

Regulation of Biologics

In the United States, most biologics are regulated by the FDA through the Center for Biologics Evaluation and Research (CBER), whereas small molecule therapeutics are regulated by the Center for Drug Evaluation and Research (CDER). However, in 2003 the FDA transferred responsibility of certain biologics from CBER to CDER. The biologic products that are now regulated under CDER include monoclonal antibodies for *in vivo* use, proteins intended for therapeutic use, including cytokines and enzymes, and immunomodulators such as proteins and peptides intended to treat disease. The types of biologics that remain regulated by CBER include cellular products such as whole cells and cell fragments, gene therapy products, human gene therapy; vaccines and vaccine-associated products; allergenic extracts used for the diagnosis and treatment of allergic diseases and allergen patch tests; blood and blood components such as albumin, immunoglobulins, and clotting factors to name a few. It is important to recognize that regulatory requirements and pathways continuously change, and it is incumbent upon the leader to understand current regulations and pathways for regulatory approval of their product in all countries where you intend to commercialize your product. Similar to traditional "therapeutics" described in the above section, the timeframe for biologic product development from idea to commercialization can require 12 to 15 years and cost upwards of $1.3 billion. Even though the costs are high and the time for development is lengthy, the value and potential payout for successful biologics is significant. Interestingly, of the top five therapeutic sales in 2012, four were biologics and three of the four were human monoclonal antibodies (Table 9.3).

Diagnostics

Diagnostics encompass a broad range of tests and testing methods. The most common term used to describe this product sector is "*in vitro* diagnostics" or IVD. The word "*in vitro*" is a Latin term that means "in glass" and refers to the test tube experimentation of samples taken and tested outside of the body, as opposed to "*in vivo*" or "in life" or in the body. The entire diagnostic testing sector is often referred to as the "*in vitro* diagnostic industry." There are many subsectors of *in vitro* diagnostic products and they can be categorized by the method that is utilized for testing (kits versus services), the purpose of the results (diagnostic versus predictive versus prognostic), whether they are paired with a specific treatment (companion diagnostics), or by the targets that they identify (molecules versus genetics versus epigenetics). More industry focus is being directed towards identifying better, faster, and more novel diagnostic methods.

TABLE 9.3 Top Five Therapeutic Annual Sales, 2012

Drug Name	Type of Product	Manufacturer	Therapeutic Category	Estimated Worldwide Sales
Humira	Human monoclonal antibody	Abbott Laboratories/Eisai	Anti-inflammatory	$9.48 billion
Enbrel	Human fusion protein	Amgen/Pfizer/Takeda	Anti- inflammatory	$8.37 billion
Advair/Seretide	Corticosteroid and beta agonist	GlaxoSmithKline	Asthma	$8 billion
Remicade	Human monoclonal antibody	Johnson & Johnson/Merck/ Mitsubishi Tanabe Pharma	Anti-inflammatory	$7.67 billion
Rituxan	Human monoclonal antibody	Roche	Cancer treatment	$6.94 billion

In this section we will discuss:

- *In vitro* diagnostics
- Molecular diagnostics
- Predictive and prognostic diagnostics
- Companion diagnostics
- Personalized medicine
- CLIA laboratory clinical testing

Most all diagnostic testing operates by determining whether a molecule, a set of molecules, or certain biochemical markers are present, absent, altered, or in higher or lower quantities than would be expected in a "normal" person. These markers are often referred to as "analytes" which are the substance being analyzed in an assay. Most often the analyte(s) being measured, whether in the body or in a specimen taken from the body, is in very low quantity. Various analytical methods and techniques have been developed to detect the smallest quantity of these analytes. Some of the methods and techniques used for *in vitro* diagnostic testing have been adopted as detection platforms from the sector of research tools and reagents. There are a variety of detection and analytical methods. Some rely on complex and expensive equipment such as mass spectroscopy and flow-cytometers, whereas others rely on visual colorimetric reading called "lateral flow assays" providing a simple "yes" or "no" result (Figure 9.7). All diagnostic tests intend to provide results that will give a clinician more information to know how to appropriately treat and/or monitor a patient's condition and or/make a proper diagnosis.

Performance Measures for Diagnostics

Although healthcare costs of diagnostics comprise only about 2 percent of healthcare costs, interestingly, diagnostics direct about 70 percent of the treatment decision costs [5]. Because of this, it is important to understand the reliability and limits of diagnostic testing results. There are several performance characteristics used to assess the value of any diagnostic test. These measures allow direct comparison of one diagnostic test to another. Although these performance measures can often be confusing and difficult to understand, knowing the reliability limits of a diagnostic test will help one assess the value of the results. Below is a brief description of the most commonly used diagnostic performance measures. The

reader is encouraged to reference additional information about these and other diagnostic performance measures as it can also help you recognize opportunities for improvements in diagnostic testing methods.

1. **Sensitivity:** This refers to the percentage of individuals who tested positive *and indeed have* the disease or condition. For instance, if a diagnostic test has a sensitivity of 87 percent it means that 87 percent of the time (in the population tested) a positive test was observed when the individuals truly had the disease or condition. These are called "true positives." However, it also means that 13 percent of the time (in the population tested) individuals who had the disease or condition, *did not* show a positive test. These are called "false negatives."

2. **Specificity:** This refers to the percentage of individuals who tested negative *and did not have* the disease or condition. For instance if a diagnostic test has a specificity of 93 percent it means that 93 percent of the time (in the population tested) a negative test was observed when the individuals, indeed, did not have the disease or condition. These are called "true negatives." However, it also means that 7 percent of the time (in the population tested) individuals who did not have the disease or condition *did not* show a negative test. These are called "false positives."

Sensitivity and specificity are two important performance measures that help assess the reliability of a diagnostic test. Knowing these values helps the clinician make a more accurate clinical diagnosis because they understand how reliable (or unreliable) the testing results are. Two other performance measures can be calculated from the same information, and these include:

1. **Positive predictive value:** This refers to the chance (percent likelihood) that a positive test would be correct. In other words, it is the percent likelihood that an individual who receives a positive test truly *would have* the disease or condition.

2. **Negative predictive value:** This refers to the chance (percent likelihood) that a negative test would be correct. In other words, it is the percent likelihood that an individual who receives a negative test result *would not have* the disease or condition.

Understanding the Data

It is not uncommon to see the data used to calculate a diagnostic test's performance in a "two-by-two" (2 × 2) table with the total population of people (or specimens) used to determine these values. A 2 × 2 typically displays a comparison of the results between the diagnostic test of interest and a "gold standard" test. The gold standard is a test that is accepted to be the most accurate diagnostic measure

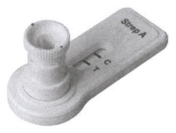

FIGURE 9.7 Lateral flow assay architecture and rapid strep test by AcuTest. (*Source: AcuTest.*)

currently available for that disease or condition irrespective of how difficult or how long it takes to perform. For instance, let's say you want to determine the performance measures of a new 15-minute point-of-care (POC) test to detect strep infections. Currently, for strep testing, the "gold standard" you would use for comparison is a laboratory culture confirmation test that would take 3 to 7 days to receive final results. The data from both of these tests would be presented in a 2 × 2 table with the sensitivity, specificity, and positive predictive and negative predictive values calculated based upon the formulas listed in Figure 9.8.

In Figure 9.9, you can see hypothetical data from our new point-of-care strep test compared to the culture confirmation gold standard. We hypothetically used 100

	Gold Standard Positive	Gold Standard Negative
New Test Positive	A	B
New Test Negative	C	D

Sensitivity = A/(A+C)
Specificity = D/(D+B)

Positive Predictive Value = A/(A+B)
Negative Predictive Value = D/(D+C)

FIGURE 9.8 Diagnostic 2 × 2 Table.

	Culture Confirmation Positive	Culture Conformation Negative
New Strep Test Positive	78	1
New Strep Test Negative	22	99

Tested with n=100 positives and n=100 negatives

New Point-of-Care Strep Test Sensitivity = 78/(78+22) = 78.0%
New Point-of-Care Strep Test Specificity = 99/(99+1) = 99.0%

Positive Predictive Value = 78/(78+1) = 98.7%
Negative Predictive Value = 99/(99+22) = 81.8%

FIGURE 9.9 Hypothetical point-of-care strep test data.

positive samples and 100 negative samples. Of the 100 positive samples (patients with the disease or condition), 78 produced positive results and 22 produced negative results in the new test; therefore the sensitivity is 78.0 percent. Of the 100 negative samples (patients without the disease or condition), 99 produced negative results and 1 produced positive results; therefore the specificity is 99.0 percent. The positive and negative predictive values are calculated as shown in Figure 9.9. A helpful reference for visually understanding diagnostic performance measures is "Understanding Sensitivity and Specificity with the Right Side of the Brain." [6]

Reliable diagnostic tests should have sensitivities and specificities in the high 80 percentile to the high 90 percentile in order for them to have significant utility. However, depending on the purpose of the test, and the alternatives available, some tests with lower specificity but high sensitivity may be utilized for rapid screening of individuals. In this type of usage, screened patients that had positive results would benefit from more accurate, or more costly and more invasive, testing. For instance, the PSA (prostate-specific antigen) blood test provides numeric scores of an individual's PSA level in the bloodstream. A cutoff score of 4.0 being positive has a reasonable sensitivity of 86 percent, whereas that cutoff is not highly specific for prostate cancer (specificity of 33 percent). What this means is that this test will generate a lot of "false positives" for individuals that really don't have prostate cancer. However, the relatively high sensitivity means that it will pick up most (86 percent) individuals who do indeed have prostate cancer. Although the specificity for current PSA testing is not great, it is an inexpensive monitoring diagnostic to identify potential prostate cancer patients who can later be screened with other tests and/or by biopsy. In applications like this, the subsequent tests are usually impractical, expensive, or unwarranted as a screening tool for the general population.

Incidence Rate and Prevalence Rate

Two values essential to properly evaluating the performance of a diagnostic test are the "*incidence rate*" and the "*prevalence rate*" of the disease or condition. Regulatory agencies will want to know these values because they affect the performance measures. If clinical testing was not performed in a manner that takes into account the disease prevalence rate, the calculated sensitivity and specificity may not be a reliable measure of the test's true performance in a real setting. For instance, if a disease or condition has a low prevalence rate, say 5 percent, meaning it is relatively infrequent among the population that will be tested, it is critical to also determine the performance measures using a similar frequency (5 percent) of positive samples. For example, suppose the sensitivity and specificity in a new test was calculated using 100 positive and 100 negative samples. If the new test only misdiagnosed 1 positive patient, this would not impact the sensitivity very much (99/100 = 99 percent sensitivity). Whereas if you clinically tested only 5 positive samples and misdiagnosed 1 positive sample, this would *significantly* impact the sensitivity results of the test (4/5 = 80 percent sensitivity).

"*Incidence*" is the number of instances of the disease or condition that occurs in a specified population *during a given period of time* (such as annually). Whereas "*prevalence*" is the number of instances of a disease or condition in a specified population *at a designated time point*. These two terms may not seem very different, but they take into account the fact that individuals may recover or die from a disease or condition and are no longer counted in the disease prevalence (see Figure 9.10).

Predictive and Prognostic Testing

For tests that are not "diagnostic" in nature, but rather predictive or prognostic, the sensitivity and specificity calculations and methods utilized will be slightly different. The performance measures for these types of tests are still evolving because these test results are predictions of outcome or predictions of who will develop a disease or condition in the future. For the reader who wants to understand these predictive and prognostic tests better, a helpful reference to review is "Systematic Review of Prognostic Tests." [7] In simple terms, for these types of tests the main premise of "sensitivity" and "specificity" is still the same:

- **Sensitivity:** Did the test correctly identify or detect those that have the disease or condition (or later contract the disease or condition).
- **Specificity:** Did the test correctly identify or detect those that do not have the disease or condition (or did not contract the disease or condition).

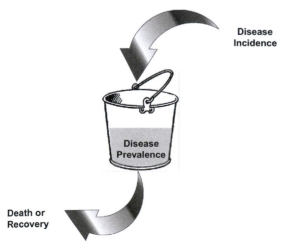

FIGURE 9.10 Disease incidence versus disease prevalence.

In Vitro Diagnostic Subsectors

The following are descriptions of the diagnostic *subsectors* and descriptions of these subcategories of diagnostic tests:

1. ***In vitro* diagnostics (IVDs):** As mentioned previously, this category can, in a general sense, include all IVDs. Broadly speaking, the FDA describes *in vitro* diagnostic products as *"those reagents, instruments, and systems intended for use in diagnosis of disease or other conditions, including a determination of the state of health, in order to cure, mitigate, treat, or prevent disease or its sequelae. Such products are intended for use in the collection, preparation, and examination of specimens taken from the human body."*[d] The size of the diagnostic market is large and growing. According to a 2013 Research and Markets report, the global IVD market was estimated at approximately $49 billion in 2012 and is expected to grow to over $69 billion by 2017. Factors likely to spur the growth include analytical laboratory automation, point-of-care testing, molecular diagnosis, immunoassays, hematology, flow cytometry, microbiology, and market expansion in emerging countries.

2. **Molecular diagnostics (MDx):** MDx comprises a category of diagnostics tests referring to the detection and analysis of nucleic acid molecules such as DNA or RNA that are used to provide clinical information. Although all IVDs measure or detect some type of "molecule," MDx is a specific category that detects and analyzes nucleic acids, DNA, and RNA as opposed to chemical, biochemical, and microbiological laboratory testing. MDx tests are available for detecting infectious diseases, cancer, genetic disease screening, human leukocyte antigen typing, coagulation, and personalized medicine.

MDx assay processes typically include:
- Extraction and purification of the nucleic acid from the sample (blood, saliva, urine, or other).
- Amplification, such as making copies of the nucleic acid of interest or attaching multiple copies of a dye to the nucleic acid.
- Detection of the amplified target using a detection platform such as real-time polymerase chain reaction (rtPCR) or end product detection including microarray platforms or DNA chips such as illumina, Agilent, Affymetirx, or flow cytometry platforms such as Luminex or various sequencing platforms.

MDx testing can be subcategorized into:
- Direct-to-consumer (DTC) tests
- Physician-ordered tests

d. Described in 21 CFR 809.3.

These categories are based upon who can order and have access to these tests. Some MDx testing companies have a business focus on DTC testing. DTC tests are generally available over the internet and *do not* require a physician to order the test, and the results go directly to the patient. Most DTC testing is performed and operated through a CLIA-certified laboratory (discussed below). As more DTC testing has become available, there have been heightened concerns by the FDA and other agencies due to the interpretation of the results and the perceived risks of some tests. Currently, there is debate on who has regulatory oversight for DTC, and no doubt there will be revised regulatory requirements soon. Conversely, physician-ordered MDx tests require a licensed physician order, and the results are sent to, and interpreted by, the physician. Although the risks for physician-ordered tests are lower than DTC testing, the same regulatory requirements may end up being applied to both. The FDA maintains a list of the FDA approved/cleared molecular diagnostic tests on their website.[e]

Medical diagnostic testing in the United States is typically paid by third-party insurance carriers and the coverage costs and coverage decisions for diagnostic tests are based upon the assigned Current Procedural Technology (CPT) codes. Beginning in early 2013, the CPT codes for MDx tests were revised and as a result there is current uncertainty surrounding the amount of reimbursement and the coverage for MDx testing (see Chapter 17 entitled "Biotechnology Product Coverage, Coding, and Reimbursement Strategies"). No doubt this will eventually be resolved; however, it reemphasizes the importance of understanding and planning for various reimbursement strategies at the beginning of any entrepreneurial endeavor.

MDx tests are categorized by the analyte measured, whereas the remaining subsectors of IVDs discussed below are categorized either by the test's purpose (prognostic or predictive), or by the method of delivery (clinical laboratory services), or by its utility (personalized medicine and companion diagnostics) rather than the analyte targeted. Because of this distinction, the remaining subsectors listed below may also include certain MDx tests if they provide the functional intent of that IVD subsector.

3. **Prognostic and predictive diagnostics:** A *prognostic test* provides information about the patient's overall disease outcome, regardless of therapy. In other words, the results tell about the likely outcome of the disease in that individual. For instance, the Prolaris®[f] test developed by Myriad Genetics for the prognosis of prostate cancer in patients that are newly diagnosed, examines an "expression signature" consisting of 31 cell cycle genes

and 15 normal genes. An expression score (Prolaris score) is provided that indicates the likelihood of prostate cancer progression based upon its genetic makeup. Whereas a *predictive test* provides information about the likelihood of an individual contracting a future disease or condition based upon their genetics. For example, BRCAnalysis®, another test developed by Myriad Genetics, examines gene mutations in the BRCA1 and BRCA2 genes and estimates the risk of women with these mutations for developing breast cancer during their lifetime. The mutations in these genes are considered highly "penetrant," meaning a high proportion of individuals carrying a particular variant (allele or genotype) of this gene will also express the associated trait (phenotype). For example, if a particular gene or gene mutation has an 85 percent penetrance, it means that 85 percent of individuals with that mutation will develop the disease, while 15 percent will not. Because mutations in the BRCA 1 and BRCA 2 gene are considered to be highly penetrant, often, women testing positive for certain BRCA mutations adopt some proactive intervention such as more frequent screening with an MRI, or in some cases, prophylactic mastectomy.

4. **Companion diagnostics:** These are tests that are paired with a particular therapeutic. Companion diagnostics are developed and utilized specifically for determining whether one particular drug is appropriate, or could be the most effective, for treatment. Companion diagnostics are often developed in partnership with a therapeutic program, or more recently within a pharmaceutical company with the specific intent to provide a single test to determine if their particular treatment would be appropriate. More pharmaceutical companies are supporting programs for the development of a companion diagnostic as these tests can assist in assuring their therapeutic will be properly prescribed when the test is positive. For instance, Her-2 testing is a good example. If it is determined that a woman's breast cancer is overexpressing Her-2, this result indicates that Herceptin (a monoclonal antibody targeted to that receptor) would be appropriate for treatment and have a great likelihood of effectiveness. The FDA maintains a list of the approved/cleared companion diagnostics on their website.[g] The category of companion diagnostics is similar in some respects to the next subcategory of personalized medicine.

5. **Personalized medicine (PM):** This refers to diagnostic tests that can tailor a treatment to the needs of each person individually. Many PM diagnostics are based upon an examination of an individual's genetics, and tailors their therapeutic dosage and frequency based upon

e.   *http://www.fda.gov/MedicalDevices/ProductsandMedicalProcedures/ InVitroDiagnostics/ucm330711.htm.*

f. Prolaris and BRC Analysis is a registered trademark of Myriad Genetics.

g.   *http://www.fda.gov/medicalDevices/ProductsandMedicalProcedures/ InVitroDiagnostics/ucm301431.htm.*

their genetic results. The availability of rapid and cost-effective DNA sequencing, along with microarray DNA chips, have made it possible to identify a set of molecular markers or genomic signatures to produce a genetic fingerprint that correlates with effective treatment options. Some examples of PM diagnostics include a broad category of tests for determining single nucleotide polymorphisms (SNPs) such as those that occur in the P450 liver enzymes. The P450 liver enzymes affect a person's ability to process a number of different drugs. Certain individuals may carry particular SNP allele (genotype) within their P450 enzymes, and as a result, it affects their ability to metabolize certain drugs. These different SNPs are correlated with normal, increased, or decreased enzyme activity. Polymorphisms in the CYP2C9*2 and/or CYP2C9*3 liver enzyme genes have been associated with decreased warfarin metabolism. Warfarin is a medication used to treat blood clots such as in deep vein thrombosis or pulmonary embolus, and to prevent new clots from forming in your body which reduces the risk of a stroke or heart attack. As a result, in August 2007, the FDA approved an update to warfarin labeling that highlighted the use of genetic testing to improve initial estimates of warfarin dosing. Personalized medicine is a very broad category and includes all tests that identify specific treatments, or determine dosages of medicines, that are optimal for the individual taking them. Another term that refers to the practice of personalized medicine is the field of "pharmacogenomics." [8] By performing PM testing prior to administering certain drugs, a physician can tailor the therapeutic dosage for safer prescribing and the most effective results for that particular patient. Whereas the traditional medical practice is to wait for individuals to present with a disease and then be diagnosed, a key goal of personalized medicine is to identify an individual's risk of future diseases and prevent it by employing risk-mitigating programs and/or early detection where treatment outcomes may be the greatest (see Figure 9.11).

6. **CLIA laboratory clinical testing:** These are laboratory tests performed in a CLIA-certified (Clinical Laboratory Improvement Amendment) laboratory as a service,

rather than a diagnostic kit which is manufactured and sold to others who perform them. All laboratories perform diagnostic tests, but the majority of the tests they perform have been developed, validated, clinically tested, achieved regulatory approval, and manufactured by a company which sells them to others who perform them. Whereas some laboratories have developed highly specialized tests on their own, validated them, and possess the unique skills internally to perform them as a testing service. These are known as laboratory-developed tests (LDTs) and they are services performed by a *single* laboratory in the United States, the one that developed it. Some advantages of LDTs are that the development time and regulatory path are usually shorter and less costly. However, the disadvantages are that the testing can only be performed by one laboratory. Examples of LDTs include Myriad Genetic's BRCA-1 and BRCA-2 test for identifying mutations in these genes that predispose for breast cancer, and Genomic Health's OncoType Dx, a prognostic test to identify a genetic signature for determining the outcome of breast cancer in women.

Regulation of Laboratory-Developed Tests and CLIA Laboratory Services

In the United States, the regulation of laboratories performing diagnostic tests is the responsibility of the Center for Medicare and Medicaid Services (CMS) by authority of the Clinical Laboratory Improvement Amendments (CLIA) of 1988. This regulation differs from IVD regulation under the responsibility of the FDA. The Food, Drug, and Cosmetic Act is a set of laws passed by Congress in 1938 that refers to the distribution of products through interstate commerce which is regulated by the FDA. Technically, laboratory services are not "distributed through interstate commerce," and there is a debate about which agency has regulatory authority in the United States for laboratory-developed tests (LDTs). The FDA has maintained that they have regulatory authority over LDTs but have exercised "enforcement discretion" and in doing so have deferred enforcement. Due in part to the of the growing number of direct-to-consumer genetic testing laboratories that have operated under the CLIA regulations, and the potential safety risk

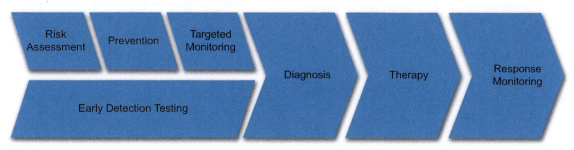

FIGURE 9.11 Personalized medicine goals. (*Source: Personalized Medicine Coalition.*)

to the public, the FDA is in the process of drafting clear regulations for LDTs. CMS operates under the Department of Health and Human Services (DHHS) and has issued a report on laboratory-developed molecular tests for the readers who are interested [9]. Recently, the FDA has coined the term "*in vitro* diagnostic multivariate index assay" (IVD-MIA) to describe a segment of the LDTs that they regulate. IVDMIAs are LDTs that have unknown or undisclosed methods for which the assay results are determined when multiple analytes are examined. Some IVDMIA tests have been successful in navigating through the FDA process and receiving regulatory clearance. An example of an IVDMIA cleared by the FDA in 2008 is AlloMap developed by XDx in Brisbane, California. This test uses a multigene expression microarray to analyze the gene expression profile of RNA isolated from peripheral blood mononuclear cells (PBMC). The results are an aid in the identification of heart transplant recipients who have a low probability of acute cellular rejection (ACR) to predict heart transplant rejection. The majority of laboratories offering IVDMIAs are not FDA cleared because at this time, clear regulations are not implemented, and these services are already compliant under the umbrella of a CLIA-certified laboratory. Based on the FDA draft guidance issued in July 2007, it is likely that some additional form of FDA regulation may be implemented in the future which may be in addition to the existing CLIA regulations already required of these laboratories.

Regulation of all In Vitro *Diagnostics*

Laboratory test systems that are sold by a manufacturer or developed by a laboratory are known as *in vitro* diagnostic devices and fall under the oversight of the Office of In Vitro Diagnostic Device Evaluation and Safety (OIVD) of the Center for Devices and Radiological Health. OIVD performs its premarket review efforts through three subordinate divisions of immunology (including hematology and pathology), microbiology, and chemistry. Premarket review of IVDs for infectious agents that involve the blood supply and for retroviral testing is usually performed within the Center for Biologics Evaluation and Research.

There are two primary routes to the marketplace for new IVDs and medical devices. These include:

- **Premarket notifications (PMN)** which are commonly referred to as "510(k)s" because it refers to that section of the law. A majority of new IVD assays enter the market through the 510(k) process.
- **Premarket approvals (PMAs).** This is a more lengthy and rigorous approval process compared to the 510(k) route. Products with greater safety risk to the public proceed through the PMA approval process.

The FDA terminology referring to commercialization and marketing approval is important to understand. Products that are authorized to be commercialized through the premarket notification route, or 510(k) route, are "cleared" for marketing. Products that reach commercialization via the PMA route are "approved" for marketing. This is an important distinction for the FDA and for labeling claims, as the FDA does not "approve" 510(k)s but rather determines them to be "substantially equivalent" to a product (a predicate device) that was placed on the market prior to May 28, 1976 (effective date of the Medical Device Amendments to the Food, Drug, and Cosmetics Act).

Regulation of IVDs through PMN and PMA allows the FDA to determine whether the device is equivalent to a device already on the market or on the market prior to 1976. Thus, "new" devices (not in commercial distribution prior to May 28, 1976) that have not been classified can be properly identified. Specifically, medical device manufacturers are required to submit a premarket notification if they intend to introduce a device into commercial distribution for the first time or reintroduce a device that will be significantly changed or modified to the extent that its safety or effectiveness could be affected. Such change or modification could relate to the design, material, chemical composition, energy source, manufacturing process, or intended use. More information is provided in Chapter 24 entitled "Development and Commercialization of *In Vitro* Diagnostics: Applications for Companion Diagnostics."

Medical Devices

A medical device is any item used to diagnose a medical condition, prevent illness, promote healing, prevent conception, alleviate incapacity, replace anatomy or physiological process, and is not a medicine, cosmetic, or a food. The legal definition of medical device within the Food Drug & Cosmetic Act is "...*an instrument, apparatus, implement, machine, contrivance, implant,* in vitro *reagent, or other similar or related article, including a component part, or accessory which is: recognized in the official National Formulary, or the United States Pharmacopoeia, or any supplement to them, intended for use in the diagnosis of disease or other conditions, or in the cure, mitigation, treatment, or prevention of disease, in man or other animals, or intended to affect the structure or any function of the body of man or other animals, and which does not achieve any of its primary intended purposes through chemical action within or on the body of man or other animals and which is not dependent upon being metabolized for the achievement of any of its primary intended purposes.*"

Examples of Medical Devices

There are a wide variety of medical devices, and many do not require biotechnology for their discovery and development. Products that are medical devices by classification

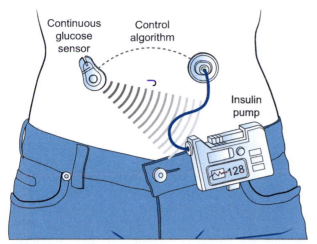

FIGURE 9.12 Integrated insulin pump with real-time glucose monitoring system. *(Image Source: Mayo Clinic.)*

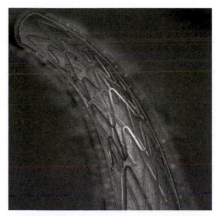

FIGURE 9.13 Combination device/therapeutic: drug-eluting stent. *(Source: Boston Scientific)*

include simple objects such as tongue depressors to complex machinery such as CAT scanners and X-ray imagers. Within the medical device industry there is a need for biotechnology applications to improve and create needed medical devices. Examples of medical devices that biotechnology is helping to create include integrated insulin pumps and monitors that simultaneously measure and monitor real-time glucose levels in the body and signal an insulin pump to administer the proper amount of insulin for maintenance of proper levels in diabetics. These medical devices function for insulin-dependent diabetics as a type of "artificial pancreas" where the individual does not need to manually test their blood sugar and inject insulin according to the blood glucose results (Figure 9.12).

Regulation of Medical Devices

The regulation of medical devices in the United States is through the FDA Center for Medical Device and Radiologic Health, the same center which regulates *in vitro* diagnostics. The FDA classifies medical devices into Class I, II, and III and regulatory control increases from Class I to Class III. The device classification regulation defines the regulatory requirements for a general device type. Most Class I devices are exempt from Premarket Notification 510(k); most Class II devices require Premarket Notification 510(k); and most Class III devices require Premarket Approval. In the UK, all medical devices that are placed on the market must comply with both European Union laws (the Medical Devices Directives and Regulations), and the UK laws (the Medical Devices Regulations). Each member state of the EU implements the Directives into their own national law.

Combination Device/Therapeutic Products

Combination devices result from the combining of medical devices with therapeutics into one product. The purpose of these devices is to enhance their effectiveness by including a therapeutic within, or in association with, the medical device. One such example of a combination device is a drug-eluting stent. Vascular stents (stainless-steel scaffolds) were created to improve the flow of blood through the blood vessels in patients with ischemic problems and arterial clogging. These stents were implanted and served the purpose, but they were found less than adequate over the longer treatment studies due to the risk of thrombosis or clotting of the stent by normal platelet aggregation. Coating the stent with platinum or gold did not seem to eliminate the problem either. However, companies found that by coating the stent with a platelet inhibitor that was released slowly (eluting) they could concentrate this drug at the site and reduce the formation of scar tissue and platelet aggregation. Today the drug-eluting stent business is approximately $4.5 billion, and operates in a product segment that did not exist about 20 years ago (Figure 9.13).

Regulation of Combination Devices

Because combination devices are considered both therapeutic and medical devices these are regulated by a section of the FDA that has access to both device and therapeutic reviewers. Combination devices require longer development times and greater amounts of capital to reach commercialization compared to typical medical devices. Combination products are assigned to a center at the FDA for review and regulation in accordance with the product's primary mode of action. When a product's primary mode of action is attributable to a type of biological product within CDER, the product will be assigned to CDER. Similarly, when a product's primary mode of action is attributable to a type of biological product assigned to CBER, the product will be assigned to CBER. For further information about combination products, see the Combination Products section[h] of the FDA website.

---

h. *http://www.fda.gov/CombinationProducts/default.htm.*

Research Tools and Reagents

The sector of research tools and reagents encompass a broad range of equipment and specialty reagents used for product development in the biotechnology industry and for academic research. The development costs for these products are typically less expensive than therapeutics, diagnostics and medical devices, and the development time is much shorter. In general, research tools and reagents are not required to receive regulatory approval from the FDA or international regulatory agencies prior to commercialization if they are used solely for research and not clinical or therapeutic purposes. The number of products within this sector are growing rapidly as they are an essential source of materials, supplies, and equipment that biotechnology companies rely upon for the development and testing of their products. Examples of some products that comprise this sector are: polymerase chain reaction (PCR) instruments, DNA sequencers, gene chip analyzers, multiplex readers using various forms of fluorescent cell sorting and laser reading devices, monoclonal antibody reagents, cytokines, cloning reagents and plasmids, and other specialty reagents used in biotechnology product development.

Sequencers

DNA sequencers play a vital role in the biotechnology industry. The ability to know the four-letter sequence of any gene or DNA segment is essential to conducting research and analyzing the genetics of individuals, organisms, plants, and animals. With the exponential improvements in sequencing DNA more rapidly and more cost effectively, there has been an explosion of genomic information which is giving us a greater understanding of disease. These astounding advances have made it possible to sequence the entire genome sequenced for about $1000 in less than a day. It is estimated that soon the cost for sequencing someone's genome can be done for about $100

and be completed within about 1 hour! Contrast this to the Human Genome Project which was launched in 1990 with multiple countries participating in sequencing the first human genome which took 15 years and cost about $3 billion.

The technology for sequencing has evolved since the initial work of Frederick Sanger in the mid-1970s, who developed techniques to sequence DNA using polyacrylamide gel electrophoresis and labeling to identify the four bases in sequence (see Figure 9.14).

With the automation of DNA sequencing in the 1980s, new methods have produced equipment that have been very effective in more rapidly sequencing DNA. Much research and development has continued to be directed toward improving the chemistry, automation, and instrumentation for DNA sequencing. The development costs and time associated with creating state-of-the art instruments can approach the lower range of costs typically associated with therapeutics.

One such example includes the Pacific Biosciences sequencer which can sequence long regions of DNA from a single DNA strand. The basic premise is a single DNA molecule is sequenced by a single polymerase molecule anchored at the bottom of a tiny micro well with a volume measured in zeptoliters (the SI unit for 10^{-21} liter). A strand of DNA is threaded to the polymerase while fluorescent labeled nucleotides are incorporated and individual color is detected when cleaved with the pyrophosphate group and a CCD camera takes video as the DNA gets polymerized (see Figure 9.15).

Microarrays

Many different methods have been developed for the study of gene interactions and gene recognition. These include microarray readers which allow the study of genes, so crucial to our understanding of the cell and its diseases (see Figure 9.16). A microarray is comprised of a small support structure, such as a small silicon wafer, on which thousands to millions of DNA sequences from different genes are attached to the support in different locations. Samples of an organism's DNA can then be incubated on the microarray and analyzed using colored florescent tags for the sequences to which they bind. These instrument readers combine chemistry, computer science, biology, and robotics, allowing us to study interactions of genes and genetic material at one time.

Regulation of Research Tools and Reagents

Because products in this category are not directly utilized as therapeutics, diagnostics, or medical devices and are primarily used in research applications, in general, there is no official regulatory approval required prior to commercialization of these products. However, there are two categories

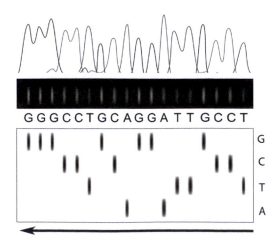

FIGURE 9.14   The Sanger method for sequencing DNA.

of reagents to be aware of, that have regulatory requirements and these are:

1. **Analyte-specific reagents (ASR).** These are raw material components or reagents used to develop assays intended for use in a diagnostic application using human biological specimens. ASRs are considered medical devices that are regulated by FDA [10].

2. **Research use only (RUO) and investigational use only (IUO).** RUO refers to a product in the laboratory research phase of development, and not represented as an IVD product. IUO refers to a product being shipped or delivered for testing prior to full commercial marketing (for example, for use on specimens derived from humans to compare the usefulness of the product with other products or procedures) [11].

The FDA has developed these reagent categories because some research reagents are utilized by companies in making their own diagnostic products or these products are utilized as an essential reagent in a diagnostic laboratory process. The primary objective was to ensure that laboratories received high-quality building blocks for their in-house-developed tests. In 1997, the FDA Center for Device and Radiologic Health (CDRH) published a final rule governing the use of ASRs in certain *in vitro* diagnostic products (IVDs) and in-house laboratory assays. Additional guidance documents have been published by the FDA since then, including: Commercially Distributed In Vitro Diagnostic Products Labeled for Research Use Only or Investigational Use Only: Frequently Asked Questions - Draft Guidance June 1, 2011 [12]. ASRs are only subject to regulation as medical devices when they are purchased by clinical laboratories for use in "Home Brews" or certain IVD tests. To control the use of ASRs, the FDA imposed a comprehensive set of restrictions. For example, ASRs may only be sold to: (1) diagnostic device manufacturers; (2) clinical laboratories

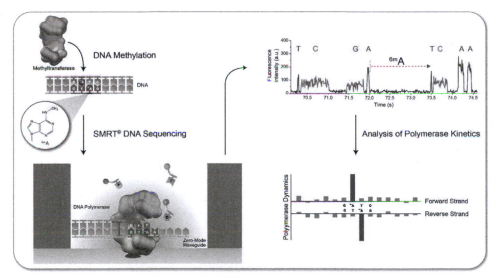

FIGURE 9.15 Pacific Biosciences sequencing method. *(Source: Pacific Biosciences)*

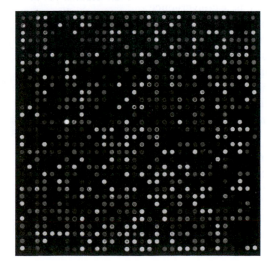

FIGURE 9.16 Microarrays. *(Image reprinted courtesy of Promega Corporation)*

that are CLIA-qualified to perform high-complexity testing or clinical laboratories regulated under the Veteran's Health Administration Directive; or (3) organizations that use the reagents to make tests for forensic, academic, research, and other nonclinical (nonmedical) uses. In addition, ASRs may be sold only for use in home-brew tests that are ordered on a prescription basis. Additional information can be found on the FDA website.[i]

The basic requirements of IUO are that all labeling for "a product being shipped or delivered for product testing prior to full commercial marketing (for example, for use on specimens derived from humans to compare the usefulness of the product with other products or procedures which are in current use or recognized as useful)" must bear the statement, prominently placed: "*For Investigational Use Only. The performance characteristics of this product have not been established.*" To be RUO, a product must be in the laboratory research phase of development and not represented as an effective *in vitro* diagnostic product. In addition, all labeling must bear the statement, prominently placed: "*For Research Use Only. Not for use in diagnostic procedures.*" Additionally, the FDA also advises manufacturers of products labeled as RUO or IUO that if they discover that one of their customers is a clinical laboratory using these IUO- or RUO-labeled products for a noninvestigational diagnostic use, "it should halt sales for such use or comply with FDA regulations for IVD products, including premarket review requirements." For more information see the FDA website.[j]

Digital Health and Healthcare Delivery IT

Digital health applications in biotechnology are diverse and expanding. With the ubiquitous nature of digital IT technology available at our fingertips and the adoption of digital IT technology in the medical and healthcare setting, more opportunities are created utilizing some aspect of biotechnology. This growing sector is a convergence of IT technologies and life science problems. Mandatory compliance in the United States for making healthcare records readily available to patients and the conversion of medical records to digital format have affected the way test results are delivered and the features imbedded within medical device products. Although every digital health and healthcare delivery IT application does not

necessarily utilize biotechnology processes per se, but they may involve biotechnology to develop, or it may lead to the utilzation of biotechnology products. As 77 million aging "baby boomers" require healthcare and maintain more active lives, more pressure has been placed on keeping healthcare costs from rising out of control. Integration of medical devices and digital health applications are one way of rapidly delivering and efficiently making healthcare decisions quicker and providing more efficient healthcare cost management.

Examples of Products

Many digital health products are methods that allow mobility and access to testing that previously could only be performed in a hospital or healthcare setting. Today, with the advancement of "smart phones" and advanced materials, an arrhythmia patient can monitor, store, and transmit their electrocardiogram (ECG) directly to their doctor in real-time from anywhere in the world. A product developed by AliveCor utilizes conductive materials, wireless transmitters in a phone case, and sophisticated programming to create an FDA-cleared product called AliveCor Heart Monitor (see Figure 9.17).

Regulation of Digital Health Products

The regulation of digital health products is determined by their usage and their claims. If a digital health product is used for, or has claims that include, diagnosis or treatment of a disease or condition, or any other claim that is listed above in the medical device section, these products will be regulated by the FDA under the same processes as therapeutics, medical devices, and diagnostics. However, if diagnosis or treatment claims are not made for these same products, FDA regulation is not required. The requirements for how these products are regulated is based upon their claims. As an example, the AliveCore ECG product was originally commercialized without a claim of usage for human health diagnosis or monitoring, but rather for a veterinary-use product. During this time the company simultaneously conducted human clinical testing and completed the necessary regulatory requirements to ultimately receive

---

i. "Guidance for Industry and FDA Staff—Commercially Distributed Analyte-Specific Reagents (ASRs): Frequently Asked Questions," FDA (Rockville, MD: 2007 [cited 22 February 2008]); available from the Internet: *http://www.fda.gov/medicaldevices/deviceregulationandguidance/guidancedocuments/ucm078423.htm.*

j. Distribution of *In Vitro* Diagnostic Products Labeled for Research Use Only or Investigational Use Only" November 25, 2013 at: *http://www.fda.gov/medicaldevices/deviceregulationandguidance/guidancedocuments/ucm253307.htm.*

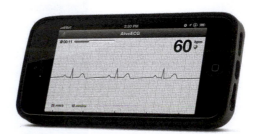

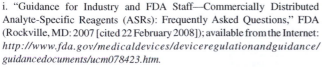

FIGURE 9.17   AliveCor Heart Monitor (digital ECG). (*Source: AliveCore, LLC.*)

a 510(k) marketing clearance from the FDA for its claims for human ECG monitoring.

BioAgriculture

Bioagriculture, or "BioAg," refers to the use of biotechnology in agricultural products (Figure 9.18). Some BioAg applications include creating crops with increased yields and insect resistance, developing biological pesticides, and microbial fertility enhancers to naturally produce healthier crops and improved yields. The benefits associated with bioagriculture not only help the farmer, but also the environment and end-consumers. For centuries, farmers have made improvements to crops through selective breeding and hybridization by controlling pollination of plants. Agricultural biotechnology is an extension of plant breeding by using genetic engineering tools to transfer beneficial traits in a more precise, controlled manner.

Bioagricultural products can be divided into three major sectors: seeds, agrochemicals, and fertilizers. The seed sector is focused on crops such as corn, soybean, and cotton to improve these varieties through breeding applications, and now through adding or modifying biotech traits. The agrochemical products include combination of a biotech trait such as herbicide tolerance and crop protection along with novel herbicides based on new targets for herbicide screening. The fertilizer sector remains a commodity sector that awaits novel products that can reduce the amount of fertilizer required or increase the nitrogen uptake of crops. This opportunity awaits novel biotechnology products that lower fertilizer requirements which would result in reduced nitrogen pollution.

The benefits of agricultural biotechnology go beyond just the farmer to include consumers and also the environment. BioAg helps the farmers by providing more cost-effective crops with lowered maintenance costs. The consumers benefit from an affordable, abundant, and safe food supply. Some examples include foods with enhanced nutrition such as tomatoes enriched with the antioxidant lycopene, rice enriched with beta-carotene (the precursor to vitamin A), cooking oils with higher levels of vitamin E,

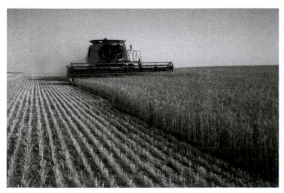

FIGURE 9.18   BioAg.

lower levels of trans-fatty acids, and increased amounts of omega-3 fatty acids. BioAg helps the environment by the utilization of less pesticides and lowered tillage needs for crop production which decreases soil erosion.

There has been controversy in some areas of agricultural biotechnology for certain products, with the predominant issue being the concept of genetically-altered food products. Like any other aspect of technology and science, including therapeutics, there are safety precautions and safety testing requirements that are performed prior to the introduction of any biotechnology product into the market. It is important for the reader and consumers to understand the issues when drawing conclusions about BioAg products. In some instances, certain BioAg products are equivalent to the way farmers and ranchers previously selected the best crops and breeds of animals, but without having to wait for stronger breeds and more hardy crops to spontaneously emerge. For more information on BioAg products see Chapter 11 entitled "Commercialization of BioAgricultural Products" which provides more information on this growing and expanding sector.

Regulation of BioAgriculture Products

BioAg products potentially have three agencies in the United States that can require approval prior to commercialization depending upon the product's use and potential safety concerns. These regulatory agencies include the Environmental Protection Agency (EPA), the Department of Agriculture (USDA), and the Food and Drug Administration (FDA).

BioFuels

Biofuels are important for a variety of reasons. The energy we use for transportation is dependent on a limited amount of fossil fuels such as oil and petroleum. Biofuels can offer an energy fuel resource that is both renewable and sustainable. Biofuels are fuels produced from living organisms such as plants or plant-derived materials and microalgae or from metabolic byproducts such as organic or food waste, often referred to as "biomass." Solar energy is first captured through photosynthesis by the plants and stored in the plants' cells. Biofuels are made by converting biomass into convenient energy containing substances in three different ways: thermal conversion, chemical conversion, and biochemical conversion. This biomass conversion can result as fuel in solid, liquid, or gas form. Another future advantage of biofuels is the reduced impact on the environment by the growth of plants used to produce biofuels. As these plants grow they absorb carbon dioxide in a process called photosynthesis. This absorbed carbon dioxide from future biofuel sources may one day balance the carbon dioxide emitted when the biofuel is combusted, thus creating a

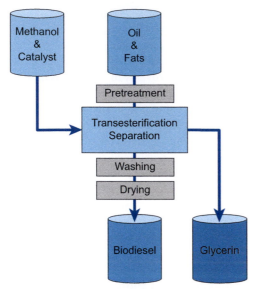

FIGURE 9.19   Production of Biodiesel. © *Hielscher Ultrasonics - www.hielscher.com.*

smaller carbon footprint than oil. Biofuels have increased in popularity because of rising oil prices and the need for energy security.

Biofuels can be categorized into the following:

- **Ethanol:** Primarily used in cars, ethanol is a type of alcohol and is most commonly made from corn or sugarcane and is based on sugars.
- **Biodiesel:** A substitute for diesel fuel, which is used mostly in trucks in the United States but is also being used in an increasing number of diesel cars. Most commonly made from soybeans and is based on oils.
- **Other biomass:** Mostly used for the generation of electricity or heat. Examples: burning wood chips to boil water and create steam, which spins turbines and creates electricity; and collecting methane from manure piles to generate heat or electricity.

Bioethanol

Bioethanol is alcohol made by fermentation typically from carbohydrates produced in sugar or starch crops such as corn or sugarcane. Biomass, derived from cellulose and nonfood sources, such as trees and grasses, is also being developed as a feedstock for ethanol production. Although ethanol can be used as a fuel for vehicles in its pure form, it is usually used as a gasoline additive to increase octane and reduce vehicle emissions.

Biodiesel

Biodiesel is made from vegetable oils and animal fats by a chemical modification process called transesterification (see Figure 9.19). Although biodiesel can be used as a fuel

for vehicles in its pure form, it is usually used as a diesel additive to reduce levels of particulates, carbon monoxide, and hydrocarbons from diesel-powered vehicles. The world's largest biodiesel producer is the European Union with an estimated production in of over 50 percent of all biodiesel production in 2010. By 2050, the International Energy Agency has a goal for biofuels to meet more than a quarter of the world demand for transportation fuels to reduce our dependence on petroleum and coal.

Regulation of Biofuels

Most regulation of biofuels is through the Environmental Protection Agency in the United States whereas in the EU the regulations that impact the EU biofuels market are the Biofuels Directive, the EU Climate and Energy Package, and the Fuel Quality Directive (FQD). Because the needs, technology, and impact of biofuels continue to advance, the regulations will also be expected to change. As the availability and technology improve for production and utilization of biofuels so will the need to adopt less restrictive legislation for the development and commercialization of biofuels.

Industrial Biotechnology

Industrial biotechnology products are applications of biotechnology used for industrial purposes such as manufacturing and production of biomaterials. The application of biotechnology to industrial processes is transforming how we manufacture products but is also providing us with new products by using cells or components of cells like enzymes to generate industrially useful products. Industrial biotechnology is referred to the third wave of biotechnology, or as referred to in Europe as *"white biotechnology,"* whereas agricultural biotechnology is referred to as *"green biotechnology,"* and pharmaceutical and medical biotechnology is referred to as *"red biotechnology."*

For instance, industrial biotechnology has produced alternative industrial products that reduce pollution that has been a problem caused by the use of phosphates in laundry and dishwashing detergents. Biotechnology companies have developed enzymes that remove stains from clothing that work better than phosphates, thus enabling the replacement of a polluting material with a nonpolluting bio-based additive while improving the performance of the end product. This innovation has dramatically reduced phosphate-related algal blooms in surface waters around the globe and simultaneously enabled consumers to get their clothes cleaner with lower wash water temperatures and concomitant energy savings.

Mechanisms Involved in Industrial Biotechnology Products

A large portion of industrial biotechnology products makes use of enzymes which are involved in the metabolic

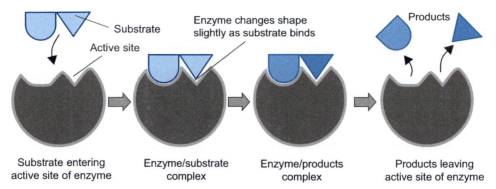

FIGURE 9.20 Enzyme reaction. *(By Tim Vickers.* Source*: Wikipedia.)*

processes of plants, animals, and humans. Enzymes are catalysts that speed chemical reactions which would take too long to accomplish normally. For example, proteases in our digestive tract are enzymes encoded by our DNA that rapidly break down proteins into their basic building blocks of amino acids from the food we eat. These building block amino acids in turn are used by other enzymes to create our body's own specific proteins. Biotechnology has utilized the genes that encode various important enzymes in plants, animals, and humans, and expressed these in large quantities to be used in industrial processes (see Figure 9.20.).

Examples of Uses of Industrial Enzymes

The capabilities of enzymes are utilized in washing and dishwashing machines. Proteases are incorporated into detergents to break down proteins responsible for soiling clothes while lipases (lipid enzymes) are added to remove fatty acid stains even at low temperatures. Enzymes have become important ingredients that reduce the energy and time required to clean with laundry and automatic dishwashing detergents. Other enzymes such as lactases (enzymes that break down lactose) are utilized in the dairy industry to turn milk, ice cream, and cheese into "lactose-free" products for those individuals who are lactose intolerant. Certain dairy enzymes are used to substitute animal-derived microbial rennets (a complex of enzymes produced in any mammalian stomach) to enhance and produce the robust flavors and textures in cheese and accelerate the ripening of naturally aged cheeses. Biotechnology has also provided a ready source of various microbial enzymes that accelerate the break down of waste products in sanitation and waste treatment plants.

Bio-based Materials

Industrial biotechnology processes are being employed to create bioplastics. Common plastics are based upon fossil fuels and are derived from petroleum and produce more greenhouse gas. Bioplastics are plastics derived from renewable biomass sources, such as vegetable fats and oils, corn starch, pea starch, or microbiota. One goal of bioplastics is to provide biodegradable bioplastics that can breakdown in either anaerobic or aerobic environments, depending on how they are manufactured. Some of the applications of bioplastics include packaging materials, dining utensils, food packaging materials, and insulation.

Regulatory Approval of Industrial Biotechnology Products

There is variation on what regulatory agency, or if any agency, requires approval of industrial biotechnology products prior to commercialization. Some agencies within the United States that may regulate industrial biotechnology products include the Food and Drug Administration (FDA), the Environmental Protection Agency (EPA), The U.S. Department of Agriculture (USDA), and others. Regulation is dependent on the product and the use of the product. For instance, products that are used in manufacturing of non-food items may not require approval, with the exception of the typical manufacturing process approvals and those that involve waste regulations from agencies such as the EPA. Whereas industrial biotechnology products such as enzymes that are used in food production may have a particular FDA route or compliance requirement since the FDA also regulates food products. Industrial biotechnology products in general do not have the lengthy or costly regulatory approvals that are encountered in the therapeutic, biologic, diagnostic, and medical device sectors. It is important, however, to determine what the standard regulatory route for commercialization is of any particular industrial biotechnology product for the United States and non-United States countries prior to beginning development.

SUMMARY

As you can see from the variety and number of products discussed, the biotechnology industry is diverse and encompasses a large number of sectors, each producing valuable products that contribute to improvements in human health, manufacturing, agriculture, and energy needs. The number of new product ideas are almost limitless as new biotechnology applications are being discovered continuously. Each of the various biotechnology sectors encompass products having distinctive costs, development timeframes, and regulatory requirements. Yet each sector yields unique products that are enabled or produced by biotechnology methods and tools. Biotechnology entrepreneurs will be well served by having a working knowledge of all these sectors. By understanding biotechnology solutions to problems in one sector, similar problems in another sector can be solved by incorporating ideas and solutions from other sectors. Should any of these sectors pique your interest, I suggest that you delve further into the broad array of opportunities and benefits of products within these diverse sectors.

REFERENCES

[1] http://www.fda.gov/RegulatoryInformation/Legislation/FederalFood-DrugandCosmeticActFDCAct/SignificantAmendmentstotheFDCAct/FoodandDrugAdministrationAmendmentsActof2007/FDAAAImplementationChart/ucm232402.htm.

[2] DeMasi JA, Grabowski HG. The Cost of Biopharmaceutical R&D: Is Biotech Different? Managerial Decis Econ 2007;28:469–79.

[3] Long G, Works J. Innovation in the Biopharmaceutical Pipeline: A Multidimensional View. The Analysis Group. *www.analysisgroup.com*; January 2013.

[4] Köhler G, Millstein C. Continuous Cultures of Fused Cells Secreting Antibody of Predefined Specificity. Nature August 7, 1975;256: 495–7.

[5] Aspinall M.G, Hamermesh R.G., "Realizing the Promise of Personalized Medicine". Harv Bus Rev October 2007;85(10): 108–17. 165.

[6] Loong T-W. Understanding Sensitivity and Specificity with the Right Side of the Brain. British Med J September 27, 2003;327(7417): 716–9.

[7] Rector TS, Taylor BC, Wilt TJ. Systematic Review of Prognostic Tests. J Gen Int Med 2012. Chaper 12. 27(Suppl. 1): 94–101.

[8] Kupiec T, Shimasaki CD. Pharmacogenomics. Remington: The Science and Practice of Pharmacy. 22nd ed. London: Pharmaceutical Press; 2013. [Chapter 57].

[9] Sun F, Bruening W, Uhl S, et al. Quality, Regulation and Clinical Utility of Laboratory-developed Molecular Tests. Rockville, MD: Agency for Healthcare Research and Quality; October 6, 2010.

[10] http://www.fda.gov/downloads/MedicalDevices/DeviceRegulation-andGuidance/GuidanceDocuments/ucm071269.pdf.

[11] http://www.fda.gov/downloads/MedicalDevices/DeviceRegulation-andGuidance/GuidanceDocuments/UCM376118.pdf.

[12] http://www.fda.gov/downloads/MedicalDevices/DeviceRegulation-andGuidance/GuidanceDocuments/UCM257460.pdf.

Chapter 10

Technology Opportunities: Evaluating the Idea

Craig Shimasaki, PhD, MBA

President & CEO, Moleculera Labs and BioSource Consulting Group, Oklahoma City, Oklahoma

Entrepreneurs in the biotechnology industry build companies based upon novel product ideas that they believe will be successful in providing value to a specific group of individuals. There are also venture capital firms that have a specific focus on identifying novel technology in which they form start-up companies themselves. How do they choose which technology concepts and product ideas may be destined for success, and which ones to reject because they may not be future winners? The answer to this question is important for entrepreneurs, company leaders and managers when determining which ideas have the best opportunity for success. This decision has long-term impact because a group of individuals will then commit an enormous amount of time and resources to the development of this product concept. The information in this chapter will provide you with a framework to more effectively evaluate new product technology ideas and understand how to assess the likelihood for future commercial success.

When one evaluates technology, an internal analysis must take place to determine whether or not the technology product concept is more than just a good research project but has potential as a valuable product. Any technology evaluation process must include an examination of the soundness of the science, an appraisal of the supporting scientific and medical literature, and an evaluation of the scientific and technical team who will be participating in the early development of the product. If the underlying technology and product concept is not sound, no amount of marketing, capital, and team talent can overcome flawed science. The research and discoveries that support the product concept must be able to stand up to criticism, naysayers, and pessimists, all of whom predictably appear when individuals move forward with a new idea. In order to complete a technology assessment, it must include more than just an examination of the technology and the research team. Once the underlying science is validated, before proceeding further, one must also evaluate whether or not this product concept will satisfy an unmet market need.

SOURCES OF BIOTECHOLOGY PRODUCT IDEAS

The majority of innovative biotechnology ideas can be traced back to basic research that began at an academic or research institution over the course of many years, possibly decades. If you examine the original source of most successful biotechnology products, you will find that the vast majority of them originated from basic research conducted by a scientist, professor, physician, or engineer at an academic or research institution. This is true because a fundamental goal of institutional research is the acquisition and discovery of new knowledge. Basic and academic research focuses on exploring new ideas, testing new concepts, and better understanding previously unknown processes in biology, science, and engineering. Unfortunately, for the commercially-minded, academic research objectives rarely include product development or commercialization goals. As you will learn in subsequent chapters about licensing and technology transfer processes at universities, increased efforts are being made to advance basic research ideas toward early stages of product development while they are still at these institutions. Nevertheless, academic and research institutions do not typically possess the depth of expertise in biotechnology product development, and are not well-equipped or experienced in assessing the potential for which technology concepts may become blockbuster products. Very few products have been fully developed within academic and research institutions. This is because their goals are not the same as in industry, and they possess limited experience in moving product concepts efficiently to product development and precommercialization prototypes. As a result, many good technology product concepts accumulate but lay dormant at these institutions.

RESEARCH TO COMMERCIALIZATION CHASM

A great chasm exists between the large body of excellent research conducted within the laboratories of academic and research institutions, and the translation of these ideas into commercial products. One reason for this chasm is that basic research expertise, and commercialization expertise, are segmented and the interface between these expertise-holders is rarely linked. While the best scientific research is most often conducted at top-notch academic and research institutions, the finest product development work is most often performed in commercial enterprises. These entities operate independently of each other and rarely overlap in any cross-functional way, and certainly not on a frequent basis. Because of this segmentation of expertise, knowledge, and ability, academic institutions may have as much as 75 percent of their entire patent portfolio sitting on their shelves with no commercial entity showing interest in these assets. During this time, these institutions are paying patent prosecution fees on pending applications and maintenance fees, translation fees, and taxes on intellectual property that remains on shelves unrecognized and unlicensed.

Because of this chasm and the abundance of technology opportunities, academic and research institutions are the best places for entrepreneurs to uncover myriads of great ideas for future biotechnology products. For those interested in pursuing a path of biotechnology entrepreneurship, one great way to "discover" potential product ideas is to talk with the staff and management at Technology Transfer Offices (TTOs) at various academic and research institutions, including federal laboratories. Here you can find some of the best life science, agricultural, and biofuel research being conducted. These institutions have numerous product opportunities for entrepreneurs who have the skill, seasoned experience, and drive to forge company opportunities based upon these technology and product concepts. When approaching a TTO, be sure to define the areas of technology expertise you are interested in, and the fields where you believe you can recruit experienced help for your product development.

Technology Transfer Offices Manage Large Portfolios of Intellectual Property

Although every academic and research institution and federal laboratory will admit that a chasm exists, it is not necessarily because the technology transfer officers are not actively soliciting potential suitors for their portfolio assets. Stanford University owns the Intellectual Property (IP) that became "Google" and in the early days attempted to out-license this IP to many of the web companies over a period of time. The inventors, then graduate students, Sergey Brin and Larry Page, were completing their Ph.D. work

and realized that none of the likely industry players were interested enough to license the IP. The inventors decided to commercialize the technology if no one else would. The TTO said that they were willing to grant a license, but they felt the pair did not really know much about commercialization. However, we all know the rest of the story.

Licensing offices at research and academic institutions are recognizing what methods work most effectively for out-licensing more of their technology assets. Stanford is one of the most prolific institutions in successfully licensing its technology and intellectual property to commercial entities. It is interesting to note that Stanford's Office of Technology Licensing (OTL) employs mostly technical staff with backgrounds in industry and often individuals with MBAs. The few J.D.'s they have on staff appear to be managing contracts rather than negotiating licenses. It has been said of the Stanford OTL office that while outside legal counsel is available, such oversight is not required if an agreement does not deviate from the university's standard practices of granting no warranty on an invention and total indemnification by the licensee. Ms. Katherine Ku has been the director of the Office of Technology Licensing since 1992. She came from a small biotechnology company and most of her associates have similar backgrounds. She has been quoted as saying "We feel we are a marketing office, not a legal office." The technical background and training of her staff have been effective in negotiating licensing agreements because successful negotiations require an understanding of the technology.

In an article by Laurence Fisher [1] about technology transfer offices, Jeffrey Labovitz, who was acting director of technology licensing at the University of California at San Francisco at the time said, "A lot of technology-transfer offices are built around patent attorneys, and they lead with the agreement as opposed to the deal, so it's very hard for them to negotiate." "Deal-making is very much a creative endeavor, so the more you know about the variables, the more creative you can be."

So Why the Gap?

I believe that there are many reasons for the accumulation of intellectual property at academic and research institutions in addition to those we discussed. These include:

1. Potential suitors who possess the ability to build a company around a technology may shy away from licensing an academic institution's IP because of the perceived, or real, issues that hamper their ability to quickly and economically license a technology from the institution.
2. The most likely licensee organizations for these patent assets may not be interested in acquiring outside technology because they have already devoted internal research and development (R&D) resources toward internal projects that already address their market interest.

3. Industry executives may not be aware of the diversity of IP opportunities available in academic, research, and federal laboratories, or they may not be willing to pay a license or royalty on future products that their company would commercialize.

4. The IP assets are based upon excellent technology concepts, but the product application chosen and tested by the scientist, engineer, or physician is not the ideal market opportunity because of existing competitive products in that market.

5. The TTO has the bulk of their resources focused on prosecuting patents currently filed with the Patent and Trademark Office (PTO) with limited resources remaining to find and solicit licensees for the IP technology they have.

6. The TTO may not have the resources or budget appropriations to hire the type of staff with the skills and expertise or the staff may not have the liberty to effectively negotiate deal structures that would attract the type of licensee partners needed for their assets.

7. Many first-time entrepreneurs that may be interested in the IP assets, do not have the skill set and experience to proceed with commercialization and may not demonstrate enough know-how for the institution to confidently license the technology to these individuals.

Because of these and other issues, the chasm remains. However, more TTOs are working to address these issues and facilitate the licensing of more of their IP assets to the best suitors. It still remains that commercial entities and entrepreneurial teams must avail themselves to these untapped opportunities because they possess the greatest ability to commercialize products from these IP assets. Together, the academic institutions and commercial entities and entrepreneurial teams must develop financial models that make licensing IP assets a viable alternative to conducting its own internal R&D. It is also helpful for entrepreneurs who are seeking to license technology from a particular institution to become acquainted with the individuals who are responsible for licensing technology. It is equally important for the potential licensee to outline their product development plans and how they intend to move a licensed product concept toward commercialization for the TTOs. There are plenty of good product ideas waiting for good homes, and TTOs will be receptive to hearing from entrepreneurs who have credible commercialization strategies.

EXPERIMENTAL PATHS: BASIC RESEARCH VERSUS TRANSLATIONAL RESEARCH

It is important to recognize that research conducted at academic research institutions by nature has a different goal than translational research performed at a biotechnology company. Academic research is performed for the purpose of gaining new knowledge, publishing discoveries, and securing grants to support further research, whereas translational research conducted at companies is performed to develop a useful product. To casual observers, academic research experiments can appear, on the surface, identical to translational research in commercial laboratories. However, basic research and translational (or applied) research programs differ markedly in their decisions on the types of experiments to be conducted and the time spent on a particular experimental direction. For instance, in basic and academic research, a team may discover a new mechanism for cell signaling that triggers a unique inflammatory response. Future research choices by the academic research scientist may include identifying the receptor, determining the crystal structure and protein sequence, elucidating the triggering mechanism for stimulation, and uncovering the precise step-wise cascade involved in this inflammatory process. However, the ultimate experiments for industry researchers would be to screen chemical compounds that inhibit this inflammatory process for the development of drugs to treat rheumatoid arthritis or other inflammatory conditions. Industry researchers do conduct similar types of experiments as do academic researchers, but the underlying purpose is different—so they can use this knowledge to ultimately produce a product. Because of the difference in goals, the entrepreneurial team or evaluator of the technology must see beyond the actual experiments and look for the best applications of this research. For instance, if the academic research has uncovered a new biological mechanism-of-action, ask the question, what potential applications would this mechanism-of-action have in other disease conditions, diagnostics, and for new medical devices? What other applications can this discovery be applied toward?

Although all academic universities and research institutions have large IP portfolios that are idle, the *research* that underlies this IP is not necessarily idle. It is the *commercial development of the product* that is idle because the scientist or professor will likely continue their focus on more basic research to uncover new discoveries and to better understand the science. This is where creative and experienced biotechnology entrepreneurs come in. There are vast technology opportunities housed within great academic institutions awaiting entrepreneurs who have the creative skill, technical expertise, and market understanding to develop desperately needed products. The academic research resource can be a treasure chest laden with valuable future biotechnology products. (See Table 10.1.)

TECHNOLOGY IS A SOLUTION SEEKING A PROBLEM TO SOLVE

Successful biotechnology entrepreneurs appreciate great scientific research, but what they keenly understand is that *technology is simply a solution seeking a problem to*

TABLE 10.1 Basic Research Versus Translational Research

	Basic Research	Translational Research
Driven by	Curiosity and questions	Developing useful products or services
Motivated by	Expanding and acquiring knowledge	Solving practical problems
Questions answered	How things work; why things work	What inventions can be developed using existing knowledge

solve. If the problem that the science and technology can solve is extremely significant, there will be great interest from customers with this unmet need. To the extent that the problem this technology solves is minor and insignificant, there will be limited customer interest. Most people are amazed at the remarkable advances in any technology field. And it is true that sophisticated, leading-edge technology can enamor us through its novelty, complexity, and the amazing things that the technology can do. However, entrepreneurs must be cautious that they do not become charmed by the technology and forget that the most critical aspect of any product's value is the *problem* that is solved. It is helpful to keep this in perspective by realizing that the customer is not principally interested in the technology or scientific method of how their problem is resolved, just that your product delivered its promise and their problem *is* solved.

HOW TO DETERMINE IF A PRODUCT CONCEPT IS WORTH PURSUING AS A COMPANY

There are many technology projects that are worthy. These projects usually have a product concept in mind that may have some value. However, the entrepreneur must determine if this is simply an interesting research project or can this establish the basis for a viable company? A research project will be considered successful if *the research idea is novel and the technology is interesting enough to be funded.* A company is not considered successful by only these criteria. Although the company's product development must also be funded, the resulting product must also provide enough value to a target market such that they would gladly purchase it and use it. Regrettably, young biotechnology companies are founded with the belief that success will follow if *the research idea is novel and the technology is interesting enough to be funded.* The criterion used for determining a successful research project is not the same criterion that produces a successful company. Research projects are considered successful if they complete their intended specific aims, whereas companies are only successful if they produce products that are successful in the market—the ultimate goals are different. The decision for the biotech entrepreneur is to carefully

assess the product idea and determine if it is simply a good research project or if it can become a great company. The decisions made when assessing the technology will result in product development that is either "doing things right" or "doing the right things." In other words, a company can be established upon *any* research project concept, but if the resulting product idea has limited market value, no amount of "right" method development or "right" project planning can change the absence of a true market need for the product.

Three Initial Criteria for Assessing Technology Product Opportunities

The biotech entrepreneur must carefully evaluate (1) the underlying science and (2) the future product concept in order to determine if it is worth pursuing. The third criteria is the people factor, which will be discussed at the end of this chapter. A scientific assessment of the technology is the first critical step and it is the foundation upon which a future company will be built. If the science is not sound then no matter how great the market interest is for such a product, it cannot be delivered. However, scientific assessment by itself will not predict the likelihood of product success. One must also evaluate the product market potential in order to determine if it has a basis for a viable business. Initially, the following criteria should be evaluated when considering a product concept or considering a technology license from an academic institution. The evaluation of future product concepts must not end with only these two criteria but incorporate additional factors such as the company business model and the five criteria for assessing a company which are discussed in Chapter 12 entitled "Understanding Biotechnology Business Models and Managing Risk." However, these two criteria should serve as the basis for the initial assessment of the science and product concept:

Initial Assessment Criteria for Technology and Product Concepts

1. Evaluate the underlying science and the technology.
2. Evaluate the product's perceived market potential.
3. Evaluate the people factor. (See Figure 10.1.)

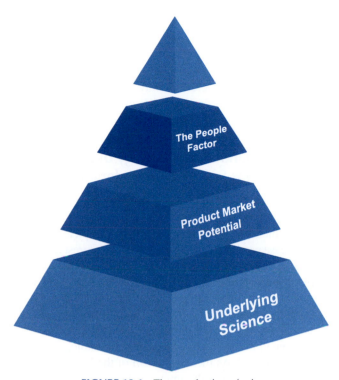

FIGURE 10.1 Three evaluation criteria.

EVALUATE THE UNDERLYING SCIENCE AND THE TECHNOLOGY TEAM

What aspects of the science and technology make it worth creating a company to support the development of this product idea? I believe there are several technology qualities that help determine its viability as a product concept. These include:

- The quality of the underlying research and the researcher's technical team.
- The degree of scientific information known about the disease or condition, or the understanding of the targeted application for the product.
- Whether or not a product is capable of being developed within the knowledge and systems available today.
- Whether this is a single product idea or a platform technology with multiple future product applications.

The Quality of the Underlying Science is Foundational

A thorough evaluation of the quality of the science and the underlying research is critical before making a decision to license or move forward with any product concept. Know that a major portion of a biotechnology company's early value is based on the science that underlies the product concept and the credentials of the inventors and researchers of the technology. Consequently, if the science is mediocre, the

company will not have much value. If the science is top-tier, then the company is perceived to possess a great asset. As the company achieves and reaches product development milestones, additional value is apportioned to the company based upon the improved likelihood that their product will be commercialized.

One good method to assess the quality of the science is by reviewing published articles on the research in peer-reviewed journals. The originating scientist, engineer, or physician can provide you with some references to begin your search. You don't need to be an expert in this research, but you do need to be able to glean whether or not the conclusions are supported by the basic tenets of the underlying research. It is also important to conduct a literature search for other researchers working in this field, as you may also find out whether others are further ahead, or if they have disproved the research conclusions. Find out to what extent others cite this inventor's research papers and whether or not the conclusions are generally believed and supported by others. One noteworthy point is that any new research concept that is a sharp departure from previous understanding is often resisted by others until enough research is published and many researchers are working in this field. When new or "radical" concepts are proposed in science, if they go against current understanding, they most often will be met with resistance. This was true for Stanley Prusiner and his proposed existence of nongenetic infectious agents called "prions." He was greatly criticized for his theory and his experiments that were later proved to be true, and he received the Nobel Prize in 1997. When peptic ulcers were proposed to be caused by bacteria, there were challenges in the medical and scientific community until enough scientific evidence supported this theory leading to the ultimate identification of *Helicobacter pylori*, the causative bacterial agent. Although countercurrent research arises, most ideas and scientific concepts are built upon stepwise and incremental research advancements expanded from previous discoveries in science, biology, medicine, engineering, or physics.

When conducting a review of the scientific research be sure to meet with the researchers and inventors themselves to assess the confidence they have in their research conclusions. Ask them about any conflicting research studies and whether the science has a controversial nature, and if so, what aspects. You can gain valuable insights by talking with them about their research. Another good way to assess the quality of the scientific research is to request to read grant applications that resulted in awards to the researchers. Also, find out how many grants and granting agencies have funded their research. Having been awarded multiple federal grants is a good indicator that both the researcher and the research are respected by their peers. In addition to the scientific review and meeting with the researchers, for medical products, you should have discussions with academic and medical opinion leaders who would be prescribing, testing with, or utilizing the proposed product. If the proposed product is in the agricultural biotechnology industry, ask farmers, consumers, and regulatory agencies for their impressions of such a product idea. Key opinion leaders' impressions of a new product concept can impact the receptivity by others in the industry. Be sure to assess the receptivity of the key opinion leaders when making a technology assessment.

If you are the inventor and you are also considering being the future entrepreneur, it is too difficult to objectively assess your own technology, so the best advice is to find assistance in obtaining an unbiased opinion about the technical merits of your research leading to your envisioned product. Most researchers tend to not be as critical of their own research as others may be, so it is advisable to recruit the help of others for feedback. If the research is performed at an academic or research institution, it is possible that your TTO may have conducted some type of technology evaluation when they were preparing invention disclosures or patent applications. If the institution does not have this type of assessment available, find a business person, consultant, or even another entrepreneur in a similar biotech sector who would be willing to assess the merit and likelihood of the research resulting in a viable product. This can help you decide whether or not to pursue the product concept, modify the product concept, or obtain a license for the technology.

The Quality of the Researcher and the Technical Team

Great scientific research is associated with talented researchers that are of high caliber and respected in the scientific community. Typically they will also have talented technicians, postdocs, and other researchers working in their laboratories. Practically speaking, the science and the scientists are not mutually exclusive. In other words, talented scientists tend to conduct impressive research. As you assess the science, you should also assess the quality of the research team who developed the underlying technology that supports the product concept you are considering. Often a good way to assess the team is to have face-to-face discussions, but when that is not possible, be sure to have plenty of telephone or video/Internet-based communications before making a decision to license a technology. Once you have concluded the underlying science is solid, and the research team is of high caliber, you must be sure that this team is willing to spend time working on the commercial application you are interested in developing. If there is limited time for this team to devote to product development due to research and teaching responsibilities, grant commitments, or other administrative duties, it will be challenging to get the momentum you need to move the company forward. In the beginning you critically need the expertise of the researchers who developed the technology so they can help train or transfer the technology to others who can continue translational development of the product.

The technology only remains viable so long as those who have developed it remain associated with its development in some capacity. It is imperative for a period of time to retain the inventors and researchers when negotiating any technology license. There are creative ways to work out arrangements with the discovering scientists even if they don't plan on being cofounders or employees of the company.

Be Sure the Underlying Biology of a Disease or Condition is Sufficiently Understood

For instance, in the medical sector, there are several technology concepts being advanced for the treatment of Alzheimer's disease, which is a debilitating albeit not completely understood disease process. There is great market interest and need for products to treat this disease condition. However, to the degree that any product correctly targets the true underlying cause, to that same degree the product will have a high likelihood of being successful. When HIV was first discovered for its association with AIDS in the early 1980s, the infectious cycle of the virus and our knowledge of immunology was not totally understood. As the mechanism of the HIV infectious cycle and its evasion of the immune system was elucidated, better and more effective treatments were developed. At the outset of any technology endeavor, you want to start with reasonable certainty that the future product is directed against the underlying pathway of the disease or condition.

Is Product Development Feasible Using Today's Knowledge and Systems?

Often a biotechnology product idea may appear initially intriguing, but as you delve deeper into the science and technology you may uncover many systems or method challenges that must also be overcome before the product can be developed. For instance, oral administration of peptide or protein-based drugs are typically degraded in the gut. If the market requires that this product must be orally administered but there is no delivery method available for the drug to become systemic except by intravenous injection, the rest of the product development process is moot. In another example, if you are developing a drug that works effectively in the brain but you do not have a method that permits it to cross the blood-brain barrier, the product development process is academic. Be sure that there is not a major road block in product development which cannot be solved or resolved by the knowledge and systems available today.

Is this a Single Product or a Core/Platform Technology with Multiple Products?

When assessing the technology, be sure to explore whether or not this is a single product or a technology platform that can produce multiple products. This may take some time to determine, but most product concepts in biotechnology have an underlying scientific basis that is applicable and transferrable to other applications. Spend some time to uncover the underlying scientific basis and work to identify additional product opportunities that have significant market value. Sometimes it is subtle which technology portion carries multiple applications. It is possible that the product development process may be the technology platform which can generate diverse products having related characteristics. For example, an innovative method for producing highly specific humanized monoclonal antibodies may be the core technology, and the original product application may be a treatment for glioblastoma. There are many other disease targets that would benefit from highly specific humanized monoclonal antibody treatments. In another example, the product application could be the development of a hepatitis vaccine, but the platform technology provides the ability to rapidly produce vaccines in mammalian cells in a fraction of the normal time. This process could be adapted to rapidly manufacture influenza vaccines for the next season's strain because part of the problem for flu vaccine manufacturers is to quickly generate product once the World Health Organization and the Centers for Disease Control predicts the next season's strain. For an example in the molecular testing industry, let's say that a product application is a combination of gene-signatures that predicts the recurrence of breast cancer. However, the know-how generated during the development of this product could be leveraged to rapidly develop another gene-signature for colon or prostate cancer recurrence. When you are searching for additional product applications, do not overlook the know-how generated during the development of the first product as an asset for accelerating other product opportunities. Often a single product application may have been the focus, but in reality all biotechnology products operate with an underlying scientific basis that enables that product application to work. The ability to attract investors increases with the likelihood that the technology can produce multiple products from the same research. Investor interest increases because they understand that follow-on products grow the future business, and a one-product company has limited long-term success. If the technology is absolutely limited to a single product, this does not mean the technology is second-rate, or that the company cannot raise capital for product development. In fact, if the product is successful, there is a high likelihood that this single product may find other uses the longer it remains in the market. Spend time talking to individuals in the field such as scientists, physicians, clinicians, medical specialists, hospital staff, and laboratory directors, because these discussions can help you identify additional useful applications even for a single product.

EVALUATING THE PRODUCT'S PERCEIVED MARKET POTENTIAL

When evaluating technology it is not uncommon to find that the research has a solid scientific basis, but sometimes the first product application is directed toward a subpar market or to a market that is already filled with competitive products adequately serving the customer's needs. To produce a successful product and company, the technology must be wisely applied to the best product opportunity that is directed toward an underserved market having a great need. The aspects of these criteria include:

1. Determining if the product application is directed toward an acute market need which is not currently being met or suitably addressed by other products or substitutes.
2. Determining whether the technology has the ability to deliver the market-needed product features.
3. Assessing if there is an existing reimbursement pathway for the product.
4. Assessing if the market is already saturated with multiple competitors having very little differentiation in value, even though all are meeting this need.

The Technology Must be Directed Toward a Product with the Greatest Market Need

As will be discussed in more detail in Chapter 16 entitled "Biotech Products and their Customers: Developing a Successful Market Strategy," understanding the market interest for a product is critical to the success of any biotechnology company. The choice of the first product application of any technology is key. Often biotechnology companies only get one chance to develop a product even though they may have a number of other good product applications using the same technology. A single product failure for a well-capitalized pharmaceutical company will quickly get shelved and another will take its place in development without missing much of a beat, whereas development-stage biotechnology companies do not have cash reserves to support multiple product development programs through to commercialization. If a biotechnology company's first product fails anywhere along the development path, they rarely can recover and have a second chance, irrespective of how great the other applications may be.

Ensuring that the first application of any technology is appropriately directed toward the best market is essential. For example, in the medical device and diagnostic sector there is an unmet need for assay methods to determine the most effective chemotherapeutic agent prior to the treatment of a patient's cancer. These chemosensitivity assays could serve a great need by predicting the most effective chemotherapy for a specific tumor biopsied from a patient without having to use treatment trial-and-error. Let's say the researcher developed a chemosensitivity test that works on a certain tumor tissue type, but the researcher selected a tumor tissue target based on the availability of tumors from collaborators, not based upon the market need (problem to be solved). This choice of a first product application may have been directed toward a suboptimal market. To explain, in some cancers there are only one or possibly two treatment choices that are effective, and a chemosensitivity device specifically targeted for that type of cancer would not solve a significant market problem. Whereas, if the device tests for a tumor type that has ten treatment options, all with varying degrees of success in different individuals, this would meet a significant market need. Be sure that the first product application of the technology is directed toward an unmet and significant need in the market.

Two additional criteria for evaluating the market potential of a product application include:

5. The acuteness of the market need for that product.
6. The competition or substitutes in the market now and in the near future.

These and other assessment criteria are essential to assess before starting a company or business based upon any product concept. Recognize that the greater the product market potential, the increased likelihood that the company can also raise the capital needed to fund development. When choosing a product concept to build a company upon, optimize your chances of success and minimize your risk of failure.

Is there Market Demand that is not Met or Addressed with Substitutes?

One key question to be answered before considering the licensing of any technology is, is there significant market demand that is not addressed by competitors or substitutes for this product? World-class technology directed toward a product that is only "useful" will not guarantee that anyone will want to purchase the product once it is developed. For many biotech entrepreneurs, the analysis of market need and substitutes does not always rise to significance at this early stage, even though it should. This is a grave mistake because the level of market interest in the product impacts a multitude of other issues—especially your ability to raise capital for the company. For example, suppose you find a novel licensing opportunity with a product application for peptides that possess powerful antibiotic properties against a limited number of gram-negative bacteria. The science may be novel and the results may be fantastic, yet there are dozens of antibiotics on the market (substitutes) that are very effective against gram-negative bacteria and certainly economical to use. This project's lackluster market appeal makes it difficult if not impossible, to generate much interest from biotech investors which hold the capital needed to develop any product through to commercialization.

However, suppose the same technology produces a peptide with antibiotic properties against methicillin-resistant staphylococcus aureus (MRSA). The market for such a product would be tremendous because of the lack of effective antibiotics that work against MRSA. Raising money for this product would be less difficult than the first. No matter how stellar, novel, exciting, or ground-breaking the science, if there is not a significant and acute market need for the resulting product which is not addressed by substitutes, the endeavor will be futile.

How Big is the Estimated Market for this Product?

Having a large market for a future product will help attract the type of investors needed to fund your product development. But there is also great interest in certain niche markets and especially those that can gain "orphan drug" status. If the product is for AgBiotech markets, the niche market strategy is not likely to be successful because of the low profit margins for most of these products. Regardless of where the technology is directed toward, whether it be AgBiotech, therapeutics, medical devices, molecular diagnostics, or industrial enzymes, be sure you know the size of the total market for this future product and the size of the "target" market which is the highest likely group of customers that have the most acute need for that product. In the end, an acute need for a product is even more important than the size of the market. The need for a product must be acute and unmet in order for a future product to have great success. The greater that the product features are needed, the greater the receptivity. Conversely, if the customers are satisfied with currently available products and substitutes, there will be minimal demand for your product.

When assessing the technology, determine if the proposed product features provide superior value to the target audience and that substitutes or alternatives are not already satisfying medical alternatives, or at least be sure the alternatives are inadequate or minimally effective in satisfying the needs of potential customers. This includes verifying that there is an existing unmet customer demand for this product because it is extremely difficult to sell a product for which you first have to create a demand. Successful products are launched to meet an existing unmet market need. If you must also create customer demand, that requires first educating the customer that they "need" the product when they don't know that they do. Creating market demand for a product is more difficult than producing a product that meets an existing unmet need.

Don't be Too Far Ahead of the Market Need

Because of the lengthy biotechnology product development time frame, it is good to anticipate future product market needs. However, there is a potential problem in being *too far ahead* of any market need because products take time to be accepted if they are too far ahead of a market need. Technology adoption, customer interest, medical practices, and societal norms constantly change, and it is difficult to predict where future demand will be far into the future. Premature products move very slowly along adoption curves. Sometimes these types of products may also create ethical concerns or face unknown consequences that would limit their market acceptance. For example, gene therapy has tremendous potential and should ultimately be effective for many debilitating conditions, but today it is too far ahead of medical adoption. Getting the timing right for a new product is just as important as choosing the right product application itself. Evaluate the market need for the future product before licensing any technology, and this will greatly improve your opportunity for success.

Is the Target Market Highly Competitive with Minimal Differentiation between Products?

You do not want to plan on entering a market that is currently saturated with products having minimal differentiating features because biotechnology products do not make good commodities. Biotech products are more complex, more expensive, and are breakthrough in nature. Companies with the most success potential are targeting markets where there are very few, if any, existing competitors, or they are targeting markets where competitor's products do not fully meet the customer's needs.

Is there a Reimbursement Pathway for the Product that is Readily Available and Accessible?

In the medical biotechnology industry there are typically three customers that must realize value in a product: the patient, the physician, and the payer. We discuss more about these three customers in Chapter 16 entitled "Biotech Products and their Customers: Developing a Successful Market Strategy." In order for a medical biotechnology product to be successful there needs to be a value proposition to the "payers" which is the third party that covers some or all of the cost of these products ordered by the physician and used on, or by, the patient. Because most countries have some form of a third-party payer system, it is critical to know if this payer system has a mechanism to cover the costs of your future product and that they would be willing and inclined to do so. More information about reimbursement issues is covered in Chapter 17 entitled "Biotechnology Product Coverage, Coding, and Reimbursement Strategies." Even though there may be an unmet market need for your product, if

there is not a reimbursement pathway that is available and accessible for your customers, this future product will have many challenges in the market.

THE PEOPLE FACTOR

Before you finally decide that you should proceed forward with this technology and product application, there is one intangible factor that also needs to be addressed and that is the "people factor," because it is the next critical predictor of success. What I mean by the people factor, is the "chemistry" between you and the stakeholders in the entire process and value chain of the technology development and the building of the company. This is something that is inwardly evaluated throughout the process when talking to the inventor, the research team, and others who are associated with the technology. This may include other individuals that have some authority and responsibility for which you will be dealing with throughout the development process.

In reality, the majority of the real know-how for any technology is not contained within the IP, but inherent within the inventor and their technical staff. If you can communicate well and understand the inventor and the technical staff, and they are enthusiastic about the commercialization of their research, this is a favorable sign. If it is challenging to communicate with the inventor and their staff, or to get answers to various issues, it is not likely to get much better when the pressure of meeting product development goals are added. The ability to communicate, work well, and to quickly resolve issues is important because there are a myriad of challenges a biotechnology entrepreneur will face during the product development, fundraising, and growth of the company. Therefore the quality of the interaction and the cohesiveness of the team is vital. If there are constant disagreements resulting in the inability to quickly resolve issues, these are what I call "artificial problems." These are internally generated issues among the team members instead of external issues between the team and the company environment. When artificial problems arise, they consume an inordinate amount of time and energy to resolve. Artificial problems detract from progress and reduce the ability to focus and resolve the true problems that face the company and its product development. The ability to work effectively and efficiently within the team is like glue for a woodworking project. You may hold all the right parts and pieces, but if they don't stick together, there will be no product. Knowing you can work well with all the stakeholders is an advantage and this will help accelerate rather than slow down the product development process.

It is rare, and highly unlikely, to find that all individuals within a group are happily cooperative and enthusiastic about every decision that is made. However, learn to recognize the situations and the individuals that create unresolvable disputes and insurmountable challenges. There are enough challenges you will face when developing a bio-technology product and building a company, so you don't want to add more by creating teams that are not meant to work together.

If you determine that the people factor is positive then before you are ready to move forward with licensing the technology, you need to have a discussion and agreement as to what level of involvement the inventors and research team will have. At a minimum, if the inventor and team are not part of the company, there needs to be an understanding that the inventors will consult for the company or possibly even conduct some product development activity within their own laboratory for a period of time, and for a fee.

WHAT TO DO NEXT?

Once you have made a decision to move forward with the technology concept and to obtain a license to the technology, you must then negotiate with the institution who owns the Intellectual Property (IP) rights. Academic institutions that conduct basic research have a Technology Transfer Office or Technology Licensing Office staffed with individuals who are trained to license their technology and to work out a deal with the licensee. As mentioned previously, there can be significant differences in the philosophies of various Technology Transfer Offices. There are standard terms and conditions when licensing technology but there are also terms that are negotiable. You may be able to find out what to expect in the deal terms from a particular institution by talking to others who have licensed technology previously from that institution. Additional information about licensing terms and licensing conventions are reviewed in Chapter 14 entitled "Licensing the Technology: Biotechnology Commercialization Strategies Using University and Federal Labs."

SUMMARY

The first step in starting a biotechnology endeavor is to be sure that the technology and product concept is foundationally sound and properly evaluated for the underlying science, literature support, and the inventor and technical team. This technology evaluation process is essential and determines whether or not the future product will provide true value to the target audience and whether the concept has a high likelihood of success scientifically. A detailed analysis of the scientific merit of a technology is essential for a scientific review. If the basic research conducted at a particular academic institution is reputable and known for excellence, the majority of their IP available for licensing should likely be of high quality. That is why one should always start with high quality and reputable institutions when seeking technology and future product concepts.

Of note, do not be misled into believing that high quality research automatically guarantees a useful or marketable biotechnology product. In other words, entrepreneurs should understand that *excellent research is not a surrogate for medically useful or marketable products*. There are multitudes of laboratories filled with excellent research, much of which never results in a successful biotechnology product. This is because there is more to producing a successful biotechnology product than conducting great science. The most successful products absolutely are predicated upon quality science; however, conducting quality science alone does not assure a successful biotechnology product. Spend adequate time evaluating the science and consulting industry and clinical experts in the field.

Next, the evaluation process must include an assessment of the future product's perceived value to the target audience. It is often the case that the technical staff and founders become enamored with the technology, but they must remember that *technology is simply a solution looking for a problem to solve*. If the problem that is selected is not because of a true unmet need, then there will be limited opportunity and interest in the future product. The final and most telling assessment is the people factor: the ability to effectively communicate each team member to address and resolve issues without creating "artificial problems" that are distracting and take away from the focus of the organization in reaching its goals.

We have discussed three initial criteria that are important when evaluating a technology product concept or idea: (1) the underlying science and technology; (2) the product's market potential: and (3) the people factor. These are critical when assessing any technology product idea and serve as the basis for screening potential technology product ideas. When considering building a company around technology owned by academic or research institutions, be sure to evaluate the underlying science, technology, and market application. When building a company and raising capital, the investor and interested partners are also looking at the product's value. If you build a company on sound science and the product addresses an acute unmet need, and the team can work together to quickly resolve problems, you will have minimized many of your early risks.

REFERENCE

[1] Fisher LM. The Innovation Incubator: Technology Transfer at Stanford University. Strategy+Business; October 1, 1998. http://www.strategy-business.com/article/13494.

Chapter 11

Commercialization of Bioagricultural Products

Neal Gutterson, PhD

President & CEO, Mendel Biotechnology, Hayward, California

It wasn't long after the early therapeutic biotechnology companies were founded that creative entrepreneurs began to develop agricultural applications of biotechnology. Not dissuaded by the lack of applicable technology, the first companies that developed biotechnology-derived crops were founded, even though methods for delivering stable DNA into plants had yet to be explored. A breakthrough came in 1983 when the first patent applications were filed on *Agrobacterium*-mediated delivery of DNA into dicotyledonous plants. *Agrobacterium* is a soil microbe commonly used to transfer DNA into plants such as a dicot, or a broad-leaved plant such as soybean and cotton. More importantly, broad patent applications for DNA delivery into monocotyledonous plants (such as corn, rice, and grasses) were not filed until the early 1990s.

At that time, I was finishing a post-doc at University of California Berkeley, and was interested in joining this emerging industry which was not yet a popular route for promising Ph.D. students in biochemistry. While I was very engaged with this emerging field and wanted to have an impact on this very practical problem, I would not have considered myself an entrepreneur. I simply wanted to apply science to solving pressing global challenges. I was influenced by the writings of Rachel Carson, whose *Silent Spring* [1] spoke to me, which inspired me to want to replace agricultural chemistries with biological solutions; whether with microbes that used natural mechanisms for controlling diseases in plants, or plants engineered to resist disease by direct gene introduction. In hindsight, perhaps I was more entrepreneurial than I realized at first because I later left the safer academic environment of basic research to join this new wave of science that could impact agriculture in ways yet unknown.

The first 5 years of my career were spent working at Advanced Genetic Sciences finding ways to improve microbial fungicides—specifically, fluorescent pseudomonads that colonize plant roots to reduce seedling diseases using genetic engineering. During this time, I and my company ran up against difficult and excessive regulatory systems including public concerns for our products which killed a promising application for improved fungicides.

From the early 1980s through the mid-1990s, I evolved from a scientist in an industrial environment into a full-blooded entrepreneur who was comfortable with the nexus of business and science, patents and products, basic research and applied outcomes. I grew to know the agricultural biotechnology (Ag Biotech) landscape intimately, working in a company that competed with teams at Monsanto but collaborated with teams at DuPont and Rohm and Haas. Those were heady days in which many of us talked about how we could change the world, change global agriculture, and do it quickly. As with any new technology, the world was not as ready as we, the developers, were for our first products. This is because Ag Biotech is a slow and cautious business serving cautious growers. Nonetheless, biotechnology has put its mark on agriculture, and will continue to do so in even more diverse ways. My hope is that at least one reader of this chapter will recognize some intriguing opportunities and challenges, and apply themselves to changing the face of global agriculture.

WHAT IS AGRICULTURAL BIOTECHNOLOGY?

Throughout the 1980s and 1990s the focus of most Ag Biotech entrepreneurs was the creation of new ways to genetically engineer crops to protect them against insects (insect resistance) and to make them more hardy in the presence of weed-killing chemicals (herbicide tolerance). Throughout much of the later 1990s and the 2000s, this focus continued along with the creation of biotech "traits" such as increased yield, stress tolerance, and increased nitrogen-use efficiency. Many small companies and entrepreneurs were instrumental in the development of these traits, although it was the large chemical companies and seed companies that brought these new products to the market. Monsanto emerged as the leading developer of Ag Biotech trait products as they quickly recognized and commercialized valuable technologies that enabled them to be a market leader.

Biotechnology has many different product applications aside from the creation of new medicines and drugs. When we talk about *agricultural* biotechnology, broadly writ, we are speaking of any application that impacts crop production as opposed to processing of the resulting grain or biomass which is the domain of *industrial* biotechnology.

The groups that serve crop production with new products that enhance or preserve the value of the crop include three major sectors (see Figure 11.1):

1. The seed sector
2. The agrochemical sector
3. The fertilizer sector

The seed, fertilizer, and chemical products commercialized by these companies are purchased by growers to assure maximum value from their land.

The Seed Sector

The seed sector, through differentiation and patent protection, can secure reliable product price premiums, and as a result it was the first sector to attract investor interest from the very beginning of the Ag Biotech industry in the early 1980s. The companies in this sector focus on producing and selling the seeds of crops such as corn, soybean, and cotton, with the regular improvement of varieties through breeding applications and periodic, but more dramatic improvements in variety that are now made through biotech traits.

The Agrochemical Sector

The agrochemical sector produces value-added products of great interest to growers, but the successful application of biotechnology to the development of novel agrochemical

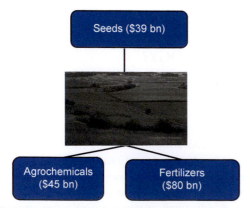

FIGURE 11.1 The estimated size of the three principal Ag Biotech sectors.

products has been much slower to materialize. Crop Solutions, founded by Erik Ward and Scott Uknes, was one of the few start-up companies that focused on the crop protection sector. Paradigm Genetics, led by John Ryals, focused on novel herbicide targets in a collaboration with Bayer Crop-Science, a combination of a biotech-trait strategy (herbicide tolerance traits) and crop-protection strategy, with novel herbicides based on new targets for herbicide screening.

The Fertilizer Sector

Fertilizers are generally commodity products and receive very little impact from biotechnology. The crop protection sector has deployed biotechnology methods but without significant change to product categories to date, in contrast to the seed sector with the introduction of the new biotech trait category. The commercial and financial value of these products are determined in part by the regulatory framework for approval in each sector and the potential for incorporating added value, as opposed to commodity products, which in turn determines the product margins and the entrepreneurial focus.

New Ag Biotech markets are emerging that are likely to rapidly increase entrepreneurial opportunities within the broader agrochemical sector. The potential of effective live biological and natural products is re-energizing this market for the first time since it was explored in the 1980s. Finally, the fertilizer sector is a commodity industry with no application to date of biotechnology and has limited scope for entrepreneurs today. Unless biotechnology can unlock new ways for fertilizers to be processed in the soil or utilized by crops, this segment will remain a lagging market for Ag Biotech entrepreneurship.

Regulation of Agricultural Biotechnology

Ag Biotech is possibly a greater challenge for entrepreneurs than medical biotechnology—an entrepreneurial challenge of its own. The time to market for Ag Biotech products is just as long as in medical biotechnology but the payout is not as compelling. Blockbuster products in the Ag Biotech sector are rare and perhaps equate to only 10 percent the value of blockbuster drugs. However, the inherent competitive advantages of major players in Ag Biotech are stronger than even those of major pharmaceutical companies. This is because biotech traits represent an inherent characteristic of a plant variety, and therefore need to be tested in a company's proprietary *germplasm* and brought to the market by that company as part of its overall product offering. Germplasm refers to a seed or a plant part such as a leaf, a stem, pollen, or even a few cells which can be turned into a whole plant. Germplasm contains the information for a species' genetic makeup and therefore can be a proprietary monopoly to a company.

In the United States, the regulatory environment for Ag Biotech can be challenging to manage, with potentially three federal agencies involved in product approval:

1. The Environmental Protection Agency (EPA)
2. The Department of Agriculture (USDA)
3. The Food and Drug Administration (FDA)

Even export market regulatory processes can be highly variable in different geographies and costly to manage. In addition to these regulatory challenges, the Ag Biotech path is fraught with risk and uncertainty given the public's adverse perceptions of biotech traits in much of the world, often driven by scientifically misinformed nongovernmental organizations (NGOs), organic growers, marketers, etc. Unwarranted fears about the safety of Ag Biotech products has made it nearly impossible for small companies to compete in the biotech trait business today. As a result, the Ag Biotech entrepreneurial ecosystem is small and fragile compared with the medical biotechnology entrepreneurial ecosystem. For instance, rather than having thousands of small biotech companies (such as in the life sciences sector) working in an ecosystem with 20 to 30 large pharmaceutical companies able to partner and fund early-stage R&D, we find perhaps 20 to 30 small Ag Biotech companies with only 6 large agricultural seed and crop protection companies with the ability to fund early stage R&D. As a result, there are fewer investors in the Ag Biotech market compared to the life science biotechnology market.

In addition, over the past decade biotech traits have proven to be ever more complicated to bring to the market, even for large companies. Regulatory uncertainty has increased, and despite the expiration of some seminal patents, the intellectual property landscape remains very complex. Due to the successes of the past 18 years, a new trait must be combined (stacked) with previous traits that already have become foundational products, and this trait must be introduced into specialized germplasm, making it much more difficult for a small company to bring a new trait to the market. With the even longer time—as of 2014, compared with 1994—to bring a trait to the market from initial conception and testing—closer to 15 years than 10 years—the opportunity for entrepreneurs to build new companies focused on the trait market has diminished. The bottleneck is the highly controlled and proprietary germplasm in which a new trait must be tested and validated. This means that biotech trait development is more and more the sole province of major seed companies.

Does that mean there is little opportunity for Ag Biotech entrepreneurs today? Not at all. Investors and entrepreneurs are focused on ways to use biotechnology and genomics to create new technologies needed by large companies and new products that improve crop production or crop protection. The financing of the start-up company AgBiome in 2013 demonstrated that biological products, such as live microbes that can colonize plant roots, which can come to the market in less than 5 years with quite limited regulatory oversight, offer a new direction for bioentrepreneurs. The recognition of the importance of the human microbiome has triggered increased interest in crop microbiomes—the collection of microbes that stably interact with plant root or leaf surfaces. Pam Marrone was able to bring her company, Marrone Bio Innovations, to the public market in 2013 based on the same basic proposition of a short and low-cost path to the market (4 to 5 years and less than $10 million), based on microbial and plant extracts that provide crop protection benefits.

One new Ag Biotech opportunity is the identification of natural products that improve crop productivity using high-throughput biotechnology-developed screens based on genomic insights, being developed by companies like my own Mendel Biotechnology. As with biopesticidal products, their development has a short and low-cost path to the market, and testing and launch of these products does not require access to proprietary germplasm or prior generations of biotech traits. Mendel Biotechnology has identified microbial extracts that are able to confer increased drought tolerance and water-use efficiency on diverse crops. These products are in an early stage of development, with first field trials expected in 2014.

Another example of using biotechnology to create new products is Ag Biotech start-up Kaiima, a company creating polyploid (having more than two copies of each chromosome, such as 4 or 6) versions of crops that have higher yields with more robust growth and development capabilities. Investors have shown favorable interest in the entrepreneurs with these ideas.

So gird your loins those of you who plan to embark on the Ag Biotech entrepreneurial road! Keep a thick skin and a strong heart. Focus on the great opportunity to help feed, fuel, and clothe the twenty-first century. Be willing to learn. Be highly focused, and yet be highly flexible, especially with the business model needed to generate value from a new technology. Be as willing to experiment with your business model as you are with your technology. More likely than not the original business model pursued will not be your final and successful business model you use. Often, even the best applications of your technology are not the original ones you started out trying to develop.

Agricultural biotechnology already has a dramatic impact on reducing the costs of producing food around the planet. More than half of all growers using biotech products are in the developing world today! [2] With this in mind, let's turn now to a brief review of the Ag Biotech product development process and associated challenges, the past accomplishments of the industry, and the opportunities that lie ahead for AgBio entrepreneurs.

THE AG BIOTECH COMMERCIALIZATION PROCESS

Early in the life of the biopharmaceutical industry, investors acquired an understanding of the stages involved in the development of new biotechnology-based drugs and the risks associated with each stage and process. The Ag Biotech industry consolidated views for a similar product development process in the early 2000s, in part to help investors understand the risk profile of biotech trait products and the reduction in risk (See Figure 11.2). Although similar terminology was adopted for Ag Biotech product development, the overall risk profile at each respective phase is not equivalent. This was important both for large companies defining their future product pipeline value as well as for small companies seeking investment from either corporate partners or venture investors.

Discovery Through to Validation

Biotech trait development begins with a discovery phase using many different research strategies to drive that process. Genomics applications in the 2000s included extensive use of *Arabidopsis*, a small weed with a short time required to produce seed and a small genome, adopted broadly as the white rat of plant science. This model plant was used for testing various DNA constructs for positive benefits in first-generation traits such as herbicide tolerance and insect resistance, and second-generation traits such as yield improvement, stress tolerance, nutrient use, and other properties. Many research strategies successfully contributed to the selection of genes to be tested.

Phase 1 Testing

With a positive result during validation, these product ideas (i.e., trait candidates) move on to Phase 1. This involves testing the same or similar construct in a target crop such as corn or soybean, first in the greenhouse then in small field plots. A number of different transgenic events (each a specific location in the genome for the delivered construct) are created in the target crop, and these events are evaluated to determine the likely benefit of the resulting biotech trait. At this stage, the likelihood that a particular trait candidate will

be commercialized is less than 25 percent. Once confirmation of that desired trait (for example, tolerance to drought, herbicide tolerance, or better use of a nutrient) is obtained at small scale, the product moves to Phase 2.

Phase 2 Testing

Phase 2 includes testing a recombinant DNA construct that conferred the trait in the target crop with a much larger number of individual transgenic events in commercial target varieties and with a construct that could pass all regulatory hurdles. With sufficient confidence in commercial performance, regulatory studies would also be initiated to begin to understand if there would be any regulatory impediments to commercial deployment of the trait. At this stage, the likelihood of commercial success increased to 50 percent. With the initial regulatory studies in hand, and selection of one or a few events that could be commercial based on molecular analysis of the integrated transgene, the product moves to Phase 3.

Phase 3 Testing

Phase 3 includes larger scale field trials in many locations in the United States that can also include South American locations to allow two sets of tests per growing season. During Phase 3 testing, the selected events are also introduced into a wider set of commercial varieties (i.e., a diverse genetic selection of the company's germplasm) for that large-scale testing. Unlike drug development, in which Phase 3 failures are *not unusual*, failure of an Ag Biotech trait in Phase 3 is relatively *uncommon*, with a 75 percent likelihood of success ascribed to this phase of development.

Ultimately, regulatory approval processes are conducted during Phases 2 and 3 development of novel biotech traits. Depending upon the functions of the trait and the crop in which it is deployed, as many as three different agencies may be involved in the United States alone: the EPA, the USDA, and the FDA. In addition, since grain or other products from crops grown in the United States are exported to other countries, and of course major crops are grown in many other countries, regulatory approval in other countries is needed prior to the commercial launch of a new biotech trait for production in the United States.

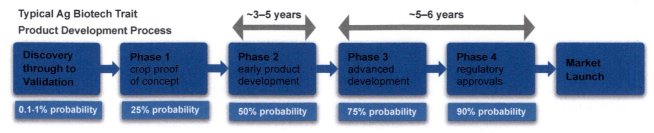

FIGURE 11.2   The typical agricultural biotechnology development cycle for the introduction of a novel biotech trait. (*Source: Phillips McDougal.*)

Phase 4 Testing

Finally, during Phase 4, regulatory submissions are made in multiple countries, including countries where the crop is grown and those countries which will receive products by importing the resulting grain or oil. The events are introduced into the commercial varieties for launch and seed is produced in large amounts preparing for the product launch. The probability of success in Phase 4, precommercial testing, is generally estimated at 90 percent. The benefits of the trait product are communicated to the market broadly and to growers specifically in the Phase 4 run-up to commercial launch.

While the development process shown in Figure 11.2 is particularly applicable to a biotech trait itself, a similar process would apply to other Ag Biotech products derived through the use of biotechnology. The application of exogenous RNAi molecules (short duplex RNA molecules of 21 to 24 nucleotides that trigger gene silencing in eukaryotic organisms) to control pests has been developed by DevGen (acquired in 2012 by Syngenta) and some other companies. Testing of such pest-targeting RNAi requires a related and lengthy development process, with RNAi treatments first conducted with pests directly, then on crops in glasshouse tests prior to testing in crops in small-scale field trials and large-scale trials in diverse environments. The regulatory process required of novel RNAi molecules is still in development globally.

Agricultural Biotechnology Product Commercialization

The wave of investments from strategic investors and some private companies in the late 1990s and early 2000s focused on the earliest phases of the development process, primarily discovery through validation, and then in some cases, proof-of-concept demonstration in relevant target crops. Companies like Mendel, Ceres, and Paradigm all ran high throughput processes of genomics-driven discovery, using primarily *Arabidopsis* as a system for testing novel-trait constructs. In most cases, these constructs used one or more different promoter sequences to program expression of a wide range of different gene sequences from *Arabidopsis* or crop plants. The premise during the earliest days of the genomics era was that although all the large companies understood the trait targets (such as increased stress tolerance, increased yield, increased nitrogen use efficiency), these companies lacked the correct genes whose expression could be modified in plants to effect these improvements. Rather than applying an academic style research program to dissect the molecular basis for a trait or process and then using that knowledge to engineer crop improvement, an unbiased approach to high throughput screening was adopted throughout the industry. This was much like a land grab, a rapid phase of investment to secure critical intellectual property (IP) positions, much like when the rail industry secured important physical locations for expansion in the mid-1800s.

The value associated with this early-stage validation would ultimately be paid to these companies via milestones and royalties upon product sales in the future. Of course most genes that pass early-stage validation still failed in later testing. The probability of success slowly increases with additional crop testing in greenhouses, then small-plot field testing, then broad-acre field testing in multiple locations. Similar to the biopharmaceutical development process where failure of a promising drug may result from variable performance in different (human) genetic backgrounds, or variable toxicity occurring in different (human) genetic backgrounds, failure of AgBio-promising leads would often occur due to either variable performances in different (crop) genetic backgrounds or in different environments or climates. Major companies invested heavily in new biotech trait-testing pipelines with a goal of identifying successful product candidates as quickly as possible, through testing in multiple geographies and crop-variety backgrounds.

The earliest products of the Ag Biotech industry were herbicide tolerance and insect resistance traits based on bacterial protein sequences, such as an EPSPS gene (encoding 5-enol-pyruvyl-shikimate-3-phosphate synthase, an early enzyme of aromatic acid synthesis) from *Agrobacterium* and insect toxin genes from *Bacillus thuringiensis*. These products were revolutionary and grower adoption followed very quickly. The EPSPS gene resistant to Monsanto's herbicide glyphosate (RoundUp) enabled the rapid expansion in the use of glyphosate, an herbicide with excellent environmental and performance properties. Until the introduction of the first RoundUp Ready trait in soybean in 1996 based on the resistant form of the EPSPS gene, glyphosate was a nonselective herbicide that could not be used in the major crops such as soybean or corn. In these major crops, glyphosate replaced older herbicides with less-desirable properties, including environmental persistence. These other herbicides rapidly lost market share after RoundUp Ready products made growers' lives much simpler. A range of different insect toxin genes enabled the replacement of synthetic insecticides applied to a crop with a crop that produced its own highly effective insecticidal activity, and ones with very good safety profiles.

These herbicide-tolerance and insect-resistance trait products performed well in a diverse set of genetic backgrounds and environments. This has contrasted with the lower probability of success for yield and stress-tolerance traits, due to required interaction with plant proteins from within an endogenous crop genome for improved crop performance. Herbicide- and insect-resistance traits are not as difficult to engineer as other desirable traits such as enhanced-yield and stress-tolerance traits, which are analogous to installing a radio in an automobile without one. In comparison, new-yield and stress-tolerance traits require re-engineering of existing functional plant systems that govern stress tolerance, analogous to trying to engineer existing automobile systems-like engines and transmissions. While small entrepreneurial companies have the wherewithal to conduct laboratory and even some greenhouse screening in *Arabidopsis* or a well-studied crop like rice (e.g., Crop Design), they do not have the financial resources to conduct the large-scale field trials required in Phases 2 and 3 development that parallel the large-scale human drug trials in similar phases of a therapeutic development program. Given the much-reduced overall value of even a high-value product (perhaps 10- to 30-fold less than a blockbuster drug), financial investors have traditionally been less interested in backing such efforts. As a result, small companies remained entirely dependent upon the large seed companies for the financing of field testing, and therefore greater value would accrue to the large seed companies rather than the small companies who initially discovered exciting new leads.

The overall regulatory approval process has become more cumbersome and complex on a global level over the past 20 years than we might have imagined when the industry emerged in the 1980s, or when the first RoundUp Ready soybean product was launched in 1996. As a result, successful entrepreneurs need to have a committed strategic partner, and probably have already been bought by them, before a trait they have initiated can come to the market. This is particularly true for the second generation biotech traits of yield increase, stress tolerance, and nutrient-use efficiency, which are more complex to test than the earlier traits of herbicide-tolerance or insect-resistance traits.

THERE IS A PATH!

So now that you have read all the disclaimers, let's get to the excitement, those few of you still wanting to read the rest of this chapter and possibly pursue an AgBio dream. What does success look like? What should your goals be as an entrepreneur! A serious technology entrepreneur will want to change how products are developed for today's markets (e.g., better marker tools for the same types of conventional varieties, a strategy developed by KeyGene in the 1990s). A serious commercial entrepreneur will want to change the face of agriculture, its practice around the planet, and the products that growers need to improve the yield and value of their products. To do this requires at least three key assets: a compelling vision; talented people; and committed capital. And once early-stage capital has been utilized by your team to demonstrate potential, much larger amounts of capital will be needed to realize the complete vision. In Ag Biotech, company financing has not traditionally come through public financial markets because of the more-limited value of agriculture compared with human health in developed countries, but rather through an acquisition by a large Ag Biotech company.

Let's examine some examples of success to understand the path. Athenix is an attractive recent model of success. Bayer CropScience acquired Athenix in 2009 to gain control of relatively early-stage but well-demonstrated crop-protection traits of insect and nematode resistance. Athenix appears to have been developed into a center of excellence within Bayer for these new trait products, with the greater resources of Bayer to realize the vision of the founders, and with a nice return for them and their investors. The founders, people like Mike Koziel, had both prior entrepreneurial as well as larger company backgrounds (people), a clear vision of their product goals (vision), and capital largely from the venture community, but also from a number of strategic deals with smaller Ag Biotech companies (capital).

The initial public offering (IPO) path is not generally available for Ag Biotech companies today, given the long timeframes to market and more-limited value of biotech trait products compared to blockbuster drugs. The primary exit has been through acquisition by a large company wanting to own and control key technologies, IP positions, or emerging products. Rarely has there been an Ag Biotech company in the public market in the past 20 years, unlike the early phase of the Ag Biotech sector where there were plenty. I believe that entrepreneurs need to focus on building capabilities that can become part of a larger enterprise, one that has already nucleated new opportunities, but knowing that the goal is to secure greater resources through incorporation into a larger corporate partner. Major venture investments, including those from strategic venture funds of major companies, remain critically important for Ag Biotech entrepreneurship, and are perhaps more important than ever before.

A recent exit for another Ag Biotech illustrates another model. GrassRoots was started through project funding by Monsanto in 2009 and was subsequently acquired by Monsanto in 2013. As a board member for most of the company's life, I worked with the company founders to navigate towards an exit without relying on venture investments of any kind. As a result, the company remained largely a financed project serving Monsanto's need for novel gene expression programs for its biotech trait business. The company's purpose was to be technology-focused, as opposed to commercially focused, working entirely within a conventional biotech trait business model. The company was able to secure additional funding through grants that enabled the development of some critical technology not owned by Monsanto. Consequently, the company developed both technologies that would be owned by Monsanto through commercial agreements, as well as new technologies developed with grant funding. GrassRoots was effectively launched through project funding. This combination drove the acquisition at a relatively early stage, after only 4 years of the strategic alliance. Philip Benfey was the key founder who learned important lessons from other companies, kept his eye on the prize, and recognized the need for technologies other than those defined entirely by the funded partnership to create high financial value in the company. Philip and the leadership team also recognized the difficulty of migrating from a technology to a commercially-driven company, as well as migrating from one major partner to other major partners. This success should be a model for modern science-driven entrepreneurial academics, especially in a world with highly focused strategic venture units at most of the major ag companies. Some strategic investors, as demonstrated by Merck in the pharmaceutical industry, are looking to create project-type venture models that build on this type of success, but which define exit value and timing based on up-front vision and milestones.

WHAT'S BEEN ACHIEVED SO FAR

The World Food Prize is generally considered the Nobel Prize for food and agriculture, with a global, feed-the-world priority. In 2013 the prize was awarded to three plant scientists each of whom contributed to the fundamental invention for the Ag Biotech industry in the 1980s, agrobacterium-mediated transformation of crops: Robb Fraley, Mary Dell Chilton, and Marc van Montagu. In fact, each of these individuals are inventors on key patent filings from 1983, the year that bore witness to the first practical means for introducing recombinant DNA into plants. The early 1980s saw the birth and growth of several companies dedicated to creating value using such technology to impact agriculture. The enthusiasm and excitement of the market for this emergent industry was remarkable given that a number of companies were able to go public without significant revenues in the near-term, and with only the first hints of how to create novel plant varieties.

Technologies of the early Ag Biotech companies spanned cell culture-based mutagenesis (somaclonal variation), genetic engineering of microbes that would prevent plant diseases or reduce frost damage when applied to crops, cell culture-based production of plant secondary metabolites, and genetic engineering of crops for a wide range of different benefits. Somaclonal variation and cell cultures proved to be too limited in utility, and consumers were clearly not ready then—nor are they now—to allow genetically engineered bacteria loose in the environment. In fact, my own first foray in the industry was an effort to use microbial genetic engineering to improve microbial colonization of plant roots and the production of antifungal secondary metabolites for effective "microbial fungicides." This effort was shut down in the late 1980s due to public resistance to releasing engineered microbes into the environment. However, biotech crops are much easier to track than microbes, and the public seemed content, initially, with the creation and commercialization of such products. Interestingly, we are seeing a new wave of interest in microbial products that offer pesticidal and growth benefits to plants, but without having to engineer them.

Many of the early Ag Biotech companies were financed through both private financing from venture investors and through the public markets. They created key enabling tools for creation of biotech traits in important commercial crops, including corn, soybean, cotton, tomato, and canola. These early companies created the first traits that would later be tested in field trials that were regulated under the Coordinated Framework. Companies like Calgene, Agracetus, Agragenetics, Mycogen, AGS, DNAP, and others raised money, went public, and thought they could change the world and create new products and entire new markets.

The science was exciting and thrilling. These new tools enabled both academics and company scientists a glimpse of the behavior of plant gene function in a way never before possible. Some companies invested heavily in the basic understanding of transgene behavior, in the context of conventional gene function in plants. We first came to understand how genes delivered by *Agrobacterium* into the genome of a plant were structured, and how variable structure influenced variable expression outcomes. These fundamental properties needed to be mastered if we were to deliver new products into the market with sufficient understanding of their behavior to give growers, and ultimately consumers, confidence in these new products of biotechnology. We learned ways to shut off gene function as well as activate gene expression. We mastered antisense silencing of gene expression, and then sense gene-mediated silencing of gene expression (cosuppression). The latter was done at DNA Plant Technology where I took on major responsibility for securing patent protection for cosuppression-mediated gene silencing. This led to major insights in plant biology, as cosuppression gave way to RNAi-mediated gene silencing, based on the designed creation of double-stranded RNA molecules (dsRNA) as opposed to incidental dsRNA produced when transgenes integrated in the genome in specific structures such as inverted repeats. The improved ability to silence plant genes for research applications, as well as the ability to silence pest genes essential for viability, has had a major impact on plant science in academia and industry.

In those days we saw few impediments and a blank canvas on which to sketch the future. Major shifts were anticipated from genetic engineering of crops. New product possibilities such as tomatoes that would not ripen and rot on the vine, but would be delivered to consumers in good shape and then ripen. Bananas that would ripen and not rot, because they no longer produced the plant hormone ethylene known to induce ripening, but which could be induced to ripen on demand. Crops resistant to viral diseases of all types. Crops with novel colors. Crops with novel flavors. Crops that failed to produce antigens that are the cause of allergenic responses in foods like peanuts. A number of such traits and improved crops were developed, but many remain "on the shelf" as opposed to in the market for a range of reasons, including public perception, regulatory and development costs that outstrip potential value, etc.

HERBICIDE-TOLERANCE AND INSECT-RESISTANCE TRAITS

Herbicide-tolerance and insect-resistance traits were high on the list of companies with a clear-eyed view of the needs of agriculture, as identified by crop-protection companies. An enormous shift in market value was driven by Monsanto's launch of RoundUp Ready soybean in 1996, and RoundUp Ready corn in 1999, as companies selling soybean and corn herbicides lost market share rapidly to Monsanto's RoundUp branded herbicide, glyphosate. Biotechnology offered a novel way to confer selective activity to a nonselective herbicide, like glyphosate, turning a useful but limited herbicide into the most important herbicide in the world over the past 20 years. Today herbicide tolerance and insect resistance traits represent more than 99 percent of the market share of the Ag Biotech industry (See Figure 11.3). Only a few crops have been successfully targeted for significant biotech trait penetration, with corn and soybean being the predominant crops in both North and South America.

The rate of penetration of insect-resistance and herbicide-tolerance traits (Figure 11.4) demonstrates the success of these biotech trait technologies, but also indicate the limitations for entrepreneurs in the biotech trait market, since these crops are dominated by a very few seed companies. In fact most of the developments in biotech traits have been financed by major companies as strategic investments focused on technologies as opposed to equity value growth. This was the case for Mendel Biotechnology's long-term relationship with Monsanto, which invested substantially over a 15-year period in research and development activities conducted at Mendel. Athenix is a rare exception to the requirement for major strategic investment, with some venture investors and a solid return in a reasonable period of time.

A few lesser-known products have come to the market, with some of these remaining in the market today. Virus-resistant papaya has been a tremendous success in Hawaii, enabling the papaya industry threatened by the devastating papaya ringspot virus to survive (well described in Brian Dick in "The Fate of a Fruit: Creating the Transgenic Papaya,"

Life Sciences Foundation Magazine, summer 2013). Virus-resistant squash, brought to the market through the efforts of Asgrow, is still commercialized by Monsanto, who acquired Seminis (which had previously acquired the vegetable seed business of Asgrow in the 1990s). Ripening-delayed tomato products were developed in the mid-1990s, by Calgene and DNAP, with Calgene's Flavr Savr tomato reaching the market in 1994, and DNAP's Endless Summer tomato unable to reach the market in 1995 through lack of obtaining licenses to recently patented technologies. Nontransgenic solutions for delayed ripening in tomatos became available in the mid-1990s, eliminating the need for the biotech product. Since then, the mainstream produce industry has abandoned biotech traits due to both costs of development as well as consumer resistance to engineered fresh food products.

Perhaps the best-known and most compelling consumer product that has never yet come to the market is Golden Rice, a product developed in the 1990s through the efforts primarily of two academic scientists, Ingo Potrykus and Peter Beyer, funded by the Rockefeller Foundation and the European Union (see *http://www.goldenrice.org/*). These scientists engineered rice with genes from both plants and a bacterium to encode proteins needed to produce substantial amounts of beta-carotene (precursor for vitamin A synthesis) in grain, leading to the golden color of the rice. Children without adequate supplies of vitamin A or a precursor like beta-carotene have a marked incidence of blindness and susceptibility to disease, leading to an increased incidence of premature death of small children, who are most susceptible to the vitamin A deficiency. Syngenta stepped up more than a decade ago to help get that product to the market, but it languishes in a convoluted global process of product approvals and testing. The potential benefit of this vitamin A-enriched rice to prevent childhood blindness and death is recognized, and yet the product languishes. This may still be one of the great humanitarian achievements through biotechnology in agriculture, if and when it finally comes to the market. It represents a systemic failure of regulatory agencies in many countries, and a demonstration of the unreasoned fear of a sound technology platform. It

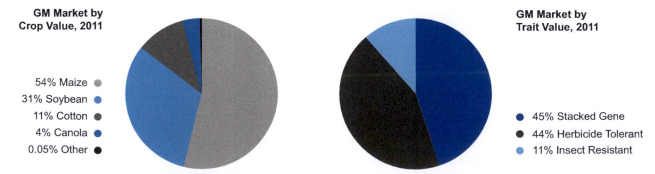

FIGURE 11.3   Biotech traits have penetrated only a few crop-production systems and seed businesses, with a focus on corn, soybean, cotton, and canola. Recently alfalfa and sugar beets have added biotech traits. Only two major trait categories have impacted the market at any substantial level in nearly 20 years, herbicide tolerance and insect resistance.

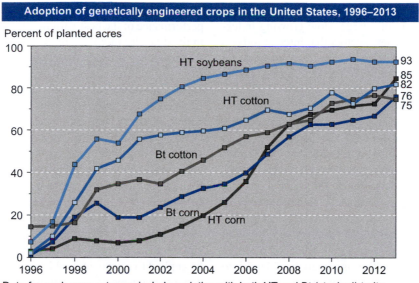

Adoption of genetically engineered crops in the United States, 1996–2013

Percent of planted acres

Data for each crop category include varieties with both HT and Bt (stacked) traits.
Sources: USDA, Economic Research Service using data from Fernandez-Cornejo and
McBride (2002) for the years 1996–99 and USDA, National Agricultural Statistics
Service, June Agricultural Survey for the years 2000–13.

FIGURE 11.4   Three crops and two traits represent greater than 98 percent of the crops and traits commercialized in the United States in 2013.

is a case-study that entrepreneurs interested in Ag Biotech would be well advised to be aware of and to know the pitfalls that they might face.

Recognizing that biotechnology applications could accelerate conventional breeding, with the result generating no biotech trait and no opposition, vegetable seed companies in Europe focused on molecular markers. Several Dutch vegetable seed companies joined together to form a company, Keygene, that they jointly owned and which would generate precompetitive markers. Keygene focused on the continued development of molecular markers and marker technologies with increasingly sophisticated biotechnology tools that would reduce the price of marker discovery and application. Technology innovation was the key to their business model, with the same market outcomes, through the same companies, but with novel and higher-value strategies for value creation. The challenges of biotech trait adoption provided an entrepreneurial context for new technologies such as amplified fragment length polymorphism (AFLP), the key platform technology at Keygene's inception. The critical context for this entrepreneurial company was the lack of competing biotech traits in markets such as vegetable seeds, and particularly in Europe. Keygene continues to innovate and find novel ways to use biotechnology to create improved crop varieties that are not themselves the subject of biotech trait regulation since they are usually based on naturally occurring alleles or alleles derived through mutagenesis and rapidly identified using modern tools of biotechnology.

As with other examples, this demonstrates the value of strategic investment as opposed to financial investment for Ag Biotech entrepreneurs. Keygene's investors were a consortium of major Dutch seed companies whose interest was the technologies to enhance value in their own companies as opposed to growing Keygene's enterprise value as an independent company. This model is fairly similar to the strategy adopted by three forestry companies to develop biotechnology applications for the forestry industry in 2000. Westvaco Corporation, International Paper Company, and Fletcher Challenge came together to form Arbor-Gen, combining R&D assets and financing development of biotech traits, that each would ultimately use in their own plantation forest business. Unlike Keygene, however, which was focused on nonbiotech applications, ArborGen focused largely on a biotech trait development model which has recently foundered due to consumer and nongovernmental organization (NGO) opposition to the incorporation of biotech traits into tree species.

HOW THE LANDSCAPE CHANGED

While fewer venture funds seem to be investing in the biopharmaceutical industry today, more venture funds are getting interested in the Ag Biotech sector. This sector is seen to have long-term, stable demand drivers that attract investment, but the lack of growth companies can be a disincentive to investment in agriculture. Given the limitations of Ag Biotech traits from a venture investor's perspective, investors in 2013 and beyond are looking for other entrepreneurial Ag Biotech opportunities, ones that can lead to products in only a few years as opposed to more than a decade hence, and ones that can lead to products that can be brought to the market directly by the entrepreneurial company itself, not by a licensee of that company. The key challenge is identifying growth sectors in a large, slow-growing industry. Recent trends point to new sectors that interest today's venture investors. Some of these may be developed using biotechnology to differentiate a product or offering; others do not require biotechnology.

One example is in agronomic practices, with the demonstration of the importance of this opportunity coming through Monsanto's acquisition of Precision Planting in 2012. This company, acquired for more than $200 million, had focused on new information tools coupled with agronomic applications and agricultural equipment, dealing with the precise planting of corn seeds to minimize yield losses from inaccurate and variable planting depth. This emphasizes an important theme: the need for very uniform practices on increasingly large acreages managed by large growers and grower groups. The aggregation of land into larger units, as well as larger management units, is a theme seen in all major agricultural regions.

Another is in the field of RNAi, where Monsanto has acquired a couple of companies in the past 2 years (Beeologics and Rosetta Green), and where Syngenta has acquired DevGen with a substantial interest in its technology for RNAi-mediated pest resistance. Both companies are seeking to build on their acquisitions with small RNA- or DNA-based products entering the market in the next few years.

PATENTLY IMPORTANT TRENDS

Intellectual property broadly, and patents specifically, are the life force for most biotechnology businesses. This is, perhaps, a truism, but for Ag Biotech the impacts are more dramatic even than for medical biotechnology. Unlike medical biotech, where the capability to bring a drug to the market may rely only on a company's solely-owned patent estate, commercialization of new Ag Biotech traits may require licenses to a broad array of enabling technology patents from others. With the stacking of biotech trait products increasingly seen in major crops, new innovations only realize value in combination with other patented technologies. Therefore a biotech trait cannot come to the market on its own; it can only do so in the context of a commercial seed or plant variety that is subject to patents and other forms of proprietary protection owned by others. This contrasts with the biopharmaceutical industry where a blockbuster drug can often come to the market relying just on its own patents.

The entire collection of varieties in a seed company, some of which are certainly trade-secrets but others the subject of an array of intellectual property protection, provide a compelling barrier to entry that makes it very difficult for an Ag Biotech entrepreneur to capture new value in this market. This collection of varieties, known as the germplasm of a seed company, represents a powerful advantage for companies like Monsanto, DuPont Pioneer, Syngenta, and other international seed companies. The power lies in the elite performance of the best varieties in the collection, as well as in the diversity of alleles represented in that collection, and the difficulty of recreating that elite performance starting from varieties readily accessible to the public through governmental variety collections, such as those managed by the USDA, for example. For crops such as corn and soybean, cotton, many vegetables, sugar beet, etc. with commercial breeding in the hands of private companies for decades if not generations, new biotech traits can only be realistically tested and evaluated by the private breeding companies. The requirement for testing, particularly for traits like yield and stress tolerance, results in a major barrier to entry. This is different for crops where the breeding is done largely in the public sector, such as wheat, but even this may change. The situation is different for chemistries or biologicals that can be applied to a crop, and which may therefore be much less dependent on specific variety performance.

Biotechnology has played an important role in a crop like soybean, enabling a new means of capturing value through traits like herbicide tolerance and insect resistance, which can be handled through patent and contractual protection. Prior to this new added value, many growers would have preferred to save seed rather than buying seed annually from major seed companies. This structural shift enabled soybean to join maize as the second most important seed crop globally in terms of value capture. Prior to this change, soybean was a required product sold by companies who made most of their money from their corn hybrids, but one from which these companies generated relatively little profit. The difference was that soybean growers could save seed from year to year, whereas corn growers relying on hybrids produced by corn seed companies, would lose the hybrid genetics in the next, save seed generation. The power of biotech traits for soybean was the ability, finally, of major seed companies to provide buyers of their seed sufficient value that they would agree not to save seed, as otherwise the grower would be infringing on a biotech trait patent incorporated into the seed genetics.

LESSONS LEARNED AND OPPORTUNITIES FOR A NEW ENTREPRENEUR

The AgBio entrepreneur developing a new technology faces a challenge that differs along many dimensions from that faced by an AgBio entrepreneur trying to introduce a new product category, or building a new market and disrupting existing markets. The critical issues differ for these two types of entrepreneurs, who also may have quite different backgrounds. The needs for Neal Carter, the CEO of Okanagan Specialty Fruits, to bring a browning-resistant apple to the market, were ones that a businessman from the orchard industry could appreciate. They are quite different from the needs for Philip Benfey, founder and CEO of Grassroots, and a highly regarded plant

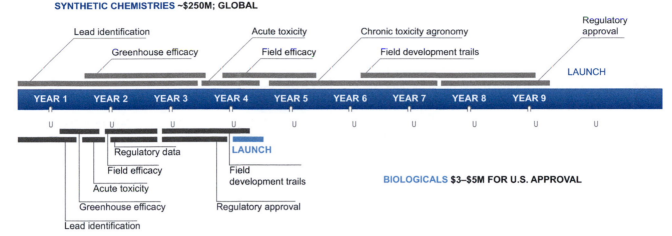

FIGURE 11.5   One driver for a new era of Ag Biotech innovation is the dramatic difference in time requirement and regulatory cost to bring a synthetic chemical versus a biological or natural product to the market. With new technologies to understand and develop biological and natural products and the recent successes of the biopesticide industry, additional new opportunities are likely to be found in the biological and natural product market segments, with biotechnology and genomics as key enablers of new innovation.

biologist, to develop a new toolbox of gene-expression tools for classical biotech trait products in major row crops. And the motivations of a commercial entrepreneur and a science entrepreneur are also often very different.

The Ag Biotech trait revolution disrupted value amongst existing crop-protection companies, as noted earlier. Monsanto leapfrogged several other crop-protection companies in herbicide sales, and has yet to look back. This was the most significant shift in industry value capture and market position from the biotech trait revolution, as only two traits continue to dominate the market. An entrepreneur in the AgBio sector sees that the era of disruptive impact of biotech traits is over, and that the leading companies have tremendous advantages in continuing incremental gains in this technology.

New and disruptive opportunities will arise in ways that leading companies today do not yet recognize! So don't be dismayed when prominent companies don't jump at the chance to partner with you on a new technology. American Cyanimid didn't see the titanic shift in value toward glyphosate-resistance soybeans, as summarized above, until it was too late. RoundUp Ready traits that enabled displacement of American Cyanimid's leading herbicides by Monsanto's RoundUp were not fully appreciated until growers themselves could test and identify the full range of benefits.

Today's new disruptive technologies and products for crop productivity improvement may lead to entirely new categories, or just be successful applications of current strategies, much as biopesticides have come of age through the work of Agraquest and Marrone Bio Innovations, the latter being one of the first ag technology companies to execute a successful public offering. The value of science well applied, and biotechnology among them, in overcoming limitations of successful biopesticides was key. New business models have also been key to this recent emergence,

for example, by securing increased product life for current synthetic pesticides, or addressing new markets. The combination of technology innovation and business model innovation for entrepreneurial success is a key lesson.

The biopesticide sector successes of the past 5 years or more suggest that the dramatic difference in cost and time to bring "bio" products to the market, now combined with new tools and better product efficacy, provides an entrepreneurial context for a new wave of Ag Biotech-derived products (see Figure 11.5). Ten years ago was likely too soon for this new direction, both for commercial and technology reasons. With a growing interest in natural solutions in the marketplace, and improving technology for understanding microbial ecosystems interacting with plants, we may be seeing the unfolding of a new chapter of Ag Biotech-enabled businesses. This could be from live microbe applications as well as natural product applications. Time will tell.

As I reflect on lessons I've learned over the past 30 years, starting with the onset of the Ag Biotech industry, my most important lesson of all is best summarized by these words of Albert Einstein: "*Out of clutter, find simplicity. From discord, find harmony. In the middle of difficulty lies opportunity.*" This has helped me numerous times remain focused despite the many challenges I've faced as a scientist entrepreneur. I offer a corollary that one should have in mind at the outset of any new venture: "*When you pursue opportunity, you will often face difficulty…when you do, seek simplicity and harmony.*" Creative solutions to difficulties can emerge when we allow ourselves time to find the simple and harmonious paths, those that enable the entrepreneur to persevere and succeed.

Ultimately how do we measure success of our ventures, or success as an entrepreneurial leader? Because failures occur in all industries, success is handling the process, knowing when to continue and when to stop, knowing how to minimize losses without missing out on big wins, and learning throughout the process. The investors with whom you partner will prize these attributes. As David Brooks noted in a recent New York Time op-ed piece, people "want to find that place, as the novelist Frederick Buechner put it, "where [their] deep gladness and the world's deep hunger meet."" If your deep gladness is satisfied by meeting the world's true hunger (for food, energy, and materials, all the key stuff of life in the modern world), then you should be a Bio Ag entrepreneur.

REFERENCES

[1] Silent Spring. Rachel Carson, Houghton Mifflin; 1962.
[2] Data from the International Service for the Acquisition of agri-biotech applications. http://www.isaaa.org/.

Chapter 12

Understanding Biotechnology Business Models and Managing Risk

Craig Shimasaki, PhD, MBA
President & CEO, Moleculera Labs and BioSource Consulting Group, Oklahoma City, Oklahoma

Biotechnology companies are started with the intent to commercialize products based upon novel technology concepts and ideas. In order to build a company that becomes profitable and generates sustainable revenue, it is critical to choose the right business model at the outset in order to give your company the best chance of success. Business models are important to both entrepreneurs and their investors, because business models are the method and manner in which a company makes, or intends to make, money. Sophisticated investors are familiar with the required components for building competitive companies that generate sustainable revenue. If the company and its founders adopt a business model that is neither competitive nor sustainable for their type of product, there will be limited investment interest in the company.

Often, eager entrepreneurs believe that decisions about company business models and commercialization methods are made *after* the company has completed product development and has an approved product to sell. Alternatively, entrepreneurs may believe they indeed "thought through" their business model choice, when in reality, they simply presumed a model which was familiar to them. Entrepreneurs must resist the erroneous belief that business model decisions are deferred far into the product development future. Rather, entrepreneurs must identify and adopt a commercialization strategy at the outset of the business because it will become part-and-parcel with the value proposition of the company. If you do not understand the strengths, weaknesses, and strategic value of any business model, the model you choose for your company may result in limited success.

WHAT IS A BUSINESS MODEL?

When describing business models, individuals often attempt to explain them in abstract concepts that are difficult to understand. In one sense, business models are abstract. However, in simpler terms, *a business model is the method by which a company makes and sells its products and services, which includes the interrelationship of all its component parts, and the manner in which the company creates value and makes money.* All companies operate within an underlying business model, whether recognized or not. Therefore, an entrepreneur should purposefully select and adopt the optimal business model for their company because a detrimental one may be entered into by default.

The building of a company around an optimal business model can be likened to an engineer who draws a set of plans, then has a construction team erect the envisioned building according to a set of prescribed architectural drawings. In this analogy, the architect conceives the structure and draws out the plans based upon the desired functions and optimized usage of the structure, long before the first steel girder is laid. Based upon the usage requirements of the envisioned building, the architect draws its "internal frame" and determines the interconnectivity of each segment to all other segments of the whole structure. The internal frame predetermines the height, width, and breadth of the structure, and it also sets its limits. (see Figure 12.1) A team of builders then follows the plans and sets the frame in place, and the final exterior construction conforms to the limits of the structural frame. If the frame does not reach a necessary height or extends in a critical direction or have connectivity to another necessary component, no exterior work can compensate for these limitations. Your business model is analogous to this "internal frame" or structure and it is the support upon which all the parts of the business (internal and external) are built and interconnected. As in this example, just as it is essential to predetermine the strategic and optimal frame prior to beginning construction, so it is vital to choose the right business model *prior* to building your business. This is because it is extremely difficult to change a business model once the organization is fully-developed. Rarely can a company successfully change its business model once it is established, and certainly not without risking forward momentum and the company's future. Some

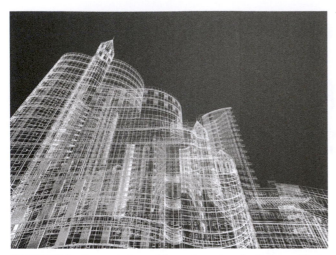

FIGURE 12.1   Just as the internal frame determines the design and limits of a building structure, so the business model predetermines the design and limits of the company functions.

companies have attempted to change their business model after commercialization with limited success; usually it is done because their current business model is not working. In reality, this is usually an attempt to salvage the most valuable parts of the business and jettison the parts that are not working. These efforts are usually survival in nature rather than plans for growth or expansion.

A development-stage biotechnology company has the opportunity to select and implement the ideal business model at their outset and it should be one that fits their technology, products, and services, and is optimized for their competitive advantage. To reiterate, a business model is simply the collective means and methods in which the company makes its products or provides its services, and the means by which the company makes money. It is the sum total of all the strategic business approaches and their interrelationship to other parts of the business and their relationship to the external world. A company selects a particular business model in order to give them a competitive advantage over other companies and their products.

In this chapter we will review representative examples of business models used in, or adapted for, different sectors within the biotechnology industry. We will discuss representative business model benefits and limitations for certain products or services. The reader should realize that there are endless permutations of business models, however, at this time we will cover a selected few. Fortunately, most business models follow a limited number of basic characteristics and these will become familiar to you as we review this in the following sections. Before we delve into the various business model examples, we want to talk about one business model that almost all biotechnology companies (irrespective of sector) should operate under for a period of time during their early development.

THE VIRTUAL COMPANY BUSINESS MODEL (A TEMPORARY START-UP MODEL)

A virtual company is an organization that outsources the majority of all its activities and owns or leases little if any physical space, and possesses few full-time employees in order to keep overhead expenses at a minimum. There are extreme variations of virtual companies. Some can be quite frugal such as one that has no full-time employees, utilizes a home address or post office box to receive business mail, borrows equipment or barters for time on equipment, and leases facilities which may be the academic laboratories of the founding scientists. Operating as a virtual company means that the company does not perform all the necessary functions internally—yet the company still completes all the necessary activities as if it was vertically integrated. I am a strong proponent of operating as a "virtual company" during the start-up phase, regardless if it is a biotherapeutic, diagnostic, medical device, Ag Biotech, or any other sector of biotechnology. The way this is accomplished is through carefully selecting outsourcing partners. For many early-stage companies, the extent of outsourcing may be significant where almost all development functions are performed under contract by outside organizations. Because of the great expense associated with research and development (R&D), preclinical, and animal testing, most early-stage biotherapeutic companies operate as a virtual company until significant funding is gained or a significant milestone is reached which can support internal staffing, equipment, and in-house activities. Sometimes the type of R&D activities required by some early-stage biotechnology companies are so unique and specialized that their only option is to perform these functions in-house; however, the more common functions can still be outsourced to keep costs down.

During start-up stages, capital is usually quite limited and a company cannot hire many full-time employees, but substantial progress must still be made in order to gain interest from investors. Operating as a virtual company during the formative stages allows entrepreneurs to extend the time horizon of their operations, and it requires much less capital to maintain and sustain the company while their product is initially being developed. I know of companies that have successfully advanced their therapeutic product through animal studies and into early human clinical testing as a virtual company. These organizations may have only one, or a few, key "employees" but they utilize many experienced consultants who are paid nominal fees, but receive stock option incentives, while the company contracts out most of their activities. For R&D outsourcing to be successful, there must be a good working relationship with the contracted R&D group. Often the laboratory that performs the R&D is the founder's/cofounder's laboratory because they have the specialized expertise and equipment to advance the translational research and advance the development of the product. R&D personnel may be contracted and operate under temporary agreements or work part-time. Typically these individuals are compensated with a combination of incentives such as stock, stock options, or restricted stock for professional services in addition to nominal salaries or fees. Be sure to discuss all employment and compensation commitments with your attorney in order to draft the necessary documents that will prevent intellectual property ownership issues in the future.

Virtual Companies Grow and Eventually Need Space

At some point in time virtual companies grow and may need dedicated laboratory and office space in order to continue their pace of progress toward product development. When making a move to dedicated space, be sure to look into the availability of space within a technology incubator, since some incubator programs will subsidize a start-up company with reduced rates that escalate later when certain financial milestones are met. Many technology incubators may also have some support services and/or shared equipment available for a small fee. When deciding on space, be sure to anticipate your needs now and growth needs into the near future, but balance that by the current funding and the timeframe to reach your next product-development milestone. As you may already know, renting biotechnology space is not cheap. Depending on the geographic location of your company and the mix of laboratory to office space, rent may cost between $30 to $75 per square foot per year. If you can, opt for month-to-month leases. If this is not possible, be sure to know the impact of any long-term lease and how these obligations may impact the overall burn rate of the company and the risk when raising another round of capital.

It is essential that most all start-up biotechnology companies initially operate as virtual companies in order to efficiently utilize capital and create early value. Being a virtual company provides time to raise start-up, seed, or Series A financing, and it also provides time for the company to increase in valuation as product development progress is made. Virtual companies conserve cash which can then be properly deployed toward advancing the technology rather than supporting overhead that limits their existence. However, a virtual company business model is not a permanent or long-term business model choice for companies. Virtual companies must still create internal value and ultimately possess some internal expertise which cannot be effectively reproduced by others. Although most companies will start as a virtual company, this business model choice should be temporary, and the company must have a commercialization business model selected and adopted that is long-term in nature.

BUSINESS MODEL EXAMPLES

In this section we will review a few business model examples that are used in the biotechnology industry. Many of these examples can be applied to different biotechnology sectors such as medical devices, agricultural and industrial biotechnology, digital health, and biofuels. These examples are presented to help understand the way in which different models are applied to different technologies and sectors. Later, we will discuss the different business model segments and how they are assembled to create new models. Some of the business models we will review include:

Therapeutic and Biologics Companies

- Fully Integrated Pharmaceutical or Biotechnology Company (FIPCO or FIBCO) business model.
- Fully Integrated Pharmaceutical or Biotechnology Network (FIPNET or FIBNET) business model.
- Research Intensive Pharmaceutical Company (RIP) business model.
- Drug Repositioning business model.
- Enabling Technology business model.

Diagnostic and Research Tool Companies

- Platform instrument/menu content business model.
- Clinical laboratory services business model.
- Subscription business model.

THERAPEUTICS AND BIOLOGICS COMPANIES

Fully Integrated Pharmaceutical Company (FIPCO) Business Model

The Fully Integrated Pharmaceutical Company (FIPCO) model is a standard business model that was previously utilized by *all* pharmaceutical companies, and is sometimes referred to as a "vertically integrated" model. In this model, the company performs (in-house) all the functions of the business—from initial R&D drug discovery, animal testing, human clinical testing, regulatory approval, manufacturing, and marketing of all their products. The advantage of the FIPCO business model is that the company can control *all* aspects of the development through to the marketing and commercialization of the product. As a result, many of the early biotechnology companies wanted to follow this model. However, successfully achieving this model was attained by venerable pharmaceutical companies with 100+ years of history and resources, but it was challenging for early-stage biotechnology companies to become a FIPCO. Regardless, in the early days of the biotechnology industry, this is what most all biotechnology companies aspired to become. As it was soon discovered, it took an enormous amount of time, resources, capital (and good fortune) for a biotechnology company to become a FIPCO. Many failed along the way trying to achieve this goal. Some fortunate ones such as Genentech, Amgen, Genzyme, and IDEC became FIPCOs. However, over time, as companies were forced to focus on capital efficiencies due to the limitations in available capital and lowered sales revenue, even the major pharmaceutical companies realized that the FIPCO business model was not the most efficient one. Pharmaceutical companies recognized that without a continual source of innovative therapeutic ideas, drug development pipelines can quickly dry up and the company is left with underutilized regulatory, clinical trials, formulation, manufacturing, and marketing capabilities.

To be more competitive and efficient, these companies modified the FIPCO business model in ways that allowed them to continue generating the types of profits expected of these multinational companies. Some of these modifications include reducing downstream capabilities to base levels that can be efficiently utilized but can be outsourced beyond that capacity, and eliminating some functions entirely in favor of using contract research organizations. In addition, instead of attempting to internally discover *all* their drug candidates, pharmaceutical companies augmented their R&D capabilities by in-licensing developing products from other biotechnology companies, or by acquiring these companies outright. This alternate business model is called a Fully Integrated Pharmaceutical Network (FIPNET) or a Virtually Integrated Pharmaceutical Company Organization (VIPCO). FIPNET and VIPCO companies have realized improved productivity and increased efficiency because they can outsource and/or contract for services at any point in their value chain and have access to complementary abilities outside the company. This model still allows a company to maintain control of the product development process and yet leverage the abilities of others at any point in the value chain. For biotechnology companies FIPCO is referred to as FIBCO where the "B" refers to "biotechnology" or "biopharmaceutical."(See Figure 12.2.)

For start-up biotechnology companies, becoming a FIPCO is not the optimal business model choice, and it is certainly not a realistic or believable one because doing this well is even difficult for major pharmaceutical companies. Though it is possible that any start-up biotechnology company could become a FIPCO sometime in the future, it is hardly a business model that an early investor would take seriously. In fact, a start-up biotechnology company that is stating a FIPCO goal would likely frighten sophisticated investors and they would disappear quickly. However, becoming a FIPNET company can be a long-term choice for biotechnology companies focused on therapeutic and biologics. Some highly innovative research-intensive companies realized their strength was in their novel research

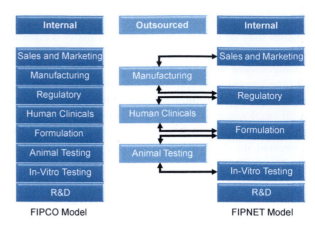

FIGURE 12.2   FIPCO and FIPNET business model structures.

functions and not their downstream activities. Hence, there arose another business model called a Research Intensive Pharmaceutical Company (RIPCO) where they focused only on the research and development, and licensed out all their product candidates to other organizations.

The Drug Repositioning Business Model

The Drug Repositioning business model is a therapeutic business model that focuses on repositioning abandoned drugs (approved or not approved) and finds alternate intended use populations or finds a population in which the drug has fewer side-effects and greater efficacy. A biotech Drug Repositioning company uses specialized know-how to identify an alternate or narrower population that can benefit from a shelved drug and that is usually based upon understanding the drug's mechanism of action. These older or unused drugs, are those that have already passed safety testing in humans. In order to speed up the development, some therapeutic biotech companies have adopted a Drug Repositioning business model to reduce the lengthy R&D timeframe and leverage the previously conducted drug safety profile. By adopting a Drug Repositioning business model, a number of biotech companies have shortened the drug development time and advanced rapidly into initial human safety testing. The support for the potential success of a Drug Repositioning business model came from the many drugs that failed for one particular indication but were later found to have success for use in another indication. One notable drug that failed as an antihypertensive drug and was later repositioned successfully was Viagra (sildenafil). Although human clinical studies did not demonstrate the desired antihypertensive effect, "side-effects" were noted by Pfizer scientists who then repositioned it as an erectile dysfunction drug. Other examples of successfully repositioned drugs include Eli Lilly's anticancer drug Gemzar (gemcitabine) which was originally developed as an antiviral agent, and Evista (raloxifene) which was originally developed as a birth control drug, then repositioned as a successful osteoporosis drug, and later, another indication as a

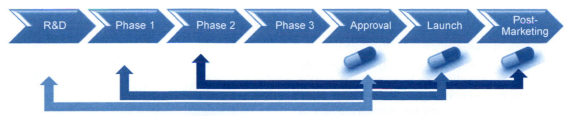

FIGURE 12.3   The Drug Repositioning business model takes drugs from later stages of testing and repositions them for other disease indications.

prophylactic for the prevention of breast cancer. Between 2007 and 2009, approximately 30 to 40 percent of the drugs and biologics that were approved or launched for the first time in the United States were drugs repositioned for new indications, reformulations, or new combinations of existing drugs [1–3] (Figure 12.3).

The advantages to a Drug Repositioning business model is that a company can leapfrog through much of the safety and *in vitro* toxicity testing and have early support for safety in *in vivo* testing. This can save literally tens of millions to hundreds of millions of dollars and multiple years of development, depending on the previous development stage and the new indication for use. However, as with any business model there are weaknesses and they must be evaluated in the context of the competition and based upon the proof that a model can be supported and become truly successful. Some of the disadvantages of this model is that a company must convince enough investors that they can continue to reposition another company's previously failed drug and biologics based upon some technology or idea that they possess. In addition, the drug repositioning business model does not *remove* drug development risks it just *reduces* them. In the early 2000s there was a large number of biotech companies that started as drug-repositioning companies because of the heightened interest and the success of several repositioned drug examples. Today there are some companies that are doing well using this business model, but there are also a fair number of companies that are no longer in business or have switched to another model. This does not mean that the Drug Repositioning business model cannot be successful, it just emphasizes that the selection of the business model is an important component, but without a good technology application, intellectual property protection, the right team, and adequate funding, no business model can guarantee success.

There are many biotechnology companies that do not operate as a Drug Repositioning Company but yet they possess a repositioned drug candidate as their company product and are having great success. For instance, the repositioned drug idea is a fantastic concept, but becoming a company whose sole mission is to identify successful candidates for repositioned drugs across a myriad of different indications may be quite challenging. However, there may be a sweet spot for an existing FIPCO therapeutic company that focuses on, for instance, rheumatoid arthritis anti-inflammatory

compounds to reposition other company's failed drugs that also carry anti-inflammatory properties and develop them for different anti-inflammatory indications. In essence, they can leverage their internal anti-inflammatory drug screening capabilities and accelerate product development for their anti-inflammatory-focused indications.

For an example, assisted a virtual therapeutic company reposition a combination drug and prepare to enter Phase 1 human clinical trials for the treatment of noise-induced hearing loss. Their technology focus had been on developing and testing novel free-radical scavenging compounds. They included in their screening another FDA-approved product used for a totally different indication which also had a mechanism-of-action as a free-radical scavenger. They combined this drug with a stroke drug (also a variation of a free-radical scavenger) that successfully completed human clinical Phase 1 and 2, but failed in Phase 3. When the combined product was tested in the new indication, the *in vitro* and animal testing showed synergistic results for the effective treatment of noise-induced hearing loss resulting from recent noise insults. This company is now advancing into Phase 1 human studies. The development of this technology to reach this point was achieved at approximately 30 to 40 percent of the typical cost and in about 50 percent of the normal drug development time. As a result, this combination product and other chemical derivatives of these compounds are the basis for a company with a technology having broad application in the treatment of hearing health. Although this company is not a "drug repositioning company" the genesis of its first product utilized one aspect of the "drug repositioning" business model, but they adopted an optimum business model for the future commercialization of the product and growth of the company.

Enabling Technology Business Models

A company operating with an Enabling Technology business model is focused on a "platform technology" and can use it to enable or improve applications of other company's products. I have categorized this business model in the Therapeutics and Biologics Company section but it can be applied to a number of other biotechnology sectors. Sometimes this business model is referred to as a "horizontal model" or a "platform model" because the company will focus on a single aspect or single segment of the value chain of a business. One example of a single value segment focus using the Enabling Technology business model is in drug delivery where a company can facilitate better methods of delivering certain drugs into the body that otherwise would not have any application, or to expand the market acceptance of current drugs through other delivery methods. ALZA, a drug delivery company formerly based in Palo Alto, California, was founded in 1968 by entrepreneur **Al**ejandro **Za**ffaroni (hence the name ALZA), had a focus on drug delivery platforms and pioneered the transdermal delivery technology. The company successfully applied its skin-patch platform technology to existing drugs such as Nicoderm® as an aid to help quit smoking, and Procardia XL® for both angina and hypertension, Duragesic® for the management of cancer pain, and Glucotrol XL® for the treatment of type 2 diabetes. In the mid-1990s the company added other segments of the vertical value chain and successfully transitioned to a FIPCO. ALZA eventually was acquired in 2001 by Johnson & Johnson for approximately $10 billion. By applying their technology to the delivery of drugs across the skin barrier, they created opportunity for their company to improve or expand access for other products of the company. Some other applications of Enabling Technology business models include servicing companies that focus on certain types of drug screening, animal testing, and even Contract Research Organizations (CRO) and Contract Manufacturing Organizations, all provide specialized services or technology as value for their business.

DIAGNOSTIC AND RESEARCH TOOLS COMPANIES

Platform Instrument/Menu Content Business Model

A successful business model in the clinical diagnostic and molecular testing industry is developing tests that run on proprietary platform instruments that are produced and manufactured by the same company. Diagnostic tools and instrument companies that use this Platform Instrument/ Menu Content business model are Luminex, Becton Dickenson, Roche, Affymetrix, and Illumina, to name a few. In this business model the company develops and markets content (different tests) that only operate on their instruments, and cannot run on a competitor's testing platform. The success of their business model works when the manufacturer can install the largest number of their platform testing equipment in the greatest number of clinical and research laboratories possible. In order for customers to have a desire to purchase these instruments the company must also develop a desirable menu of testing content that these customers want. The "Instrument and Test Menu" business model is an adaptation of the "Razor Handle and Razor Blade" business model, because the principles are

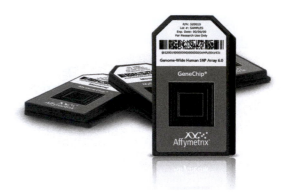

FIGURE 12.4 Affymetrix gene chip: An example of an Instrument and Menu Content business model *(Courtesy of Affymetrix, Inc., Santa Clara, CA, USA).*

identical. The company creates and sells a tool, instrument, or platform, and then perpetually sells to that same customer specialized, high margin consumables. Recall that in the shaving industry, Gillette and Schick understood they could essentially give away the razor handle and build a successful business. They understood that when a customer purchased their brand of razor handle, the customer was committed, and the company generated the majority of their profits on the reoccurring purchases of consumable razor blades. Another similar business model parallel is the inkjet printing industry. Companies such as Hewlett-Packard, Canon, and Epson compete for consumers to purchase their printers. Often they may sell their printers at a loss because they know their profits come through the perpetual selling of branded high-profit margin ink.

Another example of a biotechnology company using this type of business model is Affymetrix. The company designs, manufactures, and sells platform instruments based upon a microarray technology they have developed which performs a variety of different types of genomic analyses. The chips are consumables that are purchased to run on Affymetrix's dedicated instrument platform and operates on their proprietary software (see Figure 12.4).

The Platform Instrument/Menu Content business model can be applied to many other tools and instrument companies and also medical device and diagnostic companies. The advantages of this business model is that the company has a captive customer base with continual reoccurring revenue streams which would be proportional to the total number of instruments that are placed into the market. Often the company's consumable carries a very high profit margin and can offset even an initial loss on the instrument placement due to the long-term and perpetual purchasing of the company's consumables. One disadvantage of this business model is that competing technologies from other companies can sometimes quickly replace or even obsolete another company's platform technology, and therefore within a short period of time the reoccurring revenue streams may disappear. It is therefore imperative that companies which adopt such a model, continually invest in R&D to improve, advance, and innovate solutions that keep customers attached to their branded platforms and are wedded to their expanding test menu.

Clinical Laboratory Service Business Model

In the diagnostics sector, a company will develop a detection technology for an analyte of interest (molecule or chemical), then produce and manufacture a "kit" which is sold to others who perform these diagnostic tests. The Clinical Laboratory Service business model can be a viable alternative for these companies. In this model, molecular and diagnostic companies perform unique and proprietary tests as a *service,* operating through a single company-owned clinical laboratory, instead of manufacturing a "kit" which would be sold to others. There are several advantages to the Laboratory Service business model over the "kit" manufacturing model which include:

- A shorter timeframe from inception of test technology to product commercialization.
- Generally lower costs of product and service development.
- Usually fewer employees required to begin commercialization.
- An alternative regulatory path (CLIA) rather than the FDA regulatory approval (note that the regulatory approval route is being evaluated and may change in the future).

There are also disadvantages to this business model over the traditional diagnostic kit manufacturing model which include:

- The testing services can only be performed in one laboratory location, potentially limiting the volume of testing and creating a bottleneck.
- Testing requires specialized employees who have the expertise to perform these testing services.
- Regulatory approval includes biannual laboratory inspections and proficiency testing which, if not compliant, can shut down or restrict all services for a period of time.

Diagnostic testing companies choose one business model over the other for strategic reasons and for competitive advantages. For instance, a very complex and highly technical test that is very difficult and labor intensive to perform may be challenging to reduce to a "kit" allowing others to perform proficiently and accurately. Such a complex test may require specialized equipment that must be developed so users can adequately perform the test with consistent results. In this case, the Clinical Laboratory business model may be a better choice. Examples of companies using this business model include Myriad Genetics and Genomic Health. Myriad Genetics has research, development, marketing,

and sales functions for its clinical laboratory molecular tests which are focused on predicting risk of hereditary-based cancers. They operate a single CLIA-certified clinical laboratory which is appropriately certified and accredited to perform these laboratory testing services. Because their tests cannot be licensed to other clinical laboratories, all testing is performed at the company's sole clinical laboratory in Salt Lake City, Utah—they also control and retain all the profits. Genomic Health, based in Redwood City, California also operates as a CLIA laboratory and performs its testing services using the same business model. Both these companies have had tremendous success in using the Clinical Laboratory Services business model for their products. It is conceivable that both Myriad Genetics and Genomic Health could also create an instrument platform that could run their genetic tests and sell these instruments to multiple laboratories under the Instrument/Content business model. However, their business model choice provides them with superior financial, market, and regulatory advantages and gives them the ability to rapidly introduce new testing services or make rapid modifications or improvements to their testing menu.

Subscription Business Model

The Subscription business model has been utilized by many of the early genomic discovery companies where they sold subscriptions to their databases (ISIS Pharmaceuticals, Incyte Genomics, Millineum Pharmaceuticals, and Celera). These organizations sell information, or access to information and data, that is valuable to other companies. There are multiple options and iterations of the revenue portion of this business model which can include one or many of the following options:

- Charging an initiation fee or membership fee for initial access to data/information.
- Charging ongoing subscription fees (annual or multiple years) for access to the data/information.
- Adopting increased fees for increased number of "seats" or users that a company utilizes to access the data/information.
- Implement future royalties on products developed from the data/information.
- Charges for R&D for specialized data mining or data manipulation services.
- Increased fees for access to additional or restricted data/information that is not available to those with a "regular" membership.

The benefits of the Subscription business model is that the company has predictability of ongoing revenue and low revenue risk for the period of time that the customer is committed. Also, the company usually receives their revenue upfront, and therefore the incremental costs of servicing another customer with the same information is nominal compared to the revenue received. In other words, the gross profit margins are extremely large for the company as they add additional customers. The risks of this business model are similar to those in the Enabling Technology business model in that competing technology companies can obviate or reduce the value of your service by providing more relevant or more valuable data. However, this risk is mitigated if the company holds unique, specialized, or proprietary data such as genomic information for certain types of tissues, diseases, conditions, microbes, or analyses of specialized information such as gene methylation patterns and copy-number variations to name a few. The risk comes when competitors have access to the same or similar data (possibly because it is in the public domain) and they provide significantly improved methods of data interpretation because of their developed algorithms or better software systems. One way to mitigate this type of risk for those who adopt this particular business model is to continue advancing product improvements to the point of even displacing their current products by providing significant improvements.

ALL BUSINESS MODELS HAVE TRANSFERABLE COMPONENT PARTS OR SEGMENTS

Although we have only discussed a few representative business models, you should know that there are an endless number of models and permutations to each one. The reason the number of business models grow is that they are comprised of transposable segments each of which can be assembled in a variety of combinations to produce variations of any single model. Almost all business model segments can be "lifted" from one to create a hybrid business model for another application. A valuable tool that has been utilized by many organizations in creating, developing, or optimizing their business model is called the "Business Model Canvas" referenced in the book *Business Model Generation* [4]. The Business Model Canvas is a strategic management template for developing business models. It is a visual chart with placeholders to describe nine of a company's business model segments such as: value proposition, infrastructure, customers, and finances, to name a few. This tool has assisted firms in aligning their activities, optimizing strategy, and by illustrating potential trade-offs.

Business Model Canvas Overview of Segments

In the Business Model Canvas, there are nine business model segments that are reviewed. These include:

1. **Customer segments**—These include all the groups of people and organizations for which you are creating value, which include users and paying customers.
2. **Value proposition to each segment**—These are the values, features, and benefits provided to each customer segment.
3. **Channels to reach customers**—These are all the "touch-points" that are necessary to reach customers and deliver value to them.
4. **Customer relationships to establish**—This is a description of the type of relationship you need to establish with your customers.
5. **Revenue streams generated**—Description of how and through which pricing mechanism your business is capturing value.
6. **Key resources required to create value**—Description of the infrastructure required to create, deliver, and capture value, and the key resources that are indispensable to your business model.
7. **Key activities required to create value**—Description of which things you need to perform well.
8. **Key partners**—Description of who you need to help you leverage your business model.
9. **Cost structure of the business model**—The cost structure of the entire business model for delivering value to each customer segment.

Figure 12.5 illustrates the Business Model Canvas and the relationship of these nine segments to each other. For first-time entrepreneurs and those who are not familiar with business models and business strategies, it may be worthwhile to walk through the Business Model Canvas and familiarize yourself with each of the described segments. Once you have a working understanding of each of these segments, it is easier to formulate and select the optimum business model for your company. One great benefit of using the Business Model Canvas is that it requires that the company leaders identify and agree upon their target customers, their value proposition to each, and the manner in which they will deliver this value. These identified and optimized segments become the building blocks of the final business model. One weakness of this approach is that all the building blocks still must be assembled into an integrated model.

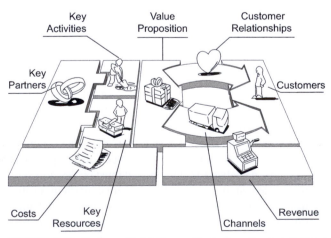

FIGURE 12.5 Business Model Canvas illustration. (Source: *Business Model Canvas.*)

In order to finalize an integrated model it requires that all the building blocks or segments be joined into one united and cohesive system where the component parts do not conflict, and the integrated whole is the most efficient and effective method for competitively delivering the product and company value. Sometimes this final integration requires that individual segments be adjusted or modified to fit within an integrated strategy. This planning exercise is valuable and essential for any start-up or development-stage biotechnology company. Having a sound and well-thought-out rationale for a company business model will help improve the likelihood of investor interest, and the potential for raising the needed capital during the formative stages of product development.

HOW DO YOU DETERMINE THE BEST BUSINESS MODEL FOR A TECHNOLOGY

Sometimes the product opportunity is straightforward and the business model is clear. However, remember there are multiple segments to a business that can result in hybrids of models which are optimized for your specific business. Don't assume that your technology or industry sector will automatically dictate the best business model strategy. Always start by first examining the unmet needs in your target market and then think about the best way your technology can help meet these needs through your choice of business model. Examine the value provided by your current or future competitors and look for better ways that your value can be provided to your target market.

In order to identify the best business model strategy for a technology, one of the first steps is to know the answers to the following questions:

- Who are the target customer groups that need and want your product?
- What are the needs your product will be satisfying for the target market? How will this be accomplished?
- Does your company have intermediaries in the value chain between itself and the end-user customers? Is there a way to leverage this relationship to improve the company's success?
- Are there any other external players in the value proposition to the customer in order to sell these products?
- How does your company intend to reach these customers?
- What is the nature of the relationship between the company and its vendors and suppliers required to produce the products or generate the services?
- Are there relationships that can be leveraged and are synergistic?
- How will the distribution of the product be carried out and by whom?
- How does the company intend to make money?

- What is the process used to develop and produce the product?
- Are there alternative ways to reduce the time, costs, or risks during development of this product?
- Does a third-party receive a benefit when the company sells its product or service to the target market? If so, can these relationships be leveraged to bring additional benefits to the company?

These questions simply represent a starting point to help you arrive at the best business model to leverage your technology and product opportunity into a market. There are a number of related questions that should be addressed when thinking about the optimum business model for your company. By knowing the answers to all of these questions, the optimal business model can be identified which maximizes the benefits of the company and efficiently delivers the product's value proposition of your target customers. Remember that some components of a business model are dynamic and these can be optimized as the market evolves or new channels and methods become available. For instance, if in the future new market channels become available or changes may occur in the regulatory environment for your product. Who would have predicted 20 years ago the market value of the Internet on advertising, social media, and on sales strategies? Even though you can refine some of these business model components and adjust them to changes and improvements in the market, you still must first identify the most strategic model at the outset because this becomes the foundation of the business strategy and all components are interconnected to this "frame."

The ultimate objectives for selecting a particular business model include the following:

- To maximize the profit potential of the company.
- To minimize or reduce the commercialization timeframe and costs of product development.
- Leverage your intellectual property (IP) protection.
- To provide a competitive advantage over other companies or products in the field.
- Long-term sustainability in a changing market or regulatory environment.

ENTREPRENEURIAL LEADERS ARE RISK MANAGERS

A key objective of the proper selection of an optimal business model is to maximize the opportunity for success of your company and to reduce the risks of failure. Throughout the process of establishing, building, leading, and managing a biotechnology company, the leaders and managers can be characterized as "risk managers." Throughout the many decisions that the leaders make, a course is chosen to reduce risk and improve success of the business. The business model selection is just one of those decisions. Every choice an individual makes, whether in business or in life, carries some measure of risk with consequences and some measure of opportunity for success. For instance, when making a decision on purchasing an automobile, deciding on a particular make and model, whether new or used, carries a risk as to reliability and repair frequency and costs as well as safety and comfort. The level of risk for these choices is usually moderate and the consequences of these decisions are usually minimal—unless of course you are in a major accident and you chose a poorly designed or poorly maintained automobile. However, choosing a cardiac surgeon to operate and perform a coronary artery bypass surgery carriers a much higher degree of risk and potentially greater consequences than the previous example. Each decision requires a risk assessment because there are differing consequences for a poor choice. The choice of a business model is critical and the proper selection will greatly reduce the future risk to the business by selecting the best one. Spend the time necessary to select the proper business model for your company.

You Cannot Manage a Risk You Do not Identify

Entrepreneurs and managers can greatly improve the odds of their success if they begin their business with a thorough understanding of the business and technology risks that they could face based upon the objectives they must accomplish. There are innumerable ways a company can fail but relatively few ways a company can succeed. One way to facilitate the success of your company is to identify and assess the risks, prioritize them as to the level of risk and impact, and address them by having mitigating plans for facilitating success. In order to do this you must have a method of risk assessment. I have found that we can group the risks of biotechnology companies into five categories that are fundamental for success. These categories are:

1. Management, leadership, and past success.
2. Technology robustness, applicability, and scientific team.
3. Market demand and positioning.
4. Regulatory hurdles and barriers to entry.
5. Future funding and financing suitability.

No doubt more than five categories of biotechnology company risks can be identified. However, if you examine the issues leading to failure of many start-up biotechnology companies, you can trace their problems back to one, or several failures within these five risk categories. Each of these risk categories is exceedingly important to success and a company must be strong in each of the five areas in order to succeed. A company that possesses exceptional strength in four of these categories must know that this

does not compensate for the weakness in the other one. A company must have strength in each of these five categories. The entrepreneur must integrate and manage all five risk categories in order to have the best opportunity for success. Integrative risk management is the ability to manage all risks simultaneously and understand how one risk impacts each of the other risks. Occasionally, activities or decisions in one area impact or cause challenges in another area as a consequence. Integrated risk management evaluates each decision in light of all the risks that must be managed.

BIOTECHNOLOGY COMPANY EVALUATION TOOL

Assessing your company's strengths and weaknesses is necessary before beginning to raise capital. Potential investors also evaluate a biotechnology business opportunity based upon similar criteria listed in the evaluation tool. Therefore, I strongly advise having an aid that may be similar to what investors may utilize when evaluating companies for investment interest. Such a tool is helpful when preparing for investor presentations and in preparation for writing your business plan. The Biotechnology Company Evaluation Tool is a worksheet I developed for assessing a company business and technology for the evaluation of investment advice, or potential for success and risks to be managed. When formally evaluating biotechnology companies one can use a more detailed set of questions and analysis, but this list serves as the basis for an initial evaluation.

The purpose of the Biotechnology Company Evaluation Tool is to objectively rate your company as compared to others and to identify its strengths and weaknesses. Use this tool with the categorized questions to determine a ranking of your business. Score your company on a 1 to 5 scale, with 1 being the worst and 5 being the best as compared to the best in the industry. After evaluating each question in each of the categories, average the scores in each section. A composite criteria score of 2.5 or below in any of these five risk categories reveals an unacceptable level of business risk that must be addressed. This tool can also measure the overall strength of the company as well as point to areas that need help, but recognize it is a snapshot in time.

Interpreting the Results

It is absolutely certain that a start-up or development-stage biotechnology company will not score well in all of these categories. When that happens, do not become discouraged—it does not mean that the company is destined to fail. Having a low score at one point in time can be transformed into a company strength years later if these risks have been addressed and overcome. It is essential to use this tool critically so you can identify your company's weaknesses because it will direct your focus on what should to be done to improve. Remember, it is impossible to deal with an unidentified weakness. Once your company's areas of weakness are identified, draft a plan on how you will overcome these shortcomings with a timeline and responsible person(s) to manage them and their progress. Entrepreneurs don't do themselves any favors by overlooking problems or by using a biased ranking in this exercise. I would encourage you to be critically objective because it is certain others evaluating your organization will. If the entrepreneur or leadership team has trouble being critically objective, enlist the help of others to give you feedback and comment on each of these categories. The opinion of outside experts can be very valuable when assessing your company's risk. This tool should also be used at regular intervals, and the results periodically assessed throughout your organization's development to evaluate improvements and assess the effectiveness of changes made. If a company's key risks are properly managed, these scores will significantly improve over time. By demonstrating you are successfully managing each of these risks, investors will be more favorable with your ability to lead your organization's development future.

Biotechnology Company Evaluation Tool

I. Management, Leadership, and Past Success

Score	Questions
	1. Does the CEO/Entrepreneur/Leader have previous successful experience in a *similar leadership capacity and demonstrated* that he/she is the right individual to *successfully* lead this organization?
	2. Is the Leadership Team passionate about their mission and work, and do they fully believe in its future success?
	3. Is the *Full Leadership Team* complete and in place with all members having directly applicable experience and success?
	4. If the management team is incomplete, are there *sound plans to bring on the remaining leaders* and are the plans sufficient to overcome current weakness?
	5. Is there a *Core Leadership Team* in place, which is a group capable of managing the current and near term company needs and has previous experience and success?
	6. Are *all* the Leadership Team members *seasoned* and do they have *directly related expertise* applicable to this type of company and in this particular industry?
	7. Does the Leadership Team collectively have *complementary abilities* and expertise and do they share common core values and work extremely well together?
	8. Is the Leadership Team accustomed to a *start-up environment* and do they have past success accomplishments in a start-up situation?
	9. Does the Leadership Team have all the ability to *fully execute the current business plan and strategy*, and have they demonstrated performing these activities successfully in the past or through previous experience?
	10. Are all the Leadership Team members *aware of their weaknesses* individually and as a collective whole, and enthusiastic and willing to seek help to fill this gap?
	TOTAL SCORE
	AVERAGE SCORE (divide by 10)

II. Technology Robustness, Applicability, and Scientific Team

Score	Questions
	1. Is the technology and product application *truly innovative* relative to other new concepts and technologies in the industry?
	2. Are the *opinion leaders* in this field *positive, complementary, and excited* about this product and technology?
	3. Does the company have a team of *top-notch scientific and technical staff* who has *demonstrated scientific leadership* in this particular field?
	4. Has the scientific team members *published multiple* proof-of-concept studies or other supporting data and studies in *top-tier peer-reviewed journals*?
	5. Has this scientific team been *awarded multiple peer-reviewed grants* (NIH, NSF, NCI, etc) which validate that their work is respected by their peers as this field?
	6. Is there universally *clear scientific understanding of the biology of the disease or condition*, such that the target or product chosen has a high likelihood of success.

II. Technology Robustness, Applicability, and Scientific Team

Score	Questions
	7. Is the underlying technology, intellectual property and product(s) protected by *issued patents*?
	8. Is there a *freedom-to-operate* opinion that has been performed that concludes the company does not have challenging intellectual property barriers?
	9. If the technology is licensed, is there a *perpetual exclusive license* having conventional royalty rates and reasonable mile-stone fees, and the freedom to sell the technology without approval from the licensee? (If the technology is wholly owned by the company outright score 5.)
	10. Is this product based upon a core technology that has the potential to *produce multiple products* rather than just a one product idea?
	TOTAL SCORE
	AVERAGE SCORE (Divide by 10)

III. Market Demand and Positioning

Score	Questions
	1. Has the company *selected the best target market* and demonstrated that there is significant *unmet demand* for their future product or service, without having to create this demand?
	2. Is the marketing strategy to the target market based upon *solid evidence* supporting that there is an *unmet market need* for this product where substitutes don't adequately satisfy the true need?
	3. Is the market *large enough* to support the types of *returns needed* for the company to become a *sustained success* once the product is commercialized?
	4. Does the company understand the *real competitors and product substitutes* which could displace market demand for their product, and is there sufficient value proposition within their product to rapidly grow the customer base?
	5. Are market forces *converging toward this product need* such that demand will increase rather than migrate away from where the product will be positioned in the future?
	6. Is there an *existing and reliable distribution channel* in place to reach this market without having to create a new one for this product to be successful?
	7. Are the *Pro forma* projections based upon *tested assumptions* and are the market penetration plans for this product realistic and reasonable?
	8. Does the company have the *necessary personnel and expertise* with the capabilities and know-how to lead and penetrate this market?
	9. Does the company have a *well-thought-out branding and positioning strategy* to successfully distinguish its product and services from others?
	10. Is the product offering *quickly scalable* and is there a world-wide need for the product offering?
	TOTAL SCORE
	AVERAGE SCORE (Divide by 10)

IV. Regulatory Hurdles and Barriers to Entry

Score	Questions
	1. Does the Leadership or Management Team have *previous experience with regulatory success* for approval of similar products or services?
	2. Does the Leadership or Management Team *know the process and the length of time* estimated to obtain regulatory approval?
	3. Does the Leadership or Management Team *know the risks for regulatory approval with this type of product*, having identified successful examples of others, without the possibility of classification into a totally new regulatory category?
	4. Has the Leadership or Management Team had recent and *direct communications with regulatory agencies or industry experts* who are intimately familiar with the current regulatory issues for their product?
	5. Are the regulations for marketing approval *clearly defined* without the possibility of dynamic and future changes anticipated for the product or the market the company is entering?
	6. Are there *impending regulation changes* for the company's product or market that are not yet completely defined?

IV. Regulatory Hurdles and Barriers to Entry

Score	Questions
	7. Does the company have a *well-developed and detailed plan* in place with the expertise in the regulatory strategy and process to assure that the regulatory steps are accomplishable by this team?
	8. Does the company possess *three or more significant barriers to entry* that have been identified such that these pose formidable challenges for competitors to successfully compete in this product market?
	9. Is the product offering free from *debatable ethical or unresolved societal issues* such that the product growth and market acceptance would not be hampered anywhere in the world?
	10. Is there *clear regulatory guidance* for the product offering in the major *countries throughout the world* such that the regulatory approval requirements are clearly understood?
	TOTAL SCORE
	AVERAGE SCORE (Divide by 10)

V. Future Funding and Financing Suitability

Score	Questions
	1. Is there very high potential for *continued funding* of the company based upon similar types of organizations and funding trends, or based upon expressed or stated interest of investors?
	2. Is the business, product or target market a *very good candidate for venture capital or institutional funding* based upon venture capital funding trends or directly expressed interest?
	3. Does the company currently have *Institutional Investors*, those with large cash investing reserves, or *Venture Capitalists* who are *positive* on the company and the product's future success potential?
	4. Is the exit strategy attractive enough to show a *potential 10× return* on investment and is there a reasonable likelihood of achieving the exit goals based upon the current economic metrics in the industry?
	5. Is there sufficient *cash on hand* to carry the company at least 18 months at its projected burn rate, or well past the next significant value-enhancing milestone?
	6. Has the company identified fundable *value-enhancing development milestones* that can be reached which will significantly improve the valuation of the company and the likelihood of securing follow-on funding?
	7. Are the *outlined use-of-proceeds* for the development of the organization reasonable and effective throughout the product development cycle?
	8. Are the current *investors supportive of the company, product, and Leadership Team* such that they would add to their investment or recommend this investment to others?
	9. Does the company reside in a geographic location that historically has access to Venture Capital or Institutional Funds and/or located in a geography that is considered a *biotechnology cluster or hub*?
	10. Does the Leadership Team have *experience in successfully raising the total amount of capital* projected to reach the exit or to reach profitability?
	TOTAL SCORE
	AVERAGE SCORE (Divide by 10)

SUMMARY

The biotechnology business model examples reviewed show how a business model can help a company become competitive with their technology or product. Recognize that there are numerous business models in the therapeutic, biologic, diagnostic, medical device, clinical laboratory, and research reagent industry, and many are adapted and modified for a company's competitive advantage. The process of selecting the optimal business model must involve the collective assessment of all the various business segments which are essential for your business, while taking into account all their associated risks. Choosing the best business model provides your company with the greatest opportunity for success and it is the first step in managing the business risk and should be selected and implemented during the company's inception stage. It is important to know the business models of your competitors in the industry and to identify what aspects of their model make them successful. There are multiple components within any single business model. Some components may be strengths and some may be weaknesses for you, so learn what they are before making a choice. Study alternate business models in adjacent sectors and in totally different industries and consider if portions of these may be adaptable and improve competitiveness or reduce business risks for your company. As with the razor-handle/razor-blade model, portions of old business models may be applicable and transferable to new products or technology depending on your needs or objectives. Identify the reasons why one model works in one particular business and why the same business model might be a failure in another business. Think about the overall strategies that give a company a sustainable competitive advantage over the competition and lead the company to sustained profitability.

As an entrepreneur or company leader, you are also the risk manager of the business. In order to manage the risk, you must first understand what they are and then actively manage them. Leaders can reduce risks by making sound decisions and identifying ways to mitigate these risks. Remember that in the early stages of any business many decisions have long-term impact such as determining your product development pathway, protecting your intellectual property, determining the method and timing of financing, deciding upon which individuals to hire, and choosing your marketing strategy. To help assess you company's risks, utilize the Biotechnology Company Evaluation Tool to rank the five risk categories. Be sure to objectively assess your strengths and weaknesses and then develop a plan for how to bring those areas to a level of excellence. This tool will be helpful when preparing to raise capital and it will also establish a reference point during your company's development that will help you gauge future progress and your overall improvement. The information gained from critically answering the questions in each of these categories will be helpful when creating your business plan as discussed in Chapter 22 entitled "Your Business Plan and Presentation: Articulating Your Journey to Commercialization."

No entrepreneur can be expected to completely eliminate risk, but it is extremely hazardous if the leader does not even know what the risks are to the company. The entrepreneurial team's objective is to understand the risks associated with accomplishing the core objectives of the company and to identify ways to mitigate these risks. It is important to recognize that success does not come solely by making the right choices when presented with decisions. Much of the success is influenced by one's creativity in finding ways to effectively and resourcefully circumvent challenges rather than simply by choosing the path holding the lowest risk.

REFERENCES

[1] Graul AI, et al. Drug News Perspect; 2010. PMID: 20155217.
[2] Graul AI, et al. Drug News Perspect; 2009. PMID: 19209296.
[3] Graul AI, et al. Drug News Perspect; 2008. PMID:18301807.
[4] Osterwalder A, Pigneur Y, Smith A, 470 practitioners from 45 countries. Business Model Generation; 2010. Self published.

The Emerging-Stage Biotechnology Company

Chapter 13

Company Formation, Ownership Structure, and Securities Issues

Craig C. Bradley, JD

Partner, Edwards Wildman Palmer LLP, Chicago, Illinois

The choice of the form of entity that is going to be used to operate the business is an important one for the biotech entrepreneur. A number of factors as described below should be carefully considered in making this decision. If the formation of the business is not properly documented, then the ownership of the entity, the ownership of the intellectual property, and tax issues can create great and sometimes insurmountable problems. Care should be taken to use a seasoned counsel who is experienced in working with technology start-up companies. You should get recommendations from successful executives in your area, and you may also get leads from accounting firms, bankers, and your nearest biotech or other technology association. It is best to interview at least two or three lawyers in order to increase your chances of finding a good "fit." Almost all attorneys will agree to a 1 hour meeting with no obligation.

Law firms charge by the hour, which can range from $200 on the low side to up to $700 for senior partners at large law firms. Of course, some start-up company needs are relatively simple and straightforward, while some can be complicated and time-consuming. A good start-up lawyer should be able to give you a fairly narrow range of estimated costs. Many firms offer discounts and deferral arrangements for promising start-up companies.

ENTITY FORMATION

Entities are formed to conduct business principally in order to limit the personal liability of the owners. It is the nature of businesses to incur liabilities. If formed and operated appropriately, creditors cannot attack the personal assets of the owners, but only the assets of the entity. These basic requirements include the formal organization of the entity in one of the states of the United States (this chapter is limited to United States law), observing certain formalities (e.g., maintaining certain company records),

avoiding being too thinly capitalized, avoiding the commingling of assets between the company and the owners, and certain other elements. As these conditions, to avoid "piercing the corporate veil" are easily met, the discussion of them is abbreviated here. One thing is for certain, it almost is never advisable to conduct business without the benefit of forming an entity to shield the personal assets of the owners – sometimes referred to as "bet your house" liability.

There are a limited number of types of entities to choose from:

1. Corporations (both C and S, and so-called "Benefit" Corporations).
2. Partnerships (both general and limited).
3. Limited Liability Companies (Limited Liability Partnerships are limited mostly to services firms and are not treated here).

Corporations

Corporations are franchises granted by a state. A corporation is formed by filing a document with the state, generally as either a "Certificate of Incorporation" or "Articles of Incorporation." The owners are issued stock and are referred to as stockholders or shareholders. The stockholders elect a board of directors who are charged with the general management of the corporation. The board of directors in turn elects the officers—usually a president, one or more vice presidents, a treasurer, and a secretary. The officers are charged with the day-to-day operation of the corporation.

The common practice in the industry of start-ups is to form entities, whether corporations or limited liability companies (LLCs) in the state of Delaware. One reason is that the Delaware statutes are well-written and the case law interpreting these laws is well-developed. It is not expensive to organize in Delaware even if the entity's operations are in another state. Another key reason is that corporate lawyers across the country are familiar with Delaware corporate law. The lawyers who represent investors prefer dealing with a company that is governed by Delaware law. Many states have quirky provisions that are traps for the unwary. The formation of a start-up technology business in a state other than Delaware is usually a red flag that the entity is not well-advised.

One of the most critical issues to consider in the formation of an entity is the fact that a corporation is subject to two levels of taxes: (1) the corporation itself is taxed at the entity level for income earned and for any gain on the sale of its assets, and (2) the stockholders are taxed on dividends (amounts received other than in liquidation) and on distributions (amounts received from the corporation as a result of the sale or liquidation of its assets). The dreaded "double tax!"

The double tax on corporations can be contrasted with the single level taxation of "pass through" entities, which are the S corporation and the LLC, as well as partnerships. Note also that an LLC or S corporation can always change to a C corporation with no adverse tax consequences. However, switching from a C corporation to an S corporation or an LLC is a deemed liquidation and a taxable event.

S Corporations

"S corporations" are the same as regular corporations, sometimes referred to as "C corporations" in all operational respects, except that an election is made under subchapter S of the Internal Revenue Code of 1986, as amended (the "IRC"), to be taxed as a partnership. Being taxed as a partnership means that the entity is disregarded for tax purposes, and all the tax attributes (e.g., profits and losses) of the entity are passed through to the owners, the stockholders. When income is earned, the S corporation owes no tax—the stockholders are liable for the income tax. When an S corporation sells its assets to a buyer, the S corporation owes no tax on the gain—the stockholders are liable for the tax.

The S election was enacted for small businesses. Accordingly, there are limitations on S corporations, namely (1) a maximum of 100 stockholders, (2) only individuals can be stockholders (other than certain trusts and charities, and also S corporations can wholly own other S corporations), (3) stockholders cannot be nonresident aliens, and (4) only one class of stock is permitted, e.g., no preferred stock is permitted (although there can be voting and nonvoting stock).

Because of these limitations, S corporations rarely are used for technology start-ups. For example, universities, which often receive some equity in exchange for the licensing of technology, cannot be stockholders in S corporations.

Most angel investors insist on a preferred equity position, and preferred stock cannot be issued by an S corporation. If a pass-through entity is desired, LLCs are invariably preferred over S corporations. Keep in mind that if the S corporation runs afoul of one of the S corporation limitations, then it is disqualified and immediately becomes, without any further condition or action, a C corporation, which can cause disastrous consequences.

Benefit Corporations

Benefit corporations, as well as so-called "L3Cs," are organizations which embed in their charters provisions that the company must legally account for nonfinancial considerations, e.g., the public good, the environment, etc. There are third-party organizations which issue certifications that a company meets certain qualifications. Very few start-up technology companies want to travel down the road of being a benefit corporation.

Partnerships

Partnerships can be general partnerships or limited partnerships. General partnerships have no limitation on personal liability. Entities can be the general partners, so most often the partners in a general partnership are corporations or LLCs. Limited partnerships require the filing of a certificate with a state. The owners of a limited partnership are comprised of a limited partner or partners and must include at least one general partner. Limited partners have limited personal liability, as long as they don't meaningfully participate in the management of the partnership. How much they can "manage" varies from state-to-state.

Partnerships are almost never used by start-ups—LLCs are invariable preferred over partnerships. These days about the only partnerships you see in the technology start-up world are long-standing venture capital firms that are limited partnerships and who have not changed over yet to an LLC structure.

Limited Liability Companies

LLCs are a hybrid of the corporation and the partnership. Most critically, LLCs are pass-through entities, taxed as partnerships (although in rare cases an LLC will elect to be taxed as a C corporation). LLCs are formed in a state by the filing of a "Certificate of Formation," and in some states "Articles of Organization." The owners are referred to as "members." The LLC can be managed by its members or the LLC can opt to be managed by a "manager" or "managers" or even by a "board of managers," analogous to a board of directors in a corporation. Ownership usually is not certificated, i.e., there are usually no paper certificates representing ownership, like a stock certificate in a corporation, although issuing certificates is permitted. Like a partnership, ownership is a percentage, with all the percentages, not surprisingly, adding up to 100 percent. Often, for ease of reference, the term "units" is employed. Like shares of stock, use of the nomenclature of units makes the calculations on a cap table much easier.

LLCs are governed by their "Limited Liability Company Agreements," also referred to as "Operating Agreements" in some states. These agreements are analogous to bylaws and stockholder agreements for corporations. These agreements, for pass-through entities such as LLCs and S corporations, should always contain a provision requiring that cash be distributed to the owners in amounts sufficient to pay their respective income tax obligations. As with stockholder agreements in corporations, they can contain:

- **Rights of first refusal**—If an owner desires to sell equity to a third party, it must first be offered to the company and/or the other owners.
- **Co-sale rights**—If rights of first refusal are not exercised, then the other owners can elect to sell a pro rata portion of their equity.
- **Drag-along rights**—If a majority (or another specified percentage) of the owners want to sell the company, then all the other owners must sell their equity too.
- **Market stand-off**—If the company does an initial public offering, then, generally, the owners can't make any transfers for 180 days.
- **Voting agreement**—The owners can agree to all vote their equity to elect a certain manager or managers.
- **Super majority voting**—The owners can agree that certain important actions require the prior written consent of a super majority percentage (e.g., two-thirds or 75 percent, or even unanimous consent), such as sale of new equity, sale of the company, sale or licensing of the company's technology, borrowing money, new hires, salaries, etc.

LLCs have none of the limitations of an S corporation. There are no limitations on the nature of its owners, on its equity structure, or with regard to how the LLC is governed. Not only can LLCs have a preferred equity structure, profits and losses can be allocated on a basis other than ownership percentage. For example, say a senior scientist started the business and invested $25,000 of his own funds but now desires to return to the lab and let others run the company. The LLC could be structured to return the first $25,000 with interest at the prime rate to the scientist, then the scientist could receive 50 percent of the first $1 million and then 10 percent after that. The scientist could retain some or all management authority until the receipt of a certain amount of funds or until the LLC raised a certain amount of investment. Cash investors can be allocated a greater amount of the losses than noncash investors (keep in mind that losses

can be taken only to the extent of "basis," i.e., cash invested plus certain recourse loans).

Making the Choice of Either a C Corporation or an LLC?

C corporations are subject to a double tax and LLCs are not. S corporations have some strict limitations and LLCs do not. An LLC or an S corporation can be changed to a C corporation with no adverse tax consequences, but not vice versa. So why ever choose to be anything other than an LLC?

If your business model requires you to obtain funding from a venture capital firm within the next 2 years, then it is likely that you should forego an LLC and start out as a C corporation. Venture capital (VC) firms only invest in C corporations and will not invest in pass-through entities, including LLCs. The investors in most VC firms include entities with 501(c)(3) status, such as pension funds, endowments, etc. These are nonprofit organizations and in order to retain their tax-free status they are not permitted to earn "unrelated business taxable income" (UBTI). Funds that pass through an LLC to the VC firm and then to the 501(c)(3) organization constitute UBTI. Funds that are distributed by a C corporation, sometimes referred to as a "blocking C corporation," do not constitute UBTI. Many investors in LLCs like the fact that they get the benefit of deducting losses, as most early-stage technology companies incur losses for several years. However, some investors don't like dealing with the K-1 tax reporting forms that are issued by LLCs. Corporations are not required to issue any tax reporting forms to stockholders unless dividends are paid, which is rare for an early-stage technology company.

Another disadvantage of an LLC is that they cannot issue "incentive stock options" (ISOs), which are options to purchase equity. ISOs have certain tax advantages which are explained below. The inability to grant ISOs is greatly ameliorated by the ability of LLCs to issue "profits interests," explained below.

Members of LLCs who also are employees are deemed to be self-employed and must pay all of their social security taxes. This is in contrast this corporations, in which the corporation pays half of these taxes. Rank-and-file employees in the lower salary ranges are often shocked to learn this and they certainly don't appreciate it. It is possible to avoid this by having the employee hold the LLC interest in an S corporation, but this is more than cumbersome. Often an LLC will pay the employee some sort of bonus to lessen the burden (although a complete "gross-up" is expensive!).

Finally, it is worth highlighting the advantage of the single level taxation of LLCs in two contexts. One is with respect to a life sciences or other technology company that is going to earn its income principally through the licensing of its technology. In this case there will be revenue streams which are far greater than minimal operating expenses resulting in the generation of significant cash income. Adopting an LLC rather than a C corporation would be much more advantageous in order for income to be distributed currently to the owners at only one level of income tax. Secondly, buyers of early-stage companies generally want to buy assets, not equity. The purchaser of the equity of an entity takes the entity subject to all of its liabilities. Buyers are afraid that there may be "wayward founders" who come out of the woodwork and claim to have an unrecorded ownership interest in the company. There could be other undisclosed liabilities that rear their ugly heads as well. The buyer of assets can specify the assets purchased and the specific liabilities assumed, and thus insulate itself from claims on equity and most other liabilities associated with the selling entity (buyers sometimes cannot escape successor liability for certain items, e.g., pension and environmental liabilities).

Because a gain on the sale of the assets of a C corporation would be subject to double taxation, an LLC is a better choice for a company that may be sold early in its history and desire to be in a better position to sell assets. Of course, sales of C corporations happen all the time, and buyers can protect themselves by insisting that the stockholders personally indemnify them from undisclosed liabilities and increased escrow funds. However, as buyers are aware, such indemnifications outside of the escrow are only as good as the wherewithal of the sellers.

Why Choose an LLC?

☑ Only one level of taxation—best if
   (1) will receive a stream of licensing revenue, or
   (2) may sell assets.
☑ Investors can deduct losses.
☑ Profits interests are a great way to grant equity to non-founders.
☑ Can change to a C corporation if needed without tax consequences.
☑ Flexible with respect to the allocation of profits and losses and governance.

Why Choose a C Corporation?

☑ If likely to get VC funding in the next 2 years.
☑ If employees won't accept paying their own half of social security taxes.
☑ If afraid employees just won't understand owning equity in an LLC.
☑ If you don't want to spend the (not much) greater expense of being an LLC.

An Interesting Life Sciences LLC Asset-Centric Paradigm

Albert Sokal, a partner of mine at Edwards Wildman, has pioneered the implementation of utilizing an asset-centric parent LLC holding company with C corporation subsidiaries. This structure is most advantageous in situations where the company owns a platform technology that can be employed in a number of separate fields and thus separate businesses. Stakeholders, including founders, employee participants, and investors, own interests in the parent LLC. A C corporation subsidiary holds the company's operating assets and is the employer. Other C corporation subsidiaries hold licenses to the technology (and may have their own separate technology). This is cutting-edge law and requires a thorough analysis of tax, governance, ownership structure, investor requirements, and other factors.

OWNERSHIP STRUCTURE

The initial issuance of equity to those who start the business, the so-called "founders' transaction," should not be taken lightly. One risk not to be overlooked is a finding by taxing authorities that the equity was issued not in consideration for payment of fair value, but in consideration for services to the company, resulting in the receipt of stock taxed as ordinary income compensation. The problem is that the value of the equity may sky rocket from almost nothing to 1 million or several million dollars (e.g., based on the pre-money value given in a financing round). If the formation papers recite only a de minimis dollar amount paid for the founders' equity, the difference between that amount and the far greater fair market value a few months later may be deemed to be compensation.

To mitigate against this, usually the tangible technology owned by the founders, such as the business plan, patentable inventions (although in a university setting these may be owned by the university), trade secrets, software, etc., can be contributed to the company in exchange for equity. This is accomplished so as to qualify as a tax-free incorporation under Section 351 of the IRC (IRC Section 701 in the case of an LLC). Tax counsel should be consulted in this regard. In any event, care should be taken to document the transfer of all pertinent technology from the founders to the company.

Restricted Stock (Corporation) or Restricted Units (LLC)

What if one of the cofounders, whom everyone assumed was going to spend a lot of time working on company matters, takes a job in another state and announces his intention to have nothing further to do with the company? Is it fair for him to retain some or all of his equity? In the case of more than one founder, it is often advisable to place restrictions on the equity so that if the owner's service to the company ceases for any reason, then the equity is forfeited or repurchased for a nominal amount. This is referred to as "reverse vesting." An example is a cofounder who received 100,000 units in an LLC, which reverse vests over a 4-year period.

A standard vesting schedule is 25 percent on the first anniversary (a so-called "1-year cliff") and equal monthly increments over the following 3 years. If service terminates prior to 1 year, then all equity is forfeited or repurchased. If service terminates after 18 months, then 18 months of equity is retained and the balance is forfeited or repurchased. These numbers are not set in stone. For example, founders often get to retain a certain percentage of their equity no matter what, say 25 percent, and only the rest is subject to vesting. Often, a portion or all of the vesting is accelerated upon a sale of the company, a so-called "single trigger," or less favorably to the stockholder upon termination by the acquiror without cause within 1 year after the acquisition, a so-called "double trigger."

These vesting provisions usually are reflected in a Restricted Stock Agreement in the case of a corporation and a Restricted Unit Agreement in an LLC. With restricted equity, the owner is the beneficial and record holder, and is entitled to voting and dividend/distribution rights. Importantly, the capital gains holding period commences upon issuance of the equity.

An election pursuant to Section 83(b) of the IRC should almost always be made by the holder of restricted equity. Without an 83(b) election, ordinary income tax is assessed at each time that restrictions lapse in the amount of the difference of the fair market value at the time of the lapse less the amount paid for the equity. Thus, an owner could find himself owing a lot in taxes due to a rapid rise in the fair market value of the company (e.g., a successful financing round) with no way to pay the tax (generally equity in a private company is illiquid until the company is sold). When an 83(b) election is made, tax is paid up front on the difference between the fair market value and the amount paid for the equity, usually a very minimal amount, and then no tax is due upon the lapsing of any restrictions. Tax is due when the equity is sold, and if that's more than a year later, then it is subject to the lower tax rate on capital gains, not ordinary income. Very critically, *an 83(b) election must be made within 30 days after the issuance of the equity*. There are no exceptions or alternatives for relief.

Profits Interests in an LLC

So called "profits interests" are a profoundly tax-efficient manner of getting equity in an LLC to nonfounders. A profits interest is an ownership interest in the LLC entitling the holder to the specified percentage of the value of the company *after* the preexisting value of the company is distributed to the prior owners. There is no tax on the grant of a profits interest (!). Like restricted equity, it is a live interest in the LLC and need be held for only over 1 year in order to receive capital gains treatment on the sale.

An example is helpful in the explanation of profits interests. Say that the founders contributed $100,000 in cash upon the start of the LLC. The company is now determined to have a fair market value of $1 million. The founders want to bring on a senior executive and grant him a 10 percent ownership interest. If a 10 percent interest were to be granted outright, then the executive would be subject to tax on $100,000 of ordinary income, representing the fair market value of the equity. With a profits interest, the executive is entitled to a 10 percent interest after the founders capital accounts have been "booked up" to the company's value at the time of the grant of the profits interest. If the company is later sold for $10 million, the executive would be entitled to 10 percent of $9 million.

Because of the advantages of the profits interest in an LLC, rarely does it make sense to grant options to purchase an LLC interest. This is because the exercise price for the option must be equal to at least the fair market value (according to IRC Section 409A), and the equity must be held for at least 1 year after the option is exercised in order to qualify for capital gains. Many tax advisors recommend filing a "protective" 83(b) filing for profits interests. Technically, an 83(b) filing is not required for a profits interest, but if for whatever reason the interest is determined not to qualify as a profits interest, then the 83(b) filing may save the day. For example, IRS Revenue Procedure 93–27 provides for a safe harbor for profits interests which, among certain other conditions, are held for at least 2 years. Profits interests held for less time do not meet this test and are susceptible to losing their status.

Incentive Stock Options and Nonqualified Stock Options

A stock option is a contract for the purchase of a certain number of shares, at a certain price, during a certain period of time, and subject to other terms and conditions. Like restricted equity, options are almost always subject to a vesting schedule. Options which qualify for treatment as "incentive stock options" under IRC Section 422 (ISOs) enjoy certain tax advantages.

An ISO can only be granted by a corporation (not an LLC and not a stockholder) to an employee (who can be full or part-time). They cannot be granted to nonemployees such as consultants or nonemployee directors. ISOs must be granted at an exercise price of at least the fair market value of the underlying stock (110 percent for owners of 10 percent or more). The maximum exercise period is 10 years (5 years for owners of 10 percent or more). The maximum value is $100,000 per year and $1 million in the aggregate (determined at the time of the grant).

There is no tax on the grant of a stock option, whether it is an ISO or a nonqualified stock option (NQO). The advantage of ISOs is that there is no tax on the exercise of an option. And if the stock which is purchased is held for a minimum of 1 year and for at least 2 years after the grant of the ISO, then a sale of the stock is entitled to capital gains. One caveat is that although the exercise of an ISO is not subject to a regular tax it is subject to the alternative minimum tax provisions of the IRC.

As alluded to above, IRC Section 409A mandates that options must have an exercise price equal to at least the fair market value of the underlying stock. If this fair market value requirement is not met, then very punitive taxes are imposed. For companies that are less than 10 years old (and are not expecting a liquidity event within 90 days or an IPO in the next 180 days), the fair market value can be determined by a written internal valuation analysis. This analysis need not be prepared by a person or entity independent from the company, but the preparer must have at least 5 years of relevant experience in business valuation, financial accounting, investment banking, private equity, secured lending, or another comparable experience.

Phantom Stock

I refer to so called "phantom stocks" as "fake equity." It's nothing more than a contract requiring the company to pay the executive money upon the occurrence of an event, usually the sale of the company. In this regard, it's more like a typical salesman commission plan. Most importantly, capital gains treatment is never available. Also, the holder of phantom stock does not really hold any equity and is not owed any fiduciary duties by the board of directors or any of the company's equity holders.

Employment and Consultant Issues

The transfer of all intellectual property rights from the founders to the company by a written Technology Assignment Agreement should not be overlooked. Also, the founders, as well as all employees and consultants, should sign an agreement, often referred to as a "Proprietary Rights Agreement," which assigns all inventions to the company and confirms that the individual will maintain the confidentiality of the company's information.

Generally, it is in the company's interest to require employees (and often consultants) to agree not to compete with the company after termination. The maximum post-termination noncompete period varies from state-to-state. The provisions of noncompetes must be carefully drafted to be enforceable, and experienced legal counsel should be consulted. It is worth noting that such noncompetes in the state of California are per se invalid.

Most start-ups can get by without formal employment agreements, although it is advisable to use written offer letters setting forth the basic terms of employment and reciting that employment is "at will," among some other basic matters.

FUNDRASING

Selling Equity Versus Convertible Debt

Most life sciences companies are birthed in university labs and often receive a healthy amount of grants and other nondilutive funding. At some point, the decision is made to spin out a company with an exclusive license from the institution (see Chapter 14 entitled "Licensing the Technology: Biotechnology Commercialization Strategies Using University and Federal Labs"). Whether or not the company was conceived in an institutional setting, in order to commercialize the technology typically outside "seed" or "angel" financing is necessary or desirable.

The first issue to confront is the "premoney" valuation of the company. In other words, what percentage of the company's ownership should the investors get for their money? For example if the premoney valuation is $2 million, and the investors pay $500,000, then the investors would receive 20 percent of the equity (500,000/2,500,000). Sophisticated investors will insist on a "preferred" instrument, meaning preferred stock in a corporation, or preferred units in an LLC. Preferred means that the investors have a preference with respect to getting their money back first—before the founders, as well as employees and consultants. In the above example, if things didn't go well and the technology was sold for $700,000, the investors would get their $500,000 back before any other distributions.

More often than not, the premoney valuation of the company is not easy to resolve between the founders, who believe the company deserves a very high valuation, and the investors, who may be optimistic but are aware of the downside risk. Convertible notes to the rescue!

The convertible note is technically debt, but typically the note is automatically converted into equity on the same terms and conditions as the next "qualified financing." A qualified financing is the next round of equity financing of at least a certain dollar amount which can range from as low as $500,000 to as high as $3 million. Qualifications can also include that it be a preferred instrument and/or that the lead investor(s) must be institutional investors. The maturity date is typically between 1 and 2 years.

If a qualified financing has not occurred by the maturity date, then alternatives may include: (1) the ability of the investors to foreclose on the assets of the company,

(2) the note is convertible into equity at a predetermined "back up" premoney valuation, or (3) the note is convertible into equity at an agreed premoney valuation or, if not agreed, then by an independent appraisal. In exchange for the risk taken by the note holders, they are given a discount on the price paid by those leading the qualified financing— a 20 percent discount is market, although it can be as low as 5 percent if a qualified financing is expected soon, or as high as 30 to 40 percent if the deal is perceived as riskier. Sometimes it's a sliding scale by the number of months it takes to complete a qualified financing.

The stated interest rate for convertible notes in years past was usually 8 percent. In recent times, with interest rates so low, the common rate has drifted down to 5 percent. A new concept, called "convertible equity" has been advanced in which no interest is payable and there is no maturity date. Another advantage to the company is that the investment is moved from the liability side of the balance sheet to the equity column, thus making the balance sheet appear in much better health to customers, suppliers, and employees. For the investor it's live equity, so the capital gains clock starts running. However, in my experience, convertible equity is just too new, and most investors resist it.

Convertible Note Checklist

☑ Amount offered, and the minimum amount, if any.
☑ Maturity date —usually 1 to 2 years.
☑ Interest rate—usually 5 to 8 percent
☑ Definition of the "qualified financing" which triggers conversion of the notes often $1 million priced round, can be more or less.
☑ Percentage discount note holders receive in the qualified financing—often 20 percent.
☑ Notes can be secured by the assets of the company.

What happens if a qualified financing has not occurred by the maturity date? It can: (1) have a "back up" premoney valuation; (2) provide for the premoney valuation to be determined by an appraisal; and (3) be silent, thus giving the note holders the right to foreclose.

What happens if the company is sold prior to conversion or the maturity date? Often, note holders are paid 2 or 3× principal.

Securities Laws

Whether it's a priced equity round or a convertible note round, the issuing company must be cognizant of federal and state securities laws. Some make the mistake of thinking that convertible notes are not securities because they are not equity instruments, or that limited liability company interests are not securities since they are not "stock." This almost always is not the case, and the securities laws apply.

Section 5 of the Securities Act of 1933, as amended (the Securities Act), requires all securities transactions to be registered with Securities Exchange Commission (SEC). Section 4(2) provides an exemption for the offering of securities in a transaction which is "not a public offering." But you can scour the Securities Act and won't find a definition of a "public offering."

The United States Supreme Court settled this question in the landmark case of *SEC v. Ralston Purina Co.*, 346 U.S. 119 (1953). In short, the holding was that in order for an offering to be private, and not public, and thus exempt from registration requirements, (1) same kind of information that otherwise generally would be available in a registration statement must be provided to investors, and (2) the investors themselves must be sophisticated—i.e., able to understand such information.

What's an entrepreneur to do, be a scholar of United States Supreme Court cases? Here, it's the SEC to the rescue in the form of Regulation D. Reg. D is not exclusive, meaning the case law of *Ralston Purina* and its progeny can be relied upon. However, if case law is relied upon then the issuing company has the burden of proof that the offering is indeed private. If a company complies with Reg. D then the presumption in a court of law is that the offering is private.

Without getting into a detailed discussion of Reg. D, the fact of the matter is that Rule 506 of Reg. D is almost always used for private offerings. One great advantage of Rule 506 is that it preempts state securities laws and has no dollar limit on the amount of funds raised. Requirements of Rule 506 include: an unlimited number of accredited investors and no more than 35 unaccredited investors; no general solicitation or advertising; and certain resale limitations and the filing of Form D within 15 days of first sale of securities (form D must also be filed in each state in which securities are sold).

Very importantly, there are rigid disclosure requirements to investors if there is even one investor who is not "accredited." Generally, it is best to offer securities only to accredited investors. Nonaccredited investors often are referred to as "widows and orphans" and have no business participating in an investment in a start-up company, by definition a very risky endeavor. The following are the categories of "accredited investor:"

● Individuals with a $1 million net worth (exclusive of primary residence) or $200,000 in income (or $300,000 with his or her spouse) in past 2 years and expected in the current year.
● Entities in which all investors are accredited investors.
● Directors and executive officers of the issuer.
● Corporations or trusts with assets in excess of $5 million (not formed for the purpose of making the investment).
● Institutional investors such as banks, savings and loans, broker-dealers, insurance companies, and investment companies.

If there are no nonaccredited investors, then no specific written disclosure is required, but the antifraud rules still apply! Because the antifraud rules always apply, it is advisable (read obligatory) to provide to investors a written disclosure document—usually referred to as a "Private Placement Memorandum," which includes the terms of the offering, risk factors, capitalization, use of proceeds, a description of the business, and the bio's of management—in other words all information material to an investment decision.

Advertising and general solicitation with regard to the sale of securities is now (since September 23, 2013) permitted under Rule 506(c) of Regulation D. This is as a result of the Jumpstart Our Business Startups (JOBS) Act and a game-changing departure. Unfortunately for entrepreneurs, the Securities and Exchange Commission (SEC) specified in the Rule that the securities can be sold to only accredited investors and that their status as accredited investors must be stringently verified—income by W-2s, 1099s, etc. and net worth by bank statements, appraisals, etc. (although an attorney, accountant, or broker-dealer can furnish a certification).

Finally, the JOBS Act permits the sale of securities through certain qualified Internet portals. To be clear, a company cannot set up its own portal to sell its securities—it must sell through an approved intermediary (SEC-registered broker-dealers and certain other registered entities). These portals are permitted to advertise and publically solicit the sale of securities. Companies are limited to raising no more than $1 million per year. Unlike Rule 506(c), *investors need not be accredited*. Individuals with less than $100,000 in income can invest up to $2000 or 5 percent of their income or net worth. Individuals with more than $100,000 can invest up to 10 percent of their income or net worth. Also unlike Rule 506(c), no strict income or net worth verification requirements are included in the proposed Regulations (although they may be included in the final Regs).

The above is not an exhaustive presentation of the United States or state securities laws, and prior to offering securities a company should obtain the advice of an experienced securities attorney.

SUMMARY

The choice of an entity for a start-up should not be made without a thorough understanding of all the implications, including tax, founder, management, and employee considerations. Invariably, the choice is between a C corporation and an LLC. An LLC most likely is the default selection, unless investment by a venture capital firm is on the near horizon. There are no tax consequences when converting from an LLC to a C corporation, but converting from an LLC to a C corporation is a taxable event.

The "founders' transaction" should be carefully considered. It almost always makes sense to institute a vesting program for founders and employees. Finally, great care should be taken to comply with federal and state securities laws. All of these matters requires sound legal advice and should be discussed with a seasoned attorney having extensive experience with start-up issues for companies in the biotechnology industry.

Chapter 14

Licensing the Technology: Biotechnology Commercialization Strategies Using University and Federal Labs

Steven M. Ferguson, CLP* and Uma S. Kaundinya, PhD, CLP**

*Deputy Director, Licensing & Entrepreneurship, Office of Technology Transfer, National Institutes of Health, Rockville, Maryland

**President & CEO, Aavishkar Innovations Inc., Bedford, Massachusetts

THE FEDERAL GOVERNMENT'S INVESTMENT IN BASIC BIOMEDICAL RESEARCH

For many years the United States has led the world in government funding of nonmilitary research and development (R&D), notably support for basic and clinical research that directly relates to health and human development. While new biotechnology entrepreneurs often rely upon the "Three Fs" of founders, friends, and family for advice, assistance, and financing during the early years of their company, they often overlook a "Fourth F" that can be of major assistance during many phases of their growth—that being Federal, especially federal labs and federally-funded research in universities and academic medical centers (AMCs), also referred to as academic medical organizations (AMOs) across the United States. A longtime focal point for such federal investment by the U.S. government in biomedical research has been the National Institutes of Health (NIH) through its intramural laboratories and the funding provided to most academic and university- or hospital-based research programs. Funding provided by the NIH alone reached $30.9 billion in fiscal year 2012; approximately 10 percent of this funding was spent on internal NIH R&D projects (intramural research) carried out by the approximately 6000 scientists employed by the NIH. The balance was distributed in the form of grants, contracts, and fellowships for the research endeavors of more than 300,000 nongovernment scientists (extramural research) at 2500 colleges, universities, and research organizations throughout the world [1]. Each year this biomedical research leads to a large variety of novel basic and clinical research discoveries, all of which generally require commercial partners in order to develop them into products for consumer, scientist, physician, or patient use. Thus, federal laboratories and universities need and actively seek corporate partners or licensees to commercialize their federally-funded research into products in order to help fulfill their fundamental missions in public health.

Academic medical centers, with their dual components of research and clinical care, are in a unique position of being at the very beginning and very end of the science-to-business and product-to-patient chain. For example Partners Health Care at Massachusetts General Hospital (MGH) and Brigham and Women's Hospital (BWH) receives about $1.4 billion in federal funding for its approximately 1300 investigators. Also, there are approximately 3000 clinicians in its core hospitals who use the very therapies and diagnostics that its researchers invent, for patient care.

TRANSLATION OF ACADEMIC RESEARCH TO PRODUCTS FOR THE PUBLIC GOOD

Most all biotechnology products have some history of their research and development that can be traced back to a basic research institution, most often funded by federal grants. Licensing and technology transfer programs at nonprofit basic research organizations provide a means for getting new inventions to the market for public use and benefit. From a research institution's perspective, this is quite desirable since the public and commercial use of inventions typically come with new recognition of the value of basic research programs at the university or organization that originated it. These inventions also serve as helpful means to attract new R&D resources and partnerships to these laboratories. Through licensing or other technology-transfer mechanisms, these institutions also receive a "return on investment" whether that is measured in terms of financial, educational or societal parameters, or some combination thereof. A recent study by the Brookings Institute [2] offers useful insights about the academic innovation enterprise.

Universities and academic medical centers are known as centers of education, patient care, and basic research. This basic research, fueled largely by the curious mind and funding from the government, has transformed our understanding of important fundamental phenomena. This research activity results in publications that dictate the careers of those in academia, and defines the institution's academic culture and spirit. Important discoveries are made at each of these institutions, but they are largely confined to the research realm. Starting from the early 1960s, the need to maximize the benefits from such intense and ground breaking research was felt thanks to Jerome Wiesner, the scientific advisor to President John F. Kennedy. He recognized that most of the innovations which impacted everyday people were left primarily to the large companies of the day—Lucent Bell Labs, Kodak, Johnson & Johnson, to name a few—which held the most patents, and their products were known the world over.

Bayh-Dole and the Birth of Technology Transfer (1980)

Picking up from the momentum of the policies of Presidents John F. Kennedy and Richard Nixon in 1980, Senators Birch Bayh and Bob Dole enacted legislation that gave universities, nonprofits, and small-businesses the *right* to own inventions made by their employees for federal government-funded research. The Bayh-Dole Act of 1980 (P.L. 96-517) reversed the presumption of title and permitted a university, small business, or nonprofit institution to elect and pursue ownership of an invention in preference to the government. The underlying spirit of this important piece of legislation was to maximally utilize the outstanding research at these universities and other nonprofits for the good of the public who funded the research through their tax dollars.

The ownership right that universities have to these inventions comes with obligations. Primarily, it is the obligation to actively market and attempt to commercialize the invention, preferably through U.S.-based business enterprises including start-ups to benefit the public. Thus, was born the field of "technology transfer" and the mushrooming of technology-transfer offices (TTOs). Prior to Bayh-Dole, 28,000 patents were owned by the U.S. government, less than 5 percent of which were commercialized. It has been reported that since the enactment of Bayh-Dole, 5000 new companies have been created, resulting in billions of dollars of direct economic impact within the United States and close to 600 products put in the market during these 30 years—all based upon university research.

Because a substantial portion of the inventions that arise from basic research programs are supported by research that is federally-funded, there are also substantial legal obligations incurred by universities and academic medical organizations to promote commercial development of such new inventions. Similarly, in the 1980s, federal intramural laboratories were also given a statutory mandate under the Stevenson-Wydler Technology Innovation Act (P.L. 96-480), the Federal Technology Transfer Act (P.L. 99-502), and Executive Order 12591 to ensure that new technologies developed in federal laboratories were similarly transferred to the private sector and commercialized.

Commercialization of inventions from nonprofit basic research institutions typically follows a multistep process as academic and federal laboratories typically do not provide technology commercialization themselves. The inventions made by these researchers are converted into products and processes by for-profit companies. The TTOs act as key liaisons to link these important connections between the academic/government and the commercial world. In some cases, these inventions, protected through intellectual property, are "transferred" to the company for product development via license agreements that give the company the rights to make the products or use these processes. In other cases, as a prelude to the license agreement or concomitant with it, a collaboration agreement or a sponsored research agreement is negotiated by the TTO that allows a period of time wherein the research institution and company researchers jointly work on the invention prior to its complete transfer to the company. In exchange, financial consideration or other benefits are received by the research institution through what is often an agreement with a small company, which may bring in a large corporate partner during a later stage of development. This process has been likened to a relay race where there may be several baton transfers!

Since the 1980s, federal labs and universities have developed a strategic focus for their technology-transfer activities and they are particularly interested in working with bioentrepreneurs. This is because revenue enhancement from licensing is no longer the sole institutional goal. Instead, institutions find themselves also looking to increase company formation and new jobs based upon academic inventiveness, support faculty recruitment and retention, enhance research funding, create an entrepreneurial culture, attract venture investment to their regions, and the like. The economic development aspects of research are being recognized as a fourth mission for such institutions—going along with education, research, and public service. Bioentrepreneurs play a key role in this "fourth mission" by establishing companies driven by new research discoveries.

ACCESSING ACADEMIC TECHNOLOGIES AND COLLABORATIONS

Generally, bioentrepreneurs can directly access research and inventions for product development from three main sources as shown in Table 14.1. For research funded by grants and contracts from NIH or other federal agencies (extramural research), the individual university or small business would control commercial rights, with only standard reporting and utilization obligations to the federal funding agency. Biomedical research conducted by the federal laboratory (intramural research program) is licensed directly through the technology transfer office at the federal lab.

According to a 2011 annual survey from the Association of University Technology Managers (AUTM) [3], this incentivized approach, which dates from the Bayh-Dole Act, has contributed to the annual formation of nearly two new products, and nearly one new company each day through university technology transfer. Table 14.2 provides trends from the 2011 annual survey and underscores the volume of licensing activity that goes on in the United States from reporting universities and AMOs.

TABLE 14.1 Federally-Funded Technologies can be Licensed from Several Sources

Federal lab research (from lab technology transfer office)

University grantee research (from specific university technology transfer offices)

SBIR and STTR (small business technology transfer) small business programs (from small business awardees)

Each of these institutions has a robust research program "pipeline" that provides novel, fundamental research discoveries available for commercial applications. NIH, for instance, as both a large-scale provider and consumer, represents a sort of "supermarket" of research products or tools for its commercial partners and suppliers. Additionally, overall product sales of all types by NIH licensees now exceed $6 billion annually. As mentioned previously, most technology transfer activities at NIH and other federal laboratories date from the Federal Technology Transfer Act of 1986 which authorized formal research partnerships with industry and provided incentives to these programs to license technology by allowing the federal laboratory to, for the first time, keep its license royalties and share them

between the individual inventors and their laboratories or institutes.

Research collaborations or research assistance with research institutions can take several forms as these researchers and clinicians can work with industry under different collaborative modalities. For example, research institutions may need to access technologies developed by industry—an imaging tool, a sequencing platform, or a drug discovered and in development by a company. The tech transfer office then works with the company to memorialize the understanding between the scientists and to allow the collaboration to happen. Of course, as with all arrangements, each party desires to obtain terms that they feel are the most equitable for the party they represent. The key components of a collaboration agreement that are often the subject of most negotiations are terms related to inventions, rights to inventions, confidentiality versus publication, managing conflicts of interest, and last but not least, indemnification. Indemnification (having one party to bear the monetary costs, either directly or by reimbursement, for losses incurred by a second party) is very important to research institutions when working with new biotech technologies that will be used in patient care.

Academic-Industry Collaborative Research Agreements

There are several types of research or collaboration-related agreements that biotech companies will commonly encounter in working with universities and federal laboratories:

Confidential Disclosure/Nondisclosure Agreements (CDA/NDA)

Prior to engaging in any collaboration, each party may need to disclose to the other party some proprietary information that if passed on to third parties might be detrimental to the interest of the disclosing party. Such a discussion is a necessary first step to determine the interest in, and the breadth and scope of any potential collaboration. The parties will negotiate a CDA/NDA that ensures the information disclosed is held confidential, is only used for the purpose of establishing the collaboration, stipulates a term of how long the information needs to be held confidential, and describes the consequences of nonadherence to the terms of the agreement.

TABLE 14.2 Volume of License Activity at Universities and Academic Medical Organizations

2011 Reporting Period	Respondents	Licenses and Options Executed To:			
		Total	Start-Ups	Small Companies	Large Companies
U.S Universities	157	5398	822	2785	1562
U.S. AMOs	28	645	65	315	265

Material Transfer Agreement (MTA), Sponsored Research Agreement (SRA), and Cooperative Research and Development Agreement (CRADA)

Companies, both small and large, have invested a lot of research and development dollars toward developing drugs or other biotech products. Research institutions have several programs that are geared towards understanding the fundamental biology underlying a wide variety of commercial products. When these two entities want to collaborate they have very different things at stake. For the company, they are hoping to learn more about their product concept, get mechanistic insights they can exploit to position their product better in the market place, and have discoveries come out of this collaboration related to their product which may extend the patent life of their eventual product. In the case of collaborations with academic medical centers, companies would like access to patient samples in addition to the valuable clinical insights they hope would guide them through the process of clinical validation of their product whether it be a drug, medical device, or diagnostic. For the academic and clinical investigator, they would like to test various drugs from various companies to build a scientific story or medical knowledge that they can publish. Even more importantly, with the dwindling of federal funds for academic research, their activities can be supported through cash from the company.

MTAs and SRAs are agreements that dictate the terms of the transfer of material and/or money from the company to the academic institution. Similarly at federal labs research projects for basic research or clinical studies are called Cooperative Research and Development Agreements (CRADAs). Because of their clinical hospitals and centers as well as other networks and facilities, the NIH and at least some universities are able to take some of their medical discoveries (or those of their partners) into clinical trials through Clinical Trial Agreements.

Key Elements of Collaborative Agreements

Provided below are key elements that are at the heart of the negotiation of these agreements:

1. **Inventions**—The definition of "invention" is crucial. Academic centers will typically require that any inventions be both conceived *and* reduced to practice during the term of the collaborative research using the company material and/or money. Companies want it to be conceived "or" reduced to practice. The problem for the TTOs with agreeing to "or", is simply that academic researchers collaborate with lots of companies, often at the same time on similar broad programs but with different individualized projects. If institutions agree to the "or" language, it creates several

issues: (a) it is nearly impossible for the TTOs to police when conception of the invention happened and when it was reduced to practice and (b) the institution may end up with conflicting arrangements with companies. Federal laboratories (by statute) use the language of "conceived or *actually* reduced to practiced" in their agreements. Practically speaking TTOs may only hear of inventions when the researchers decide to disclose them as investigators at research institutions are not under as tight control as their counterparts in industry.

2. **Ownership of inventions**—Companies may want academic researchers to assign their inventions to the companies. This is a hard one for academic TTOs to accept since in the instance of an MTA there will likely be funding from the federal government, and under the terms of the grant such assignments are prohibited without specific permission from the funding agency. Even under the terms of a sponsored research arrangement where the company is providing money in addition to providing the material, given the large amount of federal dollars that most academic institutions receive with the lab resources and several personnel being funded by the government, universities are unable to agree to the assignment of inventions to companies as it would again be in violation of the terms of the grant from the federal agency. Instead, typically the company will be granted the desired license options by the research institution to new discoveries during the collaborative or sponsored research program.

3. **Rights to inventions**—Freedom to operate (FTO) rights are very important to a company. They have invested a lot of money into their drug discovery or device-development programs. Biotech companies do not want the academic research collaborator to make important inventions that are somehow related to their drug or device in development and then not have the needed rights to the inventions that they helped with their material and money to discover. There is often no right or wrong answer to this question and it can be subject to negotiation depending on what each party feels is equitable for the specific collaboration and can vary from a royalty-bearing to a royalty-free license or license option.

4. **Confidentiality and publication**—An important aspect of the academic mission and spirit is to publish and disseminate the results of research widely to the public. This is typically at odds with the company's best interest which may need to keep things under cover until they are very sure and ready to disclose especially to their competitors. A typical compromise is for the publication/public disclosure to be provided to the company ahead of time and for the company to remove its confidential information while still providing for a meaningful publication in the journal of choice by the investigators. For example if the journal required publication of the structure of the compound to make it meaningful, then if that were not already in the

public domain through publication (journal or patent) of the company, then that constraint should be discussed at the time of the negotiation of the contract.

TECHNOLOGY TRANSFER OFFICE SET-UP AND LICENSING FROM UNIVERSITIES AND FEDERAL LABORATORIES

Technology Transfer Office (TTO) Operations

Figure 14.1 provides an overview of the core operational elements and activities of TTO offices at research institutions. There are several key areas of importance to industry. In addition, several TTOs house an internal venture group or work with some outside venture funds for commercialization of their technologies in the form of a new company/start-up. The internal funds often serve several functions including educating the investigator/inventor as they work with outside venture companies (VCs), bringing together several outside ventures, given their connections and expertise and work with the licensing staff within the TTO to help get the start-up off the ground.

Inventions and IP Strategy

Inventions made by the research center's investigators are the currency that drives the licensing operations of a TTO. As summarized later in Figure 14.2, the TTO personnel has the huge responsibility of reaching out to their research community to educate them about the process, evaluate and access patentability of inventions, devise simple to complex IP strategies for the inventions, and finally to work with attorneys to protect these inventions.

Disclosure of Inventions

When research findings are disclosed to the TTO, it typically goes through a triage process that involves accessing/scoring its scientific strength, its patentability in light of prior art, including the investigators' own prior public disclosures, its market potential, and commercial path. The TTO will also look for the investigators' availability of resources including funding as well as their commitment to work with the TTO to move the invention through the next steps of validation that would add to its commercial value.

Some key challenges that TTOs face are: (1) lack of control of the overall disclosure process since disclosure of inventions is purely voluntary—furthermore, investigators differ widely in what they would consider to be valuable inventions; (2) investigators do not sign documents assigning their inventions to their employer at the time of employment, rather they are obligated to do so under the institution's IP policies; and (3) investigators vary widely in their aptitude to work with the TTO to commercialize their inventions and get it into the market place.

Marketing of Inventions and Business Strategies

For companies looking to work with a TTO, there is both push (when the TTO reaches out to companies to license/partner the technologies) and pull (when companies contact the TTOs) marketing. Companies contact TTOs typically following a public presentation—a publication that's either in a journal or a patent. For companies seeking a license from a TTO the following outlines a good approach: (1) identify the university's technology that is of interest; (2) provide a path for diligent development of technology, if licensed, along with an estimated timeline; and (3) indicate

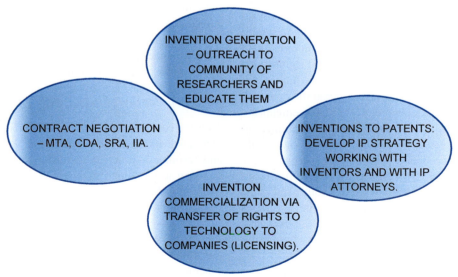

FIGURE 14.1   Core elements of a tech transfer office.

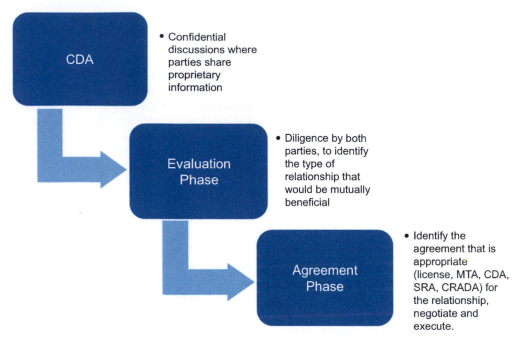

FIGURE 14.2   Fundamental steps leading to agreements with research institutions.

if the technology will add to, replace an existing product, or be a new line of products for the company. Having this basic information available will accelerate the time to a term sheet and eventually a completed license.

Licensing Technologies—Working with the Technology Transfer Offices

From Universities and Academic Medical Centers

Once the academic and company feel there is a path forward to bring the technology into the company then it proceeds to a license. Oftentimes the company is not sure and needs to bring the technology in under an evaluation license to ensure that the technology works before they can commit to a license. This is accomplished via an option agreement that would (a) obligate the academic to hold the rights to the technology for a certain period of time within which it will execute a license to the company and (b) grant the company rights to test/evaluate the technology. These agreements are accompanied by nominal fee arrangements, oftentimes to cover patent costs previously incurred and/or that would be incurred during the option period. Once the parties are engaged in negotiations, it is typical to start with a term-sheet. It is good to get all the deal-breakers addressed in the term sheet and get verbal understanding of the key terms before committing to paper. A combination of an exchange of a written draft agreement and periodic verbal communication will ensure that things are proceeding on track.

Time periods to complete these transactions can vary widely. Options agreements typically can be drawn up within

a few days to a month. License agreements for nonexclusive license agreements take on average about 2 to 6 months to finalize. For exclusive license agreements, the time period varies quite widely. If there are two committed parties that want to get a deal done it can be as quick as 3 to 4 months. An average deal would probably take 6 to 9 months to complete. In all instances of licenses, TTOs always prefer to start from their template. Given that companies' license agreements are designed for company-to-company transactions, it is very cumbersome and time-consuming for the academic licensing professional to adapt the company template to fit the academic's needs. If the institution has previously licensed the technology either nonexclusively or exclusively in another field, there would be a constraint to using terms they have agreed to with the other parties on the same technology. Also, if that company and the academic have a prior license agreement, the quickest way to a deal would be to start with that as a template for at least the nontechnology-specific terms.

From the National Institutes of Health

As is the case with universities, the NIH is not able to commercialize its discoveries even with its considerable size and resources—it relies instead upon partners. Commercializing technologies such as vaccines or drugs and then marketing them successfully in a world-wide market thus cannot be the responsibility or mission of research institutions or government agencies. Companies with access to the needed expertise and money are needed to undertake continued development of these inventions from the NIH or other research institutions into final products. Typically, a royalty-bearing exclusive license agreement with the right to sublicense is given to a company from NIH (if NIH-owned) or the university (if university-owned) to use patents, materials, or other assets to bring a therapeutic or vaccine product concept to market. Exclusivity is almost always the norm for the U.S. Food and Drug Administration (FDA)-regulated products due to the risk involved in time, money, and regulatory pathways to companies and their investors. Financial terms of the license agreement are negotiable but do reflect the nascent, high-risk nature of the discovery. Because the technologies coming from NIH or NIH-funded research are most typically preclinical inventions, most licensees are early-stage companies or start-ups rather than larger firms who typically want more proven ideas for new products. In addition to the license agreement there will often be research collaborations between the licensee and the NIH or university to assist with additional work needed on the product technology. When the licensee is able to sufficiently "de-risk" the technology through its various efforts, these companies then sublicense, partner, or get acquired by larger biotech or pharmaceutical firms for the final, most expensive stages of development with the large company expected to sell the product once it reaches the market.

Since the 1980s, federally-funded health research institutions such as the NIH and AMCs have developed an active but increasingly strategic focus on improving public health through technology-transfer activities. As such, they are particularly interested in working with start-ups and other early-stage companies in the healthcare area that are looking to develop and deliver innovative products. Rather than just seeking a financial return through revenue generation, these institutions are looking to utilize licensing of nascent inventions as a way to increase new company formation, support faculty recruitment and retention, enhance research funding, and create in general a more entrepreneurial culture within the organization, attracting venture investment and development to their specific region (universities) or to the health sector in general (NIH).

Licensing Technologies to a Start-Up

The licensing practices for most nonprofit research institutions including federal institutions and universities have changed significantly over recent years with respect to biomedical inventions [4]. With its ever-increasing consolidation, large pharmaceutical firms are typically no longer looking to directly license early-stage technologies for commercialization, whereas the number of licenses signed with start-ups as well as small- to medium-sized biotechnology companies is on the rise. Indeed as was shown in Figure 14.1, in 2011 66 percent of the total license executed by universities and AMCs were to start-ups and small biotech firms. Unlike 10 to 15 years ago, when all or most of the high-revenue medical products based on licenses from university or federal laboratory research came from direct agreements

with large pharmaceutical firms, a majority of the latest success stories tend to be from those originally partnered with biotech or other smaller companies at the time of the original license agreement. Some examples from the NIH licensing program are Kepivance® (a human growth factor used to treat oral sores arising from chemotherapy licensed to Amgen), Velcade® (a small molecule proteasome inhibitor used to treat multiple myeloma from Millennium), Synagis® (a recombinant monoclonal antibody for preventing serious lung disease caused by respiratory syncytial virus in premature infants from MedImmune), Prezista® (an HIV protease inhibitor used to treat drug-resistant AIDS patients from Tibotec) and Taxus Express® (a paclitaxel drug-eluting coronary stent used to prevent restenosis from Angiotech). Although these are all substantive, well-known companies now, at the time the underlying technology was licensed to them, they were not large corporations. Some exemplary technologies from Partners Healthcare (AMC with two leading hospitals in the Boston area under its umbrella) that fit this category are: "Coolsculpting® (an aesthetic device developed by an MGH start-up, Zeltiq) and Nvision VLE™, an *in vivo* pathology imaging system from Ninepoint Medical, Inc (another MGH start-up).

The new reality is that commercial partners, especially small, innovative ones, are essential to the goals of biomedical research institutions seeing the results of their research become novel healthcare products for the public. Another reason that licensing offices can prefer licenses to a start-up company is because unlike big companies, survival of the start-up company is dependent upon the development of the technology. Start-up companies can be highly motivated to successfully and expeditiously commercialize the licensed technology and expend all their resources towards the development of the technology. Most of the time this option is viewed more favorably to licensing the technology to a very large company where several similar technologies would typically be developed concomitantly. The risk is that the university or federal research institution's technology may get scuttled due to business factors or viewed as being of a high-risk nature. The biggest challenge licensing the technology to a start-up company, however, is "cash uncertainty," i.e., whether or not the start-up company will be able to secure future capital to develop the technology in a timely fashion. It is therefore important that bioentrepreneurs do the right thing in the right way at the right time to keep a strong relationship with the federal lab or university/AMC and its venture fund group as described in later sections of this chapter.

Basic Licensing Principles of University and Federal Laboratories

Compared to biomedical licensing from corporations, the federal laboratories and universities bring a different focus and perspective to the table when negotiating its technology transfer agreements. Because these agreements are used to further overall institutional missions, representatives from such nonprofit institutions consider the public consequences of such licenses as their first priority, not the financial terms that may be involved.

For example federally-funded nonprofit institutions, compared with their peers in industry, have the mandate to make new technology as broadly available as possible. This means that there is a strong preference to limit the scope of a particular license to only what is needed to develop specific products. Exclusive licenses are quite typical for biomedical products such as vaccines, therapeutics, and others where the underlying technologies require substantial private risk and investment (and a prior public notice and comment period in the *Federal Register* in the case of federal laboratories). In their agreements, federal laboratories and universities would also typically expect to retain the right to permit further research use of the technology whether to be conducted either in the intramural program, universities, or companies. Because the commercial rights granted represent institutional (and often public) assets, these agreements have enforceable performance benchmarks to ensure that the public will eventually receive the benefit (through commercialized products) of the research it funded. Regulations governing the license negotiation of federally-owned technologies and their mandated requirements are described in more detail at 37 Code of Federal Regulations (CFR), Part 404, while those for federally-funded technologies can be found at 37 CFR , Part 401.

Figure 14.2 illustrates the fundamental steps that lead up to a license or other types of agreements with research institutions. In a license agreement the academic entity essentially grants rights to a company to make, use, and sell products that were it not for the license, would infringe on the patent rights that the academic center owns and/or controls. In some instances the academic center also grants the company rights to use technological information/know-how or materials that goes hand-in-hand with the information in the patent application and that is valuable to the company as it hopes to commercialize the technology into products. Licensing is at the heart of operations of a university tech transfer office and is the core of its set-up, post-Bayh-Dole. However, both academic centers and federal labs function as nonprofits and do not and cannot have a product commercialization arm and so cannot themselves convert inventions into commercial products and processes. They have to partner with industry to do that. Hence these out-licensing activities are the key to fulfilling the core of Bayh-Dole and other federal mandates of commercializing inventions that arise from federal funding.

Characteristics of Typical Biotech License Agreements

Generally, it is considered good business practice in licensing from a research institution that the organization would standardize license terms to the extent possible. Standardizing nonfinancial license terms levels the playing field for licensees (an important concept for public institutions) and creates a common understanding of the balance of risks acceptable to a research institution (which may differ markedly from the for-profit sector).

Royalty rate negotiations with these institutions are influenced by factors (Table 14.3) commonly encountered in other negotiations of early-stage biomedical technologies. Unique to federal laboratory and university negotiations are factors relating to the public health interest in the technology being licensed and the products to be developed from it (so-called "white knight clauses"). Examples of this may include supply back of materials for clinical use, indigent patient access programs in the U.S., commercial benefit sharing for natural product source countries or incentives for developing world access to the licensed products.

The royalty payments themselves (Table 14.4) consist of license payments received for execution royalties, minimum annual royalties (received regardless of the amount of product sales), earned royalties (a percentage of product sales), benchmark royalties and payments for patent costs. To date the NIH has not sought equity payments in licenses or directly participated in company start-ups due to

TABLE 14.3 Factors Influencing Royalty Rate Negotiations with Research Institutions

Stage of development
Type of product
Market value of product
Uniqueness of biological materials
Scope of patent coverage
Research institution "content"
Public Health Significance

TABLE 14.4 Typical Types of Fees and Royalties in Licenses Agreements with Research Institutions

Execution fees
Minimum annual royalty (regardless of the amount of net sales)
Earned royalties (fixed percentage of net sales)
Benchmark royalties
Patent costs
Sublicense fees (percentage of income)
Equity (varies by institution)

conflict of interest concerns. Instead, in lieu of equity, the NIH can consider equity-like benchmark royalties that track successful commercial events at the company. However, many universities do take equity payments in their license agreements as a way to assist a new start-up company even though there is considerable risk in accepting equity in lieu of cash payments since such equity is illiquid and has no present value at the time license is executed.

Licensing institutions will often opt to take an equity or equity-like position when available from their licensees for several reasons. For example, equity would provide for additional revenue in addition to the licensing royalties, especially if the licensed product failed in development but the company itself later become successful. Equity also can be seen as a risk premium for the research institution that provides additional inducement to grant the license to a new start-up company verses a more-established firm. Importantly, and perhaps most important for bioentrepreneurs, equity allows a licensee who is cash poor but equity rich to substitute an ownership position for a cash payment (in full or in part) for an up-front licensing fee and/or a reduced royalty rate. Finally, research institutions accept this risk to support its mission to assist in commercialization of early-stage technologies, which may not be turned into marketable products otherwise, and to encourage small business development. However, all universities recognize that holding ownership rights in a start-up company creates potential conflict of interest and adopt various internal policies that mitigate and/or manage such conflicts.

Unlike their corporate counterparts, inventors at non-profit research institutions do receive a share of the royalties generated from the licensing of their inventions. However each institution might have a slightly different revenue-sharing policy with respect to the percent of licensing revenues that are shared with inventors. Next, we discuss what might be some of the typical license agreements that a bioentrepreneur would come across in dealings with a non-profit research institution.

Types of License Agreements

Universities and federal research institutions negotiate a variety of different types of license agreements for use and development of biomedical technologies. Besides offering exclusive and nonexclusive commercialization agreements for patented technologies, commercialization agreements are negotiated for unpatented biological materials. Being increasingly more selective as to what type of technologies they seek to patent, both types of institutions are unlikely to patent research materials or research methodologies that can be easily transferred for commercial use by biological material license agreements or publication. For patent rights or materials that are not

to be sold as commercial products but are useful in internal R&D programs, both federal research institutions and universities would typically negotiate nonexclusive internal use license agreements. Additionally, companies may obtain evaluation agreements to new technologies as well as specialized agreements relating to interference or other patent dispute settlements. Finally, for bioentrepreneurs interested in a technology that was jointly invented by two or more institutions, an interinstitutional patent/licensing management agreement would be negotiated so that the bioentrepreneur would be able to obtain an exclusive license by only dealing with one party.

Typically, federal research institutions and many universities have the types of license agreements shown in Table 14.5 and described below [5].

1. **Commercial evaluation/option license agreements** are short-term nonexclusive license agreements to allow a licensee to conduct feasibility testing but not the sale of products developed from a technology. These typically run no longer than a few months, have a modest cost associated with them, and include relevant materials that are supplied by inventor(s). Screening use is not permitted but the agreement has proven to be ideal for feasibility testing of new technologies that have a wide-variety of possible useful (but unproven) applications. "Screening use" implies use of the licensed material in the discovery or development of a different final end-product. For example, a reporter cell that expresses an oncogene can be tested to screen drug candidates that could potentially be effective in certain cancer therapeutics. Some universities may also use this type of agreement in the form of a short-term exclusive option agreement for a nascent technology with the hope that a long-term diagnostic, vaccine, or therapeutic product commercialization license agreement will later be completed.

2. **Internal commercial-use license agreements** are another nonexclusive license agreement that allows a licensee to use (but not sell) technology in its internal programs. Here materials (either patented or unpatented) are provided, and screening uses are permitted. The financial structure of this agreement can be either a "paid-up"

TABLE 14.5 Major Types of Licenses Agreements Involving Research Institutions E/OLA

Commercial evaluation/option license agreements
Internal commercial-use license agreements
Research products commercialization license agreements
Vaccine, diagnostic, therapeutic, or medical device product commercialization license agreements
Interinstitutional agreements (for joint inventions)

term license or annual royalty payments each, however, without any "reach-through" royalty obligations to other products being used or discovered by the licensee. A "paid-up term" license would be a license in which the company makes a one-time lump sum payment to obtain the rights to use the licensed technology for the duration of the license. On the other hand, "reach through" royalty provisions in a license agreement create royalties to the licensor on the future sales of downstream products that are discovered or developed through the use of licensed technology, even though the final end-product may not contain the licensed technology. In other words, reach-through royalties are royalties that are due to a licensor even though manufacture, use, or the sale of the final product does not infringe any patents claiming the licensed technology. Internal commercial-use agreements themselves historically have been very popular with medium to larger biomedical firms who are eager to acquire reagents to speed their internal development programs. Popular technologies licensed in this manner include animal models and receptors.

3. **Research products commercialization license agreements** are again another non-exclusive license agreement but allow a licensee to sell products to the research products market. Here materials (either patented or unpatented) are also generally provided with smaller firms predominating as licensees. For federal laboratories, U.S. manufacturing is required even for nonexclusive product sales in the United States unless a waiver is granted. Waivers are granted on the basis of a lack of manufacturing capacity in the United States or economic hardship for the licensee. The financial structure of these licenses generally involve low up-front royalties but relatively high earned-royalty payments since the materials provided are frequently close or very close to the finished product that is to be sold. Popular research products licensed in this manner include a wide variety of monoclonal or polyclonal antibodies or other research materials used in basic research.

4. **Vaccine, diagnostic, therapeutic, or medical device product commercialization license agreements** are agreements than can be exclusive if such is necessary for product development due to the capital and risk involved for the licensee. Important for bioentrepreneurs is that fact that by law, small, capable biomedical firms receive preference from federal laboratories and federally-funded universities as exclusive licensees. At NIH and other federal laboratories, all prospective grants of exclusive licenses (identifying the licensee and technology by name) are published in the *Federal Register* for public comment or objections. A detailed development plan with product benchmarks or milestones is expected for licenses in this area. Collaborative research with federal laboratories regarding further preclinical or clinical

development of the technology is encouraged, but not required in order to obtain a license, and is negotiated separately by the individual laboratory program. These agreements also have a requirement for U.S. manufacturing for U.S. product sales unless a waiver is granted. The federal laboratory can typically grant waivers only when U.S. manufacturing sites are unavailable or manufacturing in the United States is economically infeasible. The financial structure of these licenses can involve substantial up-front royalties, but much more moderate-earned royalties (since the technology is typically not close to a finished product) and appropriate benchmark payments. Other provisions to be negotiated include a share amount of sublicensing proceeds, any of the public health "white knight" provisions described earlier, as well as licensee performance monitoring and audit requirements.

5. **Interinstitutional agreements** are often useful for exclusive licensing as many commercializable technologies will often have inventors from more than one university or federal laboratory due to the collaborative nature of science. If a bioentrepreneur is seeking to obtain an exclusive commercialization license to a technology due to the level of investment or risk involved, it is important to obtain the rights from all of the institutions involved, especially for U.S. patent rights, as all owners have the ability to license separately. Often the joint owners of a single technology will pool their rights with a single party for patent and licensing purposes through an interinstitutional agreement. Such agreements provide significant convenience and time-saving for bioentrepreneurs since they would have to negotiate with only one research institution to secure an exclusive license to the technology.

Components of a Biotechnology License Agreement

1. **Breadth of rights**—This depends on the technology that is being licensed and the size and need of the company. If the patent rights/technology is specific to a certain company's drug, for e.g., something that arose from a sponsored research agreement (described earlier in this chapter) then it would be typical to give the company exclusive license rights to all fields available within the patent rights. For platform technologies that have broad uses in very different medical applications—for e.g., micro fluidic IP—field specific, but still exclusive licenses would be appropriate.

   a. For diagnostic technologies, the trend is to grant non-exclusive rights to the technology, if possible, but with an eye towards incentivizing the companies to invest into developing the technology. For research tool technologies, it is standard practice to give several companies nonexclusive access to use the technologies in their internal research, for example in their drug discovery, programs.

b. There is another dimension to consider in addition to the type of technology described above—the size of the company—for start-ups founded on university or federal lab technology in order for the fledgling company to attract investment, a broader field of use is appropriate. But if it is a small company, a recent start-up from another university perhaps and a second university's technology is offering a solution to a specific problem, then only narrow rights to the company from the second university would be appropriate.

2. **Signing fees and patent costs**—Having invested in the technology via supporting the protection of patent rights, the academic institution is first and foremost, eager to reimburse themselves for the patent costs incurred thus far. A license is their exit , and the minimum terms of this exit is to recoup patent costs and further, a modest signing fee is appropriate at time of signing of a license.

3. **Sublicense fees**—The statistics are that most technologies are not developed by the first licensee of the technology but by the company's further licensee (the "sublicensee"). Typically, this sublicense happens when the original company licensee has developed and validated the technology further. Depending on the situation, a fixed percentage or a sliding scale of percentage sublicense income back to the original licensor is considered equitable.

4. **Minimum annual royalties/milestone fees**—A certain percentage of royalty on net sales of the product comes back to the licensor (academic institution). To ensure diligent development, having a set annual payment is customary. Sometimes this is termed "annual maintenance fee" that is credited against royalty upon product launch. The diligent development of the product, covered next, is a key element to the contract. Payments to the academic institution upon reaching key milestones in the path to the product are customary.

5. **Diligent development of the licensed technology**—For technologies that are funded in whole or in part with federal funding this is an absolute requirement. Companies are required to give the TTOs their product development plan along with the expected timelines. The consequence of not meeting these diligence goals is termination. A key item to remember is that research institutions have flexibility to work with licensees and can accommodate changing needs. The key is to have a mechanism of communication and cooperation between both parties. If the company is really "shelving" the technology, the university or federal lab needs to be able to get it back to seek and find another licensing partner to commercialize these technologies.

6. **Reserved rights**—As per Bayh-Dole for government-funded technologies, academic centers are required to reserve rights for their continued use of the technology for further academic research. Typically, the academic center reserves rights not only for its own use but also for the research use of other academic centers. For hospitals, this would include clinical research use as well, since patient care is part of the institution mission. The reason for this clause is for licensees not to block anyone from continuing research on the technology that could benefit the public given that it was funded by the tax dollars from the public in the first place. For government labs, the reserved right is for any governmental purpose and is required by statue.

7. **Enforcement**—Patent rights are enforced by the owner or in cooperation from the owner. An "infringer" of the technology is hurting the market share of our licensee. As the patent owner, universities and federal labs are affected since the patent licensees are affected. Typically, exclusive licensees seek to get first rights to go after infringers but the actions by licensees might drag the TTOs into lawsuits and potential invalidation of the patent claims. Academic centers do not have the appetite (or the money) for lawsuits. A common approach is therefore to have the first right to pursue infringers when informed by our companies to encourage them to take a license from our licensees. Failing this, it is typical to have licensees pursue infringers.

8. **Indemnification and insurance**—Academic medical centers have to protect themselves from lawsuits that may arise from patients who may be injured by the products that companies make, market, and sell. When sponsored research is performed and broad access is given to all results that arise from the collaborations, judicious use of the results in the drug-development process is the company's responsibility and the terms of the agreement in this section are designed to protect the TTOs. Thus in their agreements, companies are required to provide evidence that they have the necessary backing via insurance protection. This is a requirement from institutional insurance carriers and therefore this term is typically nonnegotiable from the TTO's side.

9. **Conflicts of interest**—This is a very significant and real issue particularly for teaching hospitals, academic medical centers, and federal laboratories that are doing both clinical and basic research. Conflicts are managed by ensuring that at the time of the licensing of inventions to a company related to a certain drug, the medical center does not have any sponsored research collaboration on the same drug with the same investigator whose invention(s)/technology was licensed. Also, the investigator cannot consult for the company whose drugs are in clinical trials under his or her guidance. Additional

TABLE 14.6 Common Ranges of Financial Terms for Exclusive License Agreements

	Diagnostic	Therapeutic
License signing fee	$25,000 to $50,000	$50,000 to $200,000
Sublicense fees[a]	10 to 40 percent	10 to 40 percent
Annual fees or annual minimum royalties	$10,000 to $50,000	$10,000 to $100,000
Earned royalties (percentage of net sales)[b]	2 to 15 percent	2 to 6 percent
Total milestone payments[c]	$1 to 3 million	$1 to 7 million

[a]Higher percentage in payments may be appropriate if the company intends to monetize the technology through further licensing rather than through product development.
[b]The stacking of royalties to allow a company to further in-license other technologies for the development of product is typical. With stacking/offsets the lower end of the range may be applicable.
[c]Start-up or express agreements may have substantial milestones, liquidity, or equity payments in lieu of early fees.

conflict of interest rules apply to federal scientists. The conflict of interest policies of research institutions are typically available on their public websites.

Financial terms for nonexclusive license grants including license grants to research-tool technologies can vary widely. These licenses would not have all the elaborate terms described above, but rather would have a fixed annual fee-type structure or even have a one-time "fully paid-up" financial structure. Table 14.6 gives some ranges of financial terms for exclusive licenses.

ADVANTAGES FOR A BIOTECH START-UP TO WORK WITH THE NIH AND UNIVERSITIES

Why Start-Ups Should Work with NIH and Universities

NIH's New Low-Cost Start-Up License Agreements

To better facilitate this "fourth mission" of economic development in conjunction with increased development of new therapeutic products, the NIH has developed a new short-term Start-Up Exclusive Evaluation License Agreement (Start-up EELA) and a Start-up Exclusive Commercial License Agreement (Start-up ECLA) to facilitate licensing of intramural NIH and Food and Drug Administration (FDA) inventions to early-stage companies. Similar "express" or

"start-up" agreements are available at many universities as well. The new NIH Start-Up Licenses are provided to assist companies that are less than 5 years old, have less than $5 million in capital raised, and have fewer than 50 employees obtain an exclusive license from the NIH for a biomedical invention of interest arising from the NIH or FDA. NIH Start-Up Licenses are offered to companies developing drugs, vaccines, therapeutics, and certain devices from NIH or FDA patented or patent pending technologies that NIH determines will require significant investment to develop, such as those undergoing clinical trials to achieve FDA approval or Class III diagnostics. The new company must license at least one NIH- or FDA-owned U.S. patent and commit to developing a product or service for the United States market. The licensee may also obtain in the license, related NIH- or FDA-owned patents filed in other countries if the company agrees to commercialize products in those countries as well.

Financial terms for the Start-Up Licenses are designed with the fiscal realities of small firms in mind and feature either: a 1-year exclusive evaluation license with a flat $2000 execution fee (this license can be later amended to become an exclusive commercialization license) or an immediate exclusive commercialization license. The Start-Up Exclusive Commercial License includes:

- A delayed tiered up-front execution royalty, which would be due to the NIH upon a liquidity event such as an initial public offering (IPO), a merger, a sublicense, an assignment, acquisition by another firm, or a first commercial sale.
- A delayed minimum annual royalty (MAR) or a MAR that is waived if there is a Cooperative Research and Development Agreement (CRADA) with the NIH (or FDA) concerning the development of the licensed technology and providing value comparable to the MAR. Additionally, the MAR will be waived for up to 5 years during the term of a Small Business Innovation Research (SBIR) or Small Business Technology Transfer (STTR) grant for the development of the licensed technology.
- An initial lower reimbursement rate of patent expenses which increases over time to full reimbursement of expenses tied to the earliest of a liquidity event, an initial public offering, the grant of a sublicense, a first commercial sale, or upon the third anniversary of the effective date of the agreement.
- Consideration by the NIH of all requests from a start-up company to file new or continuing patent applications as long as the company is actively and timely reimbursing patent-prosecution expenses.
- A set earned royalty rate of 1.5 percent on the sale of licensed products.
- A set sublicensing royalty rate of 15 percent of the other consideration received from the grant of a sublicense.

- An antistacking royalty payment license provision can be negotiated by a company if it encounters a stacking royalty problem. A stacking royalty problem could potentially occur when a licensee's third-party royalty obligations add up to such a high total royalty percentage such that the project becomes unattractive for investment, sublicensing, or self-development due to low profit margins. Royalty stacking can especially be a problem in the development of biologics due to the breadth of a possible third party IP that may be needed compared with traditional small molecule drugs.

- Mutually agreed-upon specific benchmarks and performance milestones, which do not require a royalty payment, but rather ensure that the start-up licensee is taking concrete steps towards a practical application of the licensed product or process.

- NIH Start-Up Commercial Licenses represent a significant front-end savings in negotiation time and money for new companies. An exclusive license, for a new technology (even early-stage), might have expectations prior to negotiations (for a large-market indication) of an immediate execution fee of up to $250,000 or more, a minimum annual royalty due in the first year and beyond of up to $25,000 or more, immediate payment of all past patent expenses and ongoing payments of future patent expenses, benchmark royalties in the range of up to $1 million or more, significant sublicensing consideration, and earned royalties in the range up to 5 percent or more depending on the technology.

Because many, if not most of the technologies developed at the NIH and FDA, are early-stage biomedical technologies, the time and development risks to develop a commercial product are high. Depending on the technology and the stage of formation of the potential licensee, the company may prefer to enter into the Start-up EELA to evaluate their interest before committing to a longer-term Start-up ECLA. Bioentrepreneurs can identify technologies of interest by searching licensing opportunities on the NIH Office of Technology Transfer (OTT) website [5], by email notification via Real Simple Syndication (RSS) feed and by getting in touch with the listed licensing contact. Model template agreements for the Start-Up Licenses and other details on the licensing process are published on the OTT "Start-up Webpage." [7]

Unique Features of Biotech Start-Up Licenses

While start-ups can be seen to have the potential to produce significant opportunities for the inventors, investors, the research institution, and regional economies, such projects involve more work and are riskier than a traditional license to an existing, capitalized company. Although research conducted at federal laboratories and universities is not specifically designed to lead to a new company formation, such activities are a way for such institutions to support the economic development aspects of their licensing- and technology-transfer programs as previously described. Successful start-up companies and bioentrepreneurs are highly prized because of the direct benefits to the community, region, state, and country in terms of new employment and tax revenue. Because of this, some research institutions have in-house business development staff dedicated to working with inventors as they consider start-up opportunities for their technology. However, many institutions handle this as part of the activities of the regular technology transfer office staff.

A typical practice for a research institution that is licensing to a start-up company, is to first confirm that there is no other prior claim of rights from a commercial sponsor, and to then execute a confidentiality agreement, a letter of intent or other indication of interest, which should be followed quickly thereafter with an option agreement to a future exclusive license. If the bioentrepreneur has substantial resources already in place it may be possible to grant the license directly in place of an option when it is merited. Whatever the nature of the agreement, it is generally expected that the negotiation be with an officer of the new venture (or their attorney) and not a university faculty member who may hope to be involved in the company. Agreements should also contain clear timelines to enforce the diligent development of the technology toward commercialization. Particularly critical are deadlines for raising predetermined levels of initial funding to establish and operate the venture. To avoid conflict of interest problems at the research institution, the new company should operate separately from the inventor's lab, with local incubator or business park space being ideal. Most research institutions should also not allow their faculty inventors to serve as officers of the company without a leave of absence but should allow these companies to collaborate and/or sponsor ongoing research in the laboratories of inventors subject to conflict of interest review and approval. Generally, a federal laboratory inventor is not able to have an active role in the company without leaving federal employment. The share of equity held by a university in these circumstances can vary by the type of technology.

The actual share amount held by the research institution, or the equivalent value to be paid to it, is often not that critical as the overall goal for the university or federal laboratory to develop a robust local, regional, or national corporate research community that closely complements and interacts with ongoing research at the institution. It is also a way to support university or former federal faculty members who are themselves entrepreneurial and willing to commit their time and often their own money to bringing their inventions to the marketplace.

Advantages to Working with Universities and Federal Laboratories

Within these basic licensing structures, however, there are several advantages that bioentrepreneurs can utilize in their product development efforts since federal laboratories and universities offer favorable treatment to small businesses to create an attractive playing field for them to get into new areas of product development. For example, start-ups can utilize the expertise of the patent law firm hired by the institution to manage the patent prosecution of the licensed technology. This is particularly useful for small firms that may not yet have internal patent counsel or the resources to retain a top intellectual property (IP) law firm.

Another useful example is that license agreements with federal laboratories and universities (in contrast with corporate license agreements) do not require bioentrepreneurs to cross-license existing rights they may own, give up any product marketing rights, nor forsake any downstream developmental rights. Also research-tool licenses negotiated through the NIH and many universities carry no grant-backs or reach-through rights. For instance, when a research-tool technology is licensed to a company by the NIH, the licensee is not required to grant back any usage rights to the improvements that it may develop subsequent to the license agreement. Also the licensee is not required to share with the NIH any future profits that may be made as a result of improvements to the original discovery. In other words, intellectual property derived from new discoveries made with NIH-licensed tools will remain clear and unencumbered.

Another advantage for a bioentrepreneur to license a technology from a nonprofit institution is the flexibility in the financial terms. While the NIH and many research institutions have "Start-up" or "Express" template agreements with favorable terms already in place, these can typically be negotiated separately. For example, reimbursement of back patent expenses, which the licensee typically pays upon the signing of the license agreement, could be deferred for a certain period of time. Similarly, the license deal could be structured to be heavily back-end loaded and/or equity-based so as to allow the bioentrepreneur to apply its cash towards R&D. Unlike many research institutions that take equity in lieu of cash, federal institutions and some universities do not consider equity-based license deals but do take roughly equivalent equity-like benchmark payments. The resulting lack of equity dilution may become an important feature as the bioentrepreneur looks to raise capital through additional rounds of financing.

A bioentrepreneur could also take advantage of the capabilities and technical expertise residing in the licensor's laboratories by collaboration and/or sponsorship of the research needed to expedite the of development of the technology. While sponsoring research at the inventor's laboratory may in some circumstances raise conflict of interest issues, many institutions are willing to put together a conflict management plan with the engaged parties in order to help the start-up to exploit all the resources offered by the licensor. Many research institutions would however execute an agreement separate from a license agreement to formalize such an arrangement.

At a basic level, the success of a new biotechnology venture depends on five key ingredients: (1) technical expertise, (2) intellectual property assets, (3) business expertise, (4) physical space, and (5) money [8]. Institutional scientists or faculty entrepreneurs themselves can provide the needed technical expertise (especially if students or postdocs can be hired by the new venture) and the research institutions of course can license key patent rights to the company. But business expertise, space, and money are often more difficult to come by. Research institutions often try to help new firms bridge this gap by providing more than just IP licensing and technical expertise. This is because commercial partners, especially small, innovative ones, are essential to the role of federally-funded research institutions in delivering novel healthcare products to the market. There is now an attractive array of available options or opportunities for new biotech firms beyond just traditional licenses or start-up license agreements, and several of these options will be examined in more detail.

Research Collaboration Programs for Start-Ups

For some entrepreneurs there is a misperception that NIH scientists, (unlike their university counterparts) are not allowed to interact with private-sector firms due to the implementation of strict government ethics and conflict of interest rules. While it is true that NIH investigators, in general, cannot engage in outside consulting with biotechnology and pharmaceutical companies in their personal capacity, the fact is that technology transfer-related activities are actually among the "official duties," in which NIH scientists are encouraged to participate. These activities may include the reporting of new inventions from the laboratory and assisting technology-transfer staff with patenting, marketing, and licensing interactions with companies. NIH scientists can also officially collaborate with industry scientists through the use of various mechanisms including more complex Cooperative Research and Development Agreements (CRADAs) and Clinical Trial Agreements (CTAs) as well as simpler Confidential Disclosure Agreements (CDAs), and Material Transfer Agreements (MTAs).

In a CRADA research project, which could run for several years, NIH and company scientists can engage in mutually beneficial joint research, where each party provides unique resources, skills, and funding, and where either partner may not otherwise be able to solely provide all the resources needed for the successful completion of the project. In such an arrangement, the details of the research activity to be carried out and the scope of the license options granted to discoveries emanating from the joint research are clearly spelled out in advance. A CTA would typically involve the clinical testing of a private-sector company's small molecule compound or biologic drug. The company gains access to the clinical trial infrastructure and clinical expertise available at NIH; however, unlike what occurs with a CRADA, the company partner does not have any licensing rights to intellectual property that is generated during the clinical research project. The NIH usually enters into these agreements only in cases where such trials would be difficult or impossible to run in other places. The NIH is particularly interested in clinical trials involving rare or orphan diseases that affect 200,000 or fewer patients per year in the United States. An MTA is a popular mechanism for exchanging proprietary research reagents and is used by scientists worldwide. NIH investigators actively use this mechanism to share reagents with scientists in other nonprofit organizations. Proprietary and/or unpublished information can be exchanged between NIH researchers and company personnel in advance of making a decision to enter into a formal CRADA or CTA via the use of a CDA.

Of the collaborative mechanisms described above, a CRADA is perhaps the most comprehensive and far-reaching agreement for federal laboratories. Such agreements can provide additional funds for an NIH lab while providing the collaborating company with preferential access to the NIH scientist's future discoveries and access to scientific and medical expertise during the research or clinical collaboration. A CRADA is not, however, intended to be a means for the NIH to provide funding for a new company; in fact, the NIH cannot supply any funding to its CRADA partners. The easiest way for an entrepreneur to access this expertise is to simply approach the agency officially either by contacting a scientist directly or by contacting the institute technology-transfer office and/or technology development coordinator [9].

If an early-stage company needs access to NIH materials for commercial purposes outside a formal collaboration, this usually would be done utilizing an Internal Commercial Use License Agreement rather than a MTA. As noted before, these are nonexclusive license agreements to allow a licensee to use (but not sell) technology in its internal programs. Here, materials (either patented or unpatented) are provided, and drug screening uses are permitted. The financial structure of this agreement can be either a single payment, a paid-up term license, or annual royalty payments, though the second structure is more popular with start-up companies.

Funding Opportunities for Start-Ups—SBIR Programs

In addition to contracting opportunities, the NIH and other federal labs can provide private sector entities with nondilutive funding through the SBIR (Small Business Innovation Research) and STTR (Small Business Technology Transfer Research) programs [10]. The NIH SBIR program is perhaps the most lucrative and stable funding source for new companies and unlike a small business loan, SBIR grant funds do not need to be repaid.

Other noteworthy advantages of SBIR programs for small companies include retention by the company of any intellectual property rights from the research funding, receipt of early-stage funding that doesn't impact stock or shares in any way (e.g., no dilution of capital), national recognition for the firm, verification and visibility for the underlying technology, and the generation of a leveraging tool that can attract other funding from venture capital or angel investors.

The SBIR program itself was established in 1982 by the Small Business Innovation Development Act to increase the participation of small, high technology firms in federal R&D activities. Under this program, departments and agencies with R&D budgets of $100 million or more are required to set aside 2.6 percent (for FY 2012) of their R&D budgets to sponsor research at small companies. The STTR program was established by the Small Business Technology Transfer Act of 1992 and requires federal agencies with extramural R&D budgets over $1 billion to administer STTR programs using an annual set-aside of 0.35 percent (for FY 2012). In FY 2011 NIH's combined SBIR and STTR grants totaled over $682 million.

The STTR and SBIR programs are similar in that both seek to increase small business participation and private-sector commercialization of technology developed through federal R&D. The SBIR program funds early-stage research and development at small businesses. The unique feature of the STTR program is the requirement for the small business applicant to formally collaborate with a research institution in Phase I and Phase II (see description below).

Thus the SBIR and STTR programs differ in two major ways. First, under the SBIR program, the principal investigator must have his or her primary employment with the small business concern at the time of the award and for the duration of the project period. However, under the STTR program, primary employment is not stipulated. Second, the STTR program requires research partners at universities and other nonprofit research institutions to have a formal collaborative relationship with the small business concern. At least 40 percent of the STTR research project is to be conducted by the small business concern and at least 30 percent of the effort is to be conducted by the single "partnering" research institution.

As a major mechanism at the NIH for achieving the goals of enhancing public health through the commercialization of new technology, the SBIR and STTR grants present an excellent funding source for start-up and other small biotechnology companies. The NIH SBIR and

STTR programs themselves are structured in three primary phases:

Phase I—The objective of Phase I is to establish the technical merit and feasibility of the proposed R&D efforts and to determine the quality of performance of the small business prior to providing further federal funding in Phase II. Phase I awards are normally $150,000, provided over a period of 6 months for SBIR and $150,000 over a period of 1 year for STTR. However, with proper justification, applicants may propose longer periods of time and greater amounts of funds necessary to establish the technical merit and feasibility of the proposed project.

Phase II—The objective of Phase II is to continue the R&D efforts initiated in Phase I. Only Phase I awardees are eligible for a Phase II award. Phase II awards are normally $1 million over 2 years for SBIR and $1 million over 2 years for STTR. However, with proper justification, applicants may propose longer periods of time and greater amounts of funds necessary for completion of the project.

SBIR-TT Phase I and Phase II—Under this new program (SBIR-Technology Transfer or SBIR-TT) undertaken at the National Cancer Institute (NCI) at the NIH and in the process of being expanded to other NIH institutes, SBIR Phase I and Phase II awards are given in conjunction with exclusive licenses to selected underlying background discoveries made by an intramural research laboratory at the institute.

SBIR Phase II Bridge—The NCI SBIR program has created the Phase II Bridge Award for previously funded NCI SBIR Phase II awardees to continue the next stage of R&D for projects in the areas of cancer therapeutics, imaging technologies, interventional devices, diagnostics, and prognostics. The objective of the NCI Phase II Bridge Award is to help address the funding gap that a company may encounter between the end of the Phase II award and the commercialization stage. Budgets up to $1 million in total costs per year and project periods up to 3 years (a total of $3 million over 3 years) may be requested from the NCI. To incentivize partnerships between awardees and third-party investors and/or strategic partners, a competitive preference and funding priority will be given to applicants that demonstrate the ability to secure substantial independent third-party investor funds (i.e., third-party funds that equal or exceed the requested NCI funds). This funding opportunity is open to current and recently expired NCI SBIR Phase II projects.

Phase III—The objective of Phase III, where appropriate, is for the small business concern to pursue with non-SBIR/STTR funds the commercialization objectives resulting from the Phase I/II R&D activities.

Those who hope to receive an SBIR or STTR grant from the NIH must convince the NIH that the proposed research is unique, creates value for the general public at large through advancements in knowledge and treatment of disease, and is relevant to the overall goals of the NIH. It is important to contact the program officials ahead of time within the particular component of the NIH from where funding is sought in order to determine whether the proposed research plan fits these criteria. For start-ups, generally SBIR applications are most successful when they include an entrepreneur-founder with experience in the field, a highly innovative technical solution to significant clinical needs, an end-product with significant commercial potential, a technology in need of more feasibility data that the proposed research project would generate, and finally a project that, if successful, would have reduced risk and become more attractive for downstream investment. At the NIH, grant applications are currently reviewed three times a year (April 5, August 5, and December 5) and contract proposals the first week in November. Note that both programs were recently subject to recent reauthorization by Congress with many changes providing further assistance to companies currently in the process of implementation.

NEW AND INNOVATIVE PROGRAMS AS WE MOVE TOWARDS "V2.0" OF TECHNOLOGY TRANSFER

Basic and Clinical Research Assistance from the NIH

Basic and clinical research assistance from the NIH institutes may also be available to companies through specialized services such as drug candidate compound screening and preclinical and clinical drug development and testing services, which are offered by several programs. These initiatives are particularly targeted towards developing and enhancing new clinical candidates in the disease or health area of particular focus at various NIH institutes. The largest and perhaps best-known programs of these types at the NIH are those currently run in the National Cancer Institute (NCI) [11]. The NCI has played an active role in the development of drugs for cancer treatment for over 50 years. This is reflected in the fact that approximately one half of the chemotherapeutic drugs currently used by oncologists for cancer treatments were in some form discovered and/or developed at NCI. The Developmental Therapeutics Program (DTP) promotes all aspects of drug discovery and development before testing in humans (preclinical development), and is a part of the Division of Cancer Treatment and Diagnosis (DCTD). NCI also funds an extensive clinical (human) trials network to ensure that promising agents are tested in humans. NCI's Cancer Therapy Evaluation Program (CTEP), also a part of the DCTD, administers clinical drug development. Compounds can enter at any stage of the development process with either very little or extensive prior testing. Drugs developed through these programs include well-known products such as cisplatin, paclitaxel, and fludarabine.

Beginning in 2012 the NIH established a new center called the National Center for Advancing Translational Sciences (NCATS) that is designed to assist companies with the many costly, time-consuming bottlenecks that exist in translational product development [12]. Working in partnership with both the public and private organizations, NCATS seeks to develop innovative ways to reduce, remove, or bypass such bottlenecks to speed the delivery of new drugs, diagnostics, and medical devices to patients. The Center is not a drug development company, but focuses more on using science to create powerful new tools and technologies that can be adopted widely by translational researchers in all sectors.

NCATS was formed primarily by uniting and realigning a variety of existing NIH programs that play key roles in translational science along with adding key initiatives. Programs of particular note for bioentrepreneurs at NCATS include:

1. **Bridging Interventional Development Gaps (BrIDGs)** makes available critical resources needed for the development of new therapeutic agents. Formerly called the NIH-RAID (Rapid Access to Interventional Development) program, the BrIDGs program advances promising therapies into the clinic by providing contract services to overcome barriers faced in late-stage preclinical therapy development.

2. **Clinical and Translational Science Awards (CTSA)** fund a national consortium of 60 medical research institutions working together to improve the way clinical and translational research is conducted nationwide. These institutions will serve as a primary test bed for NCATS activities. The CTSA-Intellectual Property tool can be used to view patent and licensable technologies from institutions.

3. **Chemical Genomics Center (NCGC)** is one of the centers in the Molecular Libraries Probe Production Centers Network (MLPCN). Through this program, biomedical researchers gain access to the large-scale small molecule screening capacity, along with medicinal chemistry and informatics necessary to identify chemical probes to study the functions of genes, cells, and biochemical pathways. These chemical probes may also be used in developing of new drugs.

4. **Therapeutics for Rare and Neglected Diseases (TRND)** offers collaborative opportunities to access rare and neglected disease drug-development capabilities, expertise, and clinical/regulatory resources. Its goal is to move promising therapeutics into human clinical trials. Selected applicants can partner with TRND staff on a joint project plan and implement a drug-development program. Applicant investigators provide the drug project starting points and ongoing biological/disease expertise throughout the project. A collaboration agreement is established between TRND and successful applicants.

NCATS-supported programs and projects have also produced numerous tools to help basic and clinical researchers advance translational science. These resources include clinical research tools and resources to aid in such activities as patient recruitment, clinical study management, and public-private partnership development as well as preclinical research tools and resources to help researchers explore the functions of cells at the genome level, including more than 60 chemical probes.

There is additional assistance available from other NIH institutes to firms in a variety of disease areas including infectious diseases, drug abuse, and others—many more than can be highlighted here. All in all, such efforts can provide a wide variety of technical assistance (often at modest or no cost) for preclinical and even clinical development of novel therapies or other biomedical products by start-up firms.

Selling Products to Universities and Federal Labs

One of the most commonly overlooked opportunities by biomedical-focused companies is the ability to sell products and services to the NIH and similar research centers. Indeed, for start-up companies looking to develop new products used in conducting basic or clinical research, the NIH may be their first customer. With an intramural staff of about 18,000 employees, laboratories in several regions of the country (with the Bethesda campus in Maryland home to the majority), and an annual intramural budget of about $3 billion, the NIH is perhaps the largest individual institutional consumer of bioscience research reagents and instruments in the world. A variety of mechanisms for selling products and services to the NIH are possible, including stocking in government storerooms. Selling to the NIH can be seen as a daunting task for new companies because of the U.S. government's complex acquisition process. However, there are a few simple steps that companies can take, such as establishing a Blanket Purchase Agreement (BPA) with the NIH and getting their goods and services into the NIH stockroom. Once these hurdles are cleared, it is much easier for NIH scientists to buy from such companies, and if the quality of goods and services provided by a particular biotech company is superior, an NIH scientist can justify buying solely from that very source.

Companies that provide products and services to NIH laboratories can not only generate cash flow and revenues to fuel R&D, but also begin to demonstrate their commercial acumen to would-be partners and investors. Being a large research organization, the NIH has numerous R&D contracting opportunities. For specific information on such opportunities, visit the NIH Office of Acquisition Management and Policy website [13].

The annual NIH Research Festival is also an excellent starting point for companies hoping to sell products to the NIH [14]. This event is held every fall at the Bethesda, Maryland campus and every spring on the Frederick, Maryland campus. Part scientific, part social, part informational, and part inspirational, this 3-day event draws a variety of small- to medium-sized bioscience companies. These events attract almost 6000 NIH scientists, many of whom come to these gatherings to learn about and potentially purchase the latest research tools and services.

Translation Research Center as a V2.0 of Technology Transfer

Academic medical centers such as the Massachusetts General Hospital (MGH) are also evolving into this new model of technology commercialization that places a greater emphasis on the translational aspects of research. In the traditional technology transfer model, as you recall, the academic entity has used its intellectual capital to make break-through, cutting-edge discoveries, protecting them with patent picket-fences, and "transfers" it out to the company for them to develop these stellar scientific discoveries into products. In the case of academic medical centers there is the added component that these products would benefit the patients that are cared for in these centers. These institutions recognize that to have the best patient outcomes for these new inventions there is also a need to participate further in the translation of the early discovery to actual products.

The pictorial in Figure 14.3 illustrates this model of a "joint venture" with a company that was used at the MGH and it is evident from this depiction the huge advantages that can be had from the utilization of the complementary strengths of the two parties in such a translation research effort. As illustrated, the research center brings to the table the technology, the IP, the know-how, and deep understanding of the inner workings of the technology, and in the case of MGH, significant biological and clinical insights. The company would provide the funding, the product development expertise, the regulatory expertise, and finally and importantly the marketing and product-positioning expertise. The interesting aspect with the AMCs is that the product that is developed in such a joint venture ultimately gets used on patients, and MGH's clinical insights would tremendously help with the trial design and of course ultimately with the adoption in patient care. The advantage from the company's perspective is that the academic has simply not washed their hands off after the initial, albeit very important, discovery and are continuing to participate in translational efforts *enroute* to the product. This is an inherent derisking activity that helps the buy-in from company management for endorsing such an investment.

One such center was established at MGH with funding from a large company in the fall of 2010. The product is a next-generation diagnostic for cancer care—one that may fundamentally change therapeutic decisions for cancer patients. For this program, the TTO was instrumental right from the start in nurturing/protecting and maintaining the IP from its early days, working with the investigators to attract companies to the table, doing the deal with the company, and of course helping see this technology being translated into a product.

IMPACT OF TECHNOLOGY TRANSFER

Licensing has Spurred Biotechnology Industry Growth

As mentioned before, the economic development potential of biomedical research is being recognized as a fourth mission for research institutions—going along with education,

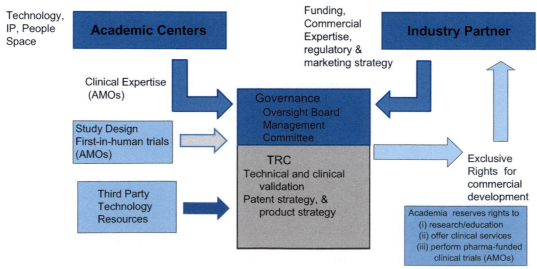

FIGURE 14.3   Newer business models for tech transfer—Translational Research Centers (TRC).

research, and public or community service. Thus it is in this "fourth mission" that bioentrepreneurs and research institutions find themselves again sharing the common goal of having new companies established based upon innovative research discoveries.

The economic importance of licensing and technology transfer has become better recognized during the recent recessionary period and some of the figures can be quite striking. For example, the overall product sales of all types by licensees of NIH intramural research is now reported by the NIH Office of Technology Transfer as being over $6 billion annually, the equivalent of midtier Fortune 500 companies. Economic development also was the focus of the October 28, 2011 U.S. Presidential Memorandum entitled "Accelerating Technology Transfer and Commercialization of Federal Research in Support of High-Growth Businesses." [14] This directive from the White House recognized the economic aspects of innovation and technology transfer for federal research in the way it fuels economic growth as well as creating new industries, companies, jobs, products and services, and improving the global competitiveness of U.S. industries. The directive requires federal laboratories such as the NIH to support high-growth entrepreneurship by increasing the rate of technology transfer and the economic and societal impact from federal R&D investments over a 5-year period. During this period, federal laboratories such as the NIH will be (a) establishing goals and measuring progress towards commercialization, (b) streamlining the technology transfer and commercialization processes, especially for licensing, collaborations, and grants to small companies, and (c) facilitating the commercialization of new technology and the formation of new start-up firms through local and regional economic development partnerships.

Taking a look at the university and academic medical center figures reported by the Association of University Technology Managers (AUTM), we find similarly strong figures for the economic impact of technology transfer. In 2011 AUTM reported that license income generated $2.5 billion and an additional $4 billion came in through industry-sponsored research. In 2011, close to 700 start-ups were formed of which approximately 500 were doing business in the same state as the university/nonprofit from which the technology arose. By the end of 2011, about 4000 start-ups (since the start of this industry) were still operational. In addition to the employment created by these start-ups, the tech-transfer industry itself has created significant employment both directly and indirectly through the related businesses it has helped to spawn.

In addition, many universities and the NIH have set up or have access to educational programs that train scientists and engineers to have a greater appreciation as to the importance of commercialization. These include entrepreneurship centers and small business assistance programs at many universities [16], and such things as the "Certificate in Technology Transfer" program given at the Foundation for Advanced Education in the Sciences (FAES) Graduate School at the NIH [17].

Maximal Leveraging of Technologies from Universities and Federal Labs

With their leading-edge research programs and focus in the healthcare market, the federal laboratory and university-based research programs have an exemplary record in providing opportunities for bioentrepreneurs to develop both high-growth companies and high-growth medical products. Indeed, a preliminary study from 2007 has shown that more than 100 drug and vaccine products approved by the U.S. FDA were based at least in part on technologies directly licensed from university and federal laboratories with federal labs (NIH) providing nearly 20 percent of the total [18]. Further, another study from 2009 has shown that university-licensed products commercialized by industry created at least 279,000 jobs across the United States during a 12-year period and that there was an increasing share of the United States GDP each year attributable to university-licensed products [19]. Additionally, a study published in the *New England Journal of Medicine* [20] in 2011 based upon the earlier 2007 preliminary study showed the intramural research laboratories at the NIH as by far the largest single nonprofit source of new drugs and vaccines approved by the FDA. This is an indication that the impact of licensing by universities and (by extension) federal laboratories will be increasingly effective and important into the future. Even with this success, there is movement towards a new, more collaborative horizon, especially with a "bench-to-beside" style collaboration as show in Figure 14.4.

With the rising costs of traditional drug discovery and mounting pressures on healthcare costs, companies are starting to adopt the model of joint venture with academia. For example, Pfizer has embarked on a novel academic-industry partnership paradigm with the establishment of its Center for Therapeutic Innovation (CTI) program. By the end of 2011, CTI has established partnerships with 20 leading academic medical centers across the United States, and supports collaborative projects from four dedicated labs in Boston, New York City, San Francisco, and San Diego. Another example is the establishment of Innovations Centers (ICs) by Johnson & Johnson in Boston, San Francisco, Shanghai, and London. Scientists from academia are embracing this model as well given the pressures of funding their research as well as their drive to see their work not only published in leading journals but also seeing the products of their research turn into a product that can benefit the public at large.

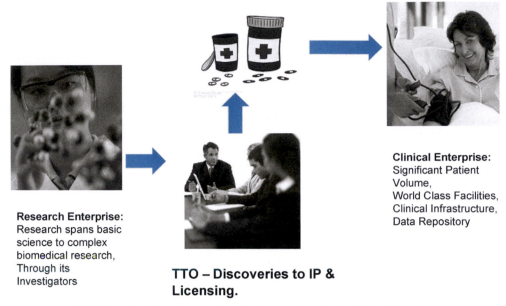

Research Enterprise:
Research spans basic
science to complex
biomedical research,
Through its
Investigators

**TTO – Discoveries to IP &
Licensing.**

Clinical Enterprise:
Significant Patient
Volume,
World Class Facilities,
Clinical Infrastructure,
Data Repository

FIGURE 14.4   NIH and academic medical centers: bench-to-bedside collaborations.

Although this commercial success has been a model in showing the value of technology transfer from federal laboratories, universities, and similar nonprofit research institutions, it is not the entire story. The final tally must include not only the full societal value and economic impact both of new companies but more importantly as well as the life-saving or enhancing therapeutics, vaccines, diagnostics, and other biomedical products on the market that have origins in this federally-funded research. This is believed to be the truest measure of the value and importance of licensing and technology transfer from research institutions.

Case Studies in Biotech Commercialization Using University and Federal Labs

Case Study 1: Licensing of HPV Vaccine Technology

The human papillomavirus (HPV) vaccine is a vaccine that prevents infection against certain species of human papillomavirus associated with the development of cervical cancer, genital warts, and some less-common cancers. Although most women infected with genital HPV will not have complications from the virus, worldwide there are an estimated 470,000 new cases of cervical cancer that result in 233,000 deaths per year. About 80 percent of deaths from cervical cancer occur in poor countries.

The research that led to the development of the vaccine began in the 1980s by groups primarily at the University of Rochester, Georgetown University, the German Cancer Center (DKFZ), Queensland University in Australia, and the NIH. This work, and the work of others, eventually became the basis of Gardasil® (sold by Merck) and Cervarix® (sold by GSK)—blockbuster products in terms of public health and market impacts.

MedImmune, Inc., then a very small development-stage vaccine company based in Gaithersburg, Maryland, licensed the HPV vaccine technology available from all U.S. institutions as well as the DKFZ in the early 1990s. GSK later received a license to all the rights held by MedImmune; Merck received a license from the NIH as well as to the Queensland rights. All of the license agreements were exclusive; those granted by NIH (who had been conducting separate clinical trials) were nonexclusive. The discoveries made at the research institutions were all very close in subject matter in what was then a relatively small research field and thus overlapping in terms of patent applications. Multiple patent interferences and patent oppositions resulted in patent offices around the world.

While patent interferences and oppositions can be expensive and difficult to resolve, the underlying technology proved to be extraordinarily successful in its clinical applications by both Merck and GSK—results that were confirmed in separate trials by the NIH. Given the strong clinical efficacy for these vaccines based upon the underlying technology discovered at the research institutions, a comprehensive settlement agreement was reached (regardless of the procedural outcomes at the patent offices around the world) whereby both Merck and GSK received coexclusive rights to the patent rights of all the research institutions, permitting the launch of similar (but slightly different) versions by both companies of these very important cervical cancer vaccines.

Discussion Questions

After reading this chapter along with others in this book:

1. Consider the role of MedImmune in the development of this vaccine. How risky was the strategy to acquire either control or access to nearly all the available license rights at a preclinical stage?

2. How did the strategy of the NIH work out, conducting some independent clinical trials and licensing both major developing parties originally on a nonexclusive basis?

Case Studies in Biotech Commercialization Using University and Federal Labs—cont'd

Case Study II—Sponsored Clinical Research Agreement

The company in this case study was providing drugs as well as money (to the tune of millions of dollars over a few years) to the hospital. The drugs were in development at the company and were poised to enter the clinic (Company's prized 'Clinical Candidates'). The collaboration with the TTO was going to be in two phases—a preclinical research collaboration and a clinical collaboration in that order. The terms below apply for the preclinical research collaboration.

Inventions were defined as those that were made during the term of the collaboration with funding from the company. Because inventorship follows U.S. patent law it was decided that ownership would follow inventorship making for three categories of inventions—company solely-owned, hospital solely-owned, and jointly-owned. The parties would work together to protect inventions via patent applications. The company would pay for patent protection for all inventions in these three categories and in exchange would receive the rights described below. If the company did not see the value in any hospital solely-owned inventions, then they would not pay for the protection of these inventions nor receive rights to these inventions.

The company retained full rights to use their own inventions. For jointly-owned inventions, they had nonexclusive rights to access the inventions for internal research and all commercial purposes by virtue of their joint ownership. For hospital solely-owned inventions, they received free rights for their internal research purposes. As compensation for paying for the patent costs to support the inventions, they also received an option to license the inventions at a later time. As the collaborative research informs them about the commercial prospects of this clinical candidate coupled with their separate on-going internal efforts in this program, they would make a decision during a defined option period about exclusive or nonexclusive licensing. The option period had a time window of 2.5 years from the time of the initial filing of the patent application to protect the invention. This coincides with an important decision point in the life of a patent application, the decision to file for patent protection in specific individual countries—a very cost-intensive decision. Notably, through the option to license, the academic center is providing a route to obtain rights to the inventions developed in the collaboration or the freedom to operate rights (FTO) that is a must-have for the company as described earlier.

The terms of the license would be standard between academia and industry for such technologies (see Table 14.6). Such a license would involve the hospital's rights in both jointly-owned inventions as well as in its solely owned inventions.

Publication Versus Confidentiality

Being clinical candidates, the company was very averse to any publications until the collaborative research was completed. This would mean publications could not happen for 2, maybe even 3 years from the start of the work. While this may be the actual timing of the publication, as an academic institution the hospital could not agree to an apparent delay of the publication for a very long time. Per the guidelines under which academic research institutions operate, they cannot "withhold" publications for longer than 2 to 3 months. This issue was resolved by tasking the steering committee that was set-up with members from both institutions with finding a reasonable solution at the time when publication of the work is imminent. It was likely that the work will be published only when it is complete which may be 2 years from the start of the research anyway, so there will be no issue to resolve. But if there was a disagreement and a long 2- to 3-year delay to provide for patent protection, then the committee will come up with a reasonable compromise.

Discussion Questions

1. What were the sensitive issues during the negotiation of the research collaboration agreement between the two parties and how did they resolve their differences?
2. Do you think either of the parties had to unnecessarily compromise on any basic principles in order to reach agreement? Discuss these points in more detail.

REFERENCES

[1] National Institutes of Health. NIH Overview. *http://www.nih.gov/about/budget.htm/* [accessed 01.12.12].

[2] Brookings Institute. University Start-ups: Critical for Improving Technology Transfer. http://www.brookings.edu/research/papers/2013/11/university-start-ups-technology-transfer-valdivia.

[3] Association of University Technology Managers (AUTM). AUTM U.S. Annual Licensing Survey Highlights. http://www.autm.net/AM/Template.cfm?Section=FY_2011_Licensing_Activity_Survey&Template=/CM/ContentDisplay.cfm&ContentID=8731/ [accessed 01.12.12].

[4] Ben-Menachem G, Ferguson S, Balakrishnan K. Doing Business with NIH. Nature Biotechnology. 2006;24(1):17–20.

[5] Ferguson S. "Products, Partners and Public Health: Transfer of Biomedical Technologies from the U.S. Government. Journal of Biolaw and Business 2002;5(2):35–9.

[6] National Institutes of Health. Office of Technology Transfer. Licensing Opportunities. *http://www.ott.nih.gov/opportunities.* [accessed 01.12.12].

[7] National Institutes of Health. Office of Technology Transfer. Start-ups. *http://www.ott.nih.gov/nih-start-exclusive-license-agreements* [accessed 01.12.12].

[8] MacWright R. The University of Virginia Patent Foundation: A Mid-sized Technology Transfer Foundation Focused on Faculty Service, Operated Using a Deal-based Business Model. AUTM Technology Transfer Practice Manual. 3rd ed.; 2010. 2(2.3a): 1–21.

[9] National Institutes of Health. Office of Technology Transfer. Public Health Service Technology Development Coordinators. http://www.ott.nih.gov/technology-development-coordinators [accessed 01.12.12].

[10] National Institutes of Health. Office of Extramural Research. Small Business Innovation Research (SBIR) and Small Business Technology Transfer (STTR) Programs. *http://grants.nih.gov/grants/funding/sbir.htm* [accessed 01.12.12].

[11] National Institutes of Health. National Cancer Institute. Developmental Therapeutics Program and Cancer Therapy Evaluation Program. *http://dtp.nci.nih.gov/.* and *http://ctep.cancer.gov/* [accessed 01.12.12].

[12] National Institutes of Health. National Center for Advancing Translational Science. http://ncats.nih.gov/ [accessed 01.12.12].

[13] National Institutes of Health. Office of Acquisition Management and Policy. http://oamp.od.nih.gov/ [accessed 01.12.12].

[14] National Institutes of Health. NIH Research Festival. http://research-festival.nih.gov/ [accessed 01.12.12].

[15] The White House. Office of the Press Secretary. Presidential Memorandum—Accelerating Technology Transfer and Commercialization of Federal Research in Support of High-Growth Businesses. http://www.whitehouse.gov/the-press-office/2011/10/28/presidential-memorandum-accelerating-technology-transfer-and-commerciali [accessed 01.12.12].

[16] Johns Hopkins University. Carey Business School. Innovate. http://carey.jhu.edu/Innovate/index.html/ [accessed 01.12.12].

[17] Foundation for Advanced Education in the Sciences (FAES). FAES Graduate School at NIH Certificate Program. http://www.faes.org/grad/advanced_studies/technology_transfer [accessed 01.12.12].

[18] Jensen, J., K. Wyller, E. London, S. Chatterjee, F. Murray, M. Rohrbaugh, and A. Stevens. The Contribution of Public Sector Research to the Discovery of New Drugs. Personal communication of poster at 2007 AUTM Annual Meeting.

[19] Roessner D, Bond J, Okubo S, Planting M. The Economic Impact of Licensed Commercialized Inventions Originating in University Research, 1996–2007. Final Report to the Biotechnology Industry Organization. http://www.bio.org/articles/economic-impact-licensed-commercialized-inventions-originating-university-research-1996-200 [accessed 01.12.12].

[20] Stevens A, Jensen J, Wyller K, Kilgore P, Chatterjee S, Rohrbaugh M. "The Role of Public-Sector Research in the Discovery of Drugs and Vaccines. New England Journal of Medicine. 2011;364:535–41.

Chapter 15

Intellectual Property Protection Strategies for Biotechnology Innovations

Gerry J. Elman, MS, JD* and Jay Z. Zhang, MS, JD**

*Elman Technology Law, P.C., Swarthmore, Pennsylvania, **Shuwen Biotech Co. Ltd., Deqing, Zhejiang Province, China and Momentous IP Ventures LLC, Salt Lake City, Utah*

Biotechnology companies typically begin with ideas for products or services that have a technological and beneficial advantage over other products in the market. As these improvements, or new product concepts and ideas, are implemented into practical commercial use, they will attract attention. The better they are, the more likely others will desire to copy them. Strategies for achieving exclusivity or at least a head start in this regard include the use of legal tools in the category of intellectual property (IP). These strategies are the focus of this chapter, wherein we provide an overview of the tools available to protect one of your company's most important assets.

Much of the early value that investors attribute to a development-stage biotechnology company is the "ownership" of these technological concepts and new product ideas as embodied in the company's IP. Also important will be your ability to communicate and collaborate with patent counsel who will be advising you about IP strategy and providing support throughout this process.

THE INTELLECTUAL PROPERTY TOOLBOX [1]

To gain a competitive advantage, your company will endeavor to provide something unique. If the technology you'll be implementing is an in-house discovery that can't be reverse-engineered by analyzing the product, the first order of business may be to keep the details secret. In that event, you'll take advantage of legal principles that protect *trade secrets* [2]. And if it's likely that, sooner or later, the technology will become publicly accessible, you'll consider other methods to fend off imitators, such as *patents* and other methods from a legal toolkit relating to *intellectual property* (*IP*) as well as regulatory regimes pertinent to the subject matter, e.g., drugs or agricultural products.

Generally, the more traditional term *industrial property* [3] (as distinguished from "intellectual property") refers to *patents*, *design patents* or *industrial designs*, *utility model patents* or *petty patents*, and *plant patents*, as well as *trademarks*, *service marks*, and layout designs of integrated circuits, commercial names and designations, geographical indications, and protection against *unfair competition*. *Intellectual property* is a more recently-coined term that subsumes the various forms of industrial property mentioned above, plus *copyright*. *Copyright*, also known in certain other jurisdictions as *authors' rights*, traditionally relates to artistic creations such as poems, novels, music, paintings, and cinematographic works, as well as photographs, the text of scientific papers, and more recently, computer software [4].

Each country, as a legal jurisdiction, has its own set of principles and practices applicable to IP. Although they have a lot in common, the details of IP law vary from jurisdiction-to-jurisdiction, and even from time-to-time. In February 2013, for example, the Federal Court of Australia ruled that isolated polynucleotides embodying naturally occurring genetic sequences are potentially patentable subject matter, whereas in June of that year, the United States Supreme Court took the opposite tack [5]. More about this later.

PATENTS

Let's take a closer look at some of these legal tools, starting with patents. The word *patent* means "open and apparent." In the present context, it is shorthand for "*letters patent*" and refers to a public document granting rights to the owner, or *holder* of the patent, to exclude others for a limited time from practicing the invention as recited in any of a series of numbered *patent claims*. Below we provide some examples of biotechnology patent claims.

Examples of U.S. Biotechnology Patent Claims:

- **Amgen's patent claims for erythropoietin:** A purified and isolated DNA sequence consisting essentially of a DNA sequence encoding human erythropoietin [6]. A nonnaturally occurring erythropoietin glycoprotein product having the *in vivo* biological activity of causing bone marrow cells to increase production of reticulocytes and red blood cells and having glycosylation which differs from that of human urinary erythropoietin.

- **Cetus/Roche's Foundation patent claim for polymerase chain reaction (PCR):** A process for amplifying at least one specific nucleic acid sequence contained in a nucleic acid or a mixture of nucleic acids wherein each nucleic acid consists of two separate complementary strands of equal or unequal length which process comprises:

  1. Treating the strands with two oligonucleotide primers for each different specific sequence being amplified under conditions such that for each different sequence being amplified an extension product of each primer is synthesized which is complementary to each nucleic acid strand, wherein said primers are selected so as to be sufficiently complementary to different strands of each specific sequence to hybridize therewith such that the extension product synthesized from one primer, when it is separated from its complement, can serve as a template for synthesis of the extension product of the other primer.
  2. Separating the primer extension products from the templates on which they were synthesized to produce single-stranded molecules.
  3. Treating the single-stranded molecules generated from step 2 with the primers of step 1 under conditions that a primer extension product is synthesized using each of the single strands produced in step 2 as a template.

- **Thomas Cech's patent for ribozymes:** An enzymatic RNA molecule not naturally occurring in nature having an endonuclease activity independent of any protein, said endonuclease activity being specific for a nucleotide sequence defining a cleavage site comprising single-stranded RNA in a separate RNA molecule and causing cleavage at said cleavage site by a transesterification reaction.

- **"Harvard Mouse" patent claim:** A transgenic nonhuman mammal all of whose germ cells and somatic cells contain a recombinant-activated oncogene sequence introduced into said mammal, or an ancestor of said mammal, at an embryonic stage.

- **University of Wisconsin Alumni Research Foundation's stem cell patent claims:**
  - A purified preparation of primate embryonic stem cells which (1) is capable of proliferation in an *in vitro* culture for over 1 year, (2) maintains a karyotype in which all the chromosomes characteristic of the primate species are present and not noticeably altered through prolonged culture, (3) maintains the potential to differentiate into derivatives of endoderm, mesoderm and ectoderm tissues throughout the culture, and (4) will not differentiate when cultured on a fibroblast feeder layer.
  - A preparation of pluripotent human embryonic stem cells comprising cells that (1) proliferate *in vitro* for over 1 year, (2) maintain a karyotype in which the chromosomes are euploid through prolonged culture, (3) maintain the potential to differentiate to derivatives of endoderm, mesoderm, and ectoderm tissues, (4) are inhibited from differentiation when cultured on a fibroblast feeder layer, and (5) are negative for the SSEA-1 cell surface marker and positive for the SSEA-4 cell surface marker.

- **A method of isolating a pluripotent human embryonic stem cell line, comprising the steps of:**
  - Isolating a human blastocyst.
  - Isolating cells from the inner cell mass of the above blastocyte.
  - Plating the inner cell mass cells on embryonic fibroblasts, wherein inner cell mass-derived cell masses are formed.
  - Dissociating the mass into dissociated cells.
  - Replating the dissociated cells on embryonic feeder cells.
  - Selecting colonies with compact morphologies and cells with high nucleus to cytoplasm ratios and prominent nucleoli.
  - Culturing the cells of the selected colonies to thereby obtain an isolated pluripotent human embryonic stem cell line.

- **Cornell University's "gene gun" patent claim:** "A method for introducing particles into cells comprising accelerating particles having a diameter sufficiently small to penetrate and be retained in a preselected cell without killing the cell, and propelling said particles at said cells whereby said particles penetrate the surface of said cells and become incorporated into the interior of said cells.

- **Merck's Fosamax patent claims:**
  - A method of treatment of urolithiasis and inhibiting bone reabsorption which consists of administering to a patient in need thereof an effective amount of 4-amino-1-hydroxybutane-1,1-biphosphonic acid.
  - A pharmaceutical composition comprising a pharmaceutically effective amount of alendronate, in a pharmaceutically acceptable carrier and a sufficient amount of a buffer to maintain a pH of the composition in the range of 2 to 8 and complexing agent to prevent the precipitation of alendronate in aqueous solution.

What is a Patent?

The patent grant is sometimes viewed as a quid pro quo exchange for the patent holder's making public the subject matter taught in the *patent specification*, which otherwise might have been kept secret indefinitely. In other words, if the inventor fully discloses to the public how to make and how to use the invention, the government grants to the patent owner a right to exclude others from making, using, selling, or importing the invention as defined by any of the *claims* recited in the patent. In the United States, patents are granted by the United States Patent and Trademark Office (PTO), an agency of the Department of Commerce, in accordance with laws passed by Congress and signed by the President. In turn, the power of Congress to enact laws governing patents and copyrights stems from the United States Constitution [7].

To seek a U.S. patent, an applicant prepares and files with the PTO a *patent application* intended to comply with various legal requirements, e.g., that it include a *disclosure* that's detailed enough to *enable* a person skilled in the technical field to make and use the invention. To provide a *written description* of the inventive subject matter, the applicant desirably has become cognizant of the characteristics that distinguish the present invention from subject matter that's already publicly known or otherwise in the legal category referred to as *prior art* [8]. Typically, this includes a *patentability search*, which seeks to uncover various forms of pertinent prior art, not only patents. Yet even if the subject of a proposed patent claim is clearly *novel*, as compared with all the prior art in the world, that isn't enough to establish that the claim fulfills the requisites of patentability.

As mentioned above, a threshold question identified by the United States Supreme Court is whether the subject matter is *patent-eligible*, that is, something which can be protected within the patent statute. For many years, a fundamental principle of patent law has been that an inventor who's merely characterized a novel composition of matter isn't entitled to a patent, regardless of whether the inventor isolated it from a natural source or synthesized it from scratch. Rather, for a newly generated composition to be patentable, the inventor would need to identify a "practical utility" for it as well.

Patent Reform Legislation

In the past few years, Congress has taken a hand in "reforming" some of the principles of U.S. patent law. Such *patent reform* was recently enshrined in the America Invents Act of 2011 (AIA), the various provisions of which took effect in stages culminating in March 2013 [9]. The most publicized of the "reforms" was to change the uniquely American practice of "first to invent"—awarding a patent sought simultaneously by two or more different inventors (or *inventive entities* composed of two or more inventors acting jointly) to the members of the entity who could prove that they were first to form a mental conception of the claimed subject matter and then act diligently to reduce it to practice, regardless of whether they beat the others in a race to file a

patent application. The administrative minitrial at the PTO to make this determination was known as an *interference proceeding*, and the dice were loaded in favor of evidence originating in the United States. In contrast, foreign patent laws favored those who first filed their patent application in the pertinent patent office, typically taking into account a *right of priority* that was accorded by the Paris Convention on Industrial Property to filings in the inventor's home patent office.

The AIA has eliminated interference proceedings for U.S. patent applications filed after May 15, 2013 that disclose new inventions. Those new applications will be examined for novelty over, and nonobviousness from, a subtly redefined universe of "prior art." Nevertheless, applications filed after that date that claim subject matter fully disclosed in previously filed applications that is with an effective filing date before May 16, 2013, will be examined under pre-AIA patent law. So during the next 20 years, some U.S. patents will have had their patentability determined against one body of prior art, whereas others will have had patentability determined by another. For patent applications filed during this transition period, an applicant should consider carefully whether to "check the box" on the application form that would direct the patent examination towards one track or the other.

Nonobviousness or Inventive Height

In addition to patent-eligibility and novelty, a valid patent claim is required to define an invention that would not have been *obvious* to a person having ordinary skill in the pertinent art. For U.S. patents governed by pre-AIA law, this hypothetical inquiry is to be performed as of the date that the patent applicant made the invention. For U.S. patents governed by post-AIA law, the obviousness question is posed as of the *effective filing date* of the patent application. In general, if a hypothetical worker having such skill, who is deemed to have assembled examples of all pertinent prior art, would arrive at the claimed invention without hindsight reconstruction but just using reason and common sense in combining different aspects of them, then the invention as claimed would fail to meet the "nonobviousness" requirement of patentability under United States law.

In some other jurisdictions, a similar analysis is performed under the rubric of "inventive height" or "inventive step."

The Patenting Process

Since 1995, there have been two kinds of U.S. patent application you could file for a useful invention: (1) a provisional patent application (PPA), and (2) the traditional, formal patent application (sometimes called a nonprovisional patent application or NPA). (See Figure 15.1.)

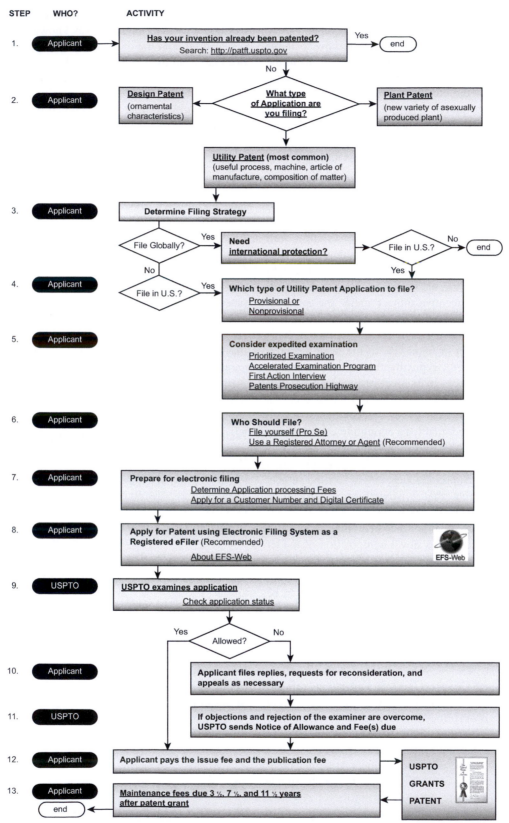

FIGURE 15.1   A flowchart for a U.S. patent application. (*From The United States Patent and Trademark Office. http://www.uspto.gov/patents/process/index.jsp.*)

The current government fee for a PPA filing is $260 plus a surcharge if it is lengthy. A 50 percent discount applies to filings by "small entities," which include businesses with fewer than 500 employees. A recently instituted discount of 75 percent applies to "micro entities" which include universities and newly minted private inventors whose income the previous year falls below a stated cap.

A PPA does not ever get published so it doesn't have to meet the stringent format requirements of an NPA. The drawings can be informal and it's okay to omit formal claims. But beware, the law requires a valid PPA to include an enabling disclosure and written description of the invention.

To get a U.S. patent on an invention disclosed in a PPA within a year from the filing of the PPA, you would typically generate and file an NPA which claims "benefit" of the PPA. If this 1-year deadline is missed, a later filed NPA would not be entitled to claim benefit of the PPA's filing date, so another year or so of prior art would become available to constrain the patentability of the NPA's claims. Each PPA automatically becomes abandoned a year after its filing date and in some circumstances it may be desirable to formally abandon a PPA before then.

As research and development (R&D) on a project progresses during the year after filing a PPA, it's likely that your technologists will make improvements to the invention(s) described in the PPA. It is often convenient to file additional PPAs that include the new information, and then to claim benefit of all of them in an NPA filed within a year of the first PPA.

Design Patents (Industrial Designs)

A different kind of patent is available to protect the "look" of useful objects. This may be a surface ornamentation or some or all of the overall configuration. Designs are examined to confirm that they are novel and not obvious from the prior art, and thereupon a design patent is granted with a term of 14 years. Design patents don't have "claims;" rather the drawings define what is protected.

Pregrant Publication of U.S. Patent Applications

Most foreign countries have been publishing patent applications 18 months from their respective priority filing dates, but until 2000, the law in the United States was that a patent would be published only when it was actually granted. However, a significant fraction of U.S. patent applications filed from then on are automatically published approximately 18 months from their respective filing or priority dates. Since March 2001, new Patent Application Publications, or "PA Pubs" have been added to the PTO website (http://www.uspto.gov/) each Thursday.

If you elect to have your patent application published, once your PA Pub appears on the PTO site, you will have certain "provisional rights" in the subject matter of your pending patent claims. That is, if a company in the United States makes, uses, sells, or imports something that infringes a published claim of your PA Pub, it would be opportune to direct your patent counsel, if appropriate, to send a formal notice to them. Then, if that claim eventually is included in your granted patent, you would be entitled to money damages not only for their infringement from the date of the patent grant, but including as well their infringement from the date of your notice up to the patent grant date. If the claims are amended to read differently from the way they have appeared in a PA Pub, it is sometimes advantageous to request the publication of the application as amended to enhance the provisional rights described above.

However, automatic pregrant publication of U.S. patent applications is subject to a certain exception. That exception is for patent applications which the applicant does *not* wish to have published, wherein the applicant states at the time of filing that he *does not intend* to file a corresponding application in any foreign countries. For such applications, the applicant can get the benefit of secrecy until the patent is granted, the same as under previous U.S. patent law. Because the PTO currently makes the docket entries and ongoing papers filed in pending applications once they are published available on the Web, some applicants prefer to forego the option to obtain provisional rights through a PA Pub and instead opt for the traditional secrecy until a U.S. patent is granted.

In the alternative, there are scenarios where it would be desirable to request early publication of an application; or others where it would be desirable to request republication, e.g., where the claims have been amended.

Patent Prosecution Strategy Affects the Scope of Patent Claims

During the past few years, the federal courts by various judicial decisions have increased the implicit "penalty" against patent applicants for presenting subject matter in patent applications that is not eventually included in granted claims. A "dedication to the public" is said to arise when an applicant includes disclosure in a patent application and does not eventually obtain claims reciting the subject matter. Similarly, an "estoppel" arises when an applicant presents a claim to the patent examiner, gets a rejection, and then acquiesces, letting the claim wither on the vine without arguing against the rejection. Such "prosecution history" is typically used in litigation by an adverse party to assert that any claims granted from the application (or a related one) are narrower than they would otherwise seem to be.

In a series of decisions on how to interpret, or "*construe*" [10], patent claims, U.S. courts developed a policy of allowing claims to "stretch" to cover certain variants that would otherwise have been outside the scope of the patent claim. This policy came to be known as the "*doctrine of equivalents*." Understand that a patent claim can be considered to recite a collection of "elements." For years, when patent claims were interpreted in court, each such element might be deemed to include not only things within its literal wording, but also some things that were outside a literal interpretation but which were still "equivalent."

Increasingly, the courts have taken heed of public outcry arising from perceptions that certain patents were overly broad. In a landmark case a few years ago, the United States Supreme Court redefined the scope of such equivalents as "mere inconsequential differences", and in another case held that there is a presumption that no equivalents would be allowed for any claim element that was amended during the prosecution of the patent. Later the court of appeals for the Federal Circuit surprisingly held that this adverse presumption applies even where the applicant merely cancels an independent claim and rewrites a preexisting dependent claim in independent form. Thus, the doctrine of equivalents is now more of an exception than a general rule.

The upshot of these cases is to increase the importance of "getting it right" as early as possible during patent prosecution. The more variations of your invention that are disclosed in the patent application, the broader the literal scope of the claims you file at the outset can be. Endeavor to set forth all the variations of the invention that you contemplate, not only what your company might provide, but also what your competitor might do if they are precluded by your patent from copying your invention.

Foreign Patent Filing

You may also be interested in making a decision regarding strategies for filing foreign counterpart patent applications either under the Patent Cooperation Treaty or otherwise. These foreign patents would be intended to provide similar rights in various foreign countries you may select. Because there is no such thing as a world-wide patent, it is necessary to obtain a patent for every country in which protection is desired. However, certain regions, namely Europe, the former USSR (Eurasia), and certain groups of countries in Africa, also have their own patent offices.

The date that a patent application is filed is important for example because anything appearing in publication after that date is not "prior art" that can be used to show that the claimed invention is not new. As mentioned above, the Paris Convention for the Protection of Industrial Property, which has been in force since 1883, created the concept of a "priority date" that could be applied to a patent application based on a previously filed application. (The Paris Convention also pertains to design patent applications and trademark applications.)

If a first patent application is filed in any of the countries that are members of the Paris Convention, then a copy of that first application that is filed in another member country (translated into the local language) can claim as a "priority date," the filing date of the first application, provided that the copy meets the requirements of the Convention. The main requirement is that the copy be filed within *12 months* of the date of the first application. (However, for *design* patents and trademarks, foreign counterparts must be filed within 6 months.)

Although the AIA has modified the "*grace period*" somewhat from what it used to be, the United States permits inventors up to 1 year from the date of their own public disclosure or placing the invention on sale before their own actions make it too late to file a U.S. patent application. After that time, we say that the patent application is "time barred." However, beware that most foreign countries *do not* provide such a "grace period." The best strategy to preserve your rights internationally is to file a U.S. patent application *before* making a nonconfidential disclosure of the invention to anyone. Then, within the prescribed period, file counterpart applications for the countries where you desire patent protection, claiming the priority date of the U.S. application.

At present 175 countries (from Albania to Zimbabwe) have signed one or more versions of the Paris Convention and thus have joined an International Union on Industrial Property. Taiwan also grants similar priority rights to applicants from the United States due to a bilateral agreement.

The Patent Cooperation Treaty

At present, 148 members of the Paris Convention also belong to the *Patent Cooperation Treaty* (*PCT*), first signed in 1970. Membership in the PCT includes the United States, Canada, virtually all European countries, Mexico, Australia, Brazil, China, Israel, Japan, Korea, India, South Africa, and many others. (Countries that are still *nonmembers* include Taiwan and various countries in the Middle East, South Asia, Africa, and Central and South America, as well as numerous island nations.)

The PCT provides a procedure whereby a single patent application in English can be filed to start the patenting process for any of the countries that are "designated" in the "PCT application" by marking a checkbox on the form and paying the requisite fee. Under the Paris Convention, a PCT application filed within 12 months of a corresponding U.S. patent application (the first of either a PPA or an NPA) could get the benefit of its priority date.

The following strategy is typical for an applicant in the United States that wishes to defer (for up to a total of 30 months) the high cost of widely filing foreign patent applications. This can provide enough time to evaluate the market and to obtain financing. The strategy is to file a U.S. patent application first (often as a PPA) and then to file a PCT application 12 months later. Typical costs of filing a PCT application range from about $3500 to about $8000, depending on the number of pages in the application and whether revisions to the previously filed text and drawings are desired.

Under PCT procedure, everything starts with the "priority date," which in this example would be the date the original U.S. application was filed, e.g., a U.S. provisional patent application. Within about 16 months from that date, an International Searching Authority examiner is supposed to issue the results of a patent search for the claimed invention (ISR) plus a preliminary "written opinion" (WO) on patentability pursuant to international standards. The PCT application is published with the ISR about 18 months after its priority date. (See Figure 15.2.)

At 18 months or 2 months from the ISR, an applicant may optionally amend the claims. At 19 months, the applicant may optionally request a supplementary international search to cover claims not searched by the ISA or to seek to turn up prior art in a language not used by the ISA. An applicant may optionally file a formal "demand" for an International Preliminary Examination pursuant to Chapter II of the PCT within 3 months after the ISR, or 22 months from the priority date, whichever is later. During the exam under Chapter II by an International Preliminary Examining Authority (typically an examiner at a selected national patent office), the applicant gets one or more chances to respond with an argument in favor of patentability and optionally submitting amendments to the claims.

For most countries, 30 months from the priority date is a crucial time. That is when the PCT procedure ends and the

application is submitted for entry into a "national phase" patent prosecution. This typically means that the application is translated into the local language and filed with the local patent office by local patent practitioners pursuant to instructions from your patent counsel.

However there are some small deviations from this rule-of-thumb. Some non-English-speaking countries such as Israel nevertheless accept English language filings, avoiding translation costs. Other patent offices, including the European Patent Office, the Eurasian Patent Office, India, and Australia, accept such filings up to 31 months from the priority date. At this point, costs for patent filings typically range from about $1500 for an English-language application in Canada or Australia to about $6000 or more for a European, Chinese, or Japanese application. Thus, to seek wide geographic coverage in, say, two dozen countries requires an investment of well over $100,000. Note, too, that most foreign countries impose annual fees ("annuities" or "maintenance fees") to maintain a patent application or patent in force, and many also require that a patent be "worked" or licensed locally. Typically a patent expires 20 years from its local or PCT filing date, provided that maintenance fees are paid for the duration.

Freedom-to-Operate Studies of Third-Party Patents

At some point your investors or board of directors may ask whether a proposed product comes within the claims of a particular patent of a competitor or other identified party. In that event, consider engaging patent counsel to determine the scope of the claims by obtaining and reviewing a copy of the prosecution history of the patent and the cited prior

PCT TIMELINE

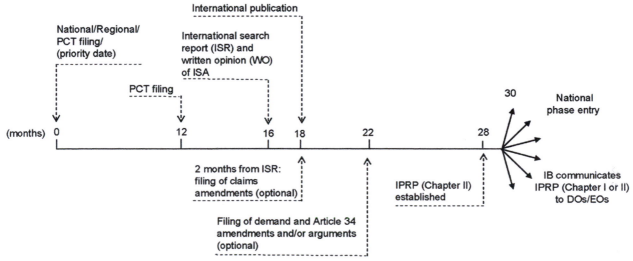

FIGURE 15.2 Patent Cooperation Treaty (PCT) timeline.

art. If the proposed product is not clearly outside the scope of the issued claims, the patent attorney would next seek to determine if any of the claims might be invalid (e.g., because of additional prior art not brought to the patent examiner's attention or perhaps due to a change in the law regarding patent-eligible subject matter since the application was examined). If counsel is able to provide an opinion that the proposed product does not infringe any valid claims of the patent, then it would benefit your company because generally a court would decline to award additional damages for "willful infringement," even if the court were to disagree with your counsel and find that the patent is infringed.

In 2007, the Federal Circuit stated in *In re Seagate* that enhanced damages for willful infringement of a patent requires clear and convincing evidence (1) that the infringer acted despite an objectively high likelihood that its actions constituted infringement of a valid patent and (2) that the infringer had knowledge (or should have known) of this risk.

Also, as part of the AIA, Congress created a variety of new pathways for a business to challenge its rivals' pending applications and granted patents. It will be advantageous for your company to monitor patent applications as they are published to the Web (PA Pubs) for optimum advantage in selecting among the available options.

Patent Expiration

It used to be relatively simple to say when a U.S. patent would expire: look at the date it was granted and add 17 years. (Except that the term could be truncated by a "*terminal disclaimer*" filed in the case to match the expiration to the term of a related patent.) But a law that took effect in 1995 has made the calculation more complicated, and another one that took effect in 2000 has created further changes.

Now, a newly issued patent generally expires 20 years after the date of filing of the earliest nonprovisional U.S. patent application on which it relies, unless it is subject to a terminal disclaimer as mentioned above or unless it is entitled to *patent term adjustment* (PTA), e.g., because the PTO took too long in some phase of patent prosecution while the applicant acted with relative diligence; or because the grant of the patent was delayed by an appeal or an interference proceeding in the PTO. Another way the patent term may have been extended would be because marketing was delayed by FDA clearance procedures—*patent term extension* (PTE) authorized under the Hatch-Waxman Act. For a drug first approved for marketing in the United States, the term of a patent covering the drug may be extended by up to 5 years provided that certain conditions are met. After the PTE, the patent term remaining at the date of FDA approval must not exceed 14 years. An application for PTE must be filed within a certain time limit after the FDA approval.

Other countries including the EU countries, Japan, and others also have similar laws to allow patent term extension for delays by regulatory approval. The PTA and PTE calculation also presumes that maintenance fees are paid within respectively 4, 8, and 12 years after the date the patent is granted. Note: it is often possible to reinstate a U.S. patent if a maintenance fee deadline is inadvertently missed.

CONTRACTS RELATING TO INTELLECTUAL PROPERTY

Who Owns the Invention?

When drafting, negotiating, or signing contracts involving your intellectual property, beware that even a single word could make the difference between owning and not owning rights to a valuable technology. For example, in 2011 the United States Supreme Court decided that Cetus Corporation, rather than Stanford University, had acquired the right to patent an invention by a Stanford faculty member that applies the PCR technique to test for HIV, the AIDS virus. When he began work for the university, the inventor had signed a form whereby he "*agree[d] to assign*" to Stanford his "right, title and interest in" inventions resulting from his employment at the University. On this basis, Stanford had filed and obtained three U.S. patents relating to the invention.

The university technology transfer office had a rude awakening when it sought patent royalties for the HIV test from Roche (the successor to Cetus). Roche asserted in court the counterintuitive argument that a Cetus document governed ownership of the invention, even though the inventor had signed it *after* he had signed the Stanford University document.

The agreement with Cetus that the inventor had signed when he started the project had included language reciting not only that the inventor "will assign" but also that he "*does hereby assign*" to Cetus his "right, title, and interest in each of the ideas, inventions, and improvements" made as a consequence of his access to Cetus. Surprising to many, the courts held that even though the inventor had originally agreed with Stanford to make a future assignment of ownership of inventions, the Cetus document, worded in the present tense, was effective, *immediately upon signing*, to transfer to Cetus the inventor's ownership of any pertinent inventions he would *thereafter* make. So although the inventor had later signed documents purporting to transfer to Stanford his ownership rights in the inventions, it was too late—he had already divested himself of those rights by the operation of the Cetus document.

The takeaway is to ask your intellectual property lawyer to review even "boilerplate" forms to ensure they embody the latest version of language that the courts have held to be effective [11].

JOINT RESEARCH PROJECTS

Most biotechnology start-ups collaborate with researchers from other companies or universities at some time during development of their inventions. Federal law includes a curious judge-made doctrine called "secret prior art" that can disqualify from protection certain inventions that involve different people contributing to the invention over a timeframe, especially if they happen to work for different employers. In September 2005, the PTO issued its regulations implementing the CREATE Act, a law passed in December 2004 that permits such inventions to avoid the pitfall, but only if a qualifying joint research agreement was in place beforehand and the agreement is properly cited in the patent application.

Although the AIA now allows a business to be named as an *applicant* for a U.S. patent, the law still requires including in the patent application as an inventor everyone who contributes materially to the subject matter of even one claim of the patent. And, as mentioned above, it may be appropriate to inform the PTO if your company has a joint research agreement in the field of the invention.

COPYRIGHTS

Good news: The *Stanford v. Roche* case (with its counter-intuitive result discussed above) doesn't apply to ownership of copyrights. Rather, your company automatically owns copyright in the works of authorship (including text, graphics, and computer code) generated by its employees in the course of their assignments, even if they haven't signed an agreement about the subject. Bad news: the same isn't true for copyrightable subject matter generated by *independent contractors*, whether individuals or at another company. If a transfer of ownership of copyrighted subject matter is desired, it must be in writing, and optionally may be recorded at the U.S. Copyright Office (an arm of the Library of Congress). Alternatively, a license, or *grant of permission* to use a copyrighted work, may be appropriate.

As soon as a work of authorship is fixed in a tangible medium of expression (e.g., written on paper or saved on a computer disk) it is protected by the U.S. Copyright Act. The protection is automatic and does not require that you take any further action. However, it's desirable to take two steps (which are optional for new works) to gain additional protection. These two steps are (1) place a copyright notice on your work, and (2) register the copyright with the U.S. Copyright Office.

A copyright notice should look like this:

Copyright © [Year of first publication] [Name of copyright owner]. All rights reserved.

If the work is not published (i.e., offered for distribution to the general public), then leave out the year of first publication. Although a copyright notice is not absolutely required for any work first published on or after March 1, 1989, it's still desirable to put copyright notices on all copyrightable works generated in the United States.

The second step is to register your company's copyrights. You aren't required to register a copyright, but the law provides additional benefits to those who do so promptly. Moreover, you can not sue an infringer in court unless and until you have received a certificate of copyright registration for your work. If you file an application for copyright registration before someone infringes your work, or within 3 months of the date your work is first published (if your work is published), then you receive two additional benefits that you would not otherwise have.

The first additional benefit is that the federal court may award you money towards your *attorney's fees*. The second additional benefit is that you may request the court to award "statutory" damages instead of any actual damages that your company proves to have suffered. *Statutory damages* are preferred when you cannot prove that you actually lost money, or when you have lost a relatively small amount. The judge may then award statutory damages somewhere between $750 and $30,000 per work. If you prove the infringer *wilfully infringed* the copyright, then the judge may award up to $150,000 of statutory damages per work.

As mentioned above, if the work of authorship is created by an independent contractor, your company does not automatically own the copyright. Make sure that agreements with independent contractors fully protect your business if you wish to own the copyright outright. Unfortunately, this fine point is frequently overlooked with independent contractors developing computer software, sometimes leading to misunderstandings and expensive litigation.

TRADEMARKS

Attorneys use the term "trademark" to refer to any design, word, or combination of words and designs used in connection with the products or services of a business. Technically, the term "service mark" is used for designations of services, but a service mark is just one type of trademark. One kind of trademark that we've mentioned above is a *brand name*, especially as contrasted with the generic name that's also adopted for the active ingredient or new chemical entity (see below for further discussion).

As soon as you start using your trademark, your company may customarily employ the symbol "TM" to designate a trademark for goods and the symbol "SM" to designate a service mark for services.

If you desire to protect your trademarks, engage your intellectual property counsel to do a search to find out if the proposed marks are available. It's typical to search not only the database of federal trademark registrations and applications, but also state trademark registrations and selected foreign jurisdictions. Many of these databases are organized for searching alphabetically for "direct hits" and also phonetic sound-alikes as well as for suffixes and prefixes. Your attorney will use the search results to initially evaluate whether your proposed trademarks are "confusingly similar" to the trademarks of your prospective competitors.

It's desirable to supplement those search results with other databases and Internet search engines to look for similar marks used by companies that haven't yet *registered* their marks. Under United States law, these companies may have developed *"common law"* rights by using their trademarks.

Bases for Filing a Trademark Application: Intent-to-Use or Actual Use

The United States trademark law was amended in 1989 to allow you to file an application based on your *bona fide* (good faith) intent to start using your trademark in the future. You may file an *"intent to use"* application even before you place your trademark on goods. By comparison, you may only file an *"actual use"* application after your company has used the trademark in interstate commerce, such as by shipping your goods to a customer in another state or by advertising your services to those in another state.

Trademark Prosecution

Within about 6 months after your application for trademark registration is filed, an attorney in the PTO searches registered marks and pending federal applications for any that may be confusingly similar to your trademark. The PTO attorney also examines the application for compliance with various technical and legal standards. Often, the PTO attorney raises questions or objections to one or more aspects of the application, and your attorney may file a response. When and if the PTO attorney finds no further barriers to granting your application, the PTO will publish your mark in the *Official Gazette of the Patent and Trademark Office*. Then, for a month or so, others who may have adopted a similar mark will have the opportunity to challenge your right to register your mark. If your mark is challenged, then the PTO conducts an administrative trial to determine the matter. If there is no challenge, your application would proceed to the next stage.

If your company has filed an "actual use" application, then the PTO registers your trademark and issues a certificate of registration. If the application is an "intent to use" application, then the PTO will not register your trademark until your attorney files your sworn statement documenting that the mark has actually gone into bona fide use in interstate commerce.

The ® Symbol

Once the PTO issues the certificate of trademark registration, your company may then use the symbol ® in connection with the mark, or alternatively the term *Reg. U.S. Pat. and T.M. Off.* (which is more cumbersome). Until you receive a certificate of trademark registration, use the *TM* and *SM* symbols.

This completes the registration process. Once the PTO issues a registration, you generally won't need to bother with this registration for another 5 years. Between the fifth and sixth anniversaries of the registration date, you would need to file an affidavit that your company is still using the trademark in connection with the same goods and services. If the "affidavit of use" is not filed during that time, the registration is canceled (although you could afterwards seek to reregister your trademark).

U.S. Trademark Affidavit of Use and Incontestability

Further, if your trademark had not been found invalid or was not in litigation at the time that you filed the affidavit of use or at the end of any 5-year period, your attorney could file an "affidavit of incontestability," either by itself or as part of the same transaction as the affidavit of use. An affidavit of incontestability provides additional rights in case your company needs to sue a trademark infringer. The infringer would have a higher standard to overcome to battle you in court as the validity of your trademark would be "incontestable."

Trademarks for Pharma/BioTech Products

There are a few additional requirements in order to clear and adopt a particular product name for the pharmaceutical industry. Drug products must satisfy not only prohibitions against deceptiveness and likelihood of confusion examined by the PTO, but they must also satisfy requirements administered by the U.S. Food and Drug Administration (FDA) [12]. Each of these agencies conducts a distinct and independent review, and only when all parties are satisfied, is the proposed mark fully cleared for use [13]. The reason for the extra scrutiny is safety. Pharmaceutical mistakes have the potential to cause serious damage, illness, or death when drug names look alike or sound alike, or there is a carelessness, lack of knowledge of drug names, poor handwriting, or human error between physicians, pharmacists, and patients.

The PTO recognizes the need for safety regarding pharmaceuticals, and applies the doctrine of greater care [14] in the prosecution of trademark applications for ethical pharmaceuticals because confusion here may have life-and-death consequences.

As the naming process runs its course, each new pharmaceutical product would acquire three names: a chemical name (the CAS registry number for the compound, e.g., 85721-33-1); a generic, nonproprietary name (e.g., ciprofloxacin); and a trademark or brand name (e.g., CIPRO).

The applicant must first propose to the United States Adopted Name (USAN) Council a *generic (or nonproprietary) name* for the product, providing chemical information and medical indications [15]. The USAN Council reviews the proposed generic name for characteristics such as: appropriateness for the drug; adherence to nomenclature rules; suitability for routine use both in the United States and internationally; not being misleading or confusing or implying efficacy or application to particular anatomical parts; and being distinctive from other drug names.

When the USAN Council assigns a generic name to the product, that name is sent for final approval to the World Health Organization (WHO) International Nonproprietary Name (INN) Committee [16]. The INN suggests that word elements from biochemical nomenclature (like *'feron* from interferon, or *'leukin* from interleukin) be used as stems for generic terms within a scheme of drug nomenclature adopted by the INN. In contrast, drug trademarks should avoid incorporating such INN stems.

The selection of trademarks for pharmaceutical products in the United States is complicated by the requirement that two different federal agencies—the PTO and the FDA— review and approve such marks. The PTO examination has been described above. The review process at the FDA starts when an applicant files a *request for proprietary name review*, coordinated by the Division of Medication Error Prevention and Analysis (DMEPA). The DMEPA would look at similar trademarks for products currently on the market and those in the development pipeline. They often perform studies with simulated prescriptions to guard against the misreading of handwritten prescriptions, and consider similar terms among common medical terminology.

As the pharmaceutical approval cycle can be a lengthy process, consider registering a trademark first for research and development services as well as for the drug product itself.

United States Trademark Renewal

A United States trademark registration is valid for 10 years. To renew the registration, a renewal application with an affidavit of continued use must be filed between 1 year before the anniversary to 6 months after the anniversary.

Foreign Trademark Registration

It's desirable to register your trademarks in other countries in which you plan to do business. There is a European Trademark Office in Alicante, Spain. In 2003, the United States became a party to the Madrid Protocol, a trademark treaty that corresponds somewhat to the PCT. There are certain advantages and disadvantages of the procedures available under the Madrid System. Also, if a trademark application is filed in a foreign country within 6 months from the day it is filed in the United States, it is generally able to get a right-of-priority under the Paris Convention based on the filing date of the United States application. Thus it is desirable to make such choices within this timeframe.

Recording Trademarks, Copyrights, and Trade Names with United States Customs

To help protect against the importation of products that infringe your intellectual property rights, your business may record your rights with the Bureau of Customs and Border Protection (CBP) in the United States Department of Homeland Security. This option is available for trademarks registered on the principal register at the U.S. Patent and Trademark Office, copyrights registered with the U.S. Copyright Office, and trade names (i.e., the names of businesses) that have been in use for at least 6 months.

An application to record your trademark, copyright, or trade name can be submitted on paper or electronically. As mentioned above, trademarks and copyrights must be federally registered before they are eligible for recordation, and the CBP automatically accepts such registrations as valid.

PHARMACEUTICAL PATENTS AND MARKET EXCLUSIVITY

Every new drug can cost hundreds of millions of dollars to develop and the risk of failure is very high. Thus, there must be adequate patent exclusivity for a new drug to incentivize investment in drug development. Indeed, that patents stimulate innovation and reward risk taking is best exemplified in the pharmaceutical area. In 1984, Congress enacted the Drug Price Competition and Patent Term Restoration Act of 1984 (a.k.a the "*Hatch-Waxman Act*") that provides the most important components of the regulatory frame for pharmaceutical exclusivity in the United States.

Notably, the Hatch-Waxman Act provides significant incentives for generic drug makers to challenge drug patents long before their expiration dates. With minimal cost associated with generic drug approval contrasted with the significant investment required for de novo drug development, it is no wonder that patent challenges by generic drug companies became the drug developers' nightmare, and are the main focus of their patent strategies.

As mentioned above, a *generic drug* is a copycat of a *brand-name drug*. It has the same active pharmaceutical ingredient (API) as the corresponding brand-name drug and is supposed to be bioequivalent to it. A generic drug is approved by the U.S. Food and Drug Administration (FDA) based on a so-called Abbreviated New Drug Application (ANDA), which relies on the preclinical and clinical data of the copied brand-name drug generated by the original developer.

In fact, the FDA requires the prescription drug labeling of the generic drug to be largely identical to that of the brand-name drug. For this reason, unlike many other technical areas, patents for an innovative drug having relatively narrow claims may provide adequate protection against generic drug competition. Innovative drug developers should not overlook incremental inventions and should endeavor to obtain patents covering as many as possible novel inventions reflected (or to be reflected) in the prescription drug labeling of a new drug.

Examples of such patentable inventions include the API and variants thereof (including advantageous racemates or enantiomers, polymorphs, salt forms, solvates, and prodrugs, as well as metabolites of the API produced in the patient's body), pharmaceutical compositions containing the API, methods of use (based on use of the API or pharmaceutical composition in specific disease indications, patient populations, lines of therapy, combination therapies, biomarkers-based or personalized treatment, dosing regimens, administration route, advantageous pharmacokinetic profiles to be achieved, etc.), formulations (immediate or extended release formulations, special delivery forms such as transdermal or buccal delivery forms and nasal spray), dosage units, coformulations for combination therapies, advantageous purity or impurity characterization of the API or pharmaceutical compositions, methods of making the API or formulations or dosage units, advantageous packaging, etc.

Even if the recent *Myriad* decision was to be read to cast doubt on the patent eligibility of purified natural products (e.g., natural proteins, isolated genes, and small molecules discovered in natural sources), pharmaceutical compositions comprising them should still be patent eligible. New drug developers should create and seize every opportunity to seek patent protection on all drug-related inventions at every stage of the drug-development process. In this way, a comprehensive patent portfolio may be established to provide multiple layers of patent protection around the new drug.

Strategically, for a new drug with a new chemical entity (NCE), it is preferable to postpone the publication of the chemical structure or identity of the NCE, typically until after completion of a Phase II trial, lest the publication be construed as prior art that interferes with patenting later incremental inventions [17]. Delaying publication of the chemical structure may also reduce the possibility that third parties experiment with the same compound and publish or seek to patent their results. Such publications by third parties would also create prior art adverse to the developer's future patent filings. In addition, third party patents may interfere with the innovator's patent strategies and even impinge upon the innovator's freedom to commercialize the drug.

To maximize patent terms, drug developers should make full use of the patent term adjustment (PTA) and patent term extension (PTE) provisions of the U.S. patent law. Specifically, the U.S. patent statute requires the PTO to adjust the term of a patent to compensate for certain delays during patent prosecution caused by the PTO. In addition, the Hatch-Waxman Act provides for an extension of a selected patent covering a newly approved drug to compensate for regulatory delay in the FDA. For a drug with an annual sale of $365 million, each extra day at the back end of the patent term means the protection of $1 million sales. It is no wonder that *The Wall Street Journal* proclaimed "The most profitable activity an NDA holder can engage in is delaying approval of a generic." [18]

Importantly, the FDA publishes the *Orange Book* listing specific patents the new drug developer certifies to cover the approved new drug [19]. A generic must overcome all patents listed in the Orange Book for a particular new drug before its ANDA for a generic drug can be approved by the FDA. So it is important to list as many drug-related patents in the Orange Book to create more barriers to generic competition. Not all kinds of patents related to a new drug can be listed in the Orange Book. Patents covering the drug compound, formulations of the drug, or methods of treating diseases by administering the drug may be listed. But patents claiming manufacturing processes, metabolites, intermediates, or packaging are not listable.

Market Protection via Regulatory Exclusivity

New drugs may also be protected by *regulatory exclusivity*, i.e., exclusive marketing rights granted by the FDA under certain conditions. Regulatory exclusivity is independent of patents and can run concurrently with patents. There are several important types of regulatory exclusivity: orphan drug exclusivity, pediatric exclusivity, and data exclusivity. *Orphan drug* exclusivity is granted by the FDA under the Orphan Drug Act of 1983 for products to treat rare diseases and conditions affecting fewer than 200,000 patients in the United States. It prohibits approval of another application "for such drug for such disease or condition" for 7 years after the initial product approval, except for a "clinically superior" product that uses the "same active moiety." *Pediatric exclusivity* (PE) is granted by the FDA to extend by 6 months the expiration dates of other forms of exclusivity (e.g., patent, orphan exclusivity, or data exclusivity) if the new drug developer conducts pediatric trials of the drug.

Data exclusivity granted by the FDA is another important aspect of the new drug protection framework. Also sometimes referred to as "*marketing exclusivity*," this form of protection prohibits, during a defined period of time after new drug approval, any reliance by a third party on the data generated for the new drug for purposes of obtaining approval of a generic. Data exclusivity is independent of, and supplements, patent protection. An NCE approved for the first time for commercial marketing in the United States is entitled to a 5-year data exclusivity.

When the FDA approval of a new drug is not the first permitted commercial marketing or use of the product in the United States, a 3-year marketing exclusivity is granted. The FDA grants a 3-year marketing exclusivity for a combination drug if one of the coformulated APIs was previously approved for marketing or use in the United States Similarly, an enantiomer drug is entitled to only 3 years of marketing exclusivity from the FDA if the racemate was previously approved for marketing in the United States. An exception to this is that an amendment to the Food Drug and Cosmetic Act in 2007 provides a 5-year marketing exclusivity for a new drug wherein the API is an enantiomer of a previously approved racemate drug, provided that the enantiomer drug has undergone independent clinical trials and is approved for a completely different indication from that of the racemate drug [20].

With a 5-year data exclusivity, a prospective competitor seeking approval of a generic may not file an ANDA during the 5 years after the FDA's approval for marketing of the brand-name drug. But if a patent covering the brand-name drug is listed in the Orange Book, a generic manufacturer may file an ANDA 4 years after the FDA's approval of the brand-name drug, certifying that the patents in the Orange Book are either invalid or not infringed, or that approval to market the generic is not sought until after the patent expiration. Once a certification of patent invalidity or patent noninfringement is made, the brand-name developer is empowered to start a patent infringement suit in a U.S.

district court against the ANDA filer. If such a patent litigation is initiated, the FDA by law must stay the approval of the ANDA for 30 months which may be extended by a court to provide a total of 7.5 years from initial NDA approval to the time of ANDA approval.

With 3-year data exclusivity, a prospective competitor may file an ANDA with the FDA, but the ANDA may not be approved until 3 years after the marketing approval of the brand-name drug. The filing of an ANDA may also trigger patent infringement litigation under the Hatch-Waxman Act as described above.

Generic drug makers have a strong incentive to challenge the relevant patents in the Orange Book, as the first filer of an ANDA who successfully challenges the patents will be entitled to a 180-day exclusivity to market the generic. So a developer of new drugs needs to implement comprehensive strategies to build a strong patent estate, erecting as many entry barriers as possible to protect market exclusivity. (See Figure 15.3.)

REGULATORY APPROVALS FOR BIOLOGICS AND BIOSIMILARS

Note that *biologics* are approved under a different regulatory regime. Biologics are biological products including, for example, recombinant proteins, antibodies, vaccines, gene and cell therapies, blood and blood components, etc. Commercial marketing of biologics requires the approval by the FDA of a *biologic license application (BLA)*. In addition to patent protection, the orphan drug exclusivity and pediatric exclusivity discussed above are applicable to biologics. The Biologics Price Competition and Innovation Act enacted in 2010 for the first time provides an abbreviated regulatory pathway for "*biosimilars*" and a regulatory framework

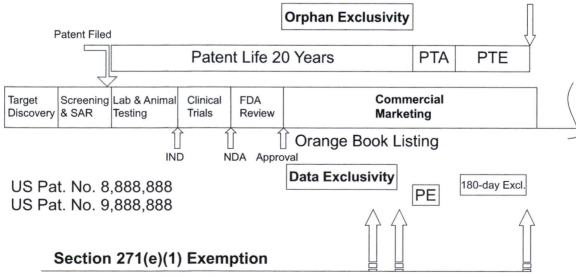

FIGURE 15.3   Market protection via regulatory exclusivity.

similar to that for new drugs under the Hatch-Waxman Act. As of this writing, the implementation of the law still awaits practical guidance to be issued by the FDA [21].

DIAGNOSTICS AND PERSONALIZED MEDICINE

The advent of personalized medicine is making the diagnostic industry ever more attractive to investors. By definition, personalized medicine requires that preventive or treatment measures be tailored to a particular patient. This customized approach necessarily depends on molecular diagnostic tests to determine a patient's genetic or molecular markers which are *correlated* to clinically useful disease characters. The significant investment and substantial risk involved in the discovery, development, and implementation of diagnostic tests mandate strong patent protection. Ironically, some recent court decisions in the United States have significantly weakened patent protection in the field and will tend to impede future efforts to patent some aspects of such tests.

Generally speaking, diagnostic tests have two fundamental components: (1) one or more biomarkers to be detected or measured, and (2) the correlation between the biomarker(s) and disease characters. Patents on the composition of matter of a biomarker molecule would essentially exclude others from making or using the same biomarker and thus would offer the strongest protection for a diagnostic test.

In addition, patent claims to the use of a correlation for diagnosis (not limited to any specific detection technique) could also provide strong protection for a diagnostic test. Many times, a biomarker can be detected by many different alternative techniques or equipment. Thus, patent claims reciting a specific detection technique or equipment often can be circumvented (*designed around*) and thus might not provide the desired exclusivity for the overall diagnostic test. See the discussion below of the U.S. Supreme Court decision in March 2012 of *Mayo Collaborative Services v. Prometheus Laboratories.*

In this post-Human-Genome-Project era, almost the entirety of the human genome, and most of its encoded proteins, as well as the general methods of analyzing such molecular markers, are public knowledge (prior art). Thus, most molecular markers, e.g., genes or proteins, wouldn't be patentable as novel molecular entities.

Exacerbating the situation, the U.S. Supreme Court's 2013 case *Association for Molecular Pathology v. Myriad Genetics, Inc.* excludes from patentable subject matter even newly discovered and isolated genes. Specifically, in *Myriad*, the Court was asked to review claims to various "isolated and purified nucleic acids" and address the question whether such molecules are eligible for patenting under the U.S. patent law [22]. In the 1990s, Myriad Genetics and its collaborators (including the NIH, the University of Utah, and others) successfully located in the human genome

the *BRCA1* and *BRCA2* genes, and identified particular mutations that are associated with the predisposition to breast and ovarian cancer. They determined the nucleotide sequences of the genes, filed patent applications, and were later granted patents for isolated nucleic acids including those gene sequences. For years, these patents provided exclusive rights for Myriad to perform mutation testing in *BRCA1* and *BRCA2* genes (i.e. its BRCAnalysis® test).

However, in 2009, a group of plaintiffs including several medical associations and clinical geneticists filed suit seeking a declaration that Myriad's patents are invalid under 35 U.S.C. §101 [23]. The plaintiffs asserted that the isolated genes have the same sequence information as the corresponding genes or mRNA in cells, and are products of nature that are ineligible for patenting. The Supreme Court, in a unanimous decision, held that while cDNA different from naturally occurring DNA is eligible for patenting, isolated genes are not eligible for patent protection because they are not "new 'with markedly different characteristics from any found in nature.'" [24] The decision concludes that: "Separating that gene from its surrounding genetic material is not an act of invention." [24] Thus, under *Myriad*, isolated, naturally occurring DNA is no longer patent eligible in the United States, and most previously granted claims to isolated genes are invalid.

Even though the *Myriad* decision applies expressly just to isolated genes, characterizing them as unique due to their information content, it also renders uncertain at this point the patent eligibility of other naturally occurring biomolecules, such as isolated or purified peptides, proteins, mRNA, miRNAs, siRNA, metabolites, antibodies, organic molecules, and others [25]. Under that rationale, mere isolation and purification of natural substances would not make such substances patent eligible.

If the courts are further misled by the arguments of those who seek freedom to profit from others' discoveries, *Myriad* will have significant negative impact on the diagnostic industry [26]. *Myriad* nonetheless is the law of the land in the United States. *Myriad* essentially precludes the patenting of molecular biomarkers as most biomarkers for diagnostic tests are molecules naturally occurring and detectable in human tissue or bodily fluid samples. Inventors and their patent attorneys would need to be really creative to gain meaningful patents on naturally occurring biomarkers. For example, if a novel protein as a biomarker has to be detected immunologically with an antibody, then a protein-antibody complex could be patent eligible if it does not exist in nature. Similarly, one may patent an artificial complex of an mRNA or miRNA with a primer or probe if the complex necessarily forms in a diagnostic test. In tests that require multiple biomarkers such as prognostic gene signatures, a composition comprising of two or more biomarkers may be claimed, although such patent claims may be circumvented by the separate measurement of the biomarkers before combining the results in the same computer analysis algorithm. Of course, one may also patent diagnostic kits containing a combination of multiple components required for performing a diagnostic test. While these patent claims are not as strong as a composition of matter claim for a single biomarker, they can provide extra layers of picket fences around the exclusive territory of a diagnostic test.

As discussed above, beside biomarkers, the other fundamental component of a diagnostic test is the correlation between the biomarker(s) and disease characters. When strong patent protection for biomarkers is unavailable, it would have been important to obtain broad patent protection for the application of the correlation in diagnosis. Before the Supreme Court decided the *Mayo v. Prometheus* case in 2012 [27], it was commonplace to obtain a patent claim to a diagnosis method based on a newly discovered correlation in the following format:

A method of diagnosing disease X, comprising determining the presence or absence [or amount] of a biomarker Y in patient, and correlating the presence [or the amount above a level W] of the biomarker Y with disease X in the patient.

Note that this patent claim would be infringed regardless of what technique is used in analyzing the biomarker Y in a patient sample. However, the *Mayo* decision made claims such as this essentially ineligible for patenting.

According to the Supreme Court, the correlation between the biomarker and the disease is an unpatentable law of nature, and "simply appending conventional steps, specified at a high level of generality, to laws of nature, natural phenomena, and abstract ideas cannot make those laws, phenomena, and ideas patentable." After *Mayo*, the method claim in the above example would most likely have to be modified to recite additional details with specificity in order to become patent eligible. Any additional specifics would necessarily narrow the scope of the claim and thereby detract from the protection that otherwise would have been afforded by the patent.

As of this writing, it appears that the PTO and courts are still struggling to articulate a clear standard to determine the patent eligibility of method claims that appear to embrace a "law of nature." We expect the case law will evolve slowly, and you'll want to seek ongoing advice from a trusted patent attorney who keeps abreast of such developments.

In the era of companion diagnostics, diagnostic method claims may be alternatively drafted in the form of method of treating diseases. The following is a hypothetical example:

A method of treating breast cancer, comprising detecting Her2 expression in a breast tumor tissue sample from a patient using an antibody immunologically reactive with Her2 protein, and administering trastuzumab to the patient if Her2 expression is detected to be positive.

Such a method-of-treatment claim may be eligible for listing in the FDA's Orange Book and thus provide an effective entry barrier against generic drug competition. Note that the above method claim includes two steps that, in reality, often are practiced by two different entities. The first step would typically be done by a diagnostic lab and the second by a doctor or patient. However, for a patent claim to be infringed, U.S. courts have generally required that all steps in the claim be performed by a single entity or at least by related entities acting in concert. Under that rubric, it would appear that none of the pertinent actors is infringing the patent claim.

This dilemma was posed in the companion cases of *Akamai Technologies, Inc. v. Limelight Networks, Inc.* Dkt. 2009-1372 and *McKesson Technologies, Inc. v. Epic Systems Corp.* Dkt. 2010-1291 (Fed. Cir. August 31, 2012 *en banc*). The U.S. Court of Appeals for the Federal Circuit applied a novel approach, holding that a party may be liable for *inducing infringement* if that party induced one or more other actors to perform steps of the claimed method, even if no single party performed all of those steps [28].

Other than biomarkers and general methods of using correlations, there may be many other patentable aspects in a new diagnostic test. Examples may include detection techniques, hardware equipment (e.g., chips, machines, magnetic beads, etc.), reagents, labeled probes and primers, synthetic primers and probes with nonnaturally occurring nucleotide sequences, and diagnostic kits. Depending on the circumstances, patents on these aspects can also provide valuable protection for a diagnostic test. One dramatic example is the original patents on the polymerase chain reaction (PCR) technique issued to Cetus Corp., which were sold in 1991 to Hoffmann-La Roche for $300 million (for all uses except DNA forensics).

It is also important to bear in mind that, although unpatentable in the United States, isolated genes and other biomolecules are still patent-eligible in almost all other major countries including the EU countries, Canada, China, Japan, South Korea, and Australia. As a generality, patent claims to methods of using correlations, although unpatentable in the United States, are routinely granted by the European Patent Office and in other countries [29]. In China, although methods of diagnosing diseases as a category are unpatentable subject matter, such method inventions may be patentable when presented in so called "Swiss use" claims. For example, if a previously known mutation in a gene is discovered to be correlated with an increased risk of cancer, then a claim may be drafted, for example, as follows:

Use of a primer or probe hybridizing to gene X for the manufacture of diagnostic reagents useful for detecting mutation Y in gene X and for diagnosing an increased risk of cancer in a human subject.

As an entrepreneur seeking to fashion a worldwide IP strategy to develop and market a novel biotechnology product or service, you may come to envy the relative certainty of the croquet match in Wonderland fantasized by Lewis Carroll, even though Alice had to use a flamingo as a mallet seeking to strike a live hedgehog as the ball [30].

In summary, recent changes in U.S. patent law have significantly weakened patent protection in the diagnostic field. Nonetheless, with creative strategies and attention to detail, entrepreneurs and businesses may still be able to obtain patents on their diagnostic tests and erect significant barriers to entry by their competitors. If foreign markets are part of the business strategies, then comprehensive foreign patent claims should be actively pursued.

CORPORATE IP MANAGEMENT

For entrepreneurs starting a biotechnology business, IP is often the most important asset that attracts investors and justifies the endeavor. Entrepreneurs should ensure that the core IP asset is adequately protected. Ideally, entrepreneurs should seek help from experts in patent law even before the formation of the business, and of course as the business grows. It is often valuable to have an experienced patent attorney as a close adviser, for example, as an interested cofounder, on the board, or as a regular consultant of the biotech start-up. Comprehensive patent strategies should be designed and implemented from the very beginning of the start-up business. A law firm or an outside attorney should be hired to advise on patent issues and prepare and prosecute patent applications. As the start-up grows, there will be an increased amount of IP-related legal work, and at some point it might be time to hire an in-house counsel. There are two main factors to consider to justify hiring an in-house IP counsel: cost saving and value creation. For example, when outside IP legal fees (excluding government fees) per year become high enough, say about $200,000 to $300,000 U.S., it might make economic sense to hire an in-house IP counsel. However, the more important factor to bear in mind is the value added by having a patent attorney stationed in the office, proactively managing IP assets and providing practical IP advice.

Indeed, an in-house IP attorney or IP department may perform a wide variety of functions within a biotechnology company. These include working with management to establish IP policies and strategies, setting up and managing necessary IP-related infrastructures and procedures, providing necessary IP-related training to the relevant company personnel, conducting patent preparation and prosecution, providing IP-related counseling to inventors and business people, resolving IP disputes and enforcing IP rights against infringers, reviewing and negotiating IP-related agreements, and in some cases, participating in business development and licensing negotiations.

To begin with, a biotechnology company should establish IP-related policies and strategies that are tailored to the business strategy and needs. For example, IP-related policies and strategies may include policies on rewarding inventors

for their inventions, ownership of inventions and patents, confidentiality obligations, invention reporting obligations, policies on scientific publication and public announcement of R&D results, patent clearance and noninfringement policies, legal fee policies, general patent filing strategies, IP dispute resolution strategies, etc. The IP department needs to set up the necessary infrastructures and procedures to implement the policies and strategies. For example, employment agreements should be prepared and signed by all employees clearly defining the ownership of inventions by employees, employees' confidentiality obligation, and, if appropriate, a noncompete covenant. Procedures should be in place to prevent the publication of valuable inventions before a patent application is filed to protect them. In addition, a company should also have a customary procedure for inventors to disclose their inventions to the IP department to be considered for patenting. The IP department may also want to conduct regular training sessions for employees to promote awareness of their IP-related obligations and ensure timely disclosure of inventions.

In many companies, in-house patent attorneys do little hands-on patent drafting and prosecution before the U.S. Patent and Trademark Office (USPTO), but farm out most of such work to outside law firms. In this approach, the in-house patent attorney acts as a liaison between the inventors within the company and the outside law firm, and supervises the outside attorneys' work. However, companies increasingly move patent preparation and prosecution work in-house. This is especially true in medium to large biotech and pharmaceutical companies whose IP departments can match small to medium patent law firms in size and functions. Biotech and pharmaceutical companies typically rely on patents much more than businesses in any other industries, and a large in-house patent preparation and prosecution group is often justifiably economical and adds substantial value: in-house patent attorneys are integrated closely with the R&D departments within the company and are narrowly focused on the company's technologies and business, and thus have a better understanding of the technologies and business goals in the company. In addition, they are not so constrained by billable hours and profit margins that outside attorneys have to be concerned about. Of course, outside counsel have their own advantages in that they deal with a wider variety of clients and gain more diverse experience which may prove beneficial in problem solving and creative patent strategies.

A biotech company should encourage in-house counsel to integrate closely with its different functional groups such as the R&D, business development, manufacturing, and marketing teams, and to have regular meetings and exchanges with these groups. In the process, in-house counsel will be able to keep up with the company business, contribute their patent expertise and perspective, and capture inventions to strengthen the company's IP portfolio. To illustrate, ideally in-house counsel should participate in R&D projects by regularly attending R&D meetings even at the project's planning stage, and follow through the entire process of the project. This way, the patent counsel will be able to gain a good understanding of the project, the technologies, and the marketing and business strategies. In turn, the counsel can advise the R&D group during the entire process, helping to further the business goals. For example, at the planning stage, the in-house counsel can help the R&D group make informed decisions for pursuing the project, e.g., by raising issues such as potential patent infringement risks associated with the technology to be used or with the expected product to be developed, competitive intelligence on patent landscape, or the patentability of the expected product. These factors may either strengthen or undermine the justification for the project. During the project, by close interaction with the R&D group, the counsel will be able to timely spot potential IP risks and capture patentable inventions that scientists might otherwise miss. Creative patent counsel should even be able to suggest certain experiments to do to generate new patents or support existing patent strategies. While some scientists might view such advice as "the tail wagging the dog," patents are so crucial to most biotech and pharmaceutical companies that sometimes the dog had better be wagged by the little tail.

Many in-house patent attorneys also spend a significant amount of time providing legal advice to the company on diverse issues such as freedom-to-operate patent clearance to avoid patent infringement, patent due diligence in business transactions, and IP-related contract negotiations. In many biotech companies, it is the patent attorneys who are put in charge of licensing and business development functions besides IP responsibilities. Indeed, as IP is the underlying basis in most licensing and business alliances in biotech, business savvy patent attorneys are a natural fit for such functions—in-house patent attorneys understand the technologies, the sophisticated IP strategies, as well as the business goals, and thus can have a better grasp of the IP-related subtleties and pitfalls in such business negotiations. Moreover, negotiation skills fostered in law school and honed by experience in the field can also be put to good use in this function.

PATENT STRATEGIES AND PRODUCT LIFECYCLE MANAGEMENT

Patents are crucial to biotechnology companies in recouping the significant investment often required to get a product developed and marketed. Patents are also critical in maintaining a competitive edge in the face of competition. Thus it is important for entrepreneurs and biotech companies to build a strong patent portfolio around their products and manage product lifecycle to maximize the exclusivity on the products. These require sophisticated patent strategies

and expertise. Close collaboration between R&D personnel and patent attorneys is also needed. Biotech businesses should avoid becoming complacent when a first patent covering a product is granted, but rather would do well to strive to build a portfolio of multiple patents and patent families covering the product. Ideally, the company will pursue multiple patents with stacked patent terms in an effort to extend the life of patent protection. Timing for filing patent applications is also important. For products that take a long time to develop, consider delaying the filing of some patents so as to maximize the overlap between the patent term and the commercialization stage of the product life. But beware that delayed patent filing incurs the risk of losing the first-to-file priority status and thus the right to obtain such a patent vis-a-vis another worker in your field. Timing in filings is also important in minimizing prior art, as well as avoiding creating prior art against the company's other patents covering the same product.

Roche's PCR patent portfolio is a good example of successful IP strategies. After Hoffmann-La Roche acquired the fundamental PCR patents from Cetus Corporation, it proceeded to acquire and file additional patents and built a comprehensive patent portfolio. In particular, this patent portfolio includes a large number of patents with different expiration dates covering different aspects of the PCR process and its various applications, including the basic PCR method, the PCR process using thermostable polymerases, purified *Taq* polymerase enzyme, recombinant *Taq* polymerase and fragments, PCR machine and method for performing automated PCR amplification, thermostable reverse transcriptase, real time PCR, *Taq*Man probes, *Taq*Man-based real-time PCR method, and others. These patents formed thick picket fences around the PCR technology since the late 1980s, with patent expiration dates between 2005 and 2017 or later. This patent portfolio has largely withstood patent challenges and generated hundreds of millions of dollars for Roche.

Merck's patent coverage on Fosamax illustrates a sound pharmaceutical patent strategy in a difficult situation. Fosamax was Merck's blockbuster drug for treating osteoporosis. Its active ingredient alendronate sodium was already publicly known by the time the Italian company Instituto Gentili, Merck's licensor, discovered its use in treating osteoporosis in 1982, and thus there was no patent available on the chemical compound itself or even a pharmaceutical composition thereof. Instituto Gentili filed for a "method-of-use" patent in 1984 and was granted a U.S. patent in 1986. After Merck licensed the program, it created multiple patents with stacked patent terms, extending exclusivity until 2008. In addition to the original method-of-use patent it licensed, Merck filed a number of patents on processes for the preparation of alendronate. It also obtained patent protection on the crystalline trihydrate form of alendronate monosodium, the final form of the active ingredient in the Fosamax drug.

A patent was also granted claiming the formulation of the oral tablet drug and the method of preparing the tablet. Moreover, a patent was also filed and granted on a weekly dosing regimen based on the discovery that a weekly dosing of a high-dose alendronate sodium was well tolerated in patients and alleviated a great deal of the side-effects associated with the original daily dosing. While some of these patents eventually were invalidated or revoked in litigation or oppositions, the portfolio as a whole was sufficient to protect Fosamax for an extended period of time even though the chemical entity of the drug was not protected by a claim to the compound itself. Of note, even before Merck lost exclusivity for Fosamax, it developed Fosamax Plus D, (a combination of alendronate sodium and vitamin D (cholecalciferol)), a second-generation product. Fosamax Plus D is covered by patents listed in the Orange Book.

Many biotechnology developments that showed promise to blossom into lifesaving products nevertheless were aborted at the research stage, never to be fully developed, largely due to lack of the patent protection that would have justified the enormous investment required. The foregoing example of Fosamax illustrates that sufficient patent protection may sometimes be established in difficult situations, provided that patent strategies are created and followed through the drug development process. Entrepreneurs and biotech managers should work closely with experienced patent counsel and stay vigilant in capturing and creating patentable inventions through the entire process of product development and even thereafter for second-generation products. Collective effort and creative strategizing among the IP, R&D, and even the marketing teams increase the likelihood of such a payoff.

SOME RESOURCES

General Information

World Intellectual Property Organization (WIPO) website: http://www.wipo.org/.

American Intellectual Property Law Association (AIPLA) website: http://www.aipla.org.

U.S. Patent and Trademark Office, Manual of Patent Examining Procedure (MPEP): http://mpep.uspto.gov.

Understanding Industrial Property (World Intellectual Property Organization—WIPO Publication No. 895(E) ISBN 978-92-805-1257-1: http://www.wipo.int/export/sites/www/freepublications/en/intproperty/895/wipo_pub_895.pdf.

Intellectual Property And Biotechnology, Arti Rai (Edward Elgar Publishing).

The Role Of Intellectual Property Rights In Biotechnology Innovation, D. Castle (Edward Elgar Publishing).

Intellectual Property And Biotechnology, M. Rimmer (Edward Elgar Publishing).

Innovation And Entrepreneurship In Biotechnology, An International Perspective, D. Hine and J. Kapeleris (Edward Elgar Publishing).

Law and Entrepreneurship, R.E. Litan and A.J. Luppino, eds. (Edward Elgar Publishing) Biotechnology And Innovation Systems, B. Göransson and C.M. Pålsson, (Edward Elgar Publishing).

Biotechnology and the Law, Revision Edition, by Iver Cooper (Clark Boardman/West Group).

Biotechnology and the Law, 2007, Hugh B. Wellons, et. al, eds. (American Bar Association Section of Science and Technology).

Biotechnology Law Report, 1982 to present, Gerry J. Elman, founding editor (Mary Ann Liebert, Inc.) http://www.liebertpub.com/blr.

The Biotech Entrepreneur's Glossary, Michael G. Pappas (M.G. Pappas & Co., Shrewsbury, MA, 1998).

Patent Searching

U.S. Patent & Trademark Office: http://www.uspto.gov/.

WIPO PatentScope: http://patentscope.wipo.int/search/en/advancedSearch.jsf.

Esp@cenet Search: http://worldwide.espacenet.com/advancedSearch.

Google Patents: http://patents.google.com.

Free Patents Online: http://freepatentsonline.com.

REFERENCES

[1] This chapter is presented for educational purposes and not as actionable legal advice. Any opinions expressed herein are those of the individual authors and not of any business, institution, or client. Due to the rapid change in this field of law and practice, the authors, editor, and publisher cannot warrant that a particular item of information is necessarily current. We recommend the reader seek up-to-date advice from counsel practicing in the relevant jurisdiction. We welcome any updates or discrepancies that readers wish to call to our attention. Direct such correspondence to elman@elman.com. We acknowledge with thanks the research assistance of Michael Donnini.

[2] Throughout this chapter, we'll present in *italics* certain "terms of art." They're the building blocks that identify concepts you'll want to keep in mind.

[3] The granddaddy international treaty on this subject was first adopted in 1883, in Paris, France. Read the "Paris Convention for the Protection of Industrial Property" at http://www.wipo.int/treaties/en/text.jsp?file_id=288514.

[4] Similarly, the major international treaty on copyrights was adopted in 1886 in Berne, Switzerland as the "Berne Convention for the Protection of Literary and Artistic Works." See http://www.wipo.int/treaties/en/text.jsp?file_id=283698.

[5] At the time of this writing, an appeal of the Australian decision is pending.

[6] This claim was granted before the U.S. Supreme Court's decision in Association for Molecular Pathology v. Myriad Genetics, Inc., June

13, 2013 Almost certainly, it wouldn't be enforceable since then. See text below in notes 17 to 20;

[7] U.S. Constitution, Art. 1, sec. 8, cl. 8: "Congress shall have the power…To promote the progress of science and useful arts, by securing for limited times to authors and inventors the exclusive right to their respective writings and discoveries."

[8] Recall that the Constitution refers to the "useful arts" for what today we'd call "technology."

[9] America Invents Act of September 16, 2011. http://www.uspto.gov/aia_implementation/index.jsp. One of the more significant changes to U.S. patent law wrought by this Act was to subtly redefine "prior art." Compare the currently amended version of § 102 of the patent law with its predecessor. Also, on December 5, 2013, yet another "patent reform" bill was introduced in Congress, as H.R. 3309, dubbed the "Innovation Act." passed the House.

[10] The process of analyzing the meaning of a patent claim, determining its legal metes and bounds, is called "*claim construction*." Note that this term does not refer to "constructing" a claim from scratch, but rather to "*construing*" its meaning after it has been written.

[11] See Supreme Court Affirms CAFC in Stanford v. Roche on Bayh-Dole, http://www.ipwatchdog.com/2011/06/06/supreme-court-affirms-cafc-in-stanford-v-roche-on-bayh-dole/id=17594/; June 6, 2011.

[12] See Sherry Flax, An Introduction to Pharma Trademarks. Available at. MSBA IP Section Newsletter, Vol.1, Mar. 2009.

[13] See Clark Lackert and Keith Sharkin, World Trademark Review, http://www.worldtrademarkreview.com/Issues/article.ashx?g=91cfc341-d571-4813-b3f4-ea3d698e16d8; October/November 2009. p. 1.

[14] See TMEP §1207.01(d)(xii) re Pharmaceuticals or Medicinal Products.

[15] See the timeline for development of a non-proprietary drug name at http://www.ama-assn.org/ama/pub/physician-resources/medical-science/united-states-adopted-names-council/drug-name-development-timeline-usan-review.page.

[16] See *Guidance on INN*, World Health Organization. Available at http://www.who.int/medicines/services/inn/innquidance/en/. The WHO created the INN based on concerns during the International conference of Drug Regulatory Authorities in 1991, thereafter adopting resolution WHA46.19 on nonproprietary names for pharmaceutical substances. For guidelines on coining generic names, see http://www.ama-assn.org/ama/pub/physician-resources/medical-science/united-states-adopted-names-council/naming-guidelines.page.

[17] If you pursue an international patent strategy, keep in mind that you won't be able to avoid having your own disclosure published 18 months from its priority date.

[18] *Wall Street Journal*, July 12, 2000.

[19] The Orange Book is available at the FDA website: http://www.accessdata.fda.gov/scripts/cder/ob/default.cfm.

[20] Public Law 110-85, codified as 21 U.S.C. § 355(u)(1) (Supp. II 2008).

[21] Information on biosimilar rules and regulations is available at the FDA website: http://www.fda.gov/Drugs/DevelopmentApprovalProcess/HowDrugsareDevelopedandApproved/ApprovalApplications/TherapeuticBiologicApplications/Biosimilars/default.htm.

[22] Section 101 of the U.S. Patent Law, 35 U.S.C. § 101, provides, in part: "Whoever invents or discovers any new and useful process, machine, manufacture, or composition of matter, or any new and useful improvement thereof, may obtain a patent therefore, subject to the conditions and requirements of [title 35 of the U.S.Code]." Court decisions interpreting this provision include man-made organisms within patent-eligible subject matter but expressly exclude laws of nature, abstract ideas, and mathematical algorithms.

[23] Powell SR, Elman GJ. ACLU Lawyers Face Off Against the U.S. Patent Office and Myriad Genetics, 29 Biotech. L. Rep 29, http://online.liebertpub.com/doi/abs/10.1089/blr.2010.9987; February 2010.

[24] Association for Molecular Pathology v. Myriad Genetics, Inc., 569 U. S. ____ (2013) (citing Diamond v. Chakrabarty, 447 U. S. 303, 310(1980)).

[25] Elman See Gerry Elman. What Subject Matter Is Patentable? Reading *Myriad Genetics* While Waiting For *Bilski*. Why is this molecule different from all other molecules? 29 Biotech. L. Rep 167, http://elman.com/2010/04/what-subject-matter-is-patentable/; Apr. 2010.

[26] In the interest of full disclosure, co-author Jay Z. Zhang was the Senior Vice President of Intellectual Property at Myriad Genetics leading the *Myriad* litigation in the district court and the Federal Circuit Court of Appeals before it was appealed to the U.S. Supreme Court.

[27] Mayo Collaborative Services v. Prometheus Laboratories, Inc., 566 U. S. ____; March 20, 2012.

[28] *Akamai Technologies, Inc. v. Limelight Networks, Inc.* Dkt. 2009-1372 and *McKesson Technologies, Inc. v. Epic Systems Corp.* Dkt. 2010-1291 (Fed. Cir. Aug. 31, 2012 *en banc*). http://www.cafc.uscourts.gov/images/stories/opinions-orders/09-1372-1380-1416-141710-1291.pdf. At the time of writing, the Supreme Court has granted certiorari and scheduled an oral argument. A final decision is expected by June 2014. http://www.supremecourt.gov/Search.aspx?FileName=/docketfiles/12-960.htm. http://www.supremecourt.gov/Search.aspx?FileName=/docketfiles/12-786.htm.

[29] See, e.g., European Patent Office Decisions *EPO* G1/04; EPO T310/99.

[30] Lewis Carroll, Alice's Adventures in Wonderland and *Though the Looking-Glass* (Signet Classics, The New America Library 1960) p. 79.

Biotechnology Market Development

Biotechnology Products and Their Customers: Developing a Successful Market Strategy

Craig Shimasaki, PhD, MBA

President & CEO, Moleculera Labs and BioSource Consulting Group, Oklahoma City, Oklahoma

In most industries, a company will discover, develop, manufacture, and then sell their products to one customer who is both the decision-maker and the end-user. In those industries, the decision-maker *decides* to purchase, then *purchases* the product, and *uses* the product directly. For instance, when Apple Computer creates and sells the latest version of the iPhone, the customer is the same individual who makes a decision to purchase the iPhone, and is the same person who pays $300 to $500 for the product, and is the same person who uses the product. This buying decision continuum is *not* how product decisions, purchasing, and utilization occurs in the medical biotechnology industry. In this industry, there are three customers, each making independent decisions for selection, purchasing, and utilization of most biotechnology products. One customer is the decision-maker who decides which product should be used, another customer makes an independent decision whether or not to pay for the product (and how much to pay for the product), and a totally different customer uses the product. This segmentation of customer decisions is an aspect that hampers the success of many biotechnology companies. It is vital to have a clear understanding of the three independent customers of biotechnology products, and to understand their motivations and responsibilities if a company expects to experience product-marketing success (see Figure 16.1). However, there are some sectors of biotechnology where products have only one or two customers, such as agricultural biotechnology, industrial biotechnology, and research tools.

In the medical biotechnology industry, the individual who makes the decision about which product to use is typically the *physician*. The entity that makes the decision on how much to pay, or whether to pay, is called the *payer*. The end-user of the product is typically the *patient*. The physician, payer, and patient each have input into the decision regarding the product, and each examines a different product value for determining their respective decision. Successful biotechnology company leaders and managers must make sure their product offering possesses a high-value proposition for each of these three customer groups. Unfortunately, young start-up companies may not consider the impact of having three different customer groups who are each responsible for a decision on their product. In countries where the government provides medical services and coverage, such as the UK and Canada, the payer and the physician are more closely aligned in their decision on the product use because the physician will be paid by the government and they know what is accepted and not accepted for usage by their government. Whereas in the United States, many of the physicians are independent of the payers of medical biotechnology products. The payers are a mix of sources, including numerous private insurance carriers in addition to the U.S. government that pays through Medicare and the state providers that pay through Medicaid. Private insurance carriers also have customers and attempt to balance the acquisition and retention of customers (the insured) who pay monthly medical insurance premiums, with the ability to offer the best medical care and still make a profit.

IDENTIFY THE PATIENT

The patient for a biotechnology product is usually easy to define, and they are identified based upon the product or service that you are providing. There are *target market* and *broader market* patients. The *target market* patients are those with the most acute need for your product and they are the customers who would have the greatest likelihood of wanting and needing your product. The *broader market* patients are those who would use the product or service but they may not be the first group to try it when the product is available. This

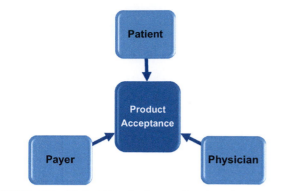

FIGURE 16.1   Medical biotechnology products have three customers.

group may have an interest in the product but their need is satisfied, albeit to a lesser degree than if they used your product. For example, if your product is a drug-eluting stent, your patient-customer is an individual with coronary artery disease wanting to avoid bypass surgery. If your product is a new statin drug, then your patient-customer is someone diagnosed with high cholesterol who fits the indications for use of this drug. If your product is a Respiratory Syncytial Virus disease diagnostic, your patient-customer is a child presenting to a clinic, hospital, or doctor's office with the disease symptoms.

IDENTIFY THE PHYSICIAN OR HEALTHCARE PROVIDER

Determining the target market physician can be a bit more complex than identifying the patient because there are multiple physician specialties and multiple service provider options where these specialty physicians provide services. There are also *target market* physician groups and *broader market* physician groups just as there is for patients. In the case of the drug-eluting stent product, the *target market* physician-customer would be an interventional cardiologist who will be inserting the stent into the appropriate patient-customer. For the statin drug product, the *target market* physician-customer would initially be a cardiologist, but the *broader market* physician-customer could be a family practice physician, a geriatrician, or even a physician's assistant. For the infectious disease diagnostic, the *target market* physician-customer would be a primary care physician, or any physician, but generally there will be a core group of them that may see more cases of this particular disease than others. For instance, if your test is for respiratory syncytial virus, this disease primarily occurs in children less than 2 years old; therefore the *target market* physician-customer would most likely be a pediatrician or hospital ER physician.

IDENTIFY THE PAYERS

There are multiple payer sources, such as private insurance (large, small, regional, national), HMOs, Medicare, Medicaid, and each have certain requirements in order to reach a

reimbursement coverage decision. In the United States we tend to have a sense of entitlement for medical care and usually do not expect to be paying much out-of-pocket for healthcare services. This means that in order to get most products or services adopted in the medical field, the company will need to secure medical reimbursement. In order to get payer coverage, your product must provide a significant benefit to the payer and to their patient. Many private insurances rely upon medical reimbursement evaluation groups for assessing reimbursement decisions—targeting these groups may save you time and money without having to deal with each payer individually. You will need to spend sufficient time examining medical reimbursement strategy issues in order to get widespread adoption of your product as this is a critical component of success for biotechnology products. Realize that these issues are *not* ones you deal with after your product is developed. Smart investors will not fund projects that have no reasonable chance of getting medical reimbursement coverage, so be sure to have a good understanding of this before you raise capital.

Multiple customers make biotech product market research and development more complex than for industries where there is only one customer. You must carefully consider each of these customers because you cannot market your product successfully without acceptance from all three. For instance, I know of a very innovative prosthetics company who created some amazing prosthetic devices for individuals with physical limitations. One medical device they created was an innovative bionic ankle that had capabilities near to a human ankle. The product was received extremely well by the patient and the physician. However, it cost about $15,000. The challenge for the successful adoption of this product was getting insurance reimbursement for such a device, as less-sophisticated ankles that still functioned adequately sold for around $3000. Without the payer realizing a value benefit, a product will not be widely accepted. For biotechnology products, all three customers must have a value proposition in order for a product to be successful.

DEVELOP A MARKETING STRATEGY FOR YOUR FUTURE PRODUCT

In order for biotechnology companies to be successful they must have a great product idea, bring together an experienced team to develop the product, and raise enough money to fund the product through development, testing, and regulatory approval. But even if a company navigates through these obstacles and overcomes these hurdles, unless there is good market strategy and their product meets an unmet medical need, there will not be commercial success of the product.

It is not enough to just develop a product—though it may seem like it should be because of the difficulty accomplishing this in the biotech industry. Before product development can be funded, the entrepreneur must prove to investors that the future product will be received by their target audience, and that the company has a marketing strategy that will accomplish this goal. It is not unusual to find that good product technology ideas do not get funded because of the wrong target market and a poor marketing strategy. A market strategy identifies the target market customers, creates a value proposition for each of the three customer groups, and identifies the optimal market channels to successfully provide the product or service to the target market.

Your company's marketing strategy has an impact well before commercialization as it inhibits or increases the company's ability to raise the needed capital to complete product development. It is the plan of how the company will provide value to the target market and make money delivering on that promise.

If you cannot develop a good marketing strategy before commercialization, then possibly that product application may not be deliverable by the underlying technology, or that product application may not be the best to undertake. Or worse, you may not know what your target market and their ultimate need. All entrepreneurs will have a "plan" or an "idea" of a marketing strategy in that they have knowledge of who the target market is and that they have a need. However, without identifying a plausible marketing strategy prior to undertaking the product development you may not be aware of the issues you will face down the road or if there is an alternate product application that should be first considered (See Figure 16.2).

When I say "marketing strategy" I am not referring to the detail of how much you will pay sales and marketing persons, or the product packaging color and who will package it. Sometimes details such as these are referred to as a "go-to-market plan" where all details are spelled out including the timing for each aspect and the responsible persons for executing that portion of the plan. What I am referring to is a strategy that includes such things as what channels will be used to get your product to the customer, what are the value drivers, what features you must minimally deliver in order to obtain acceptance, your pricing strategy, a cost/benefit analysis for the stakeholders that influence the purchase, prescribing, and product use.

I would encourage you to pick up and read some marketing strategy books to help you gain a better understanding of these concepts. Even though biotechnology products are much more complex and have greater consequences for their choices, similar marketing principles apply for most all products that are purchased and used—even medical products.

In this next section I want to share a few marketing concepts to help you understand why a well thought-out marketing strategy is critical even before product development has begun. Sometimes marketing concepts can be abstract and difficult to understand, so in these examples I will discuss familiar consumer products, then later we will apply them to biotechnology products.

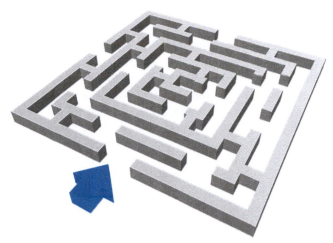

FIGURE 16.2 Product development path without first understanding needed product features.

WHAT IS MARKETING?

Marketing is an art and a science. However, most people view marketing as simply an art, yet there are sound principles that guide development of competitive marketing strategies for any product, including biotechnology products. *Merriam-Webster* defines marketing as "the act or process of selling or purchasing in a market; the process or technique of promoting, selling, and distributing a product or service; an aggregate of functions involved in moving goods from producer to consumer." In reality, marketing is not the same as "sales" which are the functions that follow good marketing.

I like to think of marketing as "meeting the acute needs of a select group of people profitably." In order to understand what marketing is, let's first discuss what market is not. Below are a few common misconceptions.

First Marketing Misconception: Marketing is not Difficult Because You Just Make It and Sell It!

Although we all know the line from the *Field Of Dreams* movie "build it and they will come," it is not a reality in business. However, most biotechnology entrepreneurs subconsciously believe their product is so revolutionary that, at some level, multitudes will clamor to get it because of its awesome technology and the great things it will do. This cannot be further from the truth. Just because a product can do many "great things," it will not be successful unless those "great things" are the exact things your target market wants and needs.

Most people do not know that Apple Computer was the first to invent a type of personal digital assistant (PDA) called the Newton. This PDA-type device was intended to keep our calendar, store our contacts, save our notes, and help keep us organized, all at our fingertips. It had a touch-screen with handwriting recognition, but was almost 1 inch thick, too large and heavy (almost 1 pound) to be considered pocket-size. The Newton was manufactured from 1993 to 1998, but discontinued because of lack of consumer interest (see Figure 16.3).

Shortly before the Newton was discontinued, an unknown competitor, Palm, Inc., launched its Palm Pilot developed by first researching the needs of their customers. Palm, Inc. successfully captured a broad market with a second generation product that was initially introduced by an unsuccessful competitor. Palm developed their product using the marketing concept which we discuss below. The rapid adoption of the PDA was often associated with Palm Pilot and the successful company Palm, Inc. These handheld devices enjoyed widespread market acceptance and were a precursor of some of the main functions incorporated into our current cell phones.

Second Marketing Misconception: If Your Technology is Better than the Competition, More People Will Buy Your Product

This is another fallacy, and definitely a slippery slope for biotechnology entrepreneurs who are captivated by their technology. A good example of this lesson occurred in the video recorder industry where two competitors, Sony and JVC, both had their own technologies for home video recording and playing devices. The first home video recorder was developed and introduced by Sony in 1975 called the Betamax format. One year later, JVC introduced their competitive VHS format. The Betamax and VHS formats were incompatible with each other, and the consumer was left to choose video formats. VHS and Betamax camera recorders were marketed and the movie industry reproduced movies in both the VHS and Betamax formats. However, JVC quickly understood the need to license their VHS format to other companies in order to gain broader market acceptance and customer adoption. Sony did not follow suit.

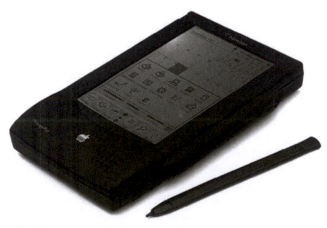

FIGURE 16.3 The Apple Newton—one of the early PDA-type devices.

Consumer demand grew for video recorders and companies that manufactured the VHS video recorders met the growing consumer demand, and more studios produced movies in the VHS format. By 1987, the VHS format held 95 percent of the video recorder market share. As could be expected, movie studios discontinued reproducing movies in the Betamax format and Sony ultimately discontinued manufacturing its Betamax video recorders. Even though Sony was one of the first movers in the home video market and their format could be considered superior to the competitor's format, the video tape format battle was won by JVC. Because of a difference in market strategy, Sony lost the opportunity to be the dominant player in home video recording. It can be estimated that hundreds of millions of dollars were spent in development and manufacturing of the Betamax format including many companies that had products supporting this format.

Between 2006 and 2008 another format war emerged for the high definition optical disk. In early 2006, Toshiba was the first mover to introduce the HD-DVD format and the first HD-DVD player. Sony followed suit with its own Blu-ray format disk player. Sony quickly secured more commitments from movie studios to offer titles in their Blu-ray format than Toshiba. In early 2008, Toshiba announced that it would discontinue its HD-DVD player. Although technology enthusiasts say that Toshiba's HD-DVD was a superior format, Sony won the DVD battle. Sony did not repeat a painful marketing lesson they previously learned. They realized that the customer is not as enamored with the technology as much as they want to be sure their needs are met by the products they purchase.

Third Marketing Misconception: It is Too Early to Have a Market Strategy because it will Get Done Once the Product is Developed

This sounds logical on the surface but fundamentally this is disastrous. Remember, a marketing strategy is not the detail of the amount of commission you pay to a sales force, but it is more about how you will reach your target customer and deliver the value that they want and need, and how you will do that strategically, competitively, and profitably. Also understand that you will not be able to attract knowledgeable investors unless you can demonstrate there is a significant unmet market need for your product and that you have a market strategy that will get your product adopted profitably. Many business plans are turned down by investors simply because the entrepreneur did not prove there was a real market need for their product. Or if the market need was evident, the entrepreneur could not show how to profitably capture this market. Investors do not invest in your company so they can fix a poor marketing strategy for your business. If you do not understand the market needs for your own product, investors conclude you will not make wise decisions in other facets of your business either. As the sophistication level of your investors increase, the more your marketing plan will be scrutinized for flaws. It is vital that you understand the market issues surrounding your product and then develop a well-thought-out market strategy to address these issues. Investors will not get excited about a biotechnology product that does not have a great marketing strategy to reach their customers. A good exercise for entrepreneurs is to ask venture capital fund managers (VCs) to name the three critical elements they need to see in a biotech company before they will invest. You can be sure that demonstrating a real market need coupled to a sensible market strategy will be high on their top three list.

ADVANCEMENT OF THE MARKETING CONCEPT

The marketing concept is an approach where the company first analyzes the needs and wants of their customers *before* making their product development decisions. It is the notion of satisfying the needs of the customer by providing solutions to the customer's problem. The marketing concept provides the foundation for a competitive advantage by first knowing who your customers are, then understanding their unique needs because it helps you develop products that satisfy these needs better than the competition.

The marketing concept evolved as a result of the need for companies to find competitive advantages over others in the same market. Understanding how this concept evolved will help entrepreneurs appreciate the value of the marketing concept in business. There were at least three major commercialization concepts that evolved during the development of products and services in the United States. These three concepts are briefly reviewed below.

The Production Concept

The production concept is the philosophy that companies simply needed to produce products at a reasonable price and in sufficient quantities then these products would sell themselves. Because there was an acute need for basic necessities at affordable prices, the production concept worked well during the Industrial Revolution. Prior to and during that time, there was a limitation for companies to produce their products efficiently and in sufficient quantity to make them affordable for everyone. As better manufacturing processes were developed and became cost-effective, these "affordable" products did indeed sell themselves. As essential consumer products were produced in larger quantities and manufacturing efficiencies continued to improve, many products that were previously unattainable by consumers suddenly became affordable to most everyone.

A statement about selling his Model T automobiles to his customers attributed to Henry Ford, summarized the production concept: "You can have it in any color you want, as long as it is black." In other words, products were manufactured that could be mass produced in sufficient quantities and at affordable prices without regard for specific customer's needs. Eventually, production capabilities for all companies improved and soon cost-effective manufacturing became the standard. By the late 1940s and early 1950s most of the basic needs of the average U.S. consumer were being met.

The Sales Concept

Once mass-production manufacturing capabilities became commonplace, there arose competition for basic necessity products and the sales concept was born. This was the philosophy of focusing on how to better persuade consumers to buy *your* product irrespective of whether your product was needed by the customer. Companies began to adopt different methods for "selling" their products to customers before competitors could reach them. This became the era of the "hard-sell" and the door-to-door salesmen. As consumers became wiser, these hard-sell tactics no longer produced the type of revenue that organizations required. It was then that clever companies searched for ways to be more competitive.

The Marketing Concept

As competition continued to increase, companies looked for more strategic ways to grow their revenue and maintain an advantage over their competitors. Companies began figuring out their customer's unmet needs before they developed products and then they created the products that satisfied them. More and more success came to the companies that better understood their customer's wants and needs and delivered the precise products they desired. This was the marketing concept.

The marketing concept is about understanding the customer's needs even if they do not express them. Proctor & Gamble (P&G) is a very successful marketing concept company. A large part of their target market is women ages 30 to 45 who purchase household goods and supplies. P&G seeks to better understand the needs of their target market in various ways, even if their customers do not clearly express these needs. P&G asks their customers questions about their household needs, but they also compensate them to visit their homes and follow them throughout their daily activities. Based upon observation and asking their target market segment about their household needs, the company then develops products to meet these needs better than their competitors.

A well-known product developed from this type of market research is the Swiffer®. The Swiffer met the target market needs so well that during the first year of introduction, sales were over $200 million. Although the target market consumers did not tell the P&G engineers that they needed something like a "Swiffer," the engineers created a product to specifically meet the needs of their customers. This solution was neither a broom nor a mop but accomplished those same functions, which was to capture dirt and clean, but was easier to use, less messy, did not require water, and could be stored in a small space.

The Swiffer example has a parallel for biotechnology companies in that this product created a brand new category that did not exist before but was successful because it met an unmet need that was not filled by any other product available. The marketing concept is the most effective marketing strategy, yet many companies neglect to first define their target market and fail to understand their specific needs.

MARKET RESEARCH AND ASSESSMENT TOOLS

When developing a market strategy it is important to first start with market research because this will be the foundation from which you will later base your assumptions. Market research is the process of gathering information to answer these questions:

1. Is there a general *market opportunity* for your product?
2. Who is your potential *target market* and what is the *total market size*?
3. What are your *target market demographics* and what are their *needs*?
4. What are your *competition's* strengths and weaknesses?

Conducting market research allows you to acquire information and gain insight about the potential market for your product and the needs of your potential customers. Market research may be gathered from medical providers, specialty physicians, insurance companies, researchers, or patients with a particular disease or condition. This information can be obtained through literature, publications, or from direct surveys and interviews.

Be sure to conduct thorough market research, gathering as much data as possible, and from as many different sources as possible. When doing market research it is important to know and understand that there can be source bias. Be sure to guard against selectively hearing information that only confirms a bias for market acceptance of your product. Be critical of your own assumptions and think of reasons why your target market may not want your product and why it may not receive medical reimbursement if it is a human health product. If you are thorough and honest with your questions you will also find the answers that investors will ask when questioning you about the market. All bias is not bad as it may help you know who your best customers may be since they may be biased in their interest of your product. A bias is bad when it is a conclusion about competition or about the risks that you will face in the market. These biases need to be uncovered as you do not want to learn something about your market after you begin commercialization. Once we obtain market research information we can then form some conclusions about the product potential, the target market needs and demographics, the market size, and the competition strengths

and weaknesses. Later, we will use this market research to formulate a market strategy. At the end of this chapter I have provided a template for formulating a market strategy and it will incorporate much of this information and other information such as market channels and competition.

Primary and Secondary Market Research

Market research is typically categorized as "primary" and "secondary" market research. Primary market research is information that comes first-hand and directly to you such as interviewing customers and their responses to your questions, conducting focus groups, or commissioning a study by a market research group. Secondary market research is any information that is gathered by and from others, and usually refers to published studies or competitive market information that is commercially available. Since all market research has some bias, it is good to know something about polling and population statistics.

Is there a General Market Opportunity for Your Product?

In order to determine this, the entrepreneur must first consider something they may not believe—that potential customers may not be as enthused about their product as they think. One of the purposes of this exercise is to determine if a strong enough market exists for your product before you develop it. Most biotech entrepreneurs have a tendency to underestimate the market risk for their product because they view marketing too simplistically. Some individuals call this a "sanity check" since we tend to focus on identifying bits of data to confirm the things that we already believe. There are many ways to do this and everyone has different ways of validating if there is a real market opportunity. Suffice it to say that it would be advantageous to first start with the notion that individuals would *not* want to purchase or use your product, then identify information that may support that premise. Check out how prevalent the information is about the negative aspects of using your proposed product and see if this may prevent future wide-spread adoption. No doubt you will find some negativity, and this is helpful at the early stages as it can assist you in directing the technology to deliver the best set of features to overcome most of these issues. In the end your goal is to be sure that there is a true market opportunity for your future product and that the subsequent steps you take will not be in vain.

Who is Your Target Market and What is the Potential Total Market Size?

Your potential total market is different from your target market in that the total market is always much larger and it is what the potential could be with the ideal product and there were no competitors and everyone that should, would

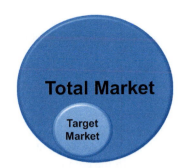

FIGURE 16.4   Total market versus target market.

want your product (See Figure 16.4). The total market is not an expectation of your future sales potential, but it does give a reference to how big a market is and how much commercial activity exists in that space. Your target market is a segment of the total market and it is identified by using various criteria discussed in the following section. Your target market will be the most homogeneous population of individuals who have the highest likelihood of initially purchasing and using your product. Market potential or market opportunity is considered to be all *potential* customers for a product. All companies and their investors would like to have the largest possible market for their product or service. Venture capital likes to see large market potentials for a biotechnology product, usually in the range of a billion dollars.

What are Your Target Market Demographics and What are Their Needs?

In order to answer this question we must review some additional tools used when defining a target market and their demographics. For the purposes of assessing who our target market would be, we need to understand the concept of segmentation.

Segmentation

No company can successfully market their product to every individual in the entire world, and every individual is not interested in purchasing your product. We must somehow divide the universe into homogeneous groups that can be reached economically with a similar message. Segmentation is how we approach and figure that out. Segmentation is the dividing of a large population into smaller customer groups based on similar needs, wants, desires, location, demographics, and purchasing habits. Segmentation allows you to identify groups of individuals that can be reasonably reached effectively because the more homogeneous the needs, wants, desires, and purchasing habits of a group, the more likely that segment will respond in a similar manner.

One of the best ways to utilize segmentation is to first know who the potential customers are for your product. This population of interested customers is rarely homogeneous but rather a conglomeration of individuals and groups

that you know have an interest in using your product. You begin segmenting this population to reduce them to the most homogeneous target market group of customers who would be the earliest and fastest adopters of your product. Your target market are potential users of your product with the highest motivation of all individuals to purchase or use a product. Without segmentation, it is impossible to target them appropriately. We segment populations of individuals by using at least three filters: geography, demographics, and behavior/usage. All of these filters may not be applicable to customers of every product because all segmentation factors may not be relevant.

Segmentation by Geographic Location

Segmentation by geography may or may not be applicable to your biotechnology product, but this is important to determine in the beginning. Some possible geographic segmentation issues could arise for services such as specialty infusion clinics. If this was the case, the customer base would be segmented by using some radius distance of the surrounding geography around all available infusion clinics. Other geographic segmentation might include transplantation services if an organ can only be transplanted at specific hospitals and if the recipients must be there within hours limiting the population of potential recipients. For the most part, usage of biotechnology products are less likely to be segmented by geography unless there are issues with worldwide markets and between countries based upon locations for manufacture, testing, or usage of a labile product or service. However, it is important to determine this at the outset.

Segmentation by Demographics

Demographic characteristics are easy to identify. These include qualities such as age, sex, family status, education level, income, occupation, and race. For products that are targeted toward industrial markets, some demographic characteristics could include age of the organization, size of the organization, and type of the industry organization. Biotechnology products targeting certain physician group practices may include demographic characteristics such as the practice specialty, the number of physicians in a practice, the number of patients seen per day/week/month/year, and the age of the practice and the age of the physicians.

Segmentation by Behavior and Usage

This can be the most difficult characteristic to identify, but often this is the most effective and the most successful means of market segmentation. This is because segmenting populations by demographics alone may not be specific enough and too broad since all customers of a particular age and gender do not have the same needs, desires, and wants. For instance all women aged 25 to 45 do not have allergies. Whereas segmenting populations by behavior *and* by demographics can target individuals with similar needs. For instance, when you segment by geography (areas with higher frequencies of pollen and mold) and include segmentation by family history of allergies, then include segmentation by age (say children between the ages of 6 and 12), you have specifically identified more homogeneous individuals with similar needs.

Patients can also be segmented by their preference for the usage of a type of medication and amount of expenditures in a particular medical category. There are many ways to use behavior and usage segmentation; it just requires that you find a method that is readily measured. Or sometimes a surrogate category is used if the real behavior pattern cannot be measured. Physicians can also be segmented by a number of prescribing and referral characteristics such as how frequently they prescribe a class of drugs, the frequency of ordering a diagnostic test, the frequency of using certain practice protocols for a particular disease, and how often and to whom they send referrals. Segmentation by behavior and usage is very powerful when coupled to other demographic criteria; however, just remember that the more detailed the segmentation, the smaller the target market, as these are opposing forces that expand or refine the segment.

What are Your Competition's Strengths and Weaknesses?

The first step is to identify who they are. If you are developing or considering developing a product where there are no direct competitors, such as is the case with many biotechnology products, don't forget to include 'substitutes.' These are products used by your future customers that "substitute" for the products they really want and need. You can be sure that if there are no direct competitors, there will be (inferior) substitutes that are used. If there are none, you seriously should reconsider if there really is a market need for your product? Because the greater the market need (in the absence of products that meet that need) there will be efforts by your future customers to use a variety of substitutes to

satisfy their need. In addition, customers must give up their substitutes when your product is available, and that is the essence of "competition." Also, do not forget to identify companies and basic research programs that are developing future products for your target market. Biotechnology product development is lengthy, therefore you must include these emerging activities in your assessment of future competition. Often these future competitors can be found in research literature, news publications about the developing opportunity, and through the company's press releases and their websites.

There are many aspects to consider about your competitors' strengths and weaknesses but we will only discuss one in this chapter, and that is *their product's features and benefits compared to yours and how much any of these align with the customer's needs.* Most biotechnology products are product innovations in some aspects and generally are not commodities, therefore the features and benefits that alignment with the customer's needs are most significant. However, in the Bio Agricultural sector, many of the products are commodities but the features and benefits they provide are novel. Therefore, the value still lies in the product's features and benefits and its alignment with the customer's needs. However, there is still pricing pressures because commodities cannot be priced too much higher than their competitors.

A helpful exercise is to begin with a matrix list of features and benefits that your product provides and that of your current or future competition, and substitutes. For example, if your product is a novel nonnarcotic pain medication, your matrix may look something like Table 16.1. Although you can add many other competitive values such as delivery, pricing, technical support, etc. I would encourage you to initially list only the features and benefits that most effectively meet the needs of the customer, and how it is better than your competitors and substitutes. Then rank these benefits on a scale of 1 to 5 with 1 being the worst and 5 being the best. This will help you determine how much superior your future product may be to the competition.

TABLE 16.1 Product Features and Benefits Matrix

Feature and Benefit	Your Product	Competitor 1	Competitor 2	Substitute 1
Relieves pain effectively at rating scale used	5	2	3	1
Requires only one dose daily	5	1	1	0
Fast acting within 1 hour	3	3	2	5
Long-term benefit after 2 weeks of use	5	3	3	1
No side-effect—Headache	4	1	3	5
No side-effect—Diarrhea	5	5	2	1

One note of caution: Do not build this matrix list based upon your *own* products features and benefits! Build this matrix list based upon the needs of the customers you are targeting. It is tempting to produce a list where your product has high rankings and the competition is inferior; but this is of no value if the features and benefits you describe have limited or no value to the customer. For instance, you may list as one feature and benefit a "10-year stability" and the others may score poorly. However, if there is no benefit to the *customer*, this is not a feature that has value to them. You can certainly include this "benefit" in an expanded matrix listing all values, as that could provide a financial value to the company in reducing the number of manufacturing runs. However, if it provides no value to the target market customer, omit it from this exercise.

OTHER MARKET TOOLS AND CONCEPTS

There are many other market tools that are essential for developing a sound market strategy, and some we want to discuss that are useful for the biotechnology entrepreneur and management team are described below. These include targeting, positioning, branding and developing future sales projections, or a pro forma.

Targeting

Targeting is everything that you do to narrow down the profile for the ideal customer. It is the next step after segmentation and it is the process of selecting *which* segment to target out of all these market segments that have been previously defined. Targeting allows you to focus and tailor your product values to the specific preferences of the best customer segment. Targeting is the rationale for choosing what market segment will be your best customers for purchasing and using your product. Targeting leads to the next step which is product positioning.

Positioning

Positioning is the way in which a company wants its target segment customers to view their product. Positioning is everything a company does to convey their product's value to the customer, and it is the way that their product solves the customer's problems. Positioning requires that you differentiate your product from other products in the market, otherwise all products will be grouped together if there is no difference in positioning. In order for potential customers to recognize your product, you have to position it in a way customers can differentiate it from all others. The more effective your product positioning, the easier it is for customers to understand your product's value to them.

Biotechnology products are positioned to associate its benefit, value, and solution to a patient's problems rather than just attributes of status, image, and the experiential benefit that

goes along with consumer products. Positioning has a lot to do with perception in the mind of the customer—you are positioning an image of value associated with your product. This is how a company creates a "brand," which we will discuss next.

Branding

Branding is often thought of as a logo, a company and product name, or a catchy phrase. However, that is not branding, but it is how companies *associate* a brand to themselves. Branding includes all the intangible attributes and thoughts in a person's mind that are associated with the company's logo, products, and other tangible aspects. Branding is more than just a product trade name and its recognizable product packaging—it is all the information evoked in the mind of the consumer when they encounter your product. Companies spend many years carefully creating a brand that suggests value in the minds of their customers. Companies sell products, but they are really marketing brands.

For biotechnology products, branding is strongly associated with the tangible medical benefit a product provides to the patient or physician or medical researcher. There are other factors that help create the brand value, and these can be enhanced if there is first a tangible medical benefit within the product. Brands convey messages about new products that an existing company develops, so it is important to determine what you want your brand to be and to manage that carefully.

Example of the Effect of a Brand

Although all companies have true capabilities to develop many types of products logically, it is important to be consistent with the brand you desire to create and the one that you have already created in the minds of customers. For instance Colgate decided to use its name on a number of food products called Colgate's Kitchen Entrees. Unfortunately, the product did not take off (see Figure 16.5). Anyone can guess what the images in the customer's minds may have been about the taste of these food items. The take-home lesson is that a brand is a powerful competitive strength and it is important to know the message it evokes in the minds of your customers.

Sales Projections Pro Forma or Management's Projections

Although this is not a tool, it is an essential component of a market strategy when building a biotechnology company and these projections will become a part of your business plan. By now you will have defined your total market potential in terms of customers and dollars, and identified your target market segment. Now you also need to project what portion of this market you anticipate your product will capture over the first 5 years of marketing. You may wonder, "Why is this important now if I am 3 to 5 years away from completing product development?" It is important because it makes you evaluate

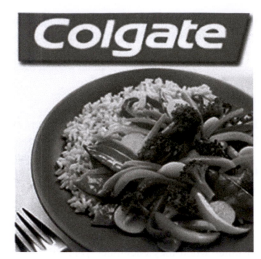

FIGURE 16.5 Power of a Brand: Colgate Kitchen Entrees.

how significantly you can (or you think you can) penetrate the market with your product. And, it is what your investors want to know to help determine if they are interested in investing in your company. In some cases, such as a biotherapeutic in discovery stages and 10 years away from potential commercialization, this exercise may not be essential yet, but irrespective, you should still have an appreciation for this process and understand the manner in which it is determined.

This financial projection is referred to as a "pro forma" or "sales projections". These projections are used to show the impact of your market strategy and the attractiveness of your product to your target market. There are two ways to develop a sales forecast, the first is the *top-down* approach and the other is a *bottom-up* approach. The top-down approach is a first approximation of potential market penetration. It is arrived at by taking the market potential and estimating a market penetration percentage based upon various assumptions including penetration rates by other companies in adjacent markets. The top-down approach is occasionally used to provide a general estimate of potential product revenue, but it is rarely taken too seriously because it is not built by the real drivers of demand. The bottom-up approach takes your key assumptions that are supported by data and builds a model based upon these and other quantified factors to estimate a resulting revenue stream.

For example, let's say your company is developing a diagnostic test for the rapid detection of ovarian cancer in women. Your market research demonstrates that the target market physicians for ordering your test will be OB/GYNs. There is more information that can refine your target market segment such as discussed in the segmentation section, but for now let's use all OB/GYNs. To develop a bottom-up financial pro forma, you will start with the total number of OB/GYNs in the country or geographic region you will be targeting. Let's say it is the United States and you find there are approximately 34,000 practicing OB/GYNs in the country. From your market

research you will know the average number of patients that one OB/GYN sees in a day, a week, a month, or a year. Your research can also tell you the age ranges of women who would likely be screened for ovarian cancer. Based upon your market strategy you can estimate the number of OB/GYNs that your technical sales can reach and recruit each year based upon a percent conversion rate per sales person per number of visits. This variable is influenced by the number of sales persons your company will hire in years 1, 2, 3, 4, and 5.

From this type of information and other key assumptions you can arrive at a plausible predictive model for your sales projections. By using the bottom-up approach, anyone can see what the key assumptions are and they can agree or disagree with any of them and you can make adjustments in your projections based upon these changes. A benefit of this method is that much of this information can be proven and demonstrated such as the number of OB/GYNs in the United States or the average number of patients that each one sees in a day, week, month, or year. Produce your revenue projections by both the bottom-up and the top-down method to arrive at the best estimates of revenue generation.

However, you should be forewarned, revenue projections are always viewed as suspect by investors because they have encountered too many instances in which entrepreneurs have produced extremely unrealistic projections. As a result, investors will rightly discount sales projections in a business plan. Unfortunately, there is no way to overcome this bias in potential investors. The best approach is to provide your key assumption and support for them, then show investors that the projections are supported with solid data and logic. Sometimes there is no data available to support a particular assumption. In this situation you can draw parallels from other markets or products; just be sure to acknowledge that these are limitations and provide the reasons you believe that the estimates are reasonable. Do not make unrealistic assumptions or provide unsupported conclusions—poor assumptions undermine your credibility in the eyes of investors.

Lastly, when building a pro forma, it is a good idea to have a worst-case scenario—one in which some of the key assumptions are not met for one reason or another. If you do not build in a worst-case scenario, and you are off in your projections, and you have not reached profitability, you may run out of money or be forced to take a lowered valuation to raise capital at an unexpected time. Build your pro forma projections using the bottom-up approach then include an additional worst-case scenario, and you will have the best estimates for your sales projections and your investors will have more confidence in your judgment.

STARTING TO DEVELOP A MARKET STRATEGY

In this section I have listed five steps to help you begin formulating a marketing strategy. There are obviously more aspects to building a marketing strategy than just these, but this will help you get started on your own marketing plan. For this process you will use much of the market research information you previously gathered and include some other important aspects such as market channels.

1. Determine Your Potential Market Size

The potential market for your product is the largest group of customers that could conceivably purchase or use your product at some time. As previously discussed, we calculate the total market opportunity for your product in terms of customers or patients (if it is in healthcare) and in dollars. The total market size represents your total market potential but it is not your sales projections. Rarely does any company's product sales approach capturing the entire market due to many limitations, including your competition.

For example, if your product is a new influenza nasal spray vaccine, since influenza is a disease that potentially affects all individuals, we would take the United States population of 314 million people and multiply that number by the price of the vaccine. Let's presume a similar but slightly higher price of $40 per vaccination—this would be a $12.6 billion market in the United States. If we calculated a UK market we would use 63 million people times $40 per person or a $2.5 billion market. For a world-wide total market we would do the same. Refinements can be made easily as needed. For instance, since we do not vaccinate infants and children under 6 months of age, we can easily exclude that population from the total market size.

In another example, if you are estimating the total market for a monoclonal antibody therapeutic that increases blood flow to an ischemic artery immediately after cardiac arrest, you would find the total number of heart attack victims per year is 920,000 (in the United States) multiplied by the estimated price of your product (presume for now at $2000); therefore the total U.S. market size would be $1.8 billion annually. For some products it is not that easy, but there are other ways to determine potential total market size such as evaluating your competitors' potential market if you have competition. If you do not have competition you can calculate the potential total market size based upon the substitute products. An important point is that you do not use actual sales of competitors or alternative products because this is not the total market potential. In this exercise you are estimating the *potential* market that could be reached with an ideal product without any competition. Most total market potential estimates are determined using demographic data.

There can be other factors included when estimating a total potential market such as the frequency of use. If your product is a diagnostic test for upper respiratory infections, and market research shows that individuals get an average of 1.7 upper respiratory infections each year, you will multiply the applicable population times the infection frequency times the product price, to arrive at the total potential market size.

One good reason we estimate the total potential market is because investors want to know if your market is large enough to support their investment and can provide them the type of return they desire. Most VC investors like to see total market potentials that exceed $1 billion annually. For instance, it would be foolish for a VC investor to put $30 million into a company if the total market potential for that product was $25 million annually.

2. Identify and Define Your Target Market Segment

Next you want to determine who is your best customer. This is a subset of your total market potential and represents the first group that you will target who has the highest likelihood of purchasing or using your product. To identify your target market segment you will use the segmentation filters described, such as geography, demographics, and behavior and usage. We are seeking homogeneous groups that have similar wants and needs regarding your product. This becomes the group with the greatest need and desire for your product and it represents the population that you must capture first in order to reach more of your potential market later.

A properly segmented target market is easier to reach than the entire potential market because the target market has many similarities and common behaviors. Products must be able to first capture their target market segment before companies can target other markets. Your target market is the most homogeneous group of individuals with similar wants, needs, and desires as it pertains to your product. Your target market segment is the first group from which you will build your market base.

As an example, let's say your product is a genetic test to determine a woman's predisposition to breast cancer, but for those without a family history of the disease. You have determined that insurance will not reimburse the patient for this genetic test, yet you still believe there is a market for it from self-paying customers. You have segmented your market through demographic and behavior characteristics and have concluded that this group has similar motivations and behaviors that it would be highly likely for them to purchase your test. So the target market segment for this genetic predisposition test would have the following characteristics:

- Women (demographic segmentation)
- Ages 40 to 69 (demographic segmentation)
- With household incomes greater than $75,000 annually (demographic segmentation)
- Seeking mammography services annually (behavior and usage segmentation).

3. Describe Your Product's Value Proposition for Your Target Market and Identify Your Competitor's

Now that you have identified your target market segment you must articulate what your value proposition is to these customers. This is what we previously described as positioning. A value proposition contains the reasons that your product is so valuable to the customer that it will make them want to purchase and use your product. In order to identify your value proposition you first want to list your product's benefits to your target market. Some helpful questions are:

- What are the features and benefits of your product that are of great value to your target market customer?
- What unmet needs are now met by your target market customers when they use your product?
- How does your target market customer benefit by using your product?
- What are the compelling points-of-difference between your product and your competition?

Simultaneously, you must also examine what value your competition or substitute products provide your target market customers. Substitute products are a form of inferior competition but you still need to determine how, in whatever way, they are meeting the needs of your customers. Compare and contrast your product to these competitors and substitutes. Determine what are the valuable points-of-differentiation between your product and competitive or substitute products.

Do not forget that for biotechnology products you have three customers and you will need a specific value proposition for each one. For the patient, some of the benefits may be related to values such as less pain, faster acting, and improved health. For the physician, some benefits may be related to values such as lower risk of adverse events and fewer complications. For the payer, some benefits may be related to pharmacoeconomic or cost benefit, quality-of-life, and survival benefit.

One example of a possible value proposition statement for the genetic predisposition test for nonfamilial breast cancer could be: genetic testing, when coupled to an actionable plan, can prevent breast cancer, or catch it at the earliest possible stages where long-term survival is the greatest.

4. Identify the Best Market Channel to Reach Your Target Market Segment

Although we did not discuss how to identify potential market channels in the previous section, it is an important component of an overall market strategy for reaching your target market segment. Market channels are the methods you will use to gain access to your target market segment customers and the way they will gain access to your product. It

is the path that the product takes to reach your customers. There are "direct market channels" where the company sells products directly to customers. There are "intermediary market channels," or third-parties, that sell and deliver your products to customers. There are "dual-distribution market channels" where you have more than one distribution method to get products to your customers. Then there are "reverse channels" that go from consumer to intermediary and then to the customer. This is the case for human blood products such as blood, plasma, platelets, and passive immunoglobulin.

All biotech products will reach their customers via some market channel and depending on what sector of biotechnology your product is in, you may not sell your product directly to the end user. Find what your best, most effective, and strategic market channel is for your product to reach your customers. Having an effective market channel is a competitive strength for your product.

Do not propose to build a new market channel as part of your market strategy, although this has been done by some biotechnology companies such as Amgen, Genentech, Genzyme, and Genomic Health. Find ways to leverage existing market channels. There are usually good market channels available to reach your target market, so pursue these first rather than developing your own. Consider collateral and alternative usages of existing market channels that are mutually beneficial to you and your partners. Ideally, you will want to leverage existing market channels because it will take time for the development of a new market channel, which is also a new market risk.

5. Validate and Refine Your Market Strategy

All marketing plans are intriguing theories but they are only good if they work for your product. Therefore, you will want to test your market strategy and your market assumptions in some way to see if they are viable and accurate.

There are endless ways you can validate your market strategy. You can hire a consultant to help, you can interview option leaders in this market, or you can hire a contract research organization (CRO) to conduct independent primary market research to see if it supports each of the assumptions you have made in your market strategy. Another way to validate the market is to test the market receptivity for your product. Market tests can be difficult and expensive to conduct, but they can provide good information and feedback to validate or refine your original market strategy. Your goal is to find some way to validate whether or not if your assumptions about your target market wanting your product are correct.

The market strategy you develop will be incorporated into your business plan. It will be modified over time and refinements will be made as you encounter obstacles and receive new information. The exercise described here will help you get started developing your own market strategy for your product using established market methods and tools.

IDENTIFY YOUR MARKET DEVELOPMENT MILESTONES

Market development milestones are important for your company in demonstrating progress in your market strategy. Just as you will have value-enhancing product development milestones, you need to identify your market development milestones. There is great diversity in marketing strategy so formulate your market development milestones with your specific product in mind. These milestones serve the same purpose as your product development milestones in that, when they are reached, they reduce the risk of your organization and they most likely will improve your company valuation.

Some examples of market development milestones could include:

- Define your target market segment.
- Determine your target market segment needs and wants and your points-of-differentiation from your competitors and substitutes.
- Complete a primary research study to validate your target market segment needs.
- Finalize your value proposition for your product to your target market customers.
- Develop and implement a branding strategy for your product and company.
- Determine product pricing.
- Complete a pharmacoeconomic assessment for your product when used in your target market.
- Conduct primary research on reimbursement codes and private insurance likelihood of reimbursement.
- Identify and secure your distribution channels for your product.
- Secure international marketing partners.

BIOTECHNOLOGY PRODUCT ADOPTION CURVE

Market adoption of biotechnology products can have many challenges because of the complexity, limited understanding of the technology, uncertainty of utility, high costs, and other factors. For those interested in understanding more about issues with technology adoption, I highly recommend *Crossing the Chasm* by Geoffrey Moore. Although his book mostly references the computer and IT industry, the adoption curve is virtually the same for biotechnology products.

The adoption stages of a target market can be subclassified into groups of individuals based upon their speed of adopting new technology.

These subcategories of individuals are ordered and labeled as: innovators, early adopters, early majority, late majority, and laggards. The first to adopt are considered innovators, followed by early adopters and a chasm to cross in order to reach the early majority and the rest of the market. Recognize that even with the best and most ideal market strategy, wide-spread product adoption will still require persistence, creativity, and adaptability in order to penetrate a market with even the best of biotechnology products.

SUMMARY

A marketing strategy is a carefully thought-out plan for how your product will bring value to, and reach its best customers. This strategy is based upon both primary and secondary market research and a segmentation analysis defining your target market which is the most homogeneous group of individuals having the highest likelihood of purchasing or using your product.

A marketing strategy is developed long before you are able to sell any product and it is a vital component of your business strategy. Be sure that your market plan is well thought-out and built upon solid data and logical with supported assumptions, not presumptions. Spend plenty of time and effort developing a solid market plan. Understand the market issues, your competitors, and substitutes; know your value proposition to your target market, and refine your market strategy as you learn new information. Unless the entrepreneur is an experienced marketing executive from a successful biotechnology or pharmaceutical company, you will need help in developing a marketing strategy. This is not an area of business in which you should pinch pennies because developing a good marketing strategy will pay for itself over time. Venture capital partners can quickly identify a poorly developed and unsupported marketing strategy.

A young biotechnology company having a solid marketing plan for their product not only helps in raising capital but also demonstrates that the entrepreneur understands the market issues. A good market development plan with milestones is equally valuable for success as is product development milestones. Don't forget that biotechnology products must meet the needs of all three of its customers in order for it to be successful, therefore you will need a value proposition for each of these stakeholders. Successful entrepreneurs demonstrate to their investors that they understand their market risks and embrace a plan to manage these risks. Your marketing strategy is an essential component of your business plan and it is a key factor in raising capital for your company.

Chapter 17

Biotechnology Product Coverage, Coding, and Reimbursement Strategies

Robert E. Wanerman, JD, MPH*a and Susan Garfield, DrPH**

*Epstein Becker Green, P.C., Washington, D.C., **Sr. Vice President, GfK Custom Research LLC, Wayland, Massachusetts

Bringing a new drug, biological, medical device, or diagnostic to market is an arduous process that can take years, cost tens of millions of dollars, and requires compliance with multiple regulatory processes. Even though inventors, investigators, manufacturers, and investors are focused on the clearance or approval of a new product by the Food and Drug Administration (FDA) or other National Regulatory Authorities (NRA) outside the United States, a successful strategy for commercializing that new products must also look beyond these regulatory agencies. Even at an early stage of development, overlooking the reimbursement processes that come into play after FDA or other national authority approval can mean the difference between ultimate success and failure. For smaller companies, a failure to develop a strategy for obtaining coverage, coding, and reimbursement can mean the difference between attracting investors and not obtaining funding at all. For a large company, the lack of a strategy can diminish or eliminate the expected return on investment. This chapter will explain these reimbursement processes. Although the challenges for each product may be different, understanding the mechanics of coverage, coding, and reimbursement is essential for identifying the issues and evaluating any potential options.

UNDERSTANDING REIMBURSEMENT AND CODING OF BIOTECHNOLOGY PRODUCTS IN THE UNITED STATES[b]

At the outset, a commercialization strategy must recognize the distinctions between the FDA regulatory framework and the regulatory processes that come into play once a product is cleared or approved for sale. Under the Federal Food, Drug, and Cosmetic Act (FDCA), the FDA's authority covers the manufacture and marketing of drugs, biologicals, medical devices, and diagnostics [1]. Since it only regulates the actions of manufacturers, its actions do not dictate the practice of medicine and do not on their own regulate the actions of third-party payers such as health plans and government programs including Medicare and Medicaid. As a result, the fact of FDA approval or clearance is a first step, but incidental to the coverage, coding, and reimbursement decisions made by third-party payers, and is not a dispositive factor [2]. Accordingly, developing a commercialization strategy should be a part of the initial planning phases to avoid significant delays in bringing the product to market [3].

A commercialization strategy in the United States market is complicated by the fact that the entities that develop a new technology and commercialize it are often not the entities that file reimbursement claims with health plans or programs. Instead, manufacturers sell products to providers or suppliers who then submit claims to health plans or programs in accordance with the reimbursement methodology that applies to the particular site of service. This problem can be illustrated in Figure 17.1.

In order to navigate through this post-FDA regulatory landscape, three fundamental concepts must be defined and understood to avoid costly errors once the organization has developed an idea. Coverage refers to terms and conditions under which a private or public health plan will pay for an item or service [4]. Coverage is not guaranteed once the FDA approves or clears a product, and a favorable coverage determination does not guarantee a particular level of reimbursement [5]. The coverage analysis typically involves a three-part inquiry:

1. Does the new technology fit into an existing benefit category?
2. Is the new technology excluded by law or by the plan's express terms?
3. Does the new technology satisfy the plan's "reasonable and necessary" or "medically necessary" criteria?

---

a. Robert E. Wanerman is a partner in the Washington, D.C. office of Epstein Becker Green, P.C. The discussion in the chapter does not constitute legal advice, as the facts and circumstances of a particular matter may involve questions of law that are not addressed here.

b. This first part of this chapter is written by Robert Wanerman.

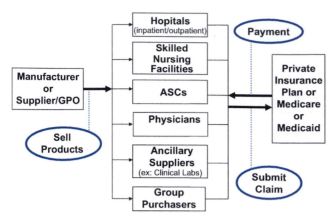

FIGURE 17.1   The United States medical reimbursement system.

Each element of this inquiry can involve significant barriers. The threshold benefit category question can usually be answered by looking to the law establishing the health benefit in the case of government-funded programs, or to a private plan's contract. For example, under the original Medicare program, screening tests such as those for colorectal cancer or glaucoma did not fit into a defined benefit category, and only became covered after Congress amended the statute to create a new screening benefit [6]. Some items such as traditional hearing aids or some forms of cosmetic surgery may be excluded by law or contract [7]. In a small number of cases, state law may mandate coverage for specific items and services in private plan offerings in their state. This is the case with 35 states and the District of Columbia that require coverage for patient costs associated with cancer clinical trials [8]. Finally, even if there is no express inclusion or exclusion, all items and services are subject to the general rule that they must meet a test for medical necessity, sometimes stated as a "reasonable and necessary" standard [9]. The conundrum for developers or investors is that this residual criterion is often undefined or vaguely defined, leaving it a moving target [10]. The converse is that it gives plans a high degree of discretion. Sometimes this discretion is exercised in a measured form. For example, some plans may initially approve coverage for a new technology or treatment only after conventional treatments have been tried and failed; in other situations, the item or service might not be covered unless quantifiable diagnostic prerequisites have been met [11]. In other cases, coverage determinations may turn on data showing improved outcomes using well-defined metrics [12].

The definition of coverage may also be subject to geographic variation. Although some large health plans may operate in multiple states, it should not be presumed that the plan's coverage will be uniform nationwide. Even the Medicare program, which was established by federal law and is administered by a federal agency, may have conflicting coverage policies in different jurisdictions due to the authority delegated to individual contractors to develop local coverage determinations

for those items and services where there is neither a statutory mandate nor a national coverage determination [13].

The second basic concept is coding. Codes and code sets are the way that the delivery of health care is identified, monitored, and ultimately paid by third-party plans. Code sets exist for, among other things, diagnoses, procedures, medical devices and supplies, and bundles of direct and indirect costs incurred in furnishing treatment. A code on its own does not guarantee either coverage or a desired reimbursement rate. The control of the relevant code sets in the United States is decentralized, as shown in Figure 17.2.

For example, the Current Procedural Terminology (CPT) code set that defines work done by physicians and other health professionals is controlled by the American Medical Association's (AMA's) CPT editorial panel with input from specialty societies, while a second AMA panel, the AMA/Specialty Society Relative Value Scale Update Committee (RUC) develops relative value recommendations to the Centers for Medicare and Medicaid Services (CMS) that, if adopted, set the reimbursement rate under the Medicare program for new CPT codes. For supplies and equipment used by physicians other health professionals, the relevant code set is the Healthcare Common Procedure Coding System (HCPCS), which is controlled by CMS with input from health plans. The process for obtaining a new code can differ among the various code sets, as does the timing of coding decisions—while the CPT process spans 2 years, the Healthcare Common Procedure Coding System (HCPCS) codes are updated on an annual cycle.

Due to the importance of codes to a commercialization strategy, stakeholders need to define the codes that apply to a new product or service using that product as well as technology in the site(s) of service where it will be used. For example, while an office-based procedure may be defined by a single diagnosis code and a single CPT code or family of CPT codes, an inpatient

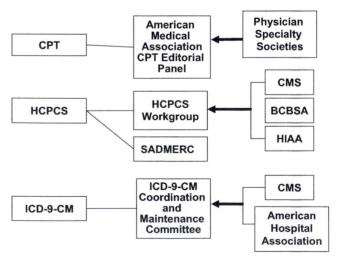

FIGURE 17.2   Process for codes used for procedures, items, and diagnoses.

procedure such as a joint replacement may involve coordinating diagnosis codes, CPT codes for physician services, and diagnosis-related group (DRG) codes for the hospital's services. Regardless of the number of codes involved in furnishing care to an individual patient, a code is, by itself, not a guarantee of coverage or payment [14]. The process of determining the correct code(s) for a new technology often includes an analysis of whether or not existing codes are sufficient to capture all of the features of that technology. However, if the existing codes are inadequate, the stakeholders may have to consider the case for creating a new code based on clinical and resource distinctions, as well as the time and effort needed to petition the coding authorities to add a new code.

The third fundamental concept is understanding the payment methodologies that apply to a particular item or service in a specific site of service. Starting from a historical model in which all items and services were paid individually on a piecework basis, health plans and government agencies have developed multiple methodologies tailored to the site of service. Depending on the site of service and the individual plan policies, payment may be made for an item or service individually, or as part of a larger bundle. Even when the payment is bundled, certain items or services may be excluded from the bundle and are separately billable; this is the case with many physicians' services that are furnished to inpatients or outpatients. In addition, the amount of payment for the same service can vary among different sites of service due to factors such as indirect costs and overhead. For example, the Medicare program assumes that when the same service is performed in an ambulatory surgical center and a hospital outpatient department, the latter will have higher overhead and labor costs and sets a higher reimbursement rate for the hospital [15]. As a result, if an existing code fits the technology, stakeholders will want to know if the resulting reimbursement associated with that code under relevant fee schedules makes it economically feasible for professionals and other users to adopt that new technology. If existing codes do not fit and a new code is warranted, the analysis shifts to a consideration of whether the data supports establishing a desirable reimbursement rate for that new code that will lead to the adoption of the technology.

The type and amount of payment a provider or supplier receives may be subject to additional thresholds or limitations, including the use of relative value scales, payment caps or ceilings, and existing payment methods and rates for comparable items and services. Depending on the facts and circumstances, one option is to fit a new technology or product into the existing coverage, coding, and reimbursement terms for a product in the same class. However, if the new technology can be considered a breakthrough or a complementary product that improves overall outcomes or results in other improvements in patient care, accepting the status quo may not be an optimal business decision. For those new technologies that substantially alter the overall cost of care, the health plan may not be able to redefine immediately or revalue a bundled payment to allow the adoption of that new technology. In these limited cases, payers such as the Medicare program will approve payment for the new technology as an "add-on" cost or as a pass-through payment while data on the new technology is compiled and the bundled payment can be reviewed [16].

THE ANALYTICAL FRAMEWORK FOR NEW TECHNOLOGIES

Regardless of the type of product or technology or the path followed by a developer of a new medical technology, once the new product is ready for testing in a clinical trial there should be a companion strategy for commercializing the product focusing on coverage, coding, and reimbursement. If the funding for the basic research and proof of the concept through a clinical trial comes from private sources, the approval of that funding (or future funding) may turn on the ability of the new product to generate a return on that investment through the three fundamental concepts described above. Therefore, the process of designing a clinical trial to prove a concept may have to be broader than just obtaining the information necessary to meet the FDA's criteria for approval or clearance. By integrating the types of outcome data that payers rely on into the trial a sponsor can save the considerable time, effort, and cost of conducting a second trial to obtain the type of information that payers will demand in order to make coverage and reimbursement determinations. This section will focus on the variables that need to be considered in crafting a commercialization strategy that is tailored to a particular item or service.

DEFINING THE TERMS OF COVERAGE

As discussed above, absent a precise statutory directive most health plans have wide discretion in determining which items and services will be covered. The Medicare statute states that items and services will be covered if they are "reasonable and necessary for the diagnosis or treatment of illness or injury," but does not explain the meaning of this term in more detail [17]. Some commercial plans rely on a general notion of medical necessity and accepted standards of practice, but they do not elaborate further [18]. In selected cases, items and services may be subject to a more rigorous evaluation process that examines improvements in outcomes and the relative benefits when compared to existing treatments [19].

Unless the terms of coverage (or an exclusion from coverage) are unambiguously defined by law or by binding policies, the threshold inquiry in developing a coverage, coding, and reimbursement strategy is to identify the type and quality of information and data that may be needed to obtain a favorable coverage determination. This analysis can be broken down to a set of basic questions:

- Does the item or service meet a plan's benefit categories or inclusion criteria?
- If professional practice guidelines exist, is the item or service consistent with those guidelines?
- Does the item or service fill an unmet clinical need?
- Who will benefit from the item or service; is it primarily one group (children or seniors), or is the benefit widely distributed?
- What is the anticipated site of service (e.g., inpatient, outpatient, office, or clinic)?
- What is (are) the expected clinical outcome(s)?
- If there are comparable covered items or services, does the new technology result in better outcomes?
- If the new technology is complex or is expected to be expensive, can it be positioned as a second-line therapy?
- Have relevant professional societies adopted the new technology as a part of their practice guidelines or other formal statements?
- Is there a potential for coverage for "off-label" indications?
- Are there any existing limits on the frequency of service(s)?
- What is the expected financial impact for the payer/consumer (ex: will adoption of the new item or service raise or lower the aggregate cost of care)?
- Are there other immediate or long-term benefits?

In answering these questions, innovators and other stakeholders should understand the existing scope of coverage. While the natural tendency is to seek coverage for any and all applications, the coverage for other competing items and services may be limited to specific clinical conditions, specific locations, or may be covered only if a first-line treatment has been tried but failed to produce results.

After these basic questions are answered, the next phase in the analysis involves a closer look at the existing environment. This may have been done in order to understand whether or not there are any potential competitors, but assuming that competitors exist, the next step is to determine if the new item or service is distinguishable and whether or not that will have any impact on coverage. One critical factor in defining the relevant coverage standard is how the item or service can be compared to other treatments for a given condition. Depending on the nature and scope of the innovation, it may be classified as (1) a breakthrough for patient health that fills a gap in treatment options or offers a treatment where none previously existed; (2) something that replaces an existing item or service; or (3) a product that adds or extends an existing technology or procedure.

Another practical consideration in developing a coverage strategy is the pace of adoption of the new technology. In a paper published in 2000, it was estimated that the average time for published clinical trial data to be translated into general medical practice was 17 years [20]. While that lag time may be shorter today for innovators and other stakeholders in new technologies, the rate of adoption of new items and services can be a significant factor in planning market entry. That rate can be highly variable from health plan to health plan; in the case of an assay used to assist in the treatment of breast cancer, the earliest adopters agreed to provide coverage approximately 1 year after the product's launch while the last adopters took up to an additional 6 years to approve coverage; the median time here was 3 years [21].

Identifying the Type and Quality of Data to Support Coverage

In the current health care environment, regardless of the pace of adoption, outcomes evidence is a paramount concern for health plans and other payers [22]. For investigators, manufacturers, and other stakeholders, identifying the type of data needed to make the strongest case for coverage can be a conundrum given the ambiguity and discretion given to health plans to make coverage determinations. The burden is usually placed on the applicant, and the type of data needed to support coverage differs from the data submitted to the FDA to meet the safe and effective standard under the Federal Food, Drug, and Cosmetic Act (FDCA). The shift toward evidence-based medical policy therefore relies on published, peer reviewed studies with sufficient statistical power to establish a given treatment hypothesis, commonly over a long term [23]. While this would call for large randomized, double-blinded studies in all circumstances, this ideal may have to be tempered by practical or ethical considerations that make other acceptable study designs feasible for their intended purpose. As a result, while it may be appropriate to conduct a drug trial involving one arm where a subject receives a placebo, in a device trial involving an implant or an invasive procedure there may be unacceptable and unethical risks if the subjects with the control arm are subjected to a sham surgical procedure; moreover, even if these hurdles could be overcome, a significant number of prospective subjects may refuse to participate under those terms, thwarting any attempt to enroll a sufficient number of subjects to ensure adequate statistical power after an expected number of dropouts. In these cases, other acceptable study designs such as case-control studies may be necessary in order to obtain any useful information at all.

Once a decision about the type of optimal study design has been made, the next step will likely involve defining the population to be studied. The Medicare program and some private payers may demand that the study population match their beneficiaries or covered lives so that the outcomes data are more accurate. This issue was central to the Medicare National Coverage Determination denying coverage for virtual colonoscopies using CT imaging [24]. Although many private health plans did offer limited coverage for CT colonographies, CMS focused its evidence review on how CT colonography compared to optical colonoscopy in the Medicare population, of whom the majority are over the age of 65. It concluded that the available evidence was deficient in part because the published studies contained only a few subjects who were eligible for Medicare, and because CMS could not determine if the results of CT colonography in younger subjects could be applied to the Medicare population [25].

A separate but related coverage issue that should be addressed arises when a new technology has multiple applications, but either the available data or the data that is anticipated is weaker for some potential applications. In these cases, the sponsor or stakeholders will need to make a business decision to focus on the one indication with the best chances for success rather than risk rejection of a request for broader coverage.

Regardless of the type of clinical data that is available or that can be obtained in a clinical trial, the presentation of that data can be enhanced through the participation of professional organizations or thought leaders in a particular specialty who can help bridge the gap between an entity seeking to commercialize an innovation and the health plans who may rely solely on the data before them. The assistance from such physician-champions can assist in educating payers and explain the reasons why a new technology should be adopted from a clinician's point of view.

The evolution of coverage into a detailed evidence-driven process begs an important question: what if this pathway will not work in an individual case? In other words, is there any middle ground between coverage or noncoverage? In a small number of cases, the new technology or a related service may have promising outcomes and hold out the prospect of cost savings but may lack the quantity or quality of data that would otherwise support a fully favorable determination. In these cases, CMS and some other payers may approve coverage on a temporary basis, typically conditioned on a manufacturer or other stakeholder agreeing to conduct additional acceptable clinical trials or establish a registry and furnish the data to be collected to the payer or plan. After a set time period, the plan can make a permanent coverage decision. In the Medicare program, this has been known as coverage with evidence development and can take one of two forms: (1) coverage with appropriateness determination, where additional clinical data is required to ensure that the item or service is being provided to appropriate beneficiaries according to established clinical criteria, and (2) coverage with study participation, where conditional coverage and reimbursement is approved subject to the enrollment of affected individuals in a clinical trial that is expected to generate sufficient data in a clinical

trial registry to allow CMS to make a final coverage determination [26].

Defining the Coding to Define the Innovation

The introduction of a new technology can have disruptive effects on the delivery of a particular treatment or therapy. One aspect of that disruption is how a provider or supplier captures the use of that technology and attempts to obtain payment. In the absence of a defined code or reimbursement rate, several interim solutions are possible, albeit with varying degrees of risk. First, a provider or supplier may submit claims using a miscellaneous code for procedures or items not otherwise defined in the relevant code set. This allows the provider, supplier, or manufacturer to negotiate a reimbursement rate. In the short run, it allows for some form of payment until a new code and a defined reimbursement rate can be established. There are several key drawbacks to this approach: claims may have to be submitted manually, reimbursement rates can vary significantly among payers, and establishing a database of payments for future use if a new code is approved may be complicated. A second option that has been used for some diagnostics is to break down the steps of the new technology and where possible assign an existing code to each step, resulting in a sequence of multiple codes in a single claim—often referred to as a "stack"—that when assembled capture all of the resources that went into the service. Once again, the benefit in the short run is that there is a positive cash flow, at the expense of an imperfect claims database to establish a reimbursement rate in the long term. In more egregious cases involving claims submitted to government-funded programs, there is always a risk that unbundling a procedure for any reason could trigger investigations and potential liability under health care fraud laws, particularly the False Claims Act [27].

What if the new technology, or a service using that technology, cannot be defined using an existing code? Once again, although there are well-defined processes for obtaining new codes, they can be cumbersome and time-consuming, and the standards for approval of a new code can be vague. For example, although the HCPCS Workgroup has developed a decision tree for code requests, the criteria applied for each step are not always transparent [28]. Similarly, while the CPT Editorial Panel has published criteria for new procedure codes, there is a wide degree of latitude in applying those criteria [29]. In general, the entities that control code sets will rely on technological distinctions, clinical improvement, and whether or not the new item or service requires a different or more intense mix of resources to deliver a service. If this is the best option for a manufacturer or stakeholder, the strategy must also factor in the lag period between a coding application and any new code: new CPT codes are assigned on a 2-year cycle and HCPCS codes follow a 1-year cycle.

POSITIONING THE PRODUCT FOR FAVORABLE REIMBURSEMENT

All of the work to obtain a favorable coverage determination and a fair coding assignment leads to the last and crucial step in commercializing any new product or service using that new product: what will health plans pay for the item or service? As with coverage and coding, this portion of the analysis does not exist in a vacuum without relevant information as a guide. As with the earlier parts of determining a commercialization strategy, several basic questions should be considered:

- What are the code(s) for similar items or services?
- What is the reimbursement methodology for the relevant site(s) of service for the new item or service?
- What is the range of reimbursement for those existing codes?
- Is that range acceptable, or are there quantative or qualitative distinctions between the current standard of care and the new technology that may justify a higher reimbursement rate?

As discussed above, the term "reimbursement" does not refer to a single concept. Depending on the site of service, reimbursement may refer to a payment amount for the new item or service on a stand-alone basis, or may refer to the same item or service as part of a bundled payment to the provider or supplier of services to an individual patient. These bundles can have different names such as a diagnosis-related group for inpatient hospital services and an ambulatory payment classification for outpatient or ambulatory surgical center services, but they typically include all items and services needed to treat a particular condition (as designated by procedure code(s) or a discharge diagnosis code) except for professional fees that are claimed separately. The actual rate for a particular condition is commonly determined based on historical claims data that is trended forward, with adjustments for variables such as case-mix intensity and relative labor costs [30]. Therefore, once all of these questions have been answered then a reimbursement strategy can begin to take shape. One potential risk for manufacturers of medical devices and diagnostics is that if FDA clearance is based on substantial equivalence under Section 501(k) of the FDCA, some health plans may attempt to apply the same code and reimbursement rate for the predicate product to the new technology. If this threatens the commercialization of the product, the rebuttal to any such proposal would have to be based on data showing superior clinical outcomes or a different cost basis. Regardless of the setting, if payment is made on a bundled basis, the manufacturer or other stakeholder must examine both its cost of doing business as well as the economic constraints placed on the provider or supplier purchasing the new product. For the prospective purchaser, the switch to a new technology may involve a trade-off between the higher cost of adopting a new technology and the expected relative efficiencies or improved outcomes that are expected. If the new technology lowers costs and improves outcomes, adoption is easy; however, if the provider's or supplier's overall costs rise too dramatically, then it may not be able to adopt the new technology without incurring losses on each patient treated. The strategy may become more complicated if the shift to the new technology also affects any related professional fee, as may be the case with implanted medical devices. In these cases, the total service must make economic sense to the facility and to the physician, who is likely to be sensitive to changes in the time and effort required to perform procedures using the new technology and how that is reflected in the applicable CPT code for that service.

Putting the Pieces of the Puzzle Together

Developing a successful commercialization strategy for a new technology, or for services using that technology requires that the coverage, coding, and reimbursement pieces fall into place. Due to the number of variables discussed in this chapter, innovators and stakeholders should anticipate some challenges and should expect that the path will be different for each new product. Coordinating and executing each part of a commercialization strategy takes patience, perseverance, excellent information, help from others, and good timing. Although these processes are difficult, thoughtful planning can be an essential tool for meeting these challenges.

EUROPEAN REIMBURSEMENT SYSTEMS OVERVIEW[c]

In Europe, reimbursement and pricing is determined on a country-by-country basis, leading to significant variations in system design, cost, and coverage. Additionally, each country has the ability to control reimbursement at the national, regional, or local level. As can be seen in Figure 17.3, significant variation in pricing, health technology assessment (HTA), and reimbursement negotiation processes exist across countries in Europe.

Regulatory Backdrop

The European Medicines Agency (EMA) is responsible for reviewing and approving all drug products sold in Europe through a centralized process. Based in London and operating as a decentralized scientific agency of the European Union, the Agency is responsible for coordinating the EU's safety-monitoring or "pharmacovigilance" system for medicines. Specifically, it coordinates the evaluation and

---

c. This second part of this chapter is written by Susan Garfield.

	National Price Negotiation	Price Referencing	IPR	National HE Evaluation	Regional HE Evaluation	Local Price Negotiation
France	✓	✓	✓	✓	✓	✓
Germany	✓	✓	✓	✓		✓
Italy	✓	✓	✓	✓	✓	✓
Spain	✓	✓	✓	✓	✓	✓
England	✓			✓	✓	✓
Scotland				✓	✓	✓
Wales				✓		✓

FIGURE 17.3 Variability in pricing, health technology assessment (HTA) and reimbursement in Europe.

monitoring of centrally authorized products and national referrals, develops technical guidance, and provides scientific advice to sponsors [31].

While drugs must go through the EMA to receive market authorization, diagnostics and devices go through a different process. These types of technologies require a CE-Mark from the European Commission, though many tests can be used prior to or without regulatory approval through a laboratory-developed test pathway. In the case of medical technologies, the CE mark denotes a product's compliance with relevant EU legislation and directives and enables commercialization of the product within the European Union.

HEALTH TECHNOLOGY ASSESSMENT (HTA)

Once a product has received marketing authorization, the reimbursement process begins. In many countries, prior to pricing and coverage, a product must go through a formal health technology assessment (HTA) process. HTAs systematically examine the short- and long-term health and cost consequences of using a specific technology or set of technologies [32]. The consequences that are considered within a HTA include the direct medical, organizational, economic, and societal impact of use to a given health system. Individuals involved in HTAs in Europe include clinical specialists, economists, policy makers, and statisticians. HTA groups use a variety of methods to consider the comparative impact use that a technology will have to affected populations. HTA analyses typically reflect a specific country's or region's perspective, including disease burden, demographics, and costs.

Elements of a national or regional HTA analysis may include considerations of equity across the population, cost-impact, cost-effectiveness, time horizon of expected benefit, and pure clinical health outcomes. HTA decision-makers are usually considering the comparative effect of a new product against the existing standard of care in that country or region.

The National Institute of Clinical Excellence (NICE) in the UK and the Institut für Qualität und Wirtschaftlichkeit im Gesundheitswesen (IQWiG) in Germany are examples of national HTA groups. The Catalan Agency for Health Information, Assessment and Quality (CAHOAQ) is an example of a regional HTA body in Spain. In many countries, affiliated institutions and academic groups conduct assessments on behalf of decision-making bodies. Italy provides a good example of this where strong regional governments allow regional HTAs to be conducted through universities or other locally founded groups. One of the more active regions, Veneto, conducts HTA assessments through the pharmacy service group, UVEF (Unita di Valutazione dell'Efficacia del Farmaco) at the University of Veneto.

PRICING

Each country in Europe has country-specific pricing and reimbursement systems. Pricing for novel pharmaceutical products is largely based on benefit (or value) assessments by payers or based on comparator products and prices in other markets (international price referencing). International price referencing (IPR) in most markets leads to a cascade effect of pricing outcomes. When one country sets a price, other countries who reference that country's prices are automatically impacted. As a result, any market that is referenced by other markets has both a significant in-country and external effect—or reference—when a price is established. Figure 17.4 depicts the complexity and the interrelated nature of the international price referencing system whereby countries set their own drug prices based on the prices established in other markets.

In several countries, such as Italy and Spain, pricing decisions are made at the national level while access is determined at the regional level. For many years, the UK and Germany were the only two European countries with free pricing for pharmaceuticals, meaning the manufacturer could set the price of the product rather than the government setting the price through price negotiation or referencing. Germany, however, recently instituted a series of reform laws that changed the pricing structure for pharmaceuticals, creating a system of initial free pricing which is then subjected to a benefits assessment by the government. Such

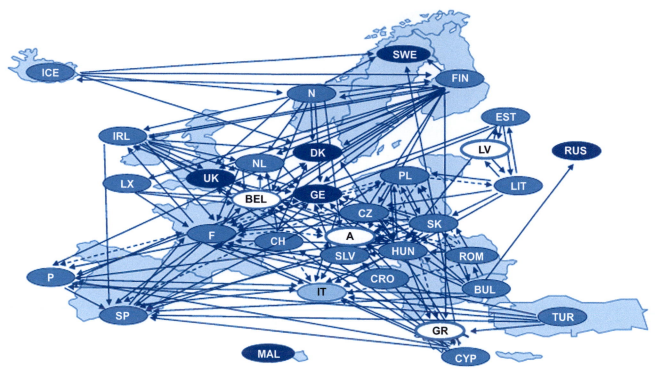

FIGURE 17.4   Complexity of the international pricing reference system.

assessments of medical and relative economic benefit are commonplace in the French market, and not too dissimilar from the new framework in Germany. The results of this process have significantly impacted pricing outcomes for new products in Germany. The UK is currently undergoing rapid change as it approaches reforms within its own national health service, soon to bring the promise of a new and unfamiliar "value-based pricing" process into routine assessment of new medical technologies.

Pricing decisions for therapies have historically been conducted separately from those related to diagnostics. While pricing for diagnostics may be related to fee schedules, tied to specific codes, or established at the hospital or laboratory level, drug pricing is usually product-specific and can have cross-border implications as a result of international referencing. Currently, no countries have an established value-based pricing pathway for novel diagnostics. Instead, companies with high value products attempt to work with payers and other decision-makers to enable access on a country-by-country, region-by-region, and in some cases hospital-by-hospital level.

Cost containment is a major priority for health systems in Europe and pharmaceuticals have been a target for budget reductions in many settings. Reforms to health systems have arisen as the result of a variety of reasons but none more visible than the drive towards austerity, judicious use of resources, and social rebalancing that is impacting many European markets. This impact has been acutely felt by manufacturers of innovative health technologies and will continue to be a major risk in most European markets. It

is expected that ongoing price pressures will be applied by European health systems as they attempt to manage escalating costs associated with an aging population. (See Figures 17.5 and 17.6.)

REIMBURSEMENT MECHANISMS

Most countries in Europe have different mechanisms to reimburse for health-related goods and services. Across countries, most hospital-related costs are reimbursed using a DRG-based system. Diagnosis-related groups (DRGs) are global payments that provide lump sum payment to hospitals to cover all goods and services provided during the course of that stay. In most settings, the DRG is based on a patient's primary diagnosis or primary procedure, and has the ability to be classified by severity to differentiate routine from complex cases. DRGs allow hospitals to manage care and purchasing decisions and offer little opportunity for separate, or product-specific reimbursement. In many markets there are routes to funding outside of the DRG for "expensive" or innovative drugs that would significantly disrupt the DRG. This includes exclusion from the T2A list (France), application for an Neue Untersuchungs- und Behandlungsmethoden (NUB Germany).

For outpatient care there is a mix of fee-for-service, global payment, capitated, and self-pay structures throughout Europe. In countries such as France and the UK, where socialized health systems guarantee citizens a minimum level of care paid for by government health insurance, there

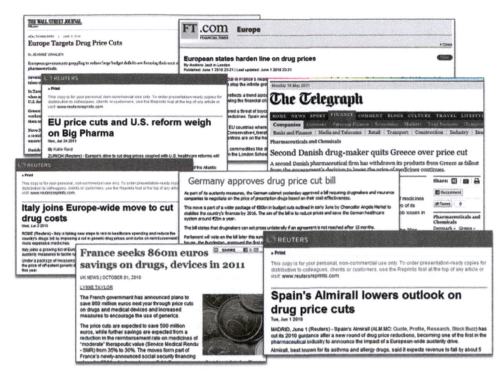

FIGURE 17.5   Illustrative examples of European initiatives to target cost control measures for pharmaceuticals.

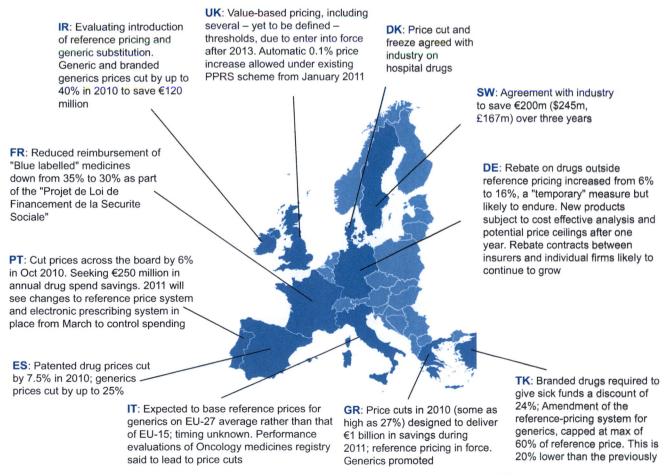

IR: Evaluating introduction of reference pricing and generic substitution. Generic and branded generics prices cut by up to 40% in 2010 to save €120 million

UK: Value-based pricing, including several – yet to be defined – thresholds, due to enter into force after 2013. Automatic 0.1% price increase allowed under existing PPRS scheme from January 2011

DK: Price cut and freeze agreed with industry on hospital drugs

SW: Agreement with industry to save €200m ($245m, £167m) over three years

FR: Reduced reimbursement of "Blue labelled" medicines down from 35% to 30% as part of the "Projet de Loi de Financement de la Securite Sociale"

DE: Rebate on drugs outside reference pricing increased from 6% to 16%, a "temporary" measure but likely to endure. New products subject to cost effective analysis and potential price ceilings after one year. Rebate contracts between insurers and individual firms likely to continue to grow

PT: Cut prices across the board by 6% in Oct 2010. Seeking €250 million in annual drug spend savings. 2011 will see changes to reference price system and electronic prescribing system in place from March to control spending

ES: Patented drug prices cut by 7.5% in 2010; generics prices cut by up to 25%

IT: Expected to base reference prices for generics on EU-27 average rather than that of EU-15; timing unknown. Performance evaluations of Oncology medicines registry said to lead to price cuts

GR: Price cuts in 2010 (some as high as 27%) designed to deliver €1 billion in savings during 2011; reference pricing in force. Generics promoted

TK: Branded drugs required to give sick funds a discount of 24%; Amendment of the reference-pricing system for generics, capped at max of 60% of reference price. This is 20% lower than the previously

FIGURE 17.6   Examples of European pricing and reimbursement cost containment initiatives.

is very little out-of-pocket cost associated with routine care. Patients do have the option to purchase noncovered services like advanced diagnostics, though practices vary by market as does access to private supplemental insurance. Diagnostics are predominantly paid for out-of-hospital and/or laboratory budgets or in some cases based on code-specific fee schedules. Surprisingly, the diagnostic reimbursement pathways in many European countries are not as clearly defined or sophisticated as those for drugs. Consequently, most diagnostic procedures are reimbursed in whole or in part by the national payer directly to hospitals, pharmacies, clinicians, or via patient reimbursement from the drugs budget.

Reimbursement Outcomes

While each European country acts independently when it comes to reimbursement decision-making, there are cross-border implications. For example, in the UK, NICE makes public their HTA decisions. It is broadly considered that NICE review standards are sophisticated and thorough and, as a result, payers and HTA organizations in other countries often refer to NICE guidance—officially and unofficially—as they develop their own perspectives and assessments. Countries are continuously evolving their reimbursement systems to meet the needs of a rapidly changing healthcare landscape. This includes healthcare technologies based on complex genetic information, products that provide remote monitoring of patients, advanced biotechnology based therapies that require specific handling and administration, advanced imaging modalities and other innovations. Each of these unique innovations and paradigm-shifting new technologies challenge the health care system's existing framework for evaluation, pricing, and payment pathways.

A Closer Look at Reimbursement in Five Key European Markets

In the United Kingdom, The National Health Service (NHS) provides health care and coverage to all citizens [33]. Individuals can purchase private insurance to supplement NHS care or for payment for noncovered treatments and services. In England, primary care trusts (PCTs), who are responsible for providing healthcare and health improvements within a local area, report to strategic health authorities which manage performance by region. Currently, the NHS awards 85 percent of their budget to PCTs to pay for healthcare products and services. Payment by PCTs is made using one of three mechanisms, payment-by-results, block contracts, or global budgeting. This arrangement is set to change, when PCTs will be replaced by a GP Commissioning Consortium.

In the UK, there is currently a system of free pricing managed through the Pharmaceutical Price Regulation Scheme (PPRS) system. Value-Based Pricing (VBP) will supplant the current system, beginning in 2014. This system will apply to all innovative medicines brought to market after the initiation of the program. "Innovative" will most likely be defined as any "new chemical entity." The process will emphasize cost-effectiveness, as measured by cost per quality-adjusted life year (QALY), reflecting a base case and additional factors (therapeutic innovation, burden of illness, therapeutic improvement, and wider societal benefit). Within the system there will be opportunities for products addressing significant unmet need to move through streamlined processes. VBP at the national level will not remove the need for local negotiation for access and uptake.

Today, many products are reviewed for inclusion within the NHS system by NICE, a system that is regarded as challenging, with a high burden of clinical, economic, and substantiation required to demonstrate successful outcomes. Thresholds are, increasingly, becoming more strict and data requirements more onerous according to many companies. Due to the rigor required to substantiate value in the eyes of NICE, advanced analysis, adept foresight, and a more than marginal clinical benefit is often required to successfully navigate HTA assessment in the UK.

The vast majority of the German population is covered by a "Bismarck" insurance fund-based system. Statutory health insurance funds (SHIs) are responsible for the costs of healthcare provision to their insured population. Private insurance coverage can only be used to supplement improved services or if an individual's yearly income exceeds a predefined level (49,950 EUR in 2010). Traditionally, hospitals are publicly funded institutions, providing only inpatient care, while ambulatory care is supplied by private practices which are paid by SHIs and private insurance. Reimbursement for diagnostics and drugs is dependent on the site of care. In the inpatient system, both are predominantly covered under a DRG global payment system. In the outpatient environment, reimbursement for drugs and diagnostics is provided based on contracted charges (drugs) and a code-based fee schedule (diagnostics). Under the new AMNOG drug pricing legislation previously mentioned, Germany has moved from free pricing to a system of benefit assessment. The Act on the Reform of the Market for Medical Products (Arzneimittelmarkt-Neuordnungsgesetz) (AMNOG) process enables drugs that are deemed to have additional clinical benefit to achieve premium pricing through a series of negotiation and arbitration processes. Figure 17.7 illustrates the process that provides opportunity to assess clinical and cost benefit against a government chosen standard.

In Italy, the national healthcare system (Servizio Sanitario Nazionale—SSN) provides healthcare coverage to the population through public financing and a mixture of public and private provision of care. The Italian system is largely decentralized and can be broken down into three levels: national, regional, and local. The responsibility for delivering hospital and community services falls to the regional level. Local health units (Azienda Sanitaria Locale—ASL)

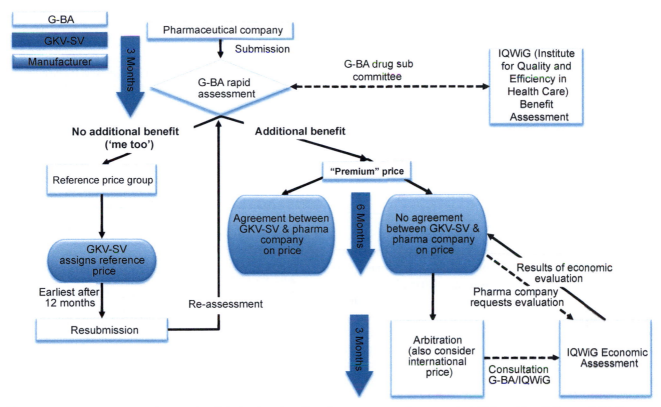

FIGURE 17.7   AMNOG process for assessing clinical and cost benefit against a government chosen standard. *(Adapted from R Skavron G-BA. Germany: Latest Developments in Pricing and Reimbursement Policy. 23 March 2011.)*

coordinate all nonemergency care and are funded by the SSN through a per capita budget. Public and private healthcare providers (whether they provide in-patient and/or out-patient care) are remunerated through a fee-for-service system based on two formulary lists, with different tariff levels. Both lists are based on the ICD-10-CM WHO Classification of Diseases and Procedures. The Italian Medicines Agency (AIFA) is the national authority responsible for drug regulation, pricing, and evaluation in Italy.

The French population is almost universally covered (99 percent of the population) by statutory health insurance (assurance-maladie), managed by the Haute Autorité de Santé (HAS). HAS is in charge of evaluating drugs, devices, diagnostics, and other products. The Commission d'Evaluation des Médicaments (Transparency Commission), within HAS, is used to assess the clinical value provided by a new product and the improvement it will provide subsequent to its use. The opinion is based on a value analysis or SMR (Service Medical Rendu)—that considers whether the product should be reimbursed and what could be the reimbursement rate, comparative assessment of clinical benefit assessment or ASMR (Amelioration du Service Medical Rendu)—the grading that provides a basis for price fixing in comparison with alternatives, and who the target population eligible for treatment should be. The Agence Française de Sécurité Sanitaire des Produits de

Santé (AFSSAPS) carries out scientific and medico-economic evaluation as part of this system. Drugs used in the outpatient setting have patient cost-sharing associated with them in most cases. This cost sharing, however, is often covered by private insurance "mutuelles," under which the vast majority of the French population is covered [34]. Since 2004, hospitals have been funded through DRGs, with most drugs and diagnostics included in the global payment system (although some high-priced drugs are funded separately).

The Spanish healthcare system (Sistema Nacional de la Salud—SNS) is compulsory and publicly funded, with administration performed at the regional level through regional health authorities (RHA). Roughly 15 percent of the population has supplemental private insurance to augment the statutory coverage, which the entire population enjoys. The RHAs fund hospitals within their regions through prospective budgets. The basis for budget allocation is largely derived from the population within the hospital area. Outpatient services are covered based on regional decision-making, largely through a fee-for-service mechanism. A national HTA agency (Instituto de Salud Carlos III-ISCIII) and several regional HTA organizations coexist in the country. Reimbursement is considered at the national level through the Spanish Ministry of Health (MSC), while pricing is determined by the Inter-Ministerial Pricing Commission CIPM (La Comisión Interministerial de Precios de los Medicamentos).

EUROPEAN PRICING AND REIMBURSEMENT SUMMARY

Tensions continue to grow as European payers attempt to manage costs and continue to improve the quality of healthcare for their constituents. Payers are increasingly relying on methods for cost containment, including:

- Increasing the role of HTAs
- Price cuts
- Comparative effectiveness requirements
- Value-based pricing
- Risk-sharing schemes
- Access with evidence development
- International price referencing

Because of this trend, innovators must plan for different approaches to product evaluation and in order to meet the needs of HTA organizations. This means that evidence development planning must be considered early in the product development lifecycle to support product value propositions and evaluation by HTAs. Additionally, the varying information requirements of regulatory agencies, HTAs, and payers across Europe must be taken into account. This can include requirements for country-specific data, varying types of health economic analyses, or analysis against a specific comparator considered the standard of care in a given context. Industry can then work with payers in each country to establish product value using the various mechanisms available.

While reimbursement systems have strict processes in place to ensure rationale use of resources, opportunities for innovation exist. Funding pathways for unmet needs and high-value treatments persist, with some preferential treatment of drugs for orphan conditions, for example, still in place. In the new world of comparative effectiveness and strict HTA-based evaluations, products most at risk for noncoverage are "me-too" treatments that cannot demonstrate significant incremental value or are significantly more expensive (and similarly or less effective) than the current standard of care.

Across markets, companies are recognizing the additional risk related to pricing and reimbursement beyond regulatory approval. This is impacting early product planning and "go" and "no go" decisions to advance products in development. The uncertainty in terms of reimbursement and pricing has impacted the valuations of many medical technologies, especially those with a significant focus on Europe. Moving forward, EU countries are expected to provide greater clarity in terms of evidence requirements and pricing expectations, which should hopefully, lead to more innovative and impactful health technologies reaching the European markets.

REFERENCES

[1] 21 U.S.C. §§ 301 et seq.; 21 C.F.R. §§ 200-299 (Drug Regulations); 21 C.F.R. §§ 300-499 (human drug regulations); 21 C.F.R. §§ 600-799 (biological regulations); and 21 C.F.R. §§ 800-1299 (medical device regulations); see also Riegel v. Medtronic, 552 U.S. 352 (2008).

[2] *Goodman v. Sullivan*, 891 F.2d 449, 451 (2d Cir. 1989) (The Medicare program was not obligated to cover a diagnostic test based only on the FDA's approval of the test.)

[3] CMS and FDA have started a pilot parallel review program under which a limited number of medical products would be considered by each agency simultaneously. 75 Fed. Reg. 57045 (2010) and 76 Fed. Reg. 62808(2011).

[4] *See, e.g., Hays v. Sebelius*, 589 F.3d 1229 (D.C. Cir. 2009).

[5] *See Goodman*, note 3, *supra*.

[6] 42 U.S.C. § 1395y(a).

[7] *Id.*

[8] http://www.cancer.org/acs/groups/cid/documents/webcontent/002552-pdf.pdf. These state laws have been supplemented by Section 10103(c) of the Patient Protection and Affordable Care Act, Pub. L. No. 111-148 (2010).

[9] *See, e.g.,* 42 U.S.C. § 1395y(a)(1)(A).

[10] See, e.g. Neumann P, Chambers J. Medicare's Enduring Struggle to Define 'Reasonable and Necessary Care. New England J Med 2012;367:1775–7.

[11] *See, e.g.,* Medicare National Coverage Determinations Manual, § 20.4 (coverage of implantable defibrillators).

[12] *Id.,* §110.8.1 (coverage of stem cell transplantation); see also Neumann P, Tunis S. Medicare and Medical Technology—The Growing Demand for Relevant Outcomes. New England J Med 2010;362:377–9.

[13] 42 U.S.C. §§ 1395y(l), 1395w–22, and 1395mm; 42 C.F.R. § 400.202.

[14] *See, e.g.,* Centers for Medicare and Medicaid Services, Innovator's Guide to Navigating Medicare, Version 2.0 (2010) at 17, available at: http://www.cms.gov/CouncilonTechInnov/01_overview.asp.

[15] *Id.* at 31—55.

[16] 42 U.S.C. § 1395ww(d)(5)(K-L) and 42 C.F.R. § 412.87(b) (inpatient); 42 U.S.C. § 1395l (t)(6) and 42 C.F.R. §§ 419.62—419.66 (outpatient).

[17] 42 U.S.C. § 1395y(a)(1)(A).

[18] *See, e.g.,* Regence Blue Cross and Blue Shield, Medical Policy Development and Review Process, available at http://blue.regence.com/trgmedpol/intro/.

[19] An example of this is the Blue Cross Blue Shield Association Technology Evaluation Center. See http://bcbs.com/blueresources/tec/.

[20] Balas E, Boren S. Managing Clinical Knowledge for Health Care Improvement. In: Bemmel J, McCray AT, editors. Yearbook of Medical Informatics; 2000. Patient-Centered Systems at 65–70.

[21] Health Advances, The Reimbursement Landscape for Novel Diagnostics 11, available at: www.healthadvances.com/pdf/novel_diag_reimbursement.pdf.

[22] *See* Neumann P. et al., supra n.13.

[23] *See, e.g.,* Eddy D. Evidence-Based Medicine: A Unified Approach. Health Affairs 2005;24(no. 1):9–17.

[24] Centers for Medicare and Medicaid Services, Decision Memo for Screening Computed Tomography Colonography for Colorectal Cancer (2009), available at: https://www.cms.gov/medicare-coverage-database/details/nca-decision-memo.aspx?NCAId=220&ver=19&NcaName=Screening+Computed+Tomography+Colonography+(CTC)+for+Colorectal+Cancer&CoverageSelection=Both&ArticleType=All&PolicyType=Final&s=All&KeyWord=colonography&KeyWordLookUp=Title&KeyWordLookUp=Title&KeyWordLookUp=Title&KeyWordSearchType=And&KeyWordSearchType=And&KeyWordSearchType=And&bc=gAAAABAAIAAA& (Accessed November 8, 2011).

[25] In addition, CMS was concerned that the data in the available studies found that the CT colonographies showed a lower sensitivity and specificity for polyps smaller than 6 mm when compared to optical colonoscopy.

[26] Centers for Medicare and Medicaid Services, Coverage with Evidence Development Solicitation (Nov. 7, 2011), available at: https://www.cms.gov/medicare-coverage-database/details/medicare-coverage-document-details.aspx?MCDId=8&McdName=National+Coverage+Determinations+with+Data+Collection+as+a+Condition+of+Coverage%3a+Coverage+with+Evidence+Development&mcdtypename=Guidance+Documents&MCDIndexType=1&bc=BAAIAAAAAAAA&. CMS is considering changes to its current policies, but has yet to publish any proposals for comment.

[27] *See, e.g.,* Carlson B. Seeking a Coding Solution For Molecular Tests. Biotech Healthcare Winter 2010:16–20.

[28] http://www.cms.gov/Medicare/Coding/MedHCPCSGenInfo/index.html?redirect=/MedHCPCSGenInfo/.

[29] http://www.ama-assn.org/ama/pub/physician-resources/solutions-managing-your-practice/coding-billing-insurance/cpt/cpt-process-faq/code-becomes-cpt.page?.

[30] *See* Medicare Payment Advisory Commission, Payment Basics: Hospital Acute Inpatient Services (2012). Available at: www.medpac.gov/documents/MedPAC_Payment_Basics_12_hospital.pdf.

[31] http://www.ema.europa.eu/ema/index.jsp?curl=pages/about_us/general/general_content_000235.jsp&mid. Accessed March 20, 2013.

[32] Henshall C, et al. Priority Setting for Health Technology Assessment: Theoretical Considerations and Practical Approaches. Int J Tech Assess Health Care 1997;13:144–85.

[33] Scotland, Wales, and Northern Ireland have separate systems for evaluation and payment for health services.

[34] OECD. Private Health Insurance in France, Thomas Buchmueller and Agnes Couffinhal; 2004.

Chapter 18

Getting the Word Out: Using Public Relations Strategies to Support Biotechnology Business Goals

Joan E. Kureczka, MSEM

Founder and Principal, Kureczka/Martin Associates and The Vivant Group, San Francisco, California

Let's say you just formed your new company. You've got a great idea, gained rights to the intellectual property around your technology or potential product, and assembled your start-up team. You've raised a small amount of money to move things forward using your own capital along with a few "friends and family" investors. Perhaps you even obtained a "seed" round of financing from some angel investors or a venture capital firm. Your research is going well. Now it's time to take things to the next level. However, you are finding that it is very competitive "out there." According to a 2012 report from Battelle and the Biotech Industry Organization (BIO), as of their 2010 census, there were over 70,000 U.S. bioscience establishments which included agricultural and industrial biotech firms; therapeutics and diagnostics developers; medical device companies; research, testing, and medical laboratories; and bioscience-related distribution companies. The vast majority of these companies are private. While each year we see some of these organizations leave the field through mergers or for various other reasons, each year also brings a new crop of start-up companies. All of these businesses are constantly competing with you for investment dollars and funding, corporate partnerships or customers, research collaborators and patients, as well as for great employees and contractors.

Early-stage biotechnology companies face communications challenges specific to their industry. If you are working in a healthcare-related field, such as therapeutics, diagnostics, or medical devices, you need to consider how regulators view your technology and products, as well as the doctors and patients who will use them. Future payers, including governmental organizations like Medicare and other large healthcare providers and insurance companies, must also be convinced of the value of your technology in order to smooth the path toward coverage and reimbursement. If your business is in a field like agricultural biotechnology

or you are introducing new technology with potential environmental or social impact, you have a special challenge of educating people about the value of your science and products to their lives. Policy makers, potential consumers, and other members of the general public—including highly vocal opposition groups—are going to need to understand the benefits of what you are doing so as not to throw up roadblocks to your ultimate success.

Moreover, no matter what business you are in, good relations with your local community, including city planners, regulators, and neighbors, are needed to smooth the path for growth. Trying to grow your business in an area hostile to your work can be costly as well as frustrating. In every case, your success will depend on reaching and clearly communicating the value of your company, products and services to a variety of audiences. Public relations is the most cost-effective method to reach each of those audiences and to create and maintain positive relationships with them.

WHAT IS PUBLIC RELATIONS AND HOW CAN IT SUPPORT YOUR BUSINESS OBJECTIVES?

Public relations (PR) is the art of creating and maintaining a positive image of your company, technology, or products in the opinions of each of your target audiences. These include investors, corporate partners, customers, current and potential employees, thought leaders, patients, the media, and others. A good PR effort will help you stand out from the crowd and give you a competitive edge by creating familiarity with your company and an understanding of your products/services and their value to target audiences. PR can help you build scientific and business credibility, especially by calling attention to, and extending the reach of, peer-reviewed research publications and presentations, as well as business milestones that validate your science and technology. PR can also help you manage your public reputation and build good relationships with those whom you do business.

Used strategically, public relations can support a wide variety of business objectives, including:

- Finding funding from investors or foundations
- Securing contracts for corporate alliances
- Attracting potential acquirers
- Creating and maintaining demand for a stock offering
- Supporting sales of products or services
- Educating or influencing policy makers
- Finding top employees, consultants and other service providers
- Creating community support for your business activities and operations.

From its formation, every start-up biotech company should be thinking about PR and when to begin applying its strategies and tactics to support your business goals.

GET READY: WHAT'S YOUR STORY?

People love stories. For example, if you talk to members of the investment community they will tell you that they invest in good people with good stories. Good stories are engaging and help the entrepreneur break through the competing noise to capture an audience's attention. They go beyond your product or technology platform to convey a message that resonates with your target audience and motivates them in some way. Ultimately, PR works by connecting your business with people through a story.

The first step in defining your story is to understand your audience in terms of how you want them to think about you, and what you want them to do. What information about you may predispose them towards you, your technology, your products, or services? Different messages have greater or lesser importance to a given audience, so it is useful to understand what motivates the people you are trying to reach with your message. Next, you will need to clearly define the key elements of your story—that is, develop a positioning statement (often alternatively described as your "elevator pitch") and the key message points that explicitly differentiate you from your competition and peers. Your positioning statement is a short paragraph—typically one to three sentences—that clearly and succinctly defines your business and says what makes it unique and why it has value. Table 18.1 gives some examples.

Your key message points are supporting statements that provide specific detail to back up your positioning. The message you define can address a specific audience's needs and wants, providing the opportunity to tailor what you want to emphasize in your communications to them.

A SWOT analysis (strengths, weaknesses, opportunities, and threats analysis) is a useful exercise when thinking about positioning, as it helps you take a hard look at

TABLE 18.1 Examples of Positioning Statements[a]

Savant HWP *develops pharmaceutical products* that improve health, maintain wellness, and prevent disease. We *identify undervalued opportunities* to create innovative products in areas where our work has the greatest impact, including *addiction medicine and neglected diseases* like Leishmaniasis and Chagas disease that are emerging in the U.S. population and endemic in other parts of the world. Our leadership team of *proven innovators has more than a century and a half of combined experience bringing new medicines to market.* Our focus is to quickly and cost-efficiently build value in the projects we undertake, to *support high-value corporate partnering and returns* for our investors.

BioSeek is *improving the success rate of pharmaceutical research and development* by *integrating human biology from the earliest stages of drug discovery onward.* Our BioMAP® systems incorporate *predictive primary human cell-based disease models* that *generate uniquely informative biological activity profiles* for each potential drug. As a result, our technology *drives the selection and development* of new drug candidates and safer chemicals.

ClinMet *provides* pharmaceutical companies with *clinically relevant insights and practical information about drug response and safety using metabolomics for diabetes, kidney disease, obesity, and cardiovascular disease.* Our unique combination of *in-depth clinical insights, proprietary metabolomics expertise,* and *computational know-how improves the speed and success rate of drug development.* ClinMet helps drug developers to efficiently transform promising compounds into safe and effective medicines.

[a]*The italic text in each example shows how each company has used important attributes and business objectives to create a well-differentiated statement of identity.*

the elements that define your business and the environment in which it operates. This exercise also helps you list specific differentiators that form the basis of your key message points. Strengths and weaknesses represent internal characteristics of your company, while opportunities and threats represent those of the overall business landscape and how they affect your business or your product sales. Performing a SWOT analysis also helps you identify individual message points that elaborate upon your positioning statement and further differentiate your company from others in the field. What are your most important business and scientific attributes? What market opportunities do you address? What will you deliver to customers, partners, or patients?

You should take the time to critically understand what sets you apart from others and how best to convey that difference to each of your targeted audiences in a clear, concise way—but without hype. The effective formulation of your positioning statement and key messages can go a long way towards building a strong brand and consistent communications as you move forward with the next step in your PR effort—preparing the various elements of your communications tool box.

GET SET: CREATING YOUR COMMUNICATIONS TOOLS

Communication tools can take many forms. The basic elements for any start-up company include a website, a corporate fact sheet, a short company presentation, and ideally, some basic graphics suitable for a variety of uses.

Your Corporate Website

Your website should make a great first impression—viewers may not know if you are a Fortune 500 company or a tiny start-up if your site is well-designed and professional looking. A good initial website need not be complex or lengthy, but it should look clean, attractive, and be easy to read. The text should also be relatively brief so it can be read quickly. The average person reads only about 20 percent of the words on a webpage so you need to make sure they efficiently and effectively convey the message you want to get across. The home page should give the visitor a brief idea of what your business is about—a version of your positioning statement will usually work well here. You may choose to include pages about your technology or products that should incorporate appropriate key messages. You also want to include brief biographies of senior management, your board of directors, and if applicable, your scientific advisors.

A contact page is also essential. Many companies like to use electronic contact forms as part of the website to cut down on unwanted phone calls and to have a record of specific contacts. However, reliance on such forms can also work against you, especially if a reporter or editor on deadline is trying to reach you. Too often, inquiries sent via website contact forms can languish for long periods of time, thus causing urgent messages to be overlooked and opportunities to be missed.

Fact Sheets and Backgrounders

As you begin to talk to potential investors, corporate partners, media, and others, you are sure to be asked to "Send me something about your company." A two-page fact sheet provides essential, nonconfidential information about your company in basic terms, and conveys what makes you unique. If you've done your positioning work ahead of writing this document, you've already created much of the useful language that can be tailored further for this use and for other specific audiences, if desired. At a minimum, a corporate fact sheet needs to briefly describe the basis of your company, its business goals, and what makes it noteworthy. You should also include a list of key management and directors, and a financing history if you have one. Don't forget to include contact information and your logo. You may additionally benefit from creating fact sheets on your platform technology or specific products under development. Remember that these documents are intended for a general audience who may not have the scientific background that you do. To ensure that your message is heard and understood, keep your language simple and nontechnical, as well as free of overstatement and hype. If graphics can more simply explain your technology than words—use them.

The Corporate Presentation

The third element in your communications tool box is a corporate presentation. Start-up companies will benefit from a basic set of slides that can then be further customized to address the information needs of specific audiences. Good presentations are simple, concise, and compelling. Forget the adjectives, buzz words, and business clichés—but do use active verbs and be concise. The best presentations are also highly visual. Audiences remember more of your message when key points are conveyed through images and charts rather than through words on a screen. In fact, research shows that we read and retain visualized messages up to 30 percent better than text because 50 percent of our brain is involved in visual processing. So if you must use words, limit their number to make the text as scannable as possible. Overcrowded slides become unreadable in the average large-scale meeting room.

Keep your audience's specific needs and interests in mind. In these days of busy schedules and ever-shortening attention spans, you need to make an impact quickly. If you have not demonstrated to your audience why they should want to learn more in the first few minutes of your presentation, you have probably lost their interest. Describe your business idea, what makes it new and exciting, and how it will deliver what your audience wants—whether that is a great product, or strong, timely investment returns. Then elaborate on that overview with the details of your science, the market opportunity, the work you've accomplished to date, and the backgrounds of your team members. If you are seeking financing, how much do you want to raise and how will you use those funds? How will you create real value out of your idea? And how will an investment in your firm or the licensing of your product bring financial returns to your listeners, and in what timeframe?

Finally, once you have your basic presentation and plenty of backup slides to respond to anticipated questions—practice your delivery. Even for the best companies with great people and stories, an under-rehearsed, ill-prepared presentation can spoil a potential financing or collaboration. One venture capital investor tells of a highly anticipated company presentation that turned into a disaster for the presenting firm. The presenters were unpolished, had inadequate slides, were unprepared for questions, and offered no financial information. As a result, the potential investors were not impressed, and the presenting company was unable to regain their interest.

Graphic Resources

Good graphics are always useful. With the rise of the Internet as a primary medium for communications, graphics have become an essential part of the communications tool box. Not only are they useful for your website, presentation, and fact sheet, but the availability of photos and other images will open the door to better Web visibility and media coverage. At a minimum, have high-resolution photos (minimum 300 dpi) available of your management and corporate logo. Visual or video representations of how your product or technology works, including animations and product photos where relevant are also a plus.

DESIGNING AND IMPLEMENTING A STRATEGIC COMMUNICATIONS PROGRAM

Now that you have the story you want to tell with the communications tools to help you tell it, it's time to think about strategy and tactics. Your aim will be to highlight key events and use a variety of communications channels to tell your story, build visibility, and develop ongoing relationships with target audiences over time.

A low-key strategy that is consistent and persistent can be more effective (and affordable in both time and dollars) than a one-time big splash—which if not followed up with additional near-term activity, will soon be forgotten. Your business objectives help prioritize your target audiences, as well as the activities you undertake and the communications channels you use to reach them. What are your business objectives for the next 8 to 12 months? Is your primary goal to raise financing? Are you looking for development partners? Or are you already seeking customers for your services or products? Generally the time to get serious about a strategic, ongoing PR program is when you can foresee a stream of potential corporate milestones building. A good starting point is to map these expected business events and important scientific communications such as peer-reviewed publications or meeting presentations, against your near-term goals. This exercise will help identify important communications opportunities as well as consideration of the timing of news releases and other activities.

NEWS RELEASES

News releases are a basic currency of a PR program but their intent has changed in recent years. Also known as "press releases," news releases were originally directed chiefly to the media who acted as the gatekeepers over what news was reported. Today, Internet dissemination via newswire services and email enables you to quickly, easily, and cost-efficiently reach your intended audiences directly, without a media filter—thus making a well-written, informative news release more important than ever. Effectively distributed for optimum visibility, news releases can help a company achieve several communications objectives. They offer a company-controlled channel to disseminate key messages, reinforce branding, and build thought leadership. They can build visibility with target audiences, especially online. They also can help drive traffic to the company website where viewers can learn more.

Many different events are suitable as the subject of a news release. Examples include:

- Successful financings
- Forming corporate partnerships or major customer relationships
- Senior management, board of directors, or scientific advisory board appointments
- Clinical or other major product development milestones, including the start of major trials as well as trial results
- Product approvals, launches, or new service offerings
- Important scientific publications and presentations
- Important patent issuances or research grants

A well-written news release should answer the standard journalistic questions: who, what, when, where, and why? They should avoid jargon, meaningless or over-used buzz-words (for example, do not use "solutions" or "solutions provider" to describe your business or technology without a stated problem unless you are talking about chemical reagents), and technical language and acronyms that go over the heads of most readers. A news release should be crafted with your readers in mind and the information they will be most interested in knowing. Quotes from company spokespersons or others relevant to your news are useful. Quotes give the news context and emphasis, allowing you to reflect on its importance to the company or target audience, or offer a brief look ahead at your business prospects. Avoid using too many quotes or tired expressions of "pleasure" (i.e. "We are pleased..." or "We are delighted...") that lack real content because they can detract from the overall impact of your news release as well as consume an unnecessary word count in the price of dissemination. Those in industry sectors overseen by the U.S. Food and Drug Administration or other regulatory agencies must also give special consideration to the rules set out by those agencies regarding communications. It is important to get the input of your regulatory and legal counsel in such cases to ensure your release remains within what is allowed. You should especially avoid making overt claims of efficacy or safety for unapproved products.

Once you have a final version of your news release and are ready to make your announcement, you have several options for its dissemination. Full-service, commercial news release distribution businesses (PR Newswire, BusinessWire, or GlobeNewswire) offer the advantages of fast, efficient, and simultaneous distribution of releases (as well as photos and other multimedia files) to media and throughout the Web. Using such services for release distribution can increase traffic to your website through search engines and can enhance your credibility as your news will appear alongside that of larger, more established companies. These services will also allow you to easily see where your release has appeared through the tracking reports they provide. However, good, effective service comes at a price, and while there are lower-cost providers for news release distribution, the quality of your results, including credibility, reach, visibility, and security is usually reflected in the price you pay.

When determining how you want to disseminate your release, you should consider the likely interest level and value of the overall news to potential readers. If it is relatively low or highly targeted (for example, a new scientific advisory board member or patent issuance), you may want to spend less money and use a much narrower newswire distribution, or just send the release via email to relevant publications directly. In some cases (for example, opening a new facility), you can just post a release to your website. For releases with greater news value, you can still limit the cost of release dissemination by restricting your wire service distribution to certain geographical areas or industry sectors. Doing so will still guarantee the release populates the Web in a comprehensive manner and reaches the industry publications most relevant to your news. For news of potential interest to general audiences, particularly scientific publications and presentations, there are two additional services that can be useful: EurekAlert (www.eurekalert.com) and Newswise (www.newswise.com). Both of these sites are designed specifically to meet the needs and interests of science and health/medical journalists, although they are also read by many of science-interested public.

MEDIA RELATIONS—WHY IT STILL MATTERS

While the true audience for your press release is not the press, media coverage of your company remains an important part of any communications program. The media are still important information gatekeepers and their coverage of your company and products is influential. They can provide context, help validate what you say about your company, and extend the reach of your communications to more people for a longer period of time. Media remains a powerful force. They bring third-party credibility by independent reporting about your business or products in newspapers, magazines, and their Internet-based counterparts, wire services, broadcast outlets, and the many other varieties of Internet-based content. Media coverage is an important tool for building recognition and reputation for a new company facing daunting competition from better known firms for funding, partners, and employees. While some start-ups are hesitant to engage with the media, a young company can benefit from a certain amount of outreach even in the early stages of its existence. There are certain audiences and publications that want to know and write about you at that formative stage. In fact, there are a few opportunities in the trade media for company profiles that are only available to early-stage

private companies, most notably with *Start-Up Magazine* and *BioCentury*.

Different types of media have different audiences, and thus, different information needs, as well as different views of what makes a story. The perspective of a pharmaceutical trade journalist will differ from that of a major news outlet like the *New York Times* or *Wall Street Journal*. A locally focused publication will differ from a national or international one and what makes a good story for a science writer may differ significantly from what serves a business reporter's audience, even if both consider the life sciences their beat. It is important to understand the target audience for each type of media outlet, and how their reporters and editors may perceive what their readers or viewers want to read or see. By doing so, you can better choose the media outlets and journalists whose interests most closely serve your own communications purposes, and frame your story and key messages in a way that those media will be most receptive to hearing it. You will want to consider:

- What is new, exciting, or different about your company, product, or technology?
- What makes the story emotionally compelling?
- Why does your story have importance outside of the small circle of your immediate scientific team?
- If you are looking for mainstream coverage, why should the broader public care about you and what you've accomplished?

You are likely to get the best reception from reporters and editors if you can identify something unique in the story you want to tell, and then tell it in a simple, straightforward, and compelling manner. On the flip side, few things are more frustrating and time-wasting to a reporter—and detrimental to building a good working relationship with them—than a wildly off-topic pitch. You will benefit from being well-prepared before embarking on a media relations effort. Your company spokespersons should be able to talk knowledgably, comfortably, and understandably about your business, technology, and products. What makes your company different, and why your products are needed? Your spokespersons should be able to communicate your positioning and key messages in a consistent fashion and tell the story in language that is understandable to a nonscientific audience.

Anticipating potential questions about your business and formulating appropriate responses is a valuable exercise before talking with the media (or indeed, all your audiences). The development of a Q&A document for internal use can be particularly helpful when you do not want to disclose all the details of a particular piece of news due to partner constraints, strategic considerations, or intellectual property reasons. Not all stories require detailed disclosure. You can work with your patent counsel, financial disclosure advisor, and other legal counsel in advance to determine the level of detail and timing of what you are willing to disclose or language that provides a simple, polite reason why you aren't going to answer a given question. Consider potential questions in advance, especially "difficult" ones where other factors affect what you might want to say. This can help ensure a smooth interview and make it easier for multiple spokespersons to communicate in a single, consistent voice.

WORKING WITH REPORTERS AND EDITORS

Developing and nurturing positive ongoing relationships with reporters requires that you understand and respect their needs throughout your interactions with them. Reporters are not your friends, but neither are they your enemies. Most just want to do their job quickly and well. Your goal is to help them do it in a way that results in fair and accurate coverage of your company. Honoring reporters' deadlines is particularly important, and those deadlines will vary with the type of publication or media outlet. With the rise of Internet journalism, much more news is reported "as it happens" on a daily basis than ever before, often requiring rapid responses within a few hours at most. Other publications maintain weekly or monthly schedules, providing a greater window for response. The bottom line: if you have announced news, make sure that a company spokesperson is available to respond in a timely fashion. If you are contacted by a journalist, one of your first questions should be, "What's your deadline?" That reply will tell you how quickly you need to respond—whether in hours or days.

A word about "embargos." An *embargo* is an agreement between you and a journalist that they will not publish or otherwise make public a piece of information until a certain date and time, or until certain conditions are met. The intent of an embargo is to give journalists more time to research and write about the news, so that their published report can coincide with the announcement date, and in theory, those reports should be more accurate. Life science companies have often employed embargoes around peer-reviewed publications or scientific meeting presentations, where the embargo date and time is mandated by the journal or meeting organizers. Embargoes have sometimes been used around major corporate or product announcements. While embargoes may be useful for helping to bring significant attention to your news, it is important to get agreement from specific media that they will honor the embargo, or you will risk having your news get out too soon. Even with such an agreement, embargoes carry significant risks. In today's world where getting a story into print or on the air first is the holy grail, embargos mean very little to some mainstream journalists. One journalist breaking your embargo and getting the news out early can anger other journalists, even though *you* did nothing wrong. Embargos may also be broken unintentionally (usually due to miscommunications

in the media outlet's newsroom). As a result, the use of embargos should be considered carefully, especially by public companies where such early "leaks" can have serious investor relations consequences.

When you are speaking with a reporter, do not say anything that you would not want to see in print. Nothing is ever really "off the record," even if you think you have an agreement with your interviewer. You are the expert on your company, technology, and products, so learn to talk comfortably and enthusiastically about them, making sure to clearly deliver the key messages you want your interviewer to take away and echo in their reporting. It's best to refrain from discussing your competition in but the most general terms (and try to redirect any questions about those companies back to your own story)—you don't want the interview to turn into a story about your competition or your feelings about them. If you don't know the answer to a question, just say so and offer to get back to the reporter with an answer later.

Obviously you may be concerned about the ultimate accuracy of any article that appears. While journalistic etiquette precludes you from asking to review and approve an article before publication (and indeed, writers for many major newspapers and magazines would be in trouble if they complied with such a request), you should offer to fact check or otherwise make yourself available for follow-up calls. You can also help the reporter by sending additional information resources, such as your fact sheet, biographies, and introductions to industry contacts who can comment knowledgably and positively about your business. Your goal should be to make it as easy as possible for the reporter to write accurately about you and your company. However, even if you have experienced a very positive interview and your reporter is enthusiastic about your story, media coverage is not guaranteed until you see it in print. Many things can affect getting a particular article published, including decisions by senior editors, competing news, and similar pieces in other publications.

Hopefully, if an article about you and your company does appear, it will be positive and accurate. If you don't like the title, in most cases you should not blame the reporter, who probably didn't write it. If you don't agree with the coverage, before you act, consider why you don't and how best to respond. If there are factual mistakes you should certainly contact the reporter to correct them in a friendly, straightforward manner. Reporters want to be accurate, and even if you are unable to get an immediate correction, you have educated them for their future coverage. If you disagree for other reasons with the coverage and seriously feel the need to respond, there may be better ways to do so than just contacting the reporter or their editor. For example, a "Letter to the Editor" or other editorial contributions to their publication will enable you to tell your own story and reinforce key message points while rebutting the points you don't agree with in the original piece.

Ultimately your goal in working with reporters is to build positive working relationships over the long-term that lead to repeated coverage in their current publication or other media outlets as well as with media outlets that employ them in the future. To that end, it helps to position yourself as a resource for the reporter: being on-topic, interesting to talk with, and quick to respond whether or not you and your company are the focus of the phone call or interview. Taking the time to meet with reporters where there is no expectation of immediate coverage is also a good way to educate them about your company in advance of news or in anticipation of future coverage. (See Table 18.2.)

TABLE 18.2 Six Myths of Media Relations

Perception	Reality
If I issue a press release, my news will be covered by the media.	Your news will only have a chance of coverage if it's understandable and relevant to a publication's particular audience. Internet feeds will pick up news releases, but edited publications choose from hundreds of news releases and story ideas every day.
A good PR agency can get me the coverage I want, any place I want.	Personal relationships may get your story a hearing. But to gain coverage, your story must fit what a publication's editors or a broadcast outlet's producers perceive as appropriate and of interest to its audience.
Every interview leads to coverage.	Many factors go into what ultimately sees print or is broadcast, even after the interview, including competing news, editorial preferences, or available space.
If I get a writer interested in my story, coverage will come quickly.	There is much competition for limited print space or broadcast capacity. Even if a reporter is interested, it can be many months before a story appears, depending on the particular publication.
If I ask for the conversation to be "off the record," then nothing I say will be printed.	Nothing is ever really off the record. Be careful when saying things or discussing topics that you do not want to appear in print.
If I give a journalist information that is embargoed for a certain date and time, nothing will appear in print until then.	Like giving "off the record" information, embargoes can be a questionable proposition and should probably be used only when necessitated by the constraints of peer-reviewed journals or major medical meetings. Even then, be prepared for possible embargo breakers to release your news before the agreed time in the heat of competition or sometimes inadvertently.

A version of this table previously appeared in *Nature Biotechnology* ("Why Media Relations Matter," by Joan Kureczka, Published online: 20 March 2006, doi:10.1038/bioent906) and appears here with permission of that publication.

BUILDING VISIBILITY WHEN YOU DON'T HAVE NEWS

Even when you don't expect to have news for many months, good opportunities exist for building visibility in the media or through other communications activities. You may be able to tap into larger news stories or business trends by showing reporters how your company fits or provides a unique and different view of the situation. There may be a strong human-interest component to your story or a particular local angle that can attract editorial interest. Your experience could serve as a successful case-study for other entrepreneurs or businesses. Round-up articles—which discuss multiple companies as part of an overview of a new field of research, technology, or therapeutic focus—provide especially good opportunities for coverage that can put you in the spotlight alongside much more prominent firms. Many trade publications publish annual editorial calendars that reveal general topics for coverage in upcoming issues that could include your company, technology, or products. You can also generate your own coverage through the contribution of articles such as opinion editorials, white papers, bylined technical articles, or commentaries on a particular topic. Such articles not only raise your company's visibility and position you as a thought-leader, but also allow you to differentiate your company from others or establish your emerging business as a peer to much bigger, more established ones. Many of these ideas for building visibility also hold beyond media relations to activities like speaking engagements on conference panels, which can often generate their own media interest, or other visibility with audiences beyond those in attendance.

CASE STUDY—STRATEGIC USE OF PR TO SUPPORT BOTH FINANCING AND PARTNERING

Here is a real-world example of how one start-up biotechnology company, Resolve Therapeutics of Seattle, Washington, used PR strategies from the time of its formation to support efforts to find both investors and a corporate partner. In the Fall of 2010, financing for most early-stage companies was near its low. Resolve Therapeutics, whose aim was to advance research on a promising potential drug for lupus, was founded with a then-unique LLC business structure aimed at giving investors a realistic chance at significant investment returns within three years. The company's objective: to raise a small amount of investment capital and sign a partnership deal as soon as possible that could pay for costly advanced clinical studies and give its founders and initial investors a substantial, relatively fast return on their investment.

Resolve used PR strategies to generate ongoing publicity for its efforts that would help create awareness and generate interest for the company's product, business strategy, and potential value as an investment. These activities included:

1. Scheduling interviews with publications targeting both the life sciences investment community and potential corporate partners that could lead within weeks to published emerging company profiles, even in the absence of specific news.
2. Using news of the company formation and initial financings to build significant business and trade media coverage of the company and its business.
3. Positioning and seeking interviews and other opportunities for Resolve's CEO to comment as a thought-leader and present a successful case study on alternative financing models for start-up life sciences companies.

The company utilized the news of its formation along with the research and product lead licensed from the University of Washington, as well as information about the Resolve's unique business structure and capitalization strategy, to interest the regional business publication *Xconomy* in writing about Resolve and the company's plans. Resolve also issued a press release and spoke with other trade publications with readership representing the company's principal audiences of corporate executives and life science investors. Additional profiles were also sought and obtained in trade publications willing to write about emerging companies.

This initial PR effort was followed up by subsequent news announcements around the company's two small financings 6 and 13 months later and again when Resolve signed its desired corporate partnership. In between news announcements, the company continued to generate a low level of coverage that helped to keep the Resolve name in the news by positioning and pitching Resolve's CEO as a thought leader on alternative financing strategies—an effort that led to multiple interviews and inclusion in several round-up articles pertaining to financing strategies.

Results: Over a period of less than 3 years, Resolve was able to generate a stream of positive press on its product and business strategy in publications that were widely read by its intended target audiences, thus supporting the company's objectives of finding a small number of new investors and signing a corporate partnership at an early stage of product development.

WHAT ABOUT DIGITAL AND SOCIAL MEDIA?

Over the past 15 years or more the media landscape has changed enormously. The rise of the Internet as a channel for providing content at any time, in any place has been accompanied by a shrinking or transformation of what were previously print and broadcast communications. The result has been both an explosion of new outlets of various qualities

and reach as well as the means for interactive communications. For companies, this change means many more ways of reaching your intended audiences, interacting directly with them, and further amplifying what is said about you and your technology or products. The number and quality of social media sites is continually changing, so this discussion is focusing on just a few prominent social media outlets that have proven to be most useful to emerging companies.

One of the earliest forms of online media to emerge was the blog—an online diary which may consist of original content, commentary on news (including other blogs), or serve as a clearinghouse for news and commentary from other sites. Today, according to Wikipedia, there are more than 150 million public blogs on a wide variety of subjects. Content includes not only text, but also artwork, photos, video or audio files, and often provide links to other websites. The majority are interactive, enabling readers to post their own comments to a site. Blog authorship ranges from single-contributor sites to those with multiple authors, and many are now sponsored by mainstream media or even individual companies who may use them to promote their own product or corporate brand. Many mainstream journalists now have their own blogs, further blurring the distinction between bloggers and reporters, thus reinforcing the need to treat them the same. Additionally, there are many blogs sponsored by patient advocacy organizations or patients themselves that can provide insight into issues that may affect a product's development or commercialization. While a company may choose not to actively comment on these sites, regular monitoring of what is said on the most influential sites closely related to your business may provide valuable insights and early warnings.

Blogs clearly offer a way for companies with products or services to interact with their customers, either through their own blogs or through those blogs or forums sponsored by others. They enable companies to receive and provide direct feedback, correct misperceptions, and put forth new ideas. They also provide opportunities for customers and other audiences to get answers directly from the company. Companies that are rapidly growing and, especially geographically dispersed ones, interested in blogging strategies may want to consider the use of internal corporate blogs to strengthen a sense of community within their own organization. Such internal sites can help create powerful conversations that open forums for education, collaboration, and teamwork, especially if contributors to the blog include frontline employees as well as senior managers. Be warned, however, if you decide to start your own blog for any purpose, blogging successfully is time-consuming and requires regular, frequent contributions in order to build an audience.

Microblogging is the posting of short pieces of content including text, photos, or video links and has become enormously popular as a way to share news and resources, interact with others and build reputation, coordinate or report on meetings, and many other uses. Twitter (www.twitter.com), the most widely used microblogging outlet for business as well as personal purposes, has an active community of those who belong to, or are interested in, the life sciences. Users include journalists, life science executives and other employees, investors, and professionals who support the industry with a variety of services, as well as interested members of the general public. While a relatively small number of companies are represented by name, the number of active corporate accounts continues to grow, and the number of individuals following those accounts is in the hundreds of thousands. Twitter has become a useful tool for those interested in reporting news as it happens, amplifying other communications (through links to press releases, news stories and video), sourcing/sharing ideas and resources, and creating a presence and network within a target community.

LinkedIn (www.linkedin.com) is another site with value for both start-up companies and individuals. Designed specifically for professional networking, users can also promote themselves and their companies by posting articles and engaging with others through specific groups assembled around both organizations and interests. At a minimum, every organization should take ownership of their company's LinkedIn page, where they can include their positioning statement and other information about their firm.

Finally, YouTube (www.youtube.com) and Vimeo (www.vimeo.com) provide opportunities for companies to post videos, which may then be promoted and shared through press releases, on the company website or on other social media.

Clearly social media has become a very useful extension of a biotechnology company's PR efforts, irrespective of the long wait for any clear guidance from the U.S. Food and Drug Administration regarding the use of social media as it pertains to therapeutic, diagnostic, and medical device products. Twitter, in particular, enables companies to reach a large audience including journalists more quickly and easily than any other medium. As a result, the return on investment for this new tool is large and growing for life sciences companies, especially for corporate communication uses, as opposed to product communications where regulatory uncertainty remains for FDA-regulated products.

SUMMARY

Public relations is an important tool for any company seeking to reach key audiences and support their business objectives, whether those include finding investors, collaborators, customers, acquirers, or employees. A critical step in reaching your target audience is to understand the story you want to tell and relate it to your audiences' needs and interests. Spend time analyzing and defining what makes you different and unique and understand where the opportunities lie in your business for creating value, then frame those attributes in a way that addresses your intended audiences' needs and interests. Utilize the language and key messages you have developed throughout all company communications, including your website, fact sheets, and corporate presentations. Once you understand and craft the story you want to tell, you can design a PR strategy to support many objectives such as raising capital, finding partners, building a customer base, or any other business goal. This campaign should not be limited to an announcement of major business milestones, but can employ a range of strategies. These can include the announcement of other important events for your company such as major scientific publications and presentations and seeking media coverage in round-up and trend stories as well as through contributed articles of various kinds. Development-stage life science companies need to know the various media and available communications channels, how they reach your desired audience, and how best to work with them. This will help you create an effective communications program that builds broad visibility and credibility for your company over time.

ADDITIONAL RESOURCES

Each of the three main full-service newswire distribution companies offer a variety of basic instructional resources on their sites including guides for writing press releases and whitepapers and other articles with more information on search engine optimization, using multimedia in press releases, and working with reporters:

1. PR Newswire: http://www.prnewswire.com/knowledge-center/
2. BusinessWire: http://www.businesswire.com/portal/site/home/education
3. GlobeNewswire: www.globenewswire.com/home/learning-support/

The Financial Capital

Chapter 19

Sources of Capital and Investor Motivations

Craig Shimasaki, PhD, MBA

President & CEO, Moleculera Labs and BioSource Consulting Group, Oklahoma City, Oklahoma

Capital is the lifeblood of every biotechnology company. Without capital, product development ceases irrespective of its potential value and market need. Because biotechnology companies require enormous amounts of capital in order to advance their product toward commercialization, it behooves the company leader to develop a well-thought-out fundraising plan tied to a detailed strategy for the use of this capital. Knowing which capital source is optimally interested in your stage of development is essential. For instance, during the inception stage when your product idea is a basic research concept and the company is without a full management team, it is unlikely that any venture capital firm would be interested in listening to a pitch about your enterprise. Your time would be wasted trying to secure a meeting with a disinterested venture capital firm. As we will discuss in more detail, most venture capital firms invest in latter-stage companies, as these managers have larger amounts of capital they need to deploy, and a $500,000 investment still requires the same amount of management time as a $5 million dollar investment.

UNDERSTANDING INVESTOR CRITERIA AND LIMITATIONS

Before we discuss these capital sources and their preferred company stages of investment, it is important to recognize that every group has investing preferences and investing limitations. These criteria include: preferences for a particular biotechnology sector (see Chapter 9 entitled "Understanding Biotechnology Sectors"), minimum and maximum investing limits, as well as a specific investing time horizon. It is an advantage to understand the interests, motivations, and limitations of each of these sources of capital prior to raising money. For instance, it would be futile to try to raise $5 to $10 million from a group of angel investors, as this amount is typically beyond their capacity and interest for investing. Possibly, some angels may appear interested in your technology and market opportunity, but if you don't know that angel investors are unlikely to collectively invest $10 million, you will be wasting your time trying to interest them in your opportunity. Late-stage investors such as venture capital (VC) firms also have preferences for specific biotechnology sectors in which their partners or principals have experience and expertise. It would be advantageous to take your medical device opportunity, for instance, to a VC group whose portfolio already contains a few medical device companies, rather than to try to interest a VC firm mostly comprised of GreenTech companies. This is because you can be sure that at least one VC partner has a preference and expertise in evaluating medical device deals and they would be more likely to consider investing in another medical device company.

Each funding source has a preferred investing time horizon in which to have their capital deployed and returned. Some investment groups have a 5- to 7-year time horizon in which they expect to see a return, whereas others have a shorter time horizon for an investment. If your business does not anticipate having an exit opportunity (exits are discussed below) until 6 years, it would be futile to spend any time trying to pitch your company to an investor group that want an exit in 3 to 4 years. When you understand the interests and limitations of different capital sources it allows you to focus your efforts on sources most interested in investing in your company. Recognize that each group's criteria may, or may not, be written down, but it is certainly understood by its principals. Always be sure to ask about a group's investing criteria and limitations before targeting an investor group; this will reduce the time you spend on fundraising and increase the likelihood of investment success.

UNDERSTANDING INVESTORS' EXPECTATIONS FOR RETURN ON INVESTMENT

Investors in biotechnology companies expect to receive a return that is significantly greater than a Certificate of Deposit or mutual fund. Most investor groups have well-defined expectations for returns on their investment, and these expectations are commensurate with the level of risk they are taking. A return on investment (ROI) is often stated as a multiple of the amount originally invested such as a 5×, 10×, or 20× return. Investment returns are also expressed as an "internal rate of return" (IRR). An IRR is the percent increase in the original investment calculated on an annual basis. IRRs are related to a specific investment timeframe without referring to that timeframe. For instance, an opportunity can be expressed as having an IRR of 25 percent, but you don't know whether the exit is in 3 years or 7 years. In general, biotech investor's interest perk up with IRRs in the range of 20 to 40 percent. When asked, most investors typically describe their expectations as a multiple of their investment, and also by the number of years in which to exit.

As we discuss in greater detail below, angel investors are early-stage investors. Because angels typically invest before VCs do, they have higher ROI expectations for their money than VCs. This is because early-stage investors bear a greater risk than a late-stage investor does. Therefore, it is not unusual for angels to have an expectation of 20× to 30× return on their investment for the higher risk they take on an investment, whereas at least a 10× return may initially get the attention of a VC. Both angels and VCs require high-return multiples because biotechnology investing is high risk, and many of the companies in their portfolio may not return any money at all. In order to compensate, investors have extremely high expectations for returns on *every* deal they make. As a manager, make sure that your product and business model supports the level of investor return necessary for the particular group you desire to interest.

UNDERSTAND WHAT COMES WITH INVESTED MONEY: MOTIVATIONS AND INTERESTS

All sources of cash invested into a company spends the same. In other words, a dollar from one investor spends the same as a dollar from another investor, and both lasts the same amount of time in a company's bank account. However, there can be vastly different ties, values, and benefits that come with each investor who puts that dollar into the company. For instance, if you need to raise $750,000 to reach your next value-enhancing milestone, this amount of capital is an amount that multiple angels can cumulatively fulfill. However, each angel investor and angel group has differing philosophies about investing, managing, and how

a business should be conducted. In addition, each investing source can have differing perceptions about how a business should be run, what is expected from a management team, and how they should be involved. Along with these varied expectations, there are different intangible benefits that accompany each investor. In other words, each capital source brings a different value to your company. For instance, some angels may be former entrepreneurs who have worked in a similar sector developing a similar product. Investors like these, if you can find them, are familiar with the issues your start-up company will face and they can advise the management about ways they overcame similar issues. Whereas, other investors who don't know about the biotechnology industry, may come with unrealistic expectations on how to develop, test, and market your future product even though they never invested in a life science deal before. The entrepreneurial leader should evaluate each investor's expectations and their perceptions of business conduct as well as their business acumen and benefit to the organization. Evaluating this prior to accepting capital can prevent or mitigate problematic issues and operational challenges that the leader may face when working and interfacing with these investors over time. In a sense, you are screening your investors for fit with the goals of your business and the core values of your company. Since most companies need capital sooner than later, all too often this "investor fit" is not evaluated, which can lead to conflicts when decisions about the methods for reaching company goals are made.

When company management and their investors are aligned, there is synergy in motivations and acceleration in the company growth and development. Harmonious alignment brings added value and enhances your ability to reach goals that may otherwise be difficult to achieve without these investors. Conversely, an incongruent investor will sooner or later precipitate inevitable conflicts between themselves and the company, taking a toll on the management, which hinders development of the company's product. When misalignment occurs, more energy is devoted to resolving internal conflicts than is expended on making product development progress. As a result, wasted energy and resources detract from the future success of the organization. I have observed in real life where investor conflicts became so severe that there was an unexpected departure of the management and entrepreneurial leaders. Always examine the interests, motivations, and core values of potential investors to be sure they are aligned with those of the company and its founders prior to closing a financing round. The entrepreneur should recognize that it is natural to have differing opinions about methods for reaching company goals, but there should still be alignment in the interests, motivations, and core values of both parties. Having value-adding investors provides an opportunity for the management to gain wisdom from like-minded individuals who have more experience and resources than they do. (Figure 19.1.)

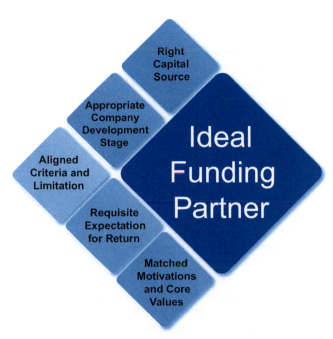

FIGURE 19.1 Funding alignment principles.

Finding the ideal funding partner is not easy but the likelihood increases in finding the right fit by following these funding alignment principles. These include:

1. Select the right capital source for your company.
2. Make sure that the target capital source has interest in the development stage of your company.
3. Make sure there is alignment with your company's financial needs and the criteria and limitations of the funding source.
4. Make sure that your opportunity can provide the necessary return that your target funding source is seeking.
5. Make sure there is alignment with the motivations and core values of the target funding source and the company.

WHAT ARE THE CAPITAL SOURCES AVAILABLE TO BIOTECHNOLOGY COMPANIES?

A variety of capital sources are available to finance product development and grow biotechnology companies. In this section we discuss the most common sources of capital available to this industry. There are additional sources of capital other than those described below, such as bank loans, but those sources are not known for investing or financing biotechnology companies. The following list contains the sources most common to this industry:

1. Personal capital
2. Friends and family
3. Government grant and financing programs
4. Angel investors
5. Foundations with a focus in your sector
6. Venture capital industry
7. Industry corporate partnerships
8. Institutional debt financing

Personal Capital

It is not unusual for the founders of a new company to initially operate for a period of time utilizing their own personal funds. Often, founders will invest some of their own money to operate their company; it shows they are serious and committed to the enterprise. Subsequent investors have a more favorable impression about the company founders knowing they have some "skin-in-the-game." Investors realize that founders are not likely to walk away or shirk their responsibilities if they have their own hard-earned capital riding on the success of their company. Depending on the stage of the company and the sector, the amount of personal money an entrepreneur invests can vary. Sometimes the amount invested can be perfunctory, like the $500 invested by both Rob Swanson and Herb Boyer when they founded Genentech. Other times, the investment can grow to tens of thousands of dollars as the founders are building the organization prior to other investors participating. A good personal rule to follow is that a capital investment of 5 percent of your net assets would be favorably viewed by other investors; whereas 20 percent or more of your personal assets invested in your start-up may seem naïve and can be viewed as a poor business decision. Even though it may sound noble to have a large portion of your assets invested in your company, it is not a financially wise thing to do. Be sure the amount committed is something you can afford to lose. Unsuspecting founders think that their investment is simply a loan to the company until new investors join and they can then be paid back. New investors, however, rarely agree to let their capital be used to pay back previous investors or company debt. New investors want their fresh capital to go toward building value into the business rather than paying off past debt obligations.

Another reason many founders will invest their own money into their company is to purchase their stock outright. Paying a nominal amount of money for founder's stock (different types of stock are discussed in Chapter 13: Company Formation, Ownership Structure and Securities Issues.) is not unusual and there can be a tax advantage to paying for your stock when the company has minimal financial value. Often, start-up entrepreneurs do not possess significant amounts of capital to contribute to their new company venture. In these cases, it is not unusual for founders to work for minimal, and sometimes no, salary for a period of time while the company matures. Underpaid or nonpaid effort is referred to as "sweat equity," and this is, in essence, a tangible contribution to the company. As the enterprise grows and additional investment capital is secured, the founders may still earn lower than average wages, but they still should be compensated by holding significant amounts of equity (stock) in their company.

Friends and Family

Early-stage capital for your venture can come from friends, family members, and close associates. These individuals may not always be sophisticated investors, and their major motivation for investing is because they know you, the entrepreneur, and they believe in what you are doing. The amount of money raised from friends and family varies, but it is usually small compared to the amount of money you need to make significant product development process. Often this capital is used along with personal capital to initiate company formation and make some progress toward product development while seeking investments from other sources of capital. Sometimes an entrepreneur may be fortunate and have very knowledgeable family members that have industry and investing experience. However, more often than not, these "experienced" family members are less experienced in the biotechnology industry than one may think. Unfortunately, sometimes friends and family may even have greater expectations than traditional investors who are knowledgeable with the risks within this industry. Although friends and family can be a ready and familiar source of capital, do not forget that Thanksgiving and Christmas are annual holidays when your friends and family may be sitting across the dinner table expecting to hear good news about their investment. If friends and family invest, it is always a good idea to be sure that it is money they can afford to lose. The amount one can expect to reasonably raise from friends and family varies from hundreds of dollars, to tens of thousands of dollars. In rare cases, you may find that the combination of your personal money and capital from friends and family could total hundreds of thousands of dollars.

Government Grant and Financing Programs

It is wise to seek and apply for various types of grant funding to help offset your research and development costs. Grant funding is competitive, but it is an excellent source of funding that can be directed toward making significant R&D progress. I know of an early-stage biotechnology company that was successfully awarded enough state and federal grants to advance their therapeutic product through animal studies and into a major portion of early human clinical trials. One medical device company has been so successful in winning federal grants that they funded almost all their research and development costs for the new products they developed and commercialized. Grant funding is also known as "nondilutive" capital. Grants are "nondilutive"

because you are not giving away equity (stock) in exchange for this capital. As will be discussed later in this chapter, each time you raise dilutive capital you must give away equity in return. When you do this you simultaneously reduce the percentage of ownership of all the existing shareholders. Even though previous shareholders, including founders, may hold the same number of shares that were originally issued, the percent ownership tied to those shares becomes "diluted" when additional shares are issued to others.

Local and federal governments are aware of the economic benefit in supporting the development and growth of technology businesses, and as such there may be new incentives in your area that support and grow biotechnology companies. Be sure to allocate time and effort finding and applying to the sources which are supportive of your business. Even though grants are "free" money, the lead time from application to receiving grant awards can be quite lengthy, on the order of 9 to 12 months. Careful planning for grant opportunities can make a difference in the success and future of your company and product development.

Academic and SBIR/STTR Grants

There are different types of grants that biotechnology companies can access. Academic professors and scientists in the United States are familiar with the National Institutes of Health (NIH) grant program which funds basic research and keeps their laboratories active with graduate students and postdocs. Traditional academic research grants are a great way for scientists, contemplating a spin-off company, to advance their product idea as far as possible on grant funding. Our most recent company, Moleculera Labs, licensed a panel of five clinical assays that were nearly ready to be commercially offered through our clinical laboratory. The product technology was advanced to near final stages because of the numerous research grants the principal investigator was awarded over the many years of development.

For-profit companies are not often recipients of academic research grants; however, there are 11 federal agencies in the United States that have other grant programs to fund scientific-based, high-risk commercial product development. This granting program is called Small Business Innovative Research (SBIR) and is operated similarly to the basic research programs that award basic research grants. These same agencies have a parallel grant program called STTR program (Strategic Technology Transfer Research), which awards grants to partnerships between the academic institutions and for-profit companies that codevelop high-technology commercial products. The SBIR and STTR programs grant money to for-profit companies that are developing products and services considered to be "high-risk" but have high potential economic payoffs. U.S. federal agencies with extramural research and development (R&D) budgets that exceed $100 million are required to allocate 2.8 percent (as of 2014) of their R&D budget to these programs. SBIR Phase I grants can provide up to $100,000 or more for 6 months, whereas SBIR Phase II grants can provide up to $1,000,000 or more for 2 to 3 years. Recently, follow-on commercialization programs awarding $500,000 to $3 million have been introduced for successful products completing Phase I and II SBIR programs. More detailed information about SBIR/STTR grants can be found in Chapter 14, Licensing the Technology: Biotechnology Commercialization Strategies Using University and Federal Labs. As an added incentive, it is not uncommon to find local government programs that will provide a one-to-one match for companies that receive SBIR and STTR funding. Even if you are not a proficient grant writer, there are free SBIR workshops to assist in improving your grant writing skills. There are also webinar-based support groups such as NCET2 [1] that offer free help to first-time grant applicants of SBIR. Alternatively, you can hire proficient grant writers to assist you in these efforts, but realize that good grant writing is not a substitute for having a top-notch research and development strategy with a novel and significant product.

Another significant value of winning peer-reviewed government grants (aside from the nondilutive benefit) is that these awards indirectly give validation from peer reviewers and scientists, especially if the company has won more than one award. Funding sources such as VCs look favorably on companies that have been successful in winning Phase II SBIR and STTR grants. More information on these government programs can be found on the Small Business Innovative Research website [2].

Local Grant Programs

Cities, states, and regional governments have become increasingly interested in creating biotechnology clusters in their locale. The biotechnology industry is attractive because it creates high technology and high-paying jobs, is a clean industry, and brings in knowledge-based and highly skilled laborers. As described in Chapter 5 entitled "Five Essential Elements for Growing Biotechnology Clusters," one of the significant universal missing elements is access to capital for these companies. As a result, local governments have created various programs, including grant programs to fund start-ups and early-development-stage technology companies as a means to jump-start their local bioscience industry. Hundreds of millions, even billions of dollars in funding initiatives have been set aside by various governments in support of local biotechnology growth initiatives. Entrepreneurs should familiarize themselves with their own local grant-support programs. These programs are usually tailored to support technology companies located in a specific region. The number

of applicants to these programs are fewer than for federal programs and as a result, they are less competitive because of the smaller pool of researchers. If you are not aware of regional government funding programs in your area, start out by asking your local Chamber of Commerce and your State Department of Commerce to find out what is available for your type of company and stage of development. Also, some municipalities have designated underdeveloped areas where the government offers financial assistance to companies that will locate in these less-commercialized areas.

As an example of local government-supported grants, the state of Oklahoma passed an Economic Development Act in 1987 creating the Oklahoma Center for the Advancement of Science and Technology (OCAST) to spur economic growth and diversity. OCAST adopted an NIH-type peer-reviewed grant system external to Oklahoma, that by the end of 2013 funded over 2455 projects with more than $250 million awarded for science and technology research that translated into companies creating technology products developed in the state of Oklahoma. At a previous company, we received over $900,000 from OCAST's competitive grant program, and at a subsequent company, we won another $850,000 to fund our company's product development. Because entrepreneurs need as much financial help as they can get, spend time learning about your local government-assistance programs. You may be pleasantly surprised at the funds which are available directly from your own state or local government.

Local Financing Programs

In your locale there may be government-backed and government-funded programs that support biotechnology and high-technology companies in a particular geographic region. The difference between government *financing* programs and government *granting* programs is that financing programs take equity in the company or have a security interest in the company in exchange for funding, whereas government grants are nondilutive and the company does not give anything in exchange. These financing programs often operate similarly to other institutional sources that take stock in exchange for capital or issue debts that must be paid back. Often these government financing programs are mission- or industry-driven and there may be some favorable terms given in order to stimulate the growth of the biotechnology industry in your local region. Other times, there may be no difference in terms compared to other sources of capital, just the fact that it is available to companies in a locale that is limited in capital resources for biotechnology companies at development stages. Check for local technology commercialization programs that may have local government-backed financing for your company. In 1997, the state of Oklahoma created a Technology Commercialization Center after the oil bust, as a means to help stimulate the organic development of new technology companies and to diversify the state's economy. The center is managed by

I2E, an acronym for Innovation-to-Enterprise, where trained staff and various funding sources are made available to shepherd and guide promising but fledgling technology companies to be successful. To date they have provided government-backed and government-financed funding of $23.8 million and leveraged an additional $402 million from private investors for Oklahoma companies. I2E has provided support services to over 500 emerging small businesses and is a recognized model organization for technology development across the country. Sometimes you may find government-backed and government-funding sources of capital that you were not aware of right in your own neighborhood.

Angel Investors

This next investor group is more purposeful in their investing than most friends and family. Private individuals who invest early in a company and meet certain investing criteria are called "angel investors." The term ascribed to these individuals is not necessarily related to their generosity or their spirituality, but rather these investors are considered to be "angelic" or "heaven-sent," in a sense, rescuing a company at critical times, providing life-supporting financing. Angel investors generally invest at early stages of product and company development which is typically before venture capital funds invest. Because of the early investment risk, their expectation for return ranges from 10× to 20× and some have higher expectations of 30× or more. Most angel investors do not co-invest with VC funds or institutional investors. The typical angel investor invests from $25,000 to $250,000 in any one deal, and in rare cases an angel investor can invest multiple millions, depending upon their interest in the technology, and their capital resources. Sometimes angel investors who want to invest less than $25,000 each will collectively pull together their investment with other angels and form a limited liability corporation (LLC) for a larger-pooled investment in a company.

The term *angel investor* is used synonymously with, or interpreted to mean, "accredited investor." The U.S. Securities and Exchange Commission (SEC) defines an accredited investor [3] as an individual (or individual and spouse) with a net worth of over $1 million, or an individual with an annual income of $200,000 or more for the past 2 years, or $300,000 with a spouse for the past 2 years, and a reasonable expectation of the same income for the current year. In the United States, there are over 400,000 active angels investing in various companies. Angels may invest in companies individually or in formalized groups called angel networks. Well-established angel networks have formal meetings with participation requirements in order to be a member. Membership dues are usually required and there are formalized structures with defined funding review systems that assist with due diligence and mechanisms for following their investments. Some examples of angel network groups that invest in life sciences include: the St. Louis Arch Angels which have about 60 active

members and have funded approximately 35 companies with approximately $30 million. The Tech Coast Angels in California is one of the largest angel networks with over 300 members who collectively invested over $120 million in over 200 companies. Tech Coast Angels invest in a broader sector of high technology, including IT and life science. The biotech entrepreneur should know that the completion for investment from these groups is high. For example, in 2012 the Tech Cost Angels received over 600 applications and funded only 17 deals. More information about Angel Investors and Angel Networks can be found in Chapter 20: Securing Angel Capital and Understanding How Angel Networks Operate.

Angel investors are motivated to invest in companies because either they are familiar with the market need for a product, have a desire to support a local company, or because they believe in the entrepreneur and their ability to make it a success. Sometimes angels may require more time to learn about the business and science if they have limited exposure to biotechnology. However, as this industry expands and matures, there are increasing numbers of experienced angels who became successful through exits from their own biotech company start-ups. In general, angels prefer to invest in local companies and they limit their investments to their local geographic region. The reason for this is a combination of the desire to see local companies succeed coupled with the lack of interest in traveling long distances to monitor their investment. Increasingly however, more angels and angel networks are branching out to "syndicate" or co-invest with other angels to diversify their portfolio, and this requires that angels consider nonlocal deals.

For the most part, for a higher likelihood of success, seek angels in your own geographic region who may know you or have heard about your company. Finding these investors can be challenging because they do not advertise their activities and investing is not their full-time job. A good way to find angel investors is by networking with people who know them and by asking them for introductions. Other ways include checking with your local university or research institution's Technology Transfer Office for names and contacts, as they may know many of the local angels. Also check with the local Chamber of Commerce, your regional economic development agency, or a technology commercialization center or equivalent—these may be good sources of angel contacts that invest in biotechnology. Do not forget that most angels are connected to other angels. Once an angel has invested, ask them for help and introductions to others. A motivated and excited angel investor telling your company story is very effective. There are many angels out there—just be persistent in locating them.

Foundations With a Focus in Your Sector

In the recent decade, nonprofit foundations focused on certain disease conditions have become an increasingly more common funder of biotechnology product development.

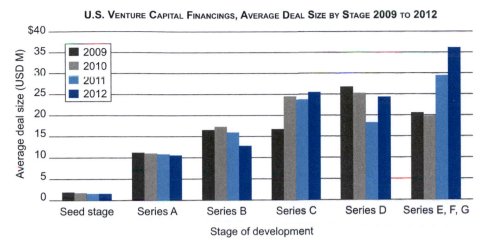

FIGURE 19.2   United States venture capital deal size by stages. *(From Burrill & Company.)*

These foundations are focused on improving the health and advancing solutions for individuals afflicted with a specific condition or disease. In the past, they have had a major focus on funding small research grants to very early-stage academic and basic research. However, these project are usually many years, possibly a decade, away from a treatment, diagnostic or solution for the constituents they are working to help. Foundations have begun to make much larger investments in individual companies that are already advancing a product, treatment or diagnostic towards commercial development. This in turn supports their mission by advancing a future commercial product by helping the company reach the market with a product sooner. Entrepreneurs should search to see if their focus is aligned with a non-profit foundation that may be interested in funding your company's product development. Some examples of disease foundations that have funded product development include: the Bill and Melinda Gates' Foundation, the Cystic Fibrosis Foundation, the Juvenile Diabetes Research Foundation, and the Michael J. Fox Foundation for Parkinson's Research.

Venture Capital Industry

Venture Capital (VC) is comprised of funds managed by professionals who invest in high-risk ventures with the expectation of producing higher than average rates of returns. Most venture capital firms raise money for their fund from institutional investors, such as foundations and endowments, pension funds, insurance companies, and high net-worth families and individuals. The investors who invest in venture capital funds are referred to as "limited partners." Venture capitalists who manage the fund are referred to as "general partners." The general partners have a fiduciary responsibility to their limited partners and are supported through a management fee from the fund. The size of any venture fund varies greatly, from $20 million to over $5

billion per fund with over 900 VC funds in existence. There are VC funds directed to most every type of industry such as life science, therapeutics, diagnostics, medical services, IT, software, and some large funds invested in all of the above. According to the National Venture Capital Association (NVCA), in 2013 over $7 billion was invested into biotechnology, healthcare, and medical device companies in the United States. VC continues to provide a large portion of the funding for the biotechnology industry, especially during the later development stages of product development where large amounts of capital are consumed during clinical trial testing. Figure 19.2 shows the average increase in funding amount from VCs (in millions of dollars) for companies as their development stage progresses.

In order to understand the motivations of venture capital, one must understand the constraints and limitations of VC funds. As shown in Figure 19.3, the venture capital firm receives money from its limited partners for a defined period of time. The limited partners have an expectation for return within that timeframe. The venture capital firm must then identify a portfolio of companies in which to invest with the hopes that these companies each return a significant profit before the fund life cycle is over. All companies are not successful nor do they all bring extraordinary returns to their investors, so the VCs must build into their plan an assumption of the number of failures while still meeting their investors' expectations for returns. There is pressure on the VC firm to have their portfolio companies perform and meet expectations. Fund managers that are not successful at this may not be able to raise a follow-on fund.

The general partners of a VC firm usually devote 100 percent of their time investing and managing their portfolio of companies, compared to angels who typically have a "day job" and invest on the side when they have time. Even though general partners work full-time at finding investments and managing their portfolio, their time is typically limited and in great demand due to the number of companies they manage and the number of issues each company faces. General partners must also answer and report to their limited partners, raise capital for their fund, find new investments, and manage their existing companies. For this reason it is vital when trying to gain the attention of a VC that you make your pitch and value proposition clear and concise so they can quickly assess their interest.

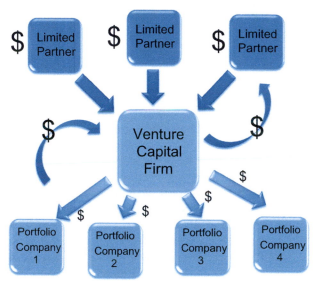

FIGURE 19.3　Understanding the venture capital cycle.

Industry Corporate Partnerships

In addition to traditional financing, another source of capital for biotechnology companies is corporate partnerships (Figure 19.4). The biotechnology company possesses something of value to the corporate partner that they cannot provide on their own. It may be that the biotechnology company's product could help increase sales of the corporate partner's existing products, or it gives them a complementary product they need in their existing market, or the new product leverages their current sales and distribution channel, or it is a way for them to remove a competitive product from their existing market. Biotechnology company partners may be pharmaceutical companies, vaccine manufacturers, medical device companies, large national laboratories, or chemical companies depending on what the biotechnology company has in development and in their pipeline. The formation of a corporate partnership most often occurs during the later stages of product development. However, it does not hurt to solicit interest from these organizations early on as they may have a special interest in the earlier stages of development. Often, a corporate partner may have a longer-term goal which may be to acquire the biotechnology company sometime in the future.

A common exchange between these partners is that the biotechnology company receives cash, milestone fees, reimbursement for development costs, and future royalties

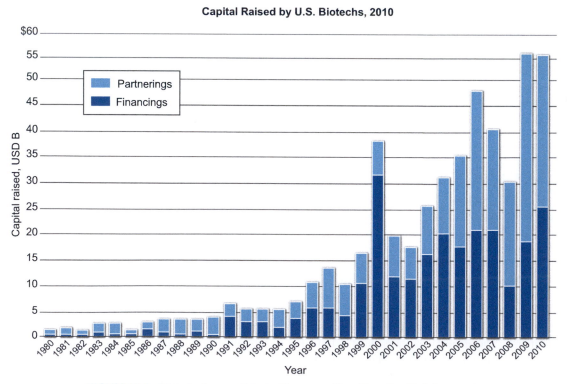

FIGURE 19.4　Biotechnology capital raised by partnerships. *(From Burrill & Company.)*

on their product (Figure 19.5). The corporate partner usually receives an exclusive license to the biotechnology company's future product and a right to market and sell that product in all countries (or selected countries). In the case of therapeutics, biologics, and vaccines, the corporate partner may also transfer responsibility for the remaining stages of human clinical testing and regulatory approval since they have the capital, resources, and the expertise.

Institutional Debt Financing

Institutional debt financing is rarely available to start-up biotechnology companies, whereas it is directed toward companies that already have a commercialized product or service, or at the very least, near-market introduction. The institutions that provide debt financing are very risk averse. Consequently, in order to provide a company with debt financing, the institution must believe that it is a very low risk that the company would not be able to pay back the debt. Lending institutions also require some form of collateral that is worth significantly more than the loan amount, should the institution have to "call" the debt because of nonpayment or default. Early-stage and development-stage biotechnology companies possess very little in the way of "tangible" assets to use as collateral. Because of this, debt financing is really only available to companies that have commercial products and services on the market and collateral becomes accounts receivable, inventory, equipment, facilities, or land. For companies that qualify, there are organizations that provide debt financing for the biotechnology industry which include Silicon Valley Bank, Comerica, and GE Capital to name a few.

Another way to free up cash for working capital is to finance existing equipment if it is already paid off and owned by the company. Cash can be given through a loan for security interest in the paid-off equipment, which would free up more cash for operations. Occasionally, other creative debt-financing methods may be possible. Sometimes an early-stage company may obtain a line of credit from a local intuitional lender if a local high-net worth investor is

willing to guarantee the loan. Obviously, the investor would need to believe there is some assurance that the company can make the payments on the note, and that there will be more value for the investor who backs the note. As a general rule, it is not advisable to use debt financing as a means of funding product development for a biotechnology company. This is because of the high risk, the long development times, and the large amount of capital needed to sustain the company through to commercialization.

DETERMINING THE VALUE OF DEVELOPMENT-STAGE BIOTECHNOLOGY COMPANIES

In order to complete a financing transaction and raise capital, all companies must address the question "how much is the company worth?" The answer to this question dictates the percentage of the company given to new investors in exchange for capital. Valuation also determines the percentage of the company retained by the founders, employees, and existing shareholders. Because of this issue, reaching agreement with potential investors on company valuation is a debated and often contentious process for the entrepreneurial management team. For every company, there is a valuation range where any amount within that range can be justified by each party. Most founders and entrepreneurial management teams want to value their company as high as possible. However, *overvaluing* your company beyond a reasonable range can be counterproductive and detrimental to attracting institutional and venture capital in the future. There are standard, universally accepted methods for determining the value of a company that has product revenue history. Unfortunately, due to the lengthy development time, development-stage biotechnology companies do not have product revenue and must raise significant amounts of capital prior to reaching commercialization.

Below is a brief overview of the various valuation methods for biotechnology companies. This will give you a reference point should you desire additional and more-detailed information on company valuation methods. When assessing the valuation of *latter development-stage companies* the following methods are utilized. Each of these methods can provide differing valuations, but the best valuation is an estimate determined by referencing all four methods.

1. **Valuation by comparables:** Identify similar organizations in similar sectors at similar development stages that have been recently valued at a financing round within the last 12 months. Although valuations of private companies are not publicly disclosed, there are available venture capital resources (for fees) you can access to obtain this information. Also, if you know or have worked with venture capital firms or institutional capital firms, an individual working there may be able to help

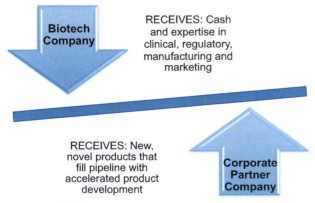

FIGURE 19.5 What do partnerships exchange?

you obtain this type of information. Ideally, one would want to have three or more comparables for reference, with those transactions being closed within the past 12 months. Frequently, exact comparables are not available but there may be related comparables in a related segment that could be used as a surrogate reference. When that occurs, one would use this valuation as a reference make appropriate adjustments (see number 4).

2. **Valuation by public and private exits:** This method is similar to the above except that the calculation is performed on mature companies that have had an exit. For instance, one would use the value of mature companies in a similar sector (therapeutic, diagnostic, medical device, clinical laboratory, bioagriculture, biofuel) determined at the time the company either completed an initial public offering (IPO) or an acquisition by a publicly-traded company. This "exit" value is then divided by the return multiples required by a typical institutional investor. For instance, if an institutional investor today requires an 8 to 10× return on their investment in order to invest, then based upon an IPO or acquisition value of $250 million for the mature company in the same sector, your company can be valued at $250 divided by 8 to 10, for an estimated valuation of $25 to $31 million.

3. **Valuation by risk-adjusted discounted cash flow (rDCF):** This is determined by first estimating the company's future revenues minus the costs associated with generating those revenues, then discounting these by an appropriate interest rate. So, starting with a *discounted cash flow* (DCF) or *net present value* (NPV) of those future earnings, the value of those future earnings is then discounted again by the risk of successfully completing the remaining phases of product development and FDA approval. This final value is called a *risk-adjusted DCF*. Although this method sounds complicated, there are good mathematical programs for calculating these values. The uncertainty comes predominately from the estimation of the risks associated with successfully completing the remaining product-development phases and regulatory success. Although this method is relatively straight-forward to calculate, it is not recognized as a reliable and trusted valuation method for pre-revenue biotechnology companies.

4. **Valuation adjustments:** There are several value-adding or value-detracting factors that warrant adjustments to an estimated valuation. Examples of valuation adjustment factors include the experience and caliber of the management team, the acuteness of the medical need for their product (e.g., HIV, Alzheimer's, cystic fibrosis), the likelihood of follow-on product applications, the strength of existing financial and development partners, and the current financing window, to name a few. There certainly are other considerations to valuation

such as if a biotech company urgently needs capital but doesn't have readily available resources, their valuation is often reduced. Conversely, an organization that is adequately funded with adequate resources to reach their next value-enhancing milestone the valuation may be enhanced.

Before performing a valuation exercise, biotechnology companys should be segmented into two separate groups: *early development-* and *latter development-stage companies*. Early development-stage companies are preseed, seed, start-up, early-stage and mid-stage organizations or those having products that are in preclinical development prior to commercialization. Latter development-stage includes later-stage, mezzanine, and publicly-traded companies, or those that have products in human clinical trials or beginning commercialization for nontherapeutics and diagnostics. For early development-stage companies, one can use all the above methods *except* the risk-adjusted discounted cash flow method (rDCF). Early development-stage companies have many more financial and scientific uncertainties that weaken the ability to confidently utilize the rDCF method. These companies lack certainty of successfully reaching the next stage of development and uncertainty in securing adequate funding to continue progress toward the clinical testing and regulatory phases. Also, the cost, risk, and time associated with the research and development phase of any one particular biotechnology product is uncertain. Once a company receives FDA approval to begin human clinical testing (for a therapeutic or medical device), there is a better understanding of the development path risks associated with these products reaching commercialization. More importantly, understand that venture capital does not use rDCF for valuation of early development-stage companies, and VCs are the most common investor at subsequent stages of development. A company's value can also decrease over time even though the valuation was fairly assessed at one point. Decreases in value can occur for a variety of reasons that are under the company's control and for reasons that are out of the control of the company. Since a biotech company's value is closely tied to its product development progress, if the company consumes much more capital than originally anticipated and does not reach any new value-enhancing milestone, this will negatively impact valuation.

Accurately determining the valuation of a development-stage biotechnology company is important for attracting investors, issuing stock at "fair-market' value and ensuring that future financing partners are not soured by an unrealistically high-valued company. The key to arriving at a fair valuation is using the appropriate method for your company's stage of development. Having a realistic valuation for your company will increase the likelihood of financing your enterprise. In reality, after utilizing all these valuation methods, never forget that valuation is ultimately determined by the investor who writes the check.

FINANCING STAGES FOR A BIOTECHNOLOGY COMPANY

All companies transition through discrete capital financing stages that are tied or related to the product development stage of the company. As discussed in the previous section, each investor group has preferred stages at which they invest and they have limitations as to the amount of capital they can invest, and for a specified timeframe. In this section we describe the most common financing stage of the company and tie them to the investor groups that most often invest at these stages. Financing stage terminology may vary but these are some of the terms most commonly used. For those that are more familiar with product development stages rather than financing stages, a product development stage is implied by the financing stage and I briefly mention the product development stage associated with these terms. I also discuss the most common order in which they occur, and review the typical exit strategies for a company.

Start-Up or Pre-Seed Capital

Start-up capital is also known as formation capital or pre-seed capital and is usually the smallest amount of money raised at any one time. Typically the funds raised are used to establish corporate operating and employment agreements, file and prosecute intellectual property, and incrementally advance the technology. Most often these are the funds that allow the full development of a business plan and marketing strategy. Sometimes these funds will be used to pay early salaries for a few individuals and pay for business cards, stationery, and a logo. Usually the company is already incorporated into an appropriate business entity or soon to be incorporated, prior to the receipt of the funds. The product that the company is based upon will be at a very early stage of inception. Sometimes the research and development may still be performed at an academic institution and it is possible that the entrepreneurs may not yet have a license to the technology. The amount of capital raised during this stage can be as little as $1000 or as much as $250,000. The sources of capital usually comes from the entrepreneurs, friends and family, and occasionally personal loans secured against personal assets of the entrepreneurs. If a large enough round of capital is raised at this stage there may not be any distinction between start-up capital and the next stage of seed capital.

Seed Capital

Seed capital is sometimes called proof-of-concept capital, and is the next larger round of capital after start-up capital.

The money raised in this round can range between $100,000 to over $1 million and is typically used to advance the technology or product to a stage that would increase the value of the company and reach a value-enhancing milestone. Other uses of capital go towards expanding the target market research, hiring consultants, subcontract to contract research organizations (CRO), and often to hire part-time or temporary employees. At this stage the entrepreneurs will take a nominal salary. Capital sources at this stage include the entrepreneurs, friends and family, government grants, existing or new angel investors, and local funding programs.

Convertible Notes

It is worthwhile to discuss at this stage what is given in exchange for cash. During these very early development stages (start-up, pre-seed, and seed rounds) when the valuation of the company is unclear, it is difficult to ascribe, or agree to, how much the company is worth to an investor, and to the company. However, the company still needs capital. The investor can still participate with the company through the use of convertible notes. A convertible note is essentially a "loan" to the company with the intent to convert that "loan" into equity at a subsequent round of financing, usually when institutional capital or VC capital is raised and the value of the company is more reasonably determined. Convertible note holders are usually given an annual accumulated interest rate, accrued but not paid, which can range from 8 to 12 percent depending on the market and need of the company, and they are given a discount into the next round (typically 20 to 40 percent) depending on the industry and the stage of the company. By issuing convertible notes, the note holder has a preferred position in the event of bankruptcy and they have the option of converting at a discount when the next round of capital is secured. Holders of convertible notes have a priority position in the event of any downturn in the company, as note holders are usually ahead of shareholders when it comes to a liquidation of the company assets in the event of bankruptcy. Although the most common method of accepting funds at this stage is through convertible notes, direct equity investments are also made at this time. A direct equity investment means that in exchange for cash, the company gives up a percentage of ownership to the new investors.

Early-Stage Capital: Series A/B Preferred Rounds

Early-stage capital rounds are considered to be Series A Preferred and Series B Preferred Rounds. This is the next significant funding round for the organization. This money may come from a syndicate of angels or a group of angels and local government funding or financing programs. Early-stage capital will occasionally come from institutional investors such as venture capital groups that focus on early-stage investing. These rounds can range from a million dollars to multiple millions of dollars; if the product is a therapeutic, a diagnostic, or a medical device it can range up to tens of millions of dollars. Money invested at this stage is exchanged for equity in the company and comes with certain "preferences" that are above all other investments previously made into the company. In other words, a Series B investment takes precedent and has preferences over Series A investors, and Series A Preferred investors have preferences over holders of common stock such as founders, management, and key employees. These "preferences" are spelled out in a "term sheet" which contains the terms of the investment. Additional preferred financing rounds are labeled alphabetically and have preferences over all previous rounds of capital raised.

Private Placements

At this point we should discuss "private placements" because raising money for a biotech company is, in essence, selling underlying securities (stock or equity) in your company. As such, these activities are regulated in the United States by the Securities and Exchange Commission (SEC). When a company raises capital, particularly when they exchange stock for capital, these offering are called "private offerings" or "private placements." Most individuals have heard of public offerings such as an IPO (initial public offering), whereas a private offering or a private placement is made to only a select group of individuals. When a private placement of stock is made, specific offering documents are required, and a good securities or corporate start-up attorney will know what documents are required and how to handle the regulatory filings after the capital is raised. There are specific exemptions in the Securities laws and the most commonly used exemption is called "Regulation D" and is a safe-harbor exemption. Under these laws, a company may be exempt from many securities requirements, but there are still obligations and legal requirements for disclosure. Your securities attorney should advise the company on how to comply with these disclosures. When raising money from individual or angel investors, it is wise to accept money only from accredited investors because this assures that your investors understand the risks associated with the investment. Also, by raising money only from accredited investors, if the company is unsuccessful, the amount the investor loses would not significantly impact their livelihood. Some of the requirements under the SEC exemptions are to provide, a "private placement memorandum" (PPM), when soliciting investments from individuals. Basically, the PPM contains your complete business plan along with your financials, your sales projections, a potential return on investment, and a lengthy list of potential risks associated with this endeavor. Your securities attorney should review these documents and ensure that the

investment risks are adequately described, whereas it is the company's responsibility to write the business plan. The business plan is a critical document that opens or closes the door to interests and investments in the company, so it is important to devote the time and effort to developing an excellent one. For more information see Chapter 22 entitled "The Business Plan and Presentation: Articulating Your Journey to Commercialization."

Mid-Stage or Development-Stage Capital: Series C/D Preferred Rounds

Series C/D preferred rounds are follow-on rounds and usually involve some or all of the investors in the previous preferred rounds plus new investors. The money that comes in at this stage is mostly institutional capital such as venture capital and corporate partners. There are more VCs that invest in mid-stage development companies than in early-stage development companies. The number and size of these rounds vary and the letter designation C and D are only examples. There are no hard and fast rules, so if the company's product has progressed far enough in development, sometimes a Series B preferred round can be considered a "mid-stage round." This may occur if the product is either a molecular test, diagnostic, or simple medical device, where the capital needs for product development are smaller and the time for development is shorter compared to human therapeutics. The amount of money usually invested in these rounds typically are in the tens of millions of dollars.

Filling the Funding Gaps with Bridge Loans

There are often gaps between funding events for a company. A development-stage company can be very close to running out of money in-between any of the above-mentioned capital rounds and still be making significant product-development progress and generating interest from investors. One simple financing instrument used to close this funding gap is a bridge loan. Bridge loans sometimes fill the funding chasm between angel funding and the receipt of venture capital and larger equity investments. Bridge loans are notes that bear a risk-appropriate interest rate, whereas convertible notes are bridge loans that have a right to convert their principle and interest into the next financing round at the same terms that the next investors determine. A company usually considers bridge loans because either they do not have long before they run out of money, or they know they will be raising a larger round later and the valuation is difficult to assess or agree upon by the company and investors. Bridge loans will often come with an extra incentive to the investor in the form of stock warrants based upon a percentage of the amount loaned. A warrant is like a stock option that gives the holder the right to purchase shares in the company over an extended period for a specific set price. Depending upon the strength of the company's product development and progress, the bridge loan holder may want it to be structured with an option for converting just like a convertible note with a discount into the next round. When a company has interested investors who cannot put up the full amount of capital needed to make all the progress a company desires, bridge loans and convertible notes provide a way to support the company and still advance product development to later gain interest from larger investors.

Later-Stage and Expansion Capital: Series E/F Preferred Rounds

Therapeutics and biologics require large capital investments and more funding rounds as compared to diagnostics, medical devices, molecular tests, and some agbiotech products. However, there are greater numbers of VC firms that invest in these later-stage rounds because fund managers can deploy more capital (tens of millions of dollars versus a few million dollars) when product-development risk is lower than at early-stage development. Usually these later-stage rounds are for therapeutics and biologics and by this funding stage the company is usually in human clinical trials and potentially for more than one indication for use. Some very complex genetic expression tests and combination medical devices may also require later-stage capital to reach commercialization. If more capital is required, preferred series designations continue alphabetically such as G, H, etc., and each subsequent round has preferences over all previous

rounds. This is one reason that previous VC investors will participate in subsequent rounds to maintain their position and ownership percentages. They will also syndicate investment participation so that responsibility for funding these subsequent and larger rounds are not borne by any one VC.

Mezzanine Capital

For companies that need it, mezzanine capital is usually the last round of capital before an IPO, an acquisition of the company, or an exit for the investors. Venture capital funds are plentiful at this stage when product development risks have been greatly reduced. Investors at this stage enjoy a shorter time from investment to exit than for those who invested at early-or development-stages. Not surprisingly, the returns on investments at this stage are lower than when investing at earlier stages of company development. For this reason VC funds may balance their portfolio with some early, later, and mezzanine capital investments. (See Table 19.1.)

Initial Public Offering (IPO) or Acquisition

An IPO or an acquisition of a company is an event where all the investors and shareholders can reap a financial reward for their work and perseverance (see exits discussed below). However, for drug-development and biologics companies, the requirement for capital is so high that an IPO really becomes another later-stage financing round for the company, rather than solely an exit for investors, although it does accomplish both. Given the tremendous amount of capital required for drug development—up to $1 billion or more—and the length

TABLE 19.1 Biotech Funding Stages, Valuation Ranges, and Amounts Raised

Stages	Product Characterization	Valuation Ranges	Amounts Raised	Funding Sources
Start-up (pre-seed)	Concept	$1 to $3 million	$1000 to $25,000	Entrepreneur/friends and family/supported by SBIR/STTR/local grants/loans
Seed	Proof-of-concept	$2 to $5 million	$0.25 to $1 million	Entrepreneur/friends and family/angels/some VC/supported by SBIR/STTR/local grants/institutions and foundations
Early and development stage Series A/B preferred	Development	$3 to $25 million	$3 to $10 million	Angels/VCs/private equity/institutions/supported by SBIR/STTR/local grants/institutions and foundations
Later stage Series C/D preferred	Development/clinical testing	$10 to $100 million	$5 to 25 million	VCs/private equity institutions supported by SBIR/STTR/local grants/institutions
Mezzanine	Market launch	$25 to $100 million	$10 to $50 million	VCs/investment banks/private equity/institutions

of time to reach the market—up to 15 years—it is not feasible for any single investor group to fund a company from start-up to commercialization without a public financing event or a corporate partnership or acquisition. Large amounts of money can be raised in an IPO with an availability for follow-on public financing rounds. This is what makes an IPO an attractive event for the company and its investors.

WHAT IS AN "EXIT" STRATEGY?

All investors invest with a purpose in mind—there will be a time when they can recoup their investment and a sizable profit. Until an exit event, all shareholder value is locked within the company and investors have no viable means to convert their shares back into cash. Although entrepreneurs may plan on staying with their company for the long haul, investors are not in it for the same reasons. Yes, your investors will believe in the mission and goals of the company; however, they are investors, and they want to know the company's exit strategy and the potential level of financial return. Investors have expectations that sometime in the not-too-distant future they will part ways with the company and receive significant monetary benefit for financing that endeavor. Therefore, before an investor commits to investing they want to know the company's exit strategy and when the company anticipates that to occur. At an exit, the investors and shareholders can exchange their shares for cash or, if desired, hold on to them anticipating that they may increase in value in the future.

Investors, by definition, invest for returns. The expectation of their level of return varies with the type of investor and the stage at which they invest in, which can range from 5× to 40× the original investment in a time period of 3 to 7 years. If your potential returns are not attractive enough to a particular investor, they will not invest. So when writing a business plan and before raising any money, the company leader should have a well-researched plan explaining how future investors will receive a return on their capital. For the entrepreneur, this exercise may seem premature and nearly impossible to calculate, but to an investor it is not an unreasonable expectation. Exit planning is essential in order to attract investors because it is simply the means by which shareholders are allowed to exchange their holdings for cash and be rewarded for their participation in the company.

What are the Exits for a Biotechnology Company?

The most likely exit options for a biotech company are a public offering through an IPO, a merger with another company (including reverse-merger), or an acquisition by a larger corporation. For a number of years there were many successful biotechnology company IPOs. When the IPO market is good, it is possible for biotech companies to get

their investors the 10× return typically sought by venture capital investors. The historic example is that of Genentech's IPO on October 14, 1980. The stock went for sale on the NASDAQ exchange at $35 a share, and within hours the share price reached $89 before closing at the end of the day at $71.25. Genentech raised $35 million that day. In its second public offering of shares on July 20, 1999, 20 million shares were sold at $97 per share raising nearly $2 billion and the closing price that day was $127 per share.

Although an IPO can seem glamorous, being a publicly-traded company also comes with certain financial governance requirements and expenses of compliance with Sarbanes-Oxley estimated to cost between $2 to $2.5 million. There are also costs of going public, it is estimated that about 15 to 30 percent of gross proceeds are consumed when a company goes public. Compliance costs annually are projected to range between $2 to $4 million for most publicly-traded companies [4]. In addition there are daily fluctuations in market value which can add pressure to make short-term decisions by the management that may be counter-productive to long-term product development and market expansion progress. Publicly-traded biotechnology companies also become subject to the same scrutiny that highly profitable Fortune 500 companies face daily. The attractiveness for a biotech IPO depends on many factors such as the general market conditions for IPOs, investor interest in the high technology sector, the success of other biotechnology companies in a similar sector, and the overall economy.

What is the Typical Sequence of Funding Events?

There is no universal funding formula for all biotechnology companies to follow. However, a typical sequence may follow something similar to this:

1. **Start-up capital** may be provided by founders, friends, and family.
2. **Seed capital** may be provided by founders, friends, and family and local government entities, and grants directed towards funding the early R&D.
3. **Series A Preferred capital** may be provided by angel investors and/or local government entities, interested foundations and possibly early-stage venture capital and grants directed toward funding the early R&D.
4. **Series B Preferred capital** may be provided by angel investors, interested foundations, and syndicated venture capital.
5. **Series C capital and later-stage capital** may be provided by syndicated venture capital and corporate partnerships.
6. **Mezzanine capital** may be provided by venture capital and large financing institutions or investment bankers.
7. **Acquisition** or **strategic partnership** with a large corporation brings capital from the parent company or **initial public offering (IPO)** capital which comes from the public and institutional investors purchasing shares on the open public market.

There are additional ways for a privately-held company to become publicly-traded, such as a reverse merger with another publicly-traded entity or a "shell" company. A reverse merger is less expensive than an IPO and is relatively easy for a company to accomplish when there is a suitable shell company to reverse merge into. This transaction provides liquidity for shareholders, as their shares would be exchanged for publicly-traded shares of the joined company. More recently it has been challenging to have an IPO and maintain a stock price well above the initial pricing, and because of this there have been more biotechnology companies opting for being acquired by larger corporations. Some investors believe that mergers and acquisitions provide a better avenue for exit and better valuation, but it also depends on the amount of corporate interest in your company and its products. Spend time researching the mergers and acquisitions (M&A) or IPO market for comparable companies in your sector. Become familiar with the valuations received for these companies and learn to calculate a potential return for investors by knowing the comparable company values at each type of exit.

HOW MUCH MONEY IS RAISED AT EACH FUNDING STAGE?

The average amount of capital raised during each funding stage can vary greatly within each biotech industry sector. The amount of money that is raised during any stage is influenced by:

1. **The type of product being developed.** Therapeutics, biologics and vaccines generally require greater amounts of capital during each round than do most medical diagnostics, medical devices, point-of-care tests, clinical laboratory tests, and many bioagriculture products. Therefore, companies developing the former products will be raising larger amounts of capital in each round compared to the latter group.

2. **The financial market's interest in a disease segment at the time of raising capital.** Investor interest in certain disease segments changes over time. In the past, antisense DNA was very popular as were antisepsis therapeutics, each being funded relatively quickly. Today it is difficult to find much interest or receive high valuations for these types of companies. More recently, genomics, proteomics and RNAi companies have received high interest and have raised great amounts of money. The success and failure of similar predecessor products influence the value placed on the company and affect the eagerness of investors to fund these companies.

3. **The strength of the IPO and acquisition market at the time of raising capital.** When financial markets as a whole increase or decline, it impacts the amount of money that can be raised for any development-stage company.

During 1999 and 2000, valuations for all biotechnology companies significantly increased because the IPO market was strong with exits available for investors that provided excellent returns, and many companies raised significant amounts of capital. Later, the stock market downturn reduced valuations of early-stage companies because the exits were not returning the profits investors expected and funding rounds were much smaller and more difficult to close. Be aware that the general condition of the economy and financial markets can impact the amount of capital you can raise at any one time.

HOW MUCH OF THE COMPANY IS GIVEN UP IN EACH ROUND?

Each time your company raises capital from investors it simultaneously gives away a portion of the ownership of the corporation. Because biotechnology companies require significant amounts of capital to reach commercialization, over time there will be significant ownership dilution of the founders, early shareholders, and management of the company who built it. Although this dilution may be undesirable, without investor financing there is little consolation in owning the majority of a company with no value.

In a survey that was completed by VentureOne with about 75 respondents, Table 19.2 shows the mean, median, minimum, and maximum percentages of the company sold on a fully-diluted basis in each round (fully-diluted basis means all stock outstanding plus any options and warrants issued or granted, such that all were converted into shares). Most companies are giving up approximately 25 to 35 percent of the company each time they raise new money. Giving up 35 percent of the company three times does not mean there is nothing left after three rounds. Ownership gets recalculated each time for everyone, so investors in the previous round also get diluted if they don't participate in the next round.

For a theoretical example, if in the first round 50 percent of the company is given away, 50 percent remains with the

TABLE 19.2 Percentages of Company Sold On a Fully Diluted Basis

	First Round	Second Round	Third and Later
Mean	41 %	35 %	27 %
Median	40 %	33 %	26 %
Minimum	8 %	6 %	4 %
Maximum	82 %	73 %	70 %
Total Respondents	97	65	79

Source: VentureOne Deal Terms Report, 4th Edition (rounded).

existing shareholders and each shareholder maintains their respective percentage of that remaining 50 percent. If the founders originally owned 70 percent, then after the first round they would own 70 percent of the remaining 50 percent, or 35 percent of the company after the first round. If the company raises capital in a second round and gives up 40 percent, then 60 percent is owned by all the prior shareholders including those that participated in the first round. After each financing round, a percentage of the company is given to the new shareholders and all subsequent shareholders are diluted. Unlike a family-owned small business where the original founders can expect to retain majority ownership of the organization, building a biotechnology company is a group project. The founder needs to realize that by the time the company is ready for an exit, they typically own a minor portion of the organization. Depending on the biotechnology sector and number of financing rounds, founder ownership can range from 5 to 15 percent by the time of an exit. This emphasizes the significance of accomplishing as much as possible with as little early money as possible and reaching significant milestones to increase valuation which reduces the equity given up in each financing round. Founders should not be too discouraged because 5 percent of hundreds of millions is much better than 100 percent of nothing.

SUMMARY

Capital for biotechnology product development comes from a variety of sources and each source has their own preference for the stage at which they invest. Each of these investor groups has different investment risk tolerances along with differing motivations and limitations for investing. Also, each group tends to focus on a particular segment or sector where they are familiar and comfortable with the investment risk. It is valuable for the management team to understand these motivations and limitations prior to a fundraising campaign. By doing so, you can decrease the time spent on raising capital and increase your likelihood of finding the right partner for your product and stage of development. At some point in development, most biotechnology companies will need VC or corporate partnership funding in order to reach commercialization. Start early and do some homework to find the ones that favor your company's technology space and target market. Be sure to target good VC and corporate partners who bring more than just money; seek a true partner who will help along the way. Connect with the right ones when the appropriate stage is reached.

The biotech entrepreneur and management team is responsible for ensuring that the company continues to make steady product development progress. Since the likelihood of raising the next round of capital is dependent upon scientific and developmental milestones made, be sure to hit most, if not all of them—on time. If your organization is consistently making progress toward its

development goals, and these milestones are significant, it will be easier to continually attract the needed capital for the company at all stages. Once capital is raised, be extremely efficient in managing capital irrespective of how much is raised or how much you have left. The efficient use of capital is one hallmark of successful biotechnology companies.

A tremendous amount of time and effort will be put forth to secure funding at the right time from the right financing partner. As a result, it may be tempting to relax when fundraising is completed. Securing funding just means the hard work can begin in earnest. The company leader must always maintain the organization's intensity toward reaching the next value-increasing milestone if they hope to have a successful biotechnology company. Never forget that a funding event is a means to an end and not an end in itself. The company goals are product development, market development, and business development milestones that increase the value and reduce the risk of the company. Keep your focus on your real goals and make progress so you won't lack for future funding.

Cash is a precious and limited commodity to a start-up company. It is like gas to a vehicle; although you may have a high-performance automobile with the most powerful engine, when it runs out of gas, you go nowhere. When you accept money from others, there is a shared level of involvement and an increased level of responsibility to others. After a funding round is completed, you will have new investors or new partners and your responsibilities broaden to more individuals than just those within the company. The hard fact is that there is not enough investment capital to fund all the good ideas conceived by every biotechnology company. Securing biotech funding requires perseverance, and the ability to learn from each investor meeting to improve the chances of funding the company at subsequent junctures. The greatest idea imagined, the most amazing drug ever conceived, or the greatest life-saving medical device dreamed, is of no consequence if one cannot finance its development to commercialization. Someone once said "a vision without execution is a hallucination." To have a vision without funds to execute it is an exercise in frustration and futility. Perseverance, flexibility, creativity, and working with exceptional people are key ingredients to successful fundraising.

REFERENCES

[1] National Council of Technology Transfer (NCET2). Research Commercialization and SBIR Center, http://center.ncet2.org/; May 7, 2013.
[2] Small Business Innovative Research, http://www.sbir.gov/; May 7, 2013.
[3] U.S. Security and Exchange Commission, Accredited Investors. http://www.sec.gov/answers/accred.htm.
[4] PriceWaterhouse Cooper. Considering an IPO: The Cost of Going Public May Surprise You?; 2012.

Chapter 20

Securing Angel Capital and Understanding How Angel Networks Operate

Robert J. Calcaterra, DSc

President, St. Louis Arch Angels, St. Louis, Missouri

WHAT IS AN ANGEL INVESTOR?

An angel investor is an individual who is willing to put some of their financial assets at risk by investing in early stage private equity companies. The term "angel investor" is often interpreted to mean an "accredited investor." The Securities and Exchange Commission (SEC) defines an accredited investor as an individual with a net worth, or joint net worth with a spouse of over $1 million excluding their home, or an individual with an annual income for the past two years of $200,000 or more, or $300,000 with a spouse, and a reasonable expectation of the same for the current year. Because angel investors tend to invest at very early stages of a company, this group will most likely be one of the first or earliest investors in a start-up biotechnology company business.

Angel investors may work alone or within organized angel networks which I will describe in more detail later. There are many well-established sophisticated angel networks throughout the United States and some have specific industry focuses. In the United States there are over 400,000 active angels investing in various companies. Most of the time an entrepreneur can find an angel network somewhere close to their geographic location. In general, most angel investors usually prefer to invest in companies within their local region to help local companies and for the convenience of monitoring their investment company.

TYPICAL BACKGROUND OF ANGEL INVESTORS

The make-up of angel investors vary depending upon where you are located. In hotbeds of entrepreneurship such as Silicon Valley, Boston, or Boulder where I lived for a number of years, the backgrounds of angels are people who have already succeeded as serial entrepreneurs and are supporting others who are trying to do the same. Unfortunately, many of these people invest independently of angel networks. They might invest as an independent syndicate, but it tends to be with others who invested in their deals. I don't know if it is their self-assuredness that motivates them to be independent or if it is not wanting to be responsible for making recommendations to a group of people they don't know very well. This is unfortunate because being exclusive and reclusive can reduce the number of sources of money available to a start-up company.

HOW MUCH DOES A TYPICAL ANGEL INVESTOR INVEST?

In a later section I will talk about teaching angel investors "to keep their powder dry." What we are talking about here is that companies you invest in will inevitably return for a second, third, and potentially fourth round of investment. You need to keep back at least two-thirds or three-fourths of the total money you ultimately want to invest in a given deal when you make your first investment. Of course that dollar amount is dependent on a particular angel investor's assets and how many companies they think they will invest in over the years.

All of that said from my experience and discussions with other angel network managers, the most common angel investment is normally around $25,000 with follow-on rounds comparable. I have seen very few investments below that and very few at $50,000 per round and higher, especially after the first year or two of the network. The amount of money invested in specific companies by one angel group varies depending on the investment round and stage of the company. Seed rounds typically are $150,000 to $300,000. With companies that have progressed through milestones and may have reached a Series A or Series B round investment, the total amount raised from a single angel group can be in the $700,000 to $2.5 million level.

ANGEL INVESTOR MOTIVATIONS

Experienced and savvy angel investors, or members of angel funds or networks, tend to want to invest in highly scalable companies (i.e. companies that can reach very high value with a relatively low level of initial investment). This is the case with agriculture and life sciences biotechnology companies. Agriculture and life science angel investors tend to be driven by motivations that include: value proposition; relative scientific risk of succeeding, and emotion. The emotional aspect of investing in agricultural and life science related deals deserves further thought. Bio agricultural investors tend to be driven by altruistic motivations related to animal health and treatment, nutrition, food safety, and feeding the world through increased yields and sustainable practices. In the life sciences, many angel investors are driven by the potential to prevent, better diagnose, treat, or cure specific illnesses. Frequently this includes having a family member suffering from a particular disease or condition where the start-up company has a product that will treat or diagnose this condition. Angel investors tend to invest in companies within their geographic region as they are interested in supporting economic growth within their city or locale. Investing in local companies also allows them to be able to follow more closely their investments and the progress the company makes.

Angel investors typically are very early investors in companies, well before most venture capital (VC) firms consider investing. Although there are some very early-stage VC firms that do invest in start-ups, the majority of the VCs invest in later stages of the company development. For those VC firms that do invest in start-ups, it is very rare to see venture capital firms co-invest in the same round as angel investors. Angels are usually willing to take more risks and as a result they have very high return expectations. In the 1970s and 1980s angels had a reputation for making ill-advised investments and not making money on the deals they invested in. The reason was that they were not concerned enough about the management team, the value proposition, marketing barriers, regulatory issues, financial needs, etc. And of course they then overvalued the company. Today, angel investors are much more sophisticated and their investing practices are much more refined.

What Does it Take for an Angel Investor to be Interested in Investing?

Angel investors are not unique in their requirements for investing in a biotech company compared with institutional investors such as venture capital. That is, we all look for unique science and/or technology that has a great value proposition, a strong experienced management team across all disciplines, a reasonable marketing and reimbursement strategy, a clear and defined regulatory path, strong intellectual property position, a well-defined timeline and financing, and an exit strategy. Companies will succeed in raising money if they present a compelling case around all of the above items. Companies commonly fail to raise money by not demonstrating the management team is knowledgable

enough during the question and answer sessions of a presentation and during due diligence. In addition, fundraising is impacted by not demonstrating that the company has a significant-enough technical and proprietary position, and value proposition. In addition investors will be looking for naïve marketing strategies versus competitive products and a reasonable path to payee status.

As a co-founder of numerous start-up companies, angel investors are of major importance to me for the following reasons:

1. They tend to be less risk-averse than institutional investors and more willing to invest at the earliest and most risky proof-of-concept stage of companies.
2. They tend to be more patient than institutional investors with respect to exit, especially in biotech-related companies where there is an emotional-related driving force.
3. They tend to be less punitive with their terms for investing in early rounds compared to institutional investors.
4. They tend to be more willing to negotiate terms in subsequent investment rounds.

There is a significant danger for entrepreneurial companies caused by items 1 and 3 above. Entrepreneurs need to be extremely cautious in the early seed stages of investment in their company. They must avoid overvaluing their company because subsequent A and B round venture capital investment terms can lead to severe negative impacts on early investors and founders for companies where this has happened. This can lead to negative feelings between founders and their most supportive stockholders.

A good solution to the overvaluation problem is to use convertible notes for early investment in companies in order to avoid the need for valuing the company at this early stage. A convertible note is simply a debt (note) that is owed to the investor but has a conversion feature that will convert the debt into equity, usually at a larger investment round. This investment vehicle will typically offer the investor a premium at conversion of 20 to 30 percent (i.e., acquiring equity during conversion for 70 to 80 percent of the stock price) interest on the investment of 8 to 10 percent per annum and a forced conversion when a qualified Series A round investment occurs. With the St. Louis Arch Angels where I have been a member for 9 years, I have actually participated in a conversion accepted by major venture capital companies for a Series A round with a 40 percent premium.

Entrepreneurs need to know that with every form of early investment there are issues that can and usually occur. For convertible notes, they work well if conversion occurs quickly. However, problems occur when conversion does not occur soon but drags on with multiple rounds of small seed investments. Many times that will lead to an unrealistic capitalization table. I always recommend in convertible notes that conversion should be forced at modest conversion prices if a qualified investment does not occur within the first year or two of seed investment. Most A and B round investors also recognize accumulated interest in convertible notes as "double dipping" and normally will negotiate elimination of the interest at conversion or a reduction of the rate in exchange for accepting the premium price. I have had both occur in investments I have made using convertible notes.

Individuals, Networks, and Funds

Angel investors come in all forms and invest through many different approaches and organizations. Each form has its own advantages and disadvantages.

Individual investors who don't participate in formal funds or networks tend to be somewhat reclusive and as a result very hard to find. Introductions to them come from very close trusted friends or through lawyers or financial advisors they have hired to manage their investments. They are reclusive because they do not want to have large numbers of people bother them with "deals" to invest in. I am aware of and have received investment into companies I have cofounded from individuals or families who have created formal funds to just invest their personal assets in early-stage companies. Their motivation is purely seeking returns on investment higher than they can get in the public markets or for personal reasons associated with family susceptibility to certain diseases (i.e., cancer, heart disease, etc.). This occurs with very wealthy individuals with a net worth at a nine-figure level. Finding individual angel investors can be challenging because they usually do not do this full-time and they certainly do not advertise. The best way to find individual angels is by networking with people who know them and by asking them for introductions. Check with your local university or research institution technology transfer office for names and contacts, as they may know some of the local angels. Also check with the local Chamber of Commerce, regional economic development agency, or a technology commercialization center or equivalent, as these may be good sources of angel contacts who invest in biotechnology. Most angels are good sources for names of other angels. Once an angel has invested, ask them for help and introductions to others, because having a motivated and excited investor first tell the story is more effective than the entrepreneur doing it cold. There are many angels out there—be persistent in locating them.

Some angel groups create and invest in *angel funds*. Angel funds are set up by people who don't have the time or inkling to get involved in the due diligence and day-to-day oversight of the companies they invest in. This requires either the hiring of professional staff to run the fund or more likely a volunteer member who does due diligence on deals and does the negotiation of investment terms with the companies. Decisions in these types of funds are commonly made by an appointed investment committee. The advantage of this approach is that angel members get their investment

spread over a large portfolio of opportunities in diverse industries much like investing in a mutual fund. The disadvantages are that you are relinquishing decision-making to a committee that may or may not be good at deciding what to invest in. Additionally, everyone participating gets a normalized return for the whole portfolio which may have some very good returns and some very bad returns.

The most common form of angel investing today occurs through *angel networks* where each member of the angel group invest only in the deals they are interested in. The Angel Capital Association (ACA) has well over 200 member groups representing over 10,000 angel investors. This is an indication of at least a minimum number of groups of people doing these types of investment nationwide. Membership in angel networks can be as low as 5 to 10 people and up to as many as 100 to 200 people in some groups in Los Angeles and Boston. In addition, some angel networks have established "side car funds" to allow members to also invest in a fund that matches investments from members; this allows members to diversify their portfolio.

Angel networks in locations that are less known for being entrepreneurial have very diverse memberships: for example, some are comprised of doctors, lawyers, accountants, and people who own their own companies that are either family or self-made. Other members come from large companies and tend to be retired from a mid-management level. We found out in our early recruiting for the St. Louis Arch Angels that the general councils of major international technology-based corporations would not allow top-level management (CEO, CSO, CIO, board of director members, etc.) to participate in angel networks because of the fear of conflicts of interest. They even strongly discouraged participation from spouses and offspring of those executives. The industry background of members also tends to be very diverse. One absolute requirement however is that there have to be a few members in the early stages of a network who have experience in investing and managing early-stage IT- and biotech-related companies. These people become the bell cows for early investments. Without their leadership angel networks will fail in the very first couple of years of formation because of lack of investment.

LOCATING ANGEL NETWORKS

Finding individual angels can be difficult because they usually have full-time jobs and do not advertise. However, locating angel networks is becoming easier as their groups are organized and more networks are emerging constantly. There are two good sources for finding angel networks in your region, these include the Angel Capital Association [1] and the Angel Resource Institute [2]. These organizations have databases containing the various angel network groups and are listed by geographic location. Another way to find interested angel networks is through Gust [3], an Internet platform that facilitates the connecting of entrepreneurs and start-up companies based upon profiles that a company creates and then sends to those groups that have an interest in investing in your sector. One important point for entrepreneurs is to learn about your audience and screen the angels and angel groups that you target. You will be wasting your time if you are working to get a meeting with a group that only invests in IT and you are in biotechnology, or the group only invests in local companies and you are out of their region.

How to Get an Audience with an Angel Group

Getting an audience with an angel fund or network is normally quite easy. They have been formed for the sole purpose to find opportunities for the group to invest in. Some groups have a much-formalized application and matriculation process and some are very informal. Whatever the process, it will be something very readily available on their website or in the local media. In both cases it is best to identify the leadership and key influencers within the organization. I have found that administrators for these organizations are very willing to identify those people for you because that is their job. Making a full PowerPoint presentation to those key people is critical to finding a champion that will help you through their process. Without someone championing your cause within the group, it is very difficult to succeed in raising money.

The advantages for entrepreneurs in engaging angel networks are numerous:

1. One point of contact to a large number of potential investors at a fairly high level of investment.
2. The ability to find knowledgeable members of your science or industry who can influence unknowledgeable members to invest in your opportunity.
3. Once invested, one point of contact that streamlines communications to your investment group.
4. Access to a very large network of people and services in your community who have been screened that might be of value to your company going forward.

THINGS TO KNOW WHEN PRESENTING TO ANGEL INVESTORS

When you, as a biotechnology entrepreneur are presenting your case to an angel network for the first time, all you are doing is trying to wet their appetite to hear more. You will only have at best 20 minutes to present. You need to remember that 90 percent of the listeners may not understand the science you are presenting. Therefore, you need a very concise and understandable lay summary of what your science is and what it does compared to current methods. Spend most of your presentation justifying the huge value

proposition over any others' approach and selling your management team's qualifications and ability to execute. Before the management team slide, which should be last, spend very little time letting your audience know that this is a huge market and that you have a proprietary position. If you have accomplished your goal of striking interest you will then have much more time in due diligence to present your plan in-depth, elaborating on all of these sections and getting into your roadmap (required tasks to complete, costs, and timing) and financial pro formas. Angels will turn down an investment if they spot certain risks because they know that companies fail because of these key reasons:

1. Poor management team.
2. No market.
3. Lack of capital.
4. Bad science.

Of course if you talk to those failed entrepreneurs, many times they feel that lack of capital and bad science was the reason they failed rather than a poor management team or the lack of a market. It's human nature *not* to blame yourself.

When I think about the hundreds of examples of companies I have observed that successfully raise money, and then assess why some succeed and others do not, it tends to be in all of the factors I have mentioned above. However, it is my impression that most companies that do not even make it through the first investment screening fail because they can't explain the value proposition of their idea well enough. Those that make it into due diligence but fail are normally because the management team does not convince the angel group that they have the ability to execute the plan. Their answers to questions don't seem to demonstrate the knowledge and experience expected. Essentially, it is a trust issue. Trust of the management team is the one thing, with everything being equal, that correlates with investment occurring. We all know the old adage "invest in companies with a top management team and average science, over a company with mediocre management and world class science." In other words, its management, management, management; good management is the biggest indicator of successful companies above all other factors. Finally, in a very few cases where companies make it through the due diligence stage and fail to close on an investment, it is usually because the management team has extreme views as to the value of their company.

UNDERSTANDING ANGEL NETWORKS AND HOW THEY ARE FORMED

Understanding how an angel network is formed may help you appreciate some of the issues, motivations, and factors that angels are dealing with to find good investments. Also, you may be a successful entrepreneur or businessperson and may consider starting your own angel network in your region. There are numerous methods for starting and developing a successful and thriving angel network. I am presenting for your consideration a case study of an approach I was intimately involved in creating—the St. Louis Arch Angels in conjunction with Bob Coy who in 2004 was an executive with the Regional Commerce and Growth Association in St. Louis. Bob is currently the President of Cincy Tech, a public private seed fund in Cincinnati, Ohio.

The St. Louis Arch Angels, where I am currently president, has succeeded beyond my fondest expectation with investments approaching $40 million over 9 years, from its founding in 2005 to 2014. We have invested in approximately 50 companies in a region where prior attempts to develop robust angel funding failed and where angel investing in 2004 was very low. Keep in mind that this investment has occurred during a 3-year recession.

Angel networks tend to be different in the types of deals they favor. The Arch Angel network, for example, are partial to IT deals that require a partnering relationship to gain traction such as retail chains, sports teams, manufacturing, or research partners with less interest in attracting direct consumer plays without a combined benefit to the partner and consumer both. With respect to agricultural and life science deals, we tend to become enamored with very big opportunities that have huge value proposition advantages over the current gold standard which is not a final solution. The process we used to build the St. Louis Arch Angel network is as follows below.

Building Consensus and Structure

A task force of approximately 10 people spent all of 2004 researching angel network structures used by others throughout the country. We agreed on a model similar to the Tech Coast Angels in Orange County, California. We rejected a fund or side car fund approach.

Key features are not insignificant: a $1500 initiation fee, $1000 annual membership fee, and a required minimum $50,000 investment yearly.

Selecting and Enlisting Key Leadership

We very deliberately hand-picked the first 10 people we sought as members because of their previous leadership and because of their successful investment history.

An Efficient Process

Our process is very structured and clear to entrepreneurs, and that process is managed by an administrator and a deal due diligence part-time employee:

1. Apply on line.
2. Initial screening and culling of applications by angel network management.

3. Presentation to selection committee of membership (invitation to all members to attend). Average of around five to eight members attend with one to two companies matriculating to membership meeting.
4. Company presenters mentored by selected volunteer members before presenting to full membership meeting.
5. Membership meeting ten times per year always on same date (i.e., last Wednesday of month). No meetings in July or December.
6. Immediate member feedback regarding interest.
7. Due diligence membership team set up with a designated leader.
8. Regular progress updates from invested companies at membership meetings.

The number of applicants to our website average five to ten each month, which would be equivalent to approximately 500 to 1000 deals over a 9-year period. We average two presentations at our monthly membership meetings so that would represent about 200 deals we listened to in 9 years, and we are now approaching 50 investments. This process continued to occur during a period of about 3 years of recession. Investments have ranged from $150,000 to $6 million per deal.

Entrepreneurs should realize that angel investing is highly dependent on building personal relationships. The smart entrepreneur should attempt to meet key members of the network to present their deal before they apply. If that member is impressed by the opportunity and management team, he or she will become champions in the selection committee and membership meetings. Accepting early coaching from angel members is key to succeeding in raising money in angel groups. Early contact between entrepreneurs and angel members can also help manage entrepreneur expectations.

The Arch Angel Network goes out of its way to participate in workshops in the community to educate entrepreneurs about our process.

Educating Angel Investors

Educating first time angel investors is very much an apprenticeship approach. However, there are numerous workshops around the country that are available. In general, the best programs are managed by the Angel Capital Association (ACA) and cover basic topics and in some cases, in-depth workshops on specialized subjects such as due diligence, term sheets, etc.

First time angels commonly make the following mistakes:

1. Becoming too enamored by the science and technology.
2. Becoming too focused on the benefit to society of the science and technology (for example a cancer cure).
3. Not concentrating enough on the qualifications of the management team.

4. Not factoring in risk and timeline in relationship to rewards associated with the investments they make.
5. Not "keeping their powder dry," i.e., investing too much of their available assets in the first seed round of the investment and not having reserves for follow on rounds.

For that very reason the Arch Angels use the initiation fee from new members to encourage them to attend angel-investing workshops. If they do so, we pay their registration and expenses from those fees. Unfortunately, not many people use this available asset. Another educational opportunity is during due diligence where we match experienced members with less experienced members on the due diligence teams.

Member Retention and Building Esprit-De-Corps

Angel networks historically have a huge amount of turnover; approximately 20 percent of the membership each year. This of course can lead to a lot of uncertainty with the networks. This has not occurred with the St. Louis Arch Angels. The members we had leave the group left very early and they were self-selected by realizing they were not comfortable with the risk profile and exit timelines for companies they were seeing. Our membership has gone from 35 in 2005 to near 80 today. We have never had to invoke the minimum investment rule. We have members who have not met the minimum $50,000 investment in a given year but they have been people who have invested substantially more money in previous or later years. I attribute our current investment success to an esprit-de-corps (feelings of loyalty) within the group and our ability to build subtle trust among members. As is normal, the quality of deals have improved with time and we have seen more deals throughout the Midwest. I believe it is also driven by our screening, training, and selection of members. We allow prospective members to attend due diligence meetings with companies as well as membership meetings numerous times before asking them to commit. Obviously, our initiation and annual fees force members to make a serious reassessment every year.

Defining Success for Angel Networks

Defining success for angel networks is very difficult because it is a constant rolling fund with no defined beginning and end. Clearly it has to be related to the return its members receive from investments they make. That could be defined by the networks total internal rate of return (IRR) over a defined period of time. I think a better measurement would be related to the number or percentage of companies invested in, that returned positive money to its investors, the number of failed companies or percentage, and a substantive number of examples of companies that can be highlighted which have returned significant multiples to member investors. During its 9 year life, the St.

Louis Arch Angels had 4 exits and 4 failed companies out of 50 investments. That is a pretty good record but we certainly can't claim success quite yet.

I personally have invested in 17 Arch Angel deals and have had two failures and one significant exit of 2.4-fold in 1.5 years which is a 40 percent ROI. I have three to four companies that may have substantial exits within the next 12 to 18 months. I have another four to five that look like very good or big exits in a longer timeframe with more risk of failure, and another six which are less promising. Of course the ace in the hole card for everyone in the investment business is that the companies that fail early have less money invested in them than the ones that look like they are good because they have had multiple investment rounds. My portfolio looks pretty good, right? We shall see. The big question is, am I representative of the other 79 members of the network or not? In other words, success of angel networks is very hard to define. It will be different for each member.

ANGEL EXPECTATIONS

In my opinion, the old venture capital model is dead. That is, portfolios populated solely with perceived high-risk, high-return (greater than 20-fold) deals with expectations of one-out-of-ten company success rates that drive the success of the fund, while dropping non-homeruns quickly from their portfolio. Many institutional investors and analysts that I have talked to recently say they have modified their strategy to invest in companies with a higher probability of success and potentially more modest (such as ten-fold or more) expectation of return. This of course necessitates an optimization strategy regarding the whole portfolio and not just the big winners. This strategy closely mirrors the strategy that has been used by angels.

Reporting and Follow-up

One of the most frustrating experiences for angel investors is the lack of communications from companies they have invested in. This can lead to the lack of follow-on investment from angels. For me, by definition, top entrepreneurs provide all of their investors, not just board members and institutional investors, quarterly updates on their companies' progress or lack thereof. This is not optional. It is required.

Risk, Reward, and Myths

If you are interested in securing angel capital, you should go through an exercise I did recently and Google "private equity investing risk vs. reward" or "VC investing risk vs. reward," or many other variations thereof. You will literally find hundreds of sites and articles. Let me summarize this for you. The general sense of what you will read is that angel investors are investing a similar total amount of money every year as are VCs. The difference is that angels are investing in ten times the number of companies as VCs and getting twice the return. Obviously this means that angel investors are investing earlier in deals at a time when the risk is much higher where VCs are being more cautious and investing at a later stage and not earning as much. Interesting! The corollary to this of course is that it is a sad indication of the lack of series A and B round money in the market and the difficulty companies are having raising money after their seed rounds. Those of us in the game of raising money for our start-ups don't need to be told this through articles on the Web or in newspapers. We are experiencing it!

Of course, another belief is that biotechnology investors typically do not make as good a return as people investing in other industries, in particular the IT industry. This of course is because of the risk of science and regulatory issues and the high cost of science. Not so according to a recent article in Forbes [4]. It turns out that investment in biotech deals on a number of fronts is not as bad as we all have been led to believe, and returns are better than in other industries. Good deals are getting funded and are succeeding and are giving great returns at exit.

I have been intimately involved in the creation, raising funds, staffing, managing, and leading as a board member for 7 companies over the last 5 years and advising over 50 companies for 24 years. It is an exhilarating experience and the most fun I have had in my whole life. I love the chase. Of course if you succeed it's all the more satisfying, as well as financially rewarding. Needless to say you don't get a financial reward from every company you invest in, however, it is still fun even if you fail. You learn from the experience and you can try again.

Therefore, if you personally have "the fire in your belly," nurture it and feed it and whatever you do—enjoy it.

REFERENCES

[1] http://www.angelcapitalassociation.org/. Last accessed January 30, 2014.

[2] http://www.angelresourceinstitute.org. Last accessed January 30, 2014.

[3] http://gust.com/. Last accessed January 30, 2014.

[4] http://www.forbes.com/sites/brucebooth/2013/05/22/debunking-myths-about-biotech-venture-capital/.

Chapter 21

Understanding and Securing Venture Capital

Craig Shimasaki, PhD, MBA

President & CEO, Moleculera Labs and BioSource Consulting Group, Oklahoma City, Oklahoma

Venture capital (VC) continues to play a vital role in the building of biotechnology businesses and the development and commercialization of innovative products. If you are an entrepreneur or work in a biotech start-up in the medical or life science industry, it is likely that you will at some point require the finances and support of venture capital. In this chapter we examine, from both the entrepreneur and the VC firm's perspective, what it takes to pair a great entrepreneurial opportunity with a great venture capital partner. The information presented in this chapter has been taken from my own experience and the advice of successful venture partners. The goal is to help entrepreneurial teams become more effective in raising capital from the right partners at the right time in their company development. As we have discussed in previous chapters, no matter how ground-breaking and world-class your technology and product opportunity, without a steady and uninterrupted source of capital no innovative products will ever be produced. Conversely, capital alone will not create these products; rather, it is the combination of skilled and experienced management, enabling technology, having a target market with an acute unmet need, and a great partnership with an experienced venture capital firm. In this chapter we will review some background information about venture capital, their objectives, how to find the right partners, how to approach them, and some of the best ways to ensure a higher likelihood of success.

WHAT IS VENTURE CAPITAL?

Venture capital funds are managed by professionals and used for the purpose of investing in high-risk ventures with the expectation of producing high rates of returns. Venture capital funds are managed by professionals called general partners (GP) and the money in these funds typically comes from institutions and high-net worth individuals and even other funds. Investors in a venture capital fund are called limited partners (LP). These funds are usually set up as limited liability companies (LLCs) for the protection of the limited partners and for certain tax treatments. The National Venture Capital Association indicates there are approximately 800 venture capital firms in the United States, defined as those funds which invest at least $5 million in companies. The size of a fund can vary widely, anywhere from $20 million to over $5 billion, with the average size of a VC fund being approximately $150 million [1]. Venture capital funds are directed toward almost every type of industry such as software, biotechnology, medical devices, media and entertainment, wireless communications, Internet and networking, and some large funds invest in all of the above. On average about $20 to $30 billion dollars are invested into companies by VC each year. (See Figure 21.1.)

For the VC firms that invest in biotechnology, their general partners will have a specialized focus on one or more sectors such as therapeutics, diagnostics, medical devices, bioagriculture, or biofuels for example. In addition to the sector focus, each firm will have a preference for investing at a particular stage of development such as start-up, early or late development stage, human clinical trials, or expansion stages. And finally, in addition, all VC firms have distinct investment philosophies that are implemented out by general partners who have different backgrounds and expertise such as cardiology, biomedical engineering, clinical laboratory, immunology, etc. An important point to remember is that there is *great* diversity among venture capital firms, not to mention their geographic focus, their fund size, and the timing and availability of investment capital. Therefore, it is critical for biotechnology entrepreneurs who are seeking a venture capital investment to understand who their most likely venture partners would be before approaching any firm.

Most VCs are extremely active in their portfolio companies and they integrate themselves in their company's strategic decisions, and even in certain operational activities as needed. These proactive VCs see themselves as part of the company rather than as simply investors. Other VCs operate somewhat passively, although I do not think the terms "venture capital" and "passive" can truthfully be used in the same

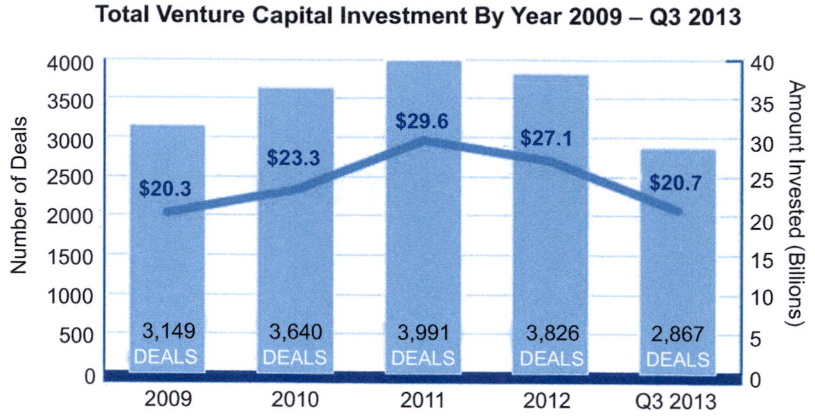

Total Venture Capital Investment By Year 2009 – Q3 2013

FIGURE 21.1 Venture capital investments through Q3 2013. (Source: *PricewaterhouseCoopers/National Venture Capital Association MoneyTree™ Report: Data Thomson Reuters.*)

sentence. However, compared to VC firms that "actively" integrate themselves into most of the company operational activities, there are others that participate predominantly through the company's quarterly board meetings. The entrepreneur should determine what type of help and participation they need from a VC partner and then seek those that provide that type of support.

CAPITAL IS A COMMODITY, WHEREAS EXPERIENCED INVESTING PARTNERS ARE NOT

Inexperienced entrepreneurs tend to view VC firms as strictly a capital resource that they need to accomplish their product development goals. In reality, a good venture capital investment will come with much more than just cash. The ideal VC investment brings valuable expertise, help in navigating product development and growth challenges, key contacts, senior management recruits, and—money. If given a choice between a $3 million investment from a band of individual investors, and $3 million from a top venture capital firm in your industry, going with the venture capital firm is usually preferable even if it means giving up more equity. A key reason for this decision is the value of their contribution, their expertise, and their resources which will improve the likelihood of success for your company. In addition, VCs have working relationships with other VCs, so if the company runs into development or market challenges that require larger financing rounds later, VCs can bring others to the table to help. Whereas, individual investors and angel networks do not typically have the funding capacity to support the next level of capital required for a growing organization with expanding financial needs.

Search for the Right Venture Capital Partnership

The way I like to describe this relationship is a "partnership." Just as a company desires to partner with the best

collaborators, they should also seek the best VCs as their partners. Finding the right venture capital partnership is critical to the ultimate success of a biotech organization. Here is some advice for those looking for the right VC partner:

- First identify all the venture firms that have funded successful deals in your technology or market space.
- Examine their track records and research the backgrounds of their partners and associates.
- Narrow this list down to your top five or ten VCs. Within each of these firms, find out which partners have the complementary backgrounds, knowledge, and expertise that will help improve the decisions your company is expected to face.
- Talk with the entrepreneurs and CEOs running companies held within their portfolio. Ask them questions about their working relationship with the VC partner to see if that partner has brought value through their participation.
- Ask these entrepreneurs if the VC partner has the patience to listen to problems and if they offer helpful solutions and sound advice.
- Ask the entrepreneurs if the VC partner has used their contacts to help with any development challenges for the company.

The Start-Up Stage and Venture Capital Investments

In general, most large venture capital firms do not focus on start-up companies unless they form them themselves. However, this can vary depending on the economy and capital markets. Some venture capital funds do allocate a portion of their fund to early-stage development. But for the most part, if your company is a start-up, focusing *all* your efforts on attracting venture capital at that stage is a time-consuming, low payoff, and disappointing endeavor. Before approaching a VC you need to have made some product development progress and you need to have reduced the scientific

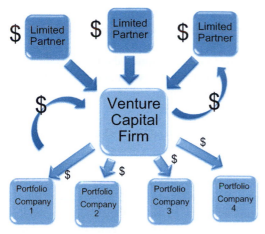

FIGURE 21.2   Understanding the venture capital cycle.

product development risks. If you are a start-up company, a good use of your time at this stage is to keep certain VCs informed of your development progress and apprise them as you move through product development stages and achieve key milestones. Let these VCs know you are not seeking funding at this time, but want to know if they would be interested in being updated on the growth and development of your organization for potential future discussions. Work on preparing prospective opportunities and establish some history and credibility with these organizations.

Another reason that most VCs do not typically invest at the start-up stage is that they have specific time horizons for their fund, and the typical fund life cycle is 10 years. Therefore, if you are a start-up company and the VC is in the last half of their fund cycle, the length of time to an exit may be beyond their ability to invest. Ideally, seek a VC fund that is in the first third of its fund cycle because they will have the longest investment horizon. A fund in the middle of its investment cycle is starting to be choosier as to the stage of investment and the potential length of time to an exit. And a fund in the final third of its life cycle is focused predominantly on follow-on investments in existing portfolio companies and liquidations, some successful and some unsuccessful. A venture capital firm receives its funds from Limited Partners to deploy into their portfolio companies, and the VC fund managers (or General Partners) are accountable to the Limited Partners. (See Figure 21.2.)

Also, be sure that your capital requirements are in sync with the VC's fund requirements because the amount of money that a VC needs to deploy is enormous. A $1 million dollar investment from a $200 million fund is not a wise decision for the VC. That is because a $1 million investment in any one company requires the same amount of time to manage as a $20 million investment.

In short, seek a venture capital partner that plays two roles— a strategic advisor *and* an investor. A good VC must possess the experience and insight to add value to growing the enterprise better than the management could without

them. Unfortunately, sometimes a company does not have a choice in venture capital partners if only one avenue for financing presents itself. This is a good reason to start a venture capital search early and target only those venture capital firms that fit with the organizational goals of your company. Ideally, search for a venture fund with general partners that share similar goals, ideals, and values because these individuals become partners who will be providing help, expertise, and guidance to your team.

VENTURE CAPITAL PARTNERS ARE TIME CONSTRAINED

It is helpful to understand the time constraints of general partners at successful venture capital firms. These individuals are extremely active and usually pressed for time. They typically sit on multiple boards of their portfolio companies, each of which have needs and problems of their own that require their help. VCs also have Limited Partners to report to and communicate the progress of their portfolio and their fund's returns. VCs also have families. VCs have limited time and attention so be sure to cut to the chase and give them the most important information about your company and product, and any other information that is of interest to them. However, do not forget the personal nature of this relationship and ultimately, if you expect to have a chance of them funding a deal, the VC partner needs to like, rather than loathe, working with you.

Dana Mead, a partner at Kleiner, Perkins, Caufield & Byers, tells listeners during a talk he gave at Stanford [2], that VC partners at his firm spend their time predominantly in the following areas:

1. **Reviewing investments**—Mead says individually they look at between 200 to 300 ventures each year. Whereas each partner invests in only one or two deals per year. The point is that all VC firms invest in a very small percentage of opportunities that they review, approximately 1 to 2 percent of all venture opportunities.
2. **Participating on boards**—Most VC partners who have an established portfolio will sit on multiple boards and therefore will have less time to focus on looking at new ventures.
3. **Networking**—Meeting many people and with other VCs that they syndicate with, or may syndicate with in the future. They have 10 to 15 select VCs that they work with out of the whole cohort of VCs. The reason is, these are the people they trust, the people they like, the people they want to work with, and it is a collaborative environment.
4. **Working with their portfolio companies**—They assist in recruiting good people for the company. They apply their network to whatever the challenge is facing the company and they help raise capital during the next round.

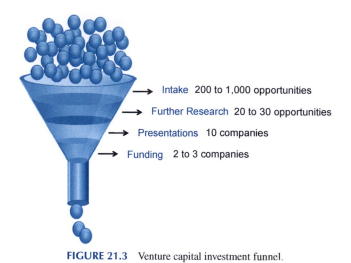

FIGURE 21.3   Venture capital investment funnel.

Intake   200 to 1,000 opportunities
Further Research   20 to 30 opportunities
Presentations   10 companies
Funding   2 to 3 companies

Supporting the point about the enormous number of opportunities reviewed, Tom Dickerson, a private equity partner, shared that they see on average 1000 business plans each year, then do further research on about 2 dozen. Of those 20 to 30 plans, they invite 10 for presentations and invest in 2 to 3 deals annually. (See Figure 21.3.)

Venture Partners are Incentivized to Build Successful Companies

Venture capital Managing Partners (also called General Partners) are the individuals who manage the funds. The success of the fund is dependent on the ability of the managing partners (MPs) to identify the opportunities that have the best success potential. They must also assist in mitigating risks and helping the company management navigate through product development and corporate development obstacles. Each VC fund typically has a 10-year cycle, which is the time expected for a return by the Limited Partner's (LP) investment. There is also an annual management fee which covers salaries and overhead that ranges from 1.5 to 2.5 percent of the fund. The fund will incentivize and align the MPs' interest by giving them a portion of the upside return which is called the "carry." The "carry" ranges between 20 and 30 percent which is a percentage of the capital realized after the original investment is returned.

What are Venture Capital Partners Looking For?

Venture capital likes to invest in big ideas that make a difference. Beth Seidenberg, another partner at Kleiner, Perkins, Caufield & Byers, in a short interview describes what she looks for in biotechnology investments [3]: "I'm looking for big ideas to disrupt the delivery of health care. KPCB is looking for people who are focused on what's possible, people who dream big and drive change. The millennial generation is frustrated and disenchanted with the current delivery

of health care. We're looking for entrepreneurs who will apply the best tools, smart business models and inventive design to connect the silos of health care in creative ways and drive the transformation of the U.S. healthcare system."

Dana Mead describes what they do when they see a venture opportunity, breaking all the different risks into the following three major areas:

1. **The technical and clinical risk and IP**—They try to figure out what the technical risks are and put some boundaries around that risk to see if there is a way with a reasonable amount of capital to mitigate those risks.
2. **The market risk**—At KPCB they are willing to take certain technical risks, but they do not like market risks. They do not want to solve a really difficult clinical problem or really difficult technical problem only to find out later that the market is only moderately interested. If they go through the time, the risk, and the hard work, they want the product to be a commercial success.
3. **The management risk**—For a young company with few management personnel, they also look at who is associated with the venture. Who are the people that have given them money? Who are people that are giving them advice? Will they be able to attract great talent as they move forward as a team?

These are the three most important things they look at in a new venture:

1. Technical and/or clinical risk and IP.
2. Market risk (unmet critical needs).
3. Management.

HOW CAN AN ENTREPRENEUR IMPROVE THEIR CHANCES OF SECURING VENTURE CAPITAL?

Dana Mead says that the number one thing that sours their interest is entrepreneurs who are imbalanced. VCs understand that early-stage companies have lots of risks, so do not be afraid to talk about what these risks are. He says to be passionate and optimistic about what you are doing, but don't be afraid to talk about the risks; but at the same time, having some balance is good. You want to show passion that is contagious and have a big vision for the company. Also, he tells listeners, entrepreneurs should really leverage their available connections and connect with experienced individuals in their locale because they want to help. In summary, his admonition to entrepreneurs is:

- Be balanced.
- Show passion for your idea and vision.
- Leverage networks and seek free counsel.
- Do not focus on the exit.
- Be persistent.
- Focus on attracting top talent and advisors.
- Have fun.

Beth Seidenberg exclaims that the biggest mistake entrepreneurs make is over-promising and under-delivering. She admonishes entrepreneurs to find the right balance between dreaming the dream and being realistic about what they can deliver within a specific timeframe. "Then do what you do best: Set up a plan and do more than anyone believed was possible." She continues, "The best entrepreneurs always meet or beat their plans—and have fun doing it. Although entrepreneurs have to be optimists and believe in their mission, they also need to highlight the risks and communicate bad news faster than good."[3]

HOW AND WHEN TO APPROACH A VENTURE CAPITAL FIRM

Know their Preferences for the Company Investment Stage

It is important to know the preferred investing stage of the VC firm that you are interested in working with. You should approach a VC firm when your development stage matches their preferred investing stage. If you are too early or too late for their fund, you will spend a lot of unproductive time resulting in little success. Most VC firms are later-stage investors, some are early-stage, and some actually participate in start-ups or even form companies around a technology themselves. However, these seed-stage VCs are rare. Most VCs that participate in early-stage investing typically participate in Series A Preferred Investment rounds. This is usually the first "institutional capital" round. Prior to this round, your company will have secured a start-up and/or a seed round of capital which typically comes from the founders themselves, friends, family, and angel investors (as discussed in Chapter 19 entitled "Sources of Capital and Investor Motivations"). Typically the company will have been established, a corporate structure formed, a talented team of scientists, advisors, consultants, and possibly partners will be working together in some capacity, but usually the company will be somewhat "virtual." There will be key proof-of-concept work or preprototypes produced and a suitable target market defined with an acute unmet need. The product will have met some early development milestones that reduce the future risk of the technology. For those interested in specific product development stages and examples of milestones, you can find more information in Chapter 6 in the book entitled *The Business of Bioscience: What Goes Into Making a Biotechnology Product* [4].

Have a Proper Introduction and Understand the VC's Financing Stage

From experience, and from talking and listening to VC partners, your introduction to a venture firm matters. The manner of introduction is a good predictor of whether or not the firm will initially have interest or even read your information. Very early on in my entrepreneurial career I erroneously presumed that the larger the number of venture firms that I contacted, the better my chances of attracting a firm that would invest. To me it was simply the "law of large numbers" the more I contacted, the higher the likelihood of success. So I purchased an expensive email contact list of all venture capital firms operating in the life science industry in the United States and overseas. I carefully crafted a (lengthy) email explaining what I was looking for and what our start-up company had plans to do, I attached what I thought was a stellar (lengthy) executive summary and sent this to over 200 VC firms I thought would be interested in my start-up. I eagerly and anxiously awaited their responses. Over a period of 1 week to as long as 4 months, I began to receive responses. Of the 200 solicitations emailed, I eventually heard from about 60 individuals and the vast majority of them gave me a very polite, and often apologetic "no." I eventually received seven "maybe" responses, but after more correspondence and an occasional phone conversation or two I received one weak interest for a presentation. I boarded an airplane and flew to their office to give the presentation, but this effort resulted in no investment. The partner I was talking with had only moderate interest which was not shared by any of his partners due to our early start-up stage. At the end of this 10-month process I had no VC partner and no money. After this disappointing but eye-opening experience, I focused on high net worth angel investors located in my geographic region and raised two rounds of capital, $1.25 million and $2.4 million each. The point of this example is to emphasize the importance of approaching VCs at the right stage of your development and to target the ones that would most likely invest. Be sure to secure an introduction from an individual who has contact with partners in the firm you are interested in. Knowing this ahead of time, could have saved me about 10 months of futile effort.

Bruce Booth, a partner at Atlas Ventures, discusses in an article on *LifeSciVC* [5], the subject of getting an introduction to a VC, and he reiterates that cold calls, or more commonly "cold emails," are ineffective in getting attention from their firm. Also, hiring a regional or boutique investment advisory firm to raise your initial round of funding is also not typically a productive way to reach a top-tier venture firm. He recommends that you be creative in finding ways to get an introduction to the venture firm partner you want, such as reaching out to the companies already within the particular VC's portfolio. These portfolio companies can be easily contacted via social media. He also says that he has had random introductions after his daughter's soccer matches. He advises *not* sending your business plan without some type of prior contact or request from a partner for it. Booth noted that Atlas has not funded a business that initially came to them via these routes. The take-home message is that qualified referrals usually attract their interest, even if just out of courtesy to the colleague that referred them.

Dana Mead describes a similar sentiment. When asked if any of the deals they did came over the "transom" or as cold calls, he indicated that although they receive a lot of investment requests over the "transom" he has not invested in any of those companies. He says that all the ones he has invested in have come through other venture capitalists that he works with and knows, or entrepreneurs or physicians or other people calling him or telling about it. Interestingly, there seems to be a reciprocating obligation as he says that "never, if I have a recommendation from one of those types of people, will I not take a meeting with the company. So it's just the way it works and a lot of it is just the comfort we have in understanding where the company came from and the people" [2].

Confidentiality

Realize that VCs see many business plans containing many different technologies. Don't expect a VC to sign a confidentiality agreement just to review your business plan. Understand that anything sent to them should be public information and nonconfidential. For confidential information that is not yet protected by patents, it is best to describe your technology in a nonconfidential manner, but be sure to demonstrate what it can do and what problem it solves. It is unrealistic to presume that any information sent to a VC will be held in confidence. It is just not possible to do so while reviewing the massive amounts of information that they receive. There are some VCs who may actually ask your permission before sending your plan or materials to others. However, you should expect that anything sent to them may be circulated to individuals from whom they may want an opinion.

What You Need to Secure a Meeting with a Venture Capital Firm

A taped interview with Brook Byers, posted on Stanford's Entrepreneurship Corner, is a valuable resource for understanding how to secure a meeting with a VC. Mr. Byers is a senior partner with Kleiner, Perkins, Caufield & Byers, and has been in the venture capital industry since 1972, and a partner with the firm since 1977. He has been closely involved with more than 60 new technology-based ventures, many of which have become public companies. Although the interview was conducted in April 2005, most of the information remains relevant today. He says that all VCs are not the same, and that all venture capital firms are idiosyncratic based upon, the firm, the limited partners, and by the individuals that are in each firm. He goes on to say that you want to connect with a person on the VC team who has the same interest and passion as you have, and someone who would become a champion or advocate for you. For those who are interested in learning more about how to improve your chances of funding from a VC firm, you should listen to his complete interview http://ecorner.stanford.edu/authorMaterialInfo.html?mid=1302.

Most all VCs are constantly inundated with proposals from companies requesting funding for their product concept. In order to get much further than simply an introduction, you will need a clear, concise, and well-written executive summary and business plan. In addition, you need to understand what a "pitch" is. A pitch is an attention-grabber that succinctly describes the technology, the market and the unmet need, to open the door for future discussions with venture capital. Because VCs are inundated with so many opportunities, it is essential that the entrepreneur present the most relevant information succinctly so that the VC partner can quickly assess if they want to hear more.

RAISING CAPITAL FOR BIOTECHNOLOGY COMPANIES

In this section, with permission, I have incorporated valuable information from Bruce Booth based upon his website *LifeSciVC* [5], I have also incorporated lessons from my own experience and offer some general guidelines about how to increase your likelihood of successful fundraising.

Know and Understand Your Investor Audience

When approaching any investor audience it is important to recognize that each investor group has varying investment requirements and motivations. Venture firms have different investing requirements and different capabilities compared with angel investors and angel networks. To begin with, be sure that the VC you are approaching has a focus that matches your product development stage. Remember, there is great diversity of VC focuses, some concentrate on seed-stage and early-development stages, whereas others concentrate on later-stage development opportunities. If you are seeking a venture firm to participate in your later-stage opportunity but they focus on early stages, you are unlikely to get their interest. Just be sure the VC firm interest matches your stage of development and, of course, your product category. In other words, if the VC firm specializes in clinical laboratory diagnostics, you are not likely to have much success if you are a therapeutic company. Pay attention to the VC's portfolio and learn what type of opportunities and at what stage they like to invest. Each individual VC partner specializes in a particular area because of their expertise and background. You can usually find information about a VC's portfolio companies and the backgrounds of their partners on their website.

Quality Science and Quality Scientists

Because biotechnology products depend on the underlying science and technology in order to develop a successful product, VCs want to invest in opportunities that are based on great science. The quality of the underlying science, the acuteness of the unmet need, and having a breakthrough application will attract the interest of VCs. This is a common theme for many venture firms as these types of opportunities support their expectations of very high returns. Do not spend much time trying to convince investors about the enormous market in cancer, heart disease, or Alzheimer's, rather focus instead on the core issues that impact the investment decision of a science-based biotechnology company. Share the scientific data that supports your claims and avoid too much conjecture, but be open about what you know and what you do not know. Always focus on data-driven evidence and good assumptions because the quality of the science is a critical component, and all data must be reproducible. As discussed in Chapter 10 entitled "Technology Opportunities: Evaluating the Idea," great science and great scientists are inseparable. The knowledge and ideas that created the discovery opportunity are inherent within the scientist, physician, engineer, or technology expert. It is important to be sure that the scientist(s) that developed the concepts be in some way associated with the company and its product development.

EXPERIENCED AND SEASONED MANAGEMENT TEAM WITH PASSION

It is always challenging to recruit great management talent for a development-stage biotechnology company, but it is easier to do so with great science and technology. In the start-up stages the management team is incomplete, yet they should be surrounded by seasoned leaders, expert scientific advisory members, experienced board members, and other quality advisors. As the company grows there is a need for an experienced and seasoned CEO to lead the organization. The best practitioners in this industry have learned through years of apprenticeship, project leadership, and real-life lessons. Make sure your team members have some of this deep experience. Also, make sure that your leadership, managers, and advisory members have a good blend of experience and enthusiasm for your product and your company. Depending on the type of product being developed, sometimes an early-stage company does not require a full-time, high-caliber CEO. However, be honest about the management gaps, and share a timeframe in which you intend to fill these positions. One great benefit of having a VC partner is their ability to recruit top management talent at the appropriate time. Therefore, it is important to get the right group of early executives and leaders when forming a solid management team. It is helpful to recognize that different management teams are often required at different stages of a company's development.

Risk Management and Risk Mitigation

The entrepreneur and management team are risk managers of both the business and the science. However, you cannot manage a risk that you don't know. Be sure to honestly evaluate and assess the risks your company will face. Then share the company and product development risks and the manner in which management has steadily reduced these risks relative to its stage of product development. As you identify the risks you are managing, be sure to include a timeline you expect to execute against and the reasons why investors should invest *before* the next risk reduction phase. Be honest with the risks you perceive because you can be sure that the investor will be looking for them. Having an honest view of these risks and the mitigating milestones that your team is working on will increase your likelihood of raising money.

DO NOT OVERVALUE YOUR COMPANY AT ANY FUNDING STAGE

Most VCs that operate in your product and technology sector will have a good idea what fair valuations are for a company at your particular stage of development. I say most, because there are some what would want to lowball your valuation. Aside from those, reputable VCs and partners will know what a current valuation is relative to the current financial markets. Understandably, most entrepreneurs will tend to overvalue their company at the start-up and early-development stages. The answer to "how much is your company worth" determines the slice of equity for the founders, employees, and current and future shareholders. However, overvaluing your company is counterproductive and detrimental to attracting institutional and venture capital during these critical stages. The right company valuation is obviously the market-clearing price at the time. Any entrepreneur that overvalues their company will also raise questions about irrational behavior in the future.

There are standard and accepted valuation methods for determining the value of companies *with* product revenue, but these methods cannot be applied accurately to an early or development-stage prerevenue biotechnology company. VCs have a good understanding of the valuation of comparable companies at your stage, in your product sector, and in your target market. This method is analogous to how real estate valuations are determined based upon comparables within a local region and based upon the past sales of comparable properties. Inherent within a VC valuation is an assessment of a return requirement at exit or a multiple expectation necessary to make the investment worthwhile for the venture firm.

Some companies at later prerevenue stages may commission a professional valuation assessment by investment bankers or other private equity firms. These firms typically estimate a company valuation using a discounted cash flow (DCF) projection of future revenue streams. This exercise may be helpful, but in reality no one can predict what actual sales will be in the future, and more importantly no one can predict the likelihood of the company successfully reaching commercialization. Even if the valuation exercise includes a risk adjustment for achieving each subsequent product development milestone (rDCF), the risk assigned to any particular development stage is a guess, and one can make an equally strong argument for a different risk adjustment. Early- and development-stage companies have many financial and scientific uncertainties that weaken the ability to confidently utilize a rDCF method. Also, the cost, risk, and time associated with the research and development (R&D) phase of any particular biotechnology product is uncertain. More importantly, venture capital does not use rDCF for valuation of early- or development-stage biotechnology companies, and they are the most common investor at this stage of development.

Accurately determining the valuation of a development-stage biotechnology company is important for attracting financing, issuing stock at "fair-market" value, and ensuring that future financing partners are not soured by an unrealistically valued company. Having a realistic valuation for your company will increase the likelihood of financing your enterprise. In reality, never forget that valuation is ultimately determined by the investor who writes the check. You can read more information about the valuation of development-stage biotechnology companies at my website [6] "How Much is Your Company Really Worth?"

Estimate the Long-Term Capital Needs and Your Likely Exit

All start-up companies should have a realistic long-term business plan that addresses how much capital is required to reach an exit or liquidity event. Such a plan should include the product-development stages and key milestones that are reached prior to each funding. As we all know there is a lot of variability in future financing plans, but these must address the amount of capital required to reach each value-enhancing milestone or product-development stage. Also, the team should know the total amount of capital needed to reach a liquidity event. For example, does the plan require $5 million, $50 million, or $100 million in equity financing to reach an exit for the investors and shareholders? VCs like to see capital-efficient organizations that are scaled appropriately for their type of product development and business strategy. The management team must know how to outsource selectively and aggressively, and leverage nondilutive sources of capital such as grants.

Utilize Experienced Corporate and Patent Counsel

Nothing hurts a start-up company's fundraising momentum more than poor corporate fundamentals, including odd company structures, convoluted capitalization tables, oversized and nonstrategic boards, a poorly drafted license option or license agreement, and a lack of intellectual property or freedom-to-operate. Remember that patents are critical to a biotech company, so be sure you retain seasoned patent counsel, preferably experienced in both prosecution and litigation of patents. Also, you must have a biotechnology industry-experienced attorney that has a history of working with start-ups. Obtaining good legal advice is very important to early-stage biotechnology companies.

Be Passionate about Your Company and Vision

Passion is an internal characteristic that is easily recognized by others. It is a requisite for success and for finding interested financial backers of your enterprise. If your product is in the medical field, be sure to tell the vision of how your product will impact patients and change medicine for the better. Be excited. Share your infectious passion because without it start-ups do not succeed.

Business Plan Contents

Fundraising is never easy, and it never has been. But focusing on the things that are most important will improve the success rate for biotechnology start-ups. As you know or will find out, your executive summary and business plan are the first documents that are needed to get the attention of any investor. Here are just a few important topics to be sure that you cover in your business plan:

- **Describe the opportunity**—Your company mission and its vision.
- **Explain the problem your product solves**—Improvements, cures, treatments, diagnostic tool.
- **Describe your target market and the acute unmet need**—Who are your target customers, how big is your market, what are the acute unmet needs.
- **Explain the technology**—How it works, what it can do, patents, reproducibility, differentiation.
- **Share your market strategy**—Your business model, market channel, pricing, partnerships, competition, substitutes.
- **List the experienced and seasoned team**—How their experience is applicable, background, board members, clinical, and scientific advisors.
- **Share financial and operating plans**—Funding and use of funds, milestones, *pro forma* projections, risk mitigations.

THE PRESENTATION TO VC PARTNERS

So now you have been invited to give a presentation and give your "pitch" to the VC partners. Here is some brief advice about how to have a great initial meeting with a venture capital firm:

1. **Know your audience**—Understand to whom you are presenting. Are they scientists, physicians, engineers,

business, or marketing professionals? Depending on the audience, be sure to speak to the aspects that are important to those listening. Do not forget to explain the science in terms that everyone can understand. However, if the partners are scientists, do not gloss over the science, but present the relevant data and discuss the risks and implications.

2. **Share relevant information about the market need**—Spend time on any aspect of your target market that may be unique or unappreciated for that particular disease condition or market for your product. Clearly describe the problem that your product will solve. It is not necessary to spend too much time describing general knowledge about markets such as cancer, heart disease, or diabetes. Help your audience know and appreciate key features of your market that make your product ideally suited to meet those needs.

3. **Point out strengths of team members succinctly**—As mentioned before, management is critical to the success of any company. Share past accomplishments that are relevant to your current and future needs but you do not need to go into great detail because all venture capital firms can recognize great teams when they see them. Point out the strengths that may not be obvious in your founding team members, scientific advisors, and board members—but do not spend more than a few minutes on these.

4. **Share your vision but be realistic**—Share your vision for success, especially how your product will impact and change the lives of those that use them. If you are a biotherapeutic company, share how your patient's lives will be helped by using your product. If you are a medical device company, share how your device will affect the well-being of those that will use it. Do not over-promote and over-promise. But there needs to be clear scientific evidence supporting the market value of your product and the ability of the technology to deliver these key features and benefits.

5. **Conclude with realistic exit scenarios**—Be prepared to discuss how much equity capital you think it will take to bring this deal to a liquidity event. Most biotechnology companies will have an exit by acquisition. It is important to list some of the likely acquirers and those organizations that acquired similar companies in the past. Unless you are confident that your company has a special story that Wall Street and the public market will love, you should not consider including an initial public offering (IPO) in the exit scenario.

6. **Engage in questions and answers (Q&A)**—Be engaging when answering the questions from your listeners. Do not become defensive about any question but rather explain the information and data that has led you to your conclusions. If you do not know the answer to a question, share what you do know and propose to return with an answer later. Do not make up answers when you really do not know them. This is a sure way for your listeners to lose confidence in you. As with all investor presentations, expect to receive some hard questions, but remember this is beneficial because they are helping you to uncover risks, and you cannot manage a risk that you do not know.

7. **Manage the meeting's agenda and time**—At the outset, be sure to explicitly ask how much time has been allotted for your meeting. If it is a 1-hour meeting, plan to talk for no more than 30 minutes. If it is interesting, the VC partners will easily be pushing an hour. You do not want to find out that you do not have time to finish your presentation or that you have not managed your allotted time well. Plan to save time for the most important part of the meeting and that is the discussion at the end.

NEXT STEPS IN THE INVESTMENT COMMITMENT PROCESS

The Term Sheet

Once the partners at the VC firm have expressed a favorable interest for investing in your company, they will send you a "term sheet." Although this is a "nonbinding" commitment, it is a significant step towards funding and it indicates that if everything presented holds to be true, the VC firm will make an investment in your company. The term sheet contains a list of terms and conditions under which the VC firm is willing to invest. These terms include the amount of capital that will be invested, the premoney valuation of the company (the value of the company prior to the VC investment), and many addition terms. Some of the more common terms include:

- Type of stock to be issued: preferred, junior preferred, common, warrants
- Liquidation preferences
- Dividend preferences
- Redemption rights and price
- Conversion rights
- Antidilution provisions
- Rights of first refusal
- Price protection
- Voting rights
- Registration rights

This by no means is an exhaustive list of terms, but includes some of the most common ones seen in a venture capital term sheet. Some of these terms may be negotiable and some may not. This is where your attorney can assist by helping you understand the impact of these terms on your company and future fundraising efforts. The definitions of these terms can be found through many resources on the Internet. You can also find an example of a standard term sheet at the National Venture Capital Association's website, in their Resources Section under "Model Legal Documents" [7].

The Next Step is Due Diligence

Once a term sheet is received, accepted, and signed, the next step is for the VC firm to perform due diligence on the company. Due diligence is a detailed and thorough examination of all the issues and risks of the company including technology issues, intellectual property, market assumptions, and corporate structure and agreements. Completing due diligence requires considerable time and effort from both the company and the interested investment group. This process can consume between 4 to 6 months for the management team and their corporate counsel depending on the stage of the company and the size of the transaction. Once due diligence is completed there may be outstanding issues that need to be remedied if they can. If all outstanding issues are successfully resolved, a closing date can be set for funding. Closing is a joyous event and the actual process not too dissimilar to a closing when purchasing a new home—just more paperwork. Upon closing you will receive a check or wire transfer for the committed funds. This is a significant milestone and it is a good time to celebrate! However, do not forget that funding simply means the work begins in earnest. Keep in mind that you must reach each successive product-development milestone to ensure continued funding and commercialization success.

SUMMARY

Starting a biotechnology company is challenging and requires continuous sources of capital over long periods of time. At some stage most biotechnology companies will need the financial assistance of venture capital. Finding the right VC partner can assist the entrepreneurial team in successfully overcoming product development and growth issues. Every VC firm will have a focus on a particular development stage, technology, and market. It is advantageous for the company leaders to understand the interests and motivations of these firms, as it will increase the likelihood of securing funding. Biotechnology product development is a high-risk endeavor and many product ideas do not always work out as envisioned. However, finding the right VC partnership with expertise in your area can assist in overcoming development obstacles that previously seemed insurmountable. Spend time researching the best VC partners for your company and work on mitigating the early development risks, which will increase interest from the best VC firms.

Additional information about venture capital in the United States can be obtained from the National Venture Capital Association (www.nvca.org). Venture capital information in the UK can be obtained from the British Venture Capital Association (www.bvca.co.uk), in Europe from the European Venture Capital Association (ww.evca.com), in Canada at Canada's Private Equity and Venture Capital Association (www.cvca.ca), and in Japan at the Japan Venture Capital Association (www.jvca.jp). Links to venture capital in other countries can be found at the National Venture Capital Association's website [8].

REFERENCES

[1] National Venture Capital Association. http://www.nvca.org/index. php?option=com_content&view=article&id=119&Itemid=621. Last accessed on November 16, 2013.

[2] Stanford University's Entrepreneurship Corner. http://ecorner. stanford.edu/authorMaterialInfo.html?mid=2811. Last accessed on November 16, 2013.

[3] Silicon Beat. http://www.siliconbeat.com/2013/11/08/elevator-pitch-beth-seidenberg-on-the-shakeup-at-kleiner-perkins/. Last accessed on November 16, 2013.

[4] Shimasaki CD. "The Product Development Pathway: Charting the Right Course." The Business of Bioscience: What Goes Into Developing a Biotechnology Product. Springer; 2009. Chapter 6.

[5] Life Sci VC. http://lifescivc.com/category/general-venture-capital/. Last accessed on November 16, 2013.

[6] BioSource Consulting Group Bioblog. http://biosourceconsulting. com/bio-blog/how-much-is-your-company-really-worth/. Last accessed on November 16, 2013.

[7] National Venture Capital Association. http://www.nvca.org/index. php?option=com_content&view=article&id=108&Itemid=136. Last accessed March 16, 2014.

[8] National Venture Capital Association. http://www.nvca.org/index. php?option=com_content&view=article&id=106&Itemid=592. Last accessed on March 16, 2014.

Chapter 22

Your Business Plan and Presentation: Articulating Your Journey to Commercialization

Lowell W. Busenitz, PhD, MBA

Academic Director, Price College Center for Entrepreneurship, University of Oklahoma, Norman, Oklahoma

PITCHING TO INVESTORS AND PARTNERS

If a venture is to be successful, entrepreneurs always need to be able to sell their concept to potential stakeholders by letting them know they have a viable venture. Such stakeholders usually involve financial investors, but they can also involve suppliers, buyers, or key partnerships with other firms who will add value to the venture. Stakeholders typically want to learn about your venture and its viability before commitments are made. Potential financial partners in particular are noted for probing deeply for information about the foundations and direction of the venture. Whenever potential stakeholders inquire about the nature, viability, and direction of the venture, entrepreneurs need to be ready. Having a written business plan is an excellent and frequently expected way for entrepreneurs to signal the depth of their understanding of, and commitment to, the venture. A written business plan is the most common document used to start attracting outside stakeholders. Furthermore, a well-written business plan is a great foundation in which to show the viability of a business concept.

In addition to having a written business plan to offer to stakeholders, there are a couple of key reasons that encourage building a business plan. First, starting a venture involves putting together a team. Internally, the founding entrepreneur or team will inevitably need to make some key hires. Without a clear articulation of: what the venture is about, specifications of resources already in place, the proposed direction, and targeted directions for the venture, effective hires becomes increasingly unlikely. A written business plan is a valuable tool to help lead the founders through this process. Building the "team" may also involve external stakeholders such as key suppliers or buyers. When financing is involved, such inquirers will typically want extensive information about

the venture. Also, and perhaps most importantly, many financial investors will generally want to be considered part of the team giving meaningful input on the strategic direction and operations of the venture going forward. The more people that get involved with the venture, the more a business plan becomes a valuable tool for communicating what the venture is really about and to get the key individuals involved pulling together in the same direction.

The likelihood of potential investors or other stakeholders asking for a written business plan is what generally motivates entrepreneurs to develop such a document. However, no one will gain more from writing the business plan than the entrepreneurs who put it together. It is the building of all the different components of the plan and their new insights that make the process so rich. As I discuss below, much learning and realignment are all integral parts of a quality-evolving business plan and the maturing of the concept.

Feasibility Analysis Versus Business Plans

Before we move further into the business planning process, we will address the purpose of a feasibility analysis compared with that of a business plan. A feasibility analysis is about an idea that an entrepreneur is interested in pursuing, but he or she does not yet know if it is a viable opportunity. In its simplest form, feasibility work is most relevant for the very earliest stages of concept development and is for internal validation purposes about whether this venture concept has potential. Such analyses typically involves determining if the technology is feasible, if there is real demand for the product or service, if prospective customers feel a pain that would make the proposed product desirable to them, and if so, what is the best way for them to gain access to the product? Financial feasibility, such as how much will customers pay is also important. How much will it cost to make? How much start-up capital will be needed? Doing further research by developing hypotheses about technology and markets and prospective customers and finances are all part of the feasibility analysis. Then doing extensive research to see if the initial hypotheses are substantiated. Some of this work may be done through access to research databases; but there are very few substitutes for hitting the pavement to interview industry experts and prospective customers. A feasibility analysis helps the founding team evaluate if this is a potential "go" or "no go" concept.

A business plan comes after the entrepreneurs are satisfied that the venture concept is feasible. At least some of the information gleaned from the research for a feasibility analysis will become foundational for the business plan. A business plan starts with the assumption that the venture concept has significant viability and that the entrepreneur is now in the process of putting the building blocks into place in pursuit of commercialization. Since the research of a feasibility analysis is rarely conclusive, more validation is invariably needed to verify various parts of the commercialization process. Furthermore, while a business plan is a selling document, it should always be seen as a "living" document that continues to take shape based on learning and further input. See Table 22.1 for a summary comparison of the differences between feasibility analysis and the business plan. The following section addresses the dynamic learning process of putting together a business plan in greater depth.

THE BUSINESS PLANNING PROCESS

Business plans are a communication tool between the entrepreneur and outside investors such as venture capitalists for example. There are many good things that come from putting together a well-crafted business plan. It can be of great assistance in facilitating the support and collaborations of partners and outside investors. Unfortunately, many entrepreneurs find the research and writing process to be challenging. The major resistance to putting together a quality business plan usually comes from the time and effort that it takes to assemble such a product. The research, revisions, reiterations, and time are generally substantial.

With the goal of having a viable business plan in hand to help communicate with prospective investors, let's take a closer look at the value that the process can add. In preparing for battle, General Dwight Eisenhower once said, "I have always found that plans are useless but planning is indispensable." Preparing to launch a new venture is a major undertaking that almost always encounters significant obstacles. In response to the risks and unknowns that new ventures face, business plans can be perceived as irrelevant. The new venture start-up process usually involves

TABLE 22.1 Comparisons of Feasibility Analysis and Business Plans

	Feasibility Analysis	Business Plan
Central intent	To determine if a business concept has the potential to become a viable business opportunity.	To specify the commercialization plan and sell the business concept to prospective investors and stakeholders.
Key decisions	Is this venture concept a "go" or "no go?"	What resources are needed to take this concept to the next level? How much capital do we need to raise? From whom will we raise it? What will we give up in return?
For whom	For the nascent entrepreneurs. If it is a "go," then am I the right person to lead this venture?	For prospective investors and potential stakeholders. A form of strategic planning for the entrepreneurs.
Data to be gathered	Gathering data from prospective customers to assess market need.	Gathering data from experts and prospective customers about how best to launch and implement this venture.
Commitment level	Everything is tentative.	Fully committed to pressing forward with the venture.
Business models	Evaluating different ways that this business could potentially operate.	Adopting a specific business model and the specific resources needed to launch the venture.

significant adjustments, thus it is sometimes argued that a written business plan quickly becomes out-of-date and thus is an irrelevant process. While there are some truths to this, such a perspective completely misses the point. As Eisenhower noted, the planning process itself is indispensable when preparing for a significant and uncertain action ahead, even when it involves uncharted territory. So let's explicitly observe some of the benefits of the business plan process for an entrepreneurial team.

First, the process of writing the business plan gives the entrepreneurs another *communication tool* with which to reach the desired stakeholders. As entrepreneurs move out and start selling their business concept to prospective investors, possible suppliers, and potential customers, they will often need multiple communication tools. In putting together a written business plan, entrepreneurs will be challenged to obtain a better understanding of the issues that are important to the investment community. Furthermore, as the writing process unfolds, entrepreneurs will develop special communication mediums and terminology associated with unique characteristics of the industry. The process of developing special and unique language then becomes a tool for helping entrepreneurs communicate their venture to the needed parties. The writing process facilitates more effective communication.

Second, writing a plan helps entrepreneurs build a *logical whole*. By definition, a solid business plan brings together multiple components into one package. It is like a puzzle in which all the pieces need to fit together. A solid plan will effectively address the following:

- Identify the technology
- Analyze competition
- Segment the serviceable market and entry points
- Address the venture's competitive advantage
- Develop a strategy for entering the market
- Cover implementation and operation strategies
- Specify the management team
- Explain the company structure
- Identify the critical risks
- Build the revenue model
- Offer key investment considerations

Without being challenged to integrate all these components into a larger whole, it is unlikely that entrepreneurs would effectively think through the package deal in sufficient depth. This represents a fairly comprehensive set of issues that are interlinked and build from one to another. It is very easy to lose focus in fitting all the pieces of a business plan together. With a well-developed business plan, the various pieces fit together like a puzzle integrated nicely into one cohesive package. The process of writing a business plan facilitates this process.

Third, the business plan writing process encourages the development of *creative insights*. The writing and assembling of the business plan into a whole package often leads to fresh insights into things that previously were not apparent. Most entrepreneurs pursuing a new venture think about it all day, every day. There are many good things to say about that kind of energy and passion. However, with such focus and intensity can also come gaps and tunnel vision. Entrepreneurs need tools that will give them a different perspective on various parts of their venture. Entrepreneurs in this process often come to see and understand their venture in a way they previously had not. Such insights can lead to follow-on opportunities, new ways to deal with potential competitors, or a creative approach to entering the market.

Fourth, the writing process establishes a *foundation* for the ongoing strategic development of the venture. Without writing down how one is actually thinking about their venture, one can easily become blown around by different conversations and ideas. Entrepreneurs sometime respond to suggestions for the venture by saying "yes" we can do that without understanding the implications for the entire venture. However, without established foundations in place, they are in no position for true and meaningful learning about what may be wrong, and what, and how much needs to be changed. The current paradigm and business plan that is in place for a venture is, in essence, the thought foundation of the venture. Right or wrong, from this paradigm the venture moves forward. The emerging logic represented in a business plan will almost always need to be adjusted, sometimes substantially. Failure to do so often means a failed venture. Having a logical plan gives entrepreneurs the foundation from which to evaluate their current logic—where it is strong and where it is flawed. Without this baseline in place, the entrepreneurial team will be tossed about like a ship without a rudder. Assuming that a written business plan is not set in concrete, it can serve as a great vehicle for strategic thinking. Stated differently, a business plan should always be a working or "living" document!

These four points suggest that writing a business plan can be a very constructive activity on the way to building a viable venture. The thought process needed to build a venture is substantial. Putting together a business plan and continuing to revise it is an amazing process that many thousands of entrepreneurs have found to be beneficial. Most entrepreneurs find putting a business plan together is a challenging process, but it usually pays dividends many times over. We now move to discuss in greater detail what actually goes into the making of a quality business plan.

THE CONTENTS OF THE BUSINESS PLAN

Among prospective investors who regularly review business concepts and business plans, an "industry standard" of the key issues that should be covered and also to a lesser extent, the order in which the various components should be covered has emerged. Sometimes entrepreneurs, being the creative individuals that many of them tend to be, try to change things around to bring some innovation to the business plan. While there is some room for variation, and most business concepts usually call for some tweaking to capture the nuances of that specific venture, business plans as a whole are not the place to get overly creative. I strongly suggest you largely follow an established outline using the norms for the building of business plans.

The outline and guidelines for building a business plan are found below. The suggested outline offers enough detail to give significant guidance. Also, clear distinctions are made between industry, market, and competitive advantage components—issues that are often confused and intermingled. The industry addresses the competitors who are currently in the space now and who are likely to be the key competitors for the venture going forward. The market addresses the prospective customers, the size of the serviceable market, how can the serviceable market be segmented, and where is the sweet spot of all the potential customers.

As you dig into the details of building a wonderful business plan, it is helpful to keep in mind the following bigger picture that most prospective investors want to know about every business they consider:

1. What is the customer pain and is the motivation likely to be strong enough for prospective customers to buy the offered solution?
2. What sets this venture apart from existing competitors and will it be able to build and protect its competitive advantage?
3. How big is the market and is there significant growth in this space?
4. Has a quality team been assembled to lead this venture and why are they the right people to lead this concept forward?

5. How will the business make money? The expenses and potential revenues will need to be shown to be realistic and lead to long-term profitability. Are the potential revenues and profits large enough to adequately reward the type of investors that you will be pitching too?

With that introduction, I now suggest the following outline. It starts with the executive summary. This section, while first in the business plan, is usually written last. The writing of the business plan starts in earnest with Section II on the venture opportunity. Remember that in writing your business plan and following the outline, it is important to tell your story. The path to this concept is unique and it has the possibility of changing the world that is relevant to the business concept. Starting with the name of the business, the mantra, product name, section titles, and body content, the business plan should communicate a great story about a great business venture that is in development and is going to resolve a critical customer pain while returning a nice return for your prospective investors. Keep the central theme of your story as a common thread throughout. Always work towards building your *story*!

Business Plan (Bplan) Outline

Cover Page and Table of Contents

I. Executive summary (to be written last).
  A. The executive summary must make a great *first impression*.
  B. Potential investors should be provided enough relevant information in the executive summary to convince them to inquire further, identifying such central issues as:
   - The specific product or service offering.
   - The reasons a customer would buy this product or service.
   - The reasons a customer would buy it from this venture.
   - The reasons a customer would buy it right now.
   - The manner in which the company name, logo, mantra, and tag line help to communicate the company's strategy, goals, etc.
  C. The executive summary should be brief and should clearly describe the offering to investors. Briefly specify the type of funding you seek, the amount you want, the use of the funds, and the length of time the funds are needed. Also mention how much of the company *you are prepared to offer* in exchange for financing and the role you would like a potential investor to have.

II. Venture Opportunity (opportunity context)
  A. Business description
   - The company (name/form/logo) and industry category.
   - The specific product/service offering.
   - The goals, mission (mantra), strategy, objectives.

   - How your business will work (consider using a visual model).
   - Explain your interest in this business concept.
  B. Financial cost/benefit analysis for the venture.
   - What will be the source(s) for revenue? Provide some meaningful estimations of how much revenue each source will provide for the first 3 years of anticipated revenue.
   - What are the main anticipated variable costs required to launch the venture? What are the major anticipated fixed costs required to launch the venture?
   - Show that the financial benefits outweigh the costs.
  C. Customer value proposition:
   - What are specific benefits that you will deliver to your principal customers? These will most likely involve financial benefits, but psychological benefits could *also* be noted.
   - Develop quantitative numbers comparing and contrasting the way your targeted customer is currently spending time/money with how your new offered product will improve production and/or financial gains for your customer.
  D. The innovation/technology.
   - Identify your technology innovation.
   - Show how it compares to the currently accepted practice.
   - Include helpful diagrams that inform the investor.
   - Emphasize the benefits the end-users will experience.

Business Plan (Bplan) Outline—Cont'd

- Put together a "product matrix" to show comparisons with currently existing products (see sample worksheet in Table 22.2).
- Any key industry standards or requirements?
- If applicable, put technical specifications in an appendix.

III. Industry Examination

A. Macro factors impacting the overall industry trends: What emerging macro-trends suggest the traditional way of doing business is changing? Substantiate your arguments with changes *starting to appear,* or are projected to appear, in the economic, political, regulatory, demographic, technological, socio-cultural, or global arenas. The focus here is on macro-level trends (why the time may be right for your concept).

B. Industry analysis.
- Description (type, size, segmentation, major players).
- Demand conditions (life cycle, profitability, history, trends).
- Industry attractiveness (Porter's 5 forces).

C. Current industry models/competitors/trends.
- Develop a "competitor matrix" (see sample worksheet in Table 22.3).
- What business models are currently used by established firms?
- How are new products typically introduced in this space?
- Provide examples of successful start-ups in this industry.
- Provide examples of unsuccessful start-ups in this industry.

IV. Market Examination

A. Macro-level analysis.
- Market segmentation of serviceable market.
- Size (must be large enough to sustain a business).
- Demographics (income, habits, personal characteristics, standard of living, etc., for major segments).
- Trends in the various segments.
- Psychographic profile (interests, activities, opinions).

B. Your customers (micro-level analysis).
- Identify multiple target segments; compare and evaluate them.
- Identify your initial target customer segment.
- Motivations for target customers to purchase.
- Timing (why is the timing right).
- Where is your projected "sweet spot" in the market?
- Scalability—can success in one area lead to success in another?
- Develop a matrix table that summarizes and distinguishes the different customer segments. Conclude with justifying your chosen entry segment

and why you think that this is your starting "sweet spot."
- Include customer testimonials that validate your market.

Most top quality business plans build customer analysis from *primary data* collected by the team. This typically includes structured interviews or survey data (details of data collected are typically included in an appendix). Secondary data can also provide rich sources of customer information.

V. Competitive Advantage

A. What resource(s) will be used to seek a competitive advantage?

B. Can the resources to be used be considered as "valuable," "rare," and/or hard to "imitate?"
- Are there patents, trademarks, and/or copyrights involved?
- Is there intellectual property to be developed?
- What other resources should be considered?

C. For a new venture, it can be very effective to articulate one or two resource-based advantages and by what means you plan to build these competitive advantages down the road assuming that you have a successful launch.

VI. Pricing, Marketing, and Supply Chain

Based on your industry and market analyses and your competitive advantage, explicitly develop and state your overall marketing strategy. (Your pricing, distribution, promotion, sales and service operations should all flow from your overall marketing strategy.)

The *fundamental purpose of this section* is to design a plan for how you are going to sell your *first* customers (remember to approach this with a bottom-up approach). Rarely is it appropriate for a new venture to initially focus on appealing to the mass market.

A. Pricing operations (e.g., quantity discounts? Premium price?). Pricing strategies:
- Keystone pricing—many businesses double their costs.
- Cost-plus pricing—mark-up based on the cost of the unit sold.
- Competitive pricing—based on what competitors are selling for.
- Market pricing—charging the highest price that customers will bear. *Pricing can be based on more than one of the above as appropriate.*

B. Promotion and advertising operations.

C. Distribution operations (wholesaler channels, use of Internet, retail sales, combination, etc.).

D. Sales approach. Who will develop leads, work with prospects, and close the sale? How will sales people be compensated? Describe the sales cycle. Demonstrate interest by potential buyers.

Continued

Business Plan (Bplan) Outline—Cont'd

E. Service operations (how will customer service be offered?).

VII. Implementation and Operating Strategies

Explaining how and when you will execute your Bplan strategy.

A. Identify what has already been accomplished. Focus particularly on specifying the specific steps that need to be accomplished between now and the point of the first sale.

B. Provide a timeline with milestones to show projected timing and the sequence of key events. While one to three significant accomplishments may be included, the focus should be on the six to ten most significant future milestones, usually spanning the next 2 to 3 years (major milestones in years 4 to 5 may also be included).

C. Critical operational issues to potentially address might include:
- Facility requirements—leased, purchased, or both.
- Labor requirements.
- Supply chain track and alternatives.
- Capital requirements—equipment list, financing, etc.
- Seasonality—production planning, inventory turnover and control, lead-times, storage, etc.

Overall, this section should accomplish the following:
- Specify key future steps to be accomplished in establishing proof-of-concept and launching this venture.
- Do you anticipate rolling out additional products or services in the next 3 to 5 years?
- Signal funding needs for the early phases of the venture.

VIII. Company Structure and Management

A. Company structure.
- Legal form of the organization (LLC, LLP, C-Corp. etc.).
- Ownership structure of the business.

B. Management Team
- Training, work experience, and the personal capabilities.
- Supporters of the team.
- Profile key future hires needed in the future.

C. The extended team:
- Advisory board
- Board of directors?

IX. Critical Risks

A. Identify three to six of the most critical risk factors. Where might the venture hit obstacles going forward?

B. Possible internal critical risks—market adoption and acceptance, cost/time over runs, key personnel issues, etc.

C. Possible external critical risks—environmental shifts, market shifts, competitors' actions, etc.

D. For each risk factor, how will you mitigate these risks in the event that they emerge?

X. The Revenue Model and Key Investment Considerations

A. Specify your financial assumptions (most likely make these explicit in an Appendix).

B. An "average unit economic analysis" should show revenue to be received from the first year of sales on a per unit basis, the costs associated with start-up, and ongoing costs in year one.

C. Summary financials in one table for years 1 to 5 to include units sold, COGS, revenue, operating income.
- Include a "Valley of Death" chart (capital required, B/E, etc.).

D. Financial analysis schedules (cash flow statement; income statement, balance sheet). The detailed schedules should be monthly for at least 1 year, quarterly for first 2 years, and annually through 5 years. Put in an Appendix.

E. Required funding (type of funding and the deal structure).
- "Use of funds" statement identifying main expenditures.
- Timing of funds being sought and key milestones.
- Terms to be offered to investors (equity percent).

F. Future growth opportunities (scalability).
- Leveraging developed capabilities for further expansion.
- Follow-on customer market opportunities.

G. Key reasons to invest (develop two to four reasons to invest).
- Unique product, service, use of new (existing) technology.
- Any usually qualified individuals, perhaps with linkages?
- Do you have a particularly strong competitive advantage?
- Realistic assessment of ROI potential
- What kind of exit is likely within 5 years?

Appendix

The appendix is the last section of the business plan. It is used to communicate supplemental and supporting information.
- Detailed financial statements or worksheets.
- Detailed product or technical description and patent grants.
- Published articles and/or technical reports.
- Primary research detailing competitor or customer feedback.
- Business agreements.
- Letters of intent connected to the business.
- Sample of marketing or promotional materials.
- Accolades/awards/commendations/testimonials.
- Purchase orders for your product/service.

Business Plan (Bplan) Outline—Cont'd

Miscellaneous Information on Writing your BPlan

- Business plans should be long enough to effectively tell your story. This will most likely be between 20 and 30 pages plus appendices. Longer Bplans tend to have too many details that potential investors are unlikely to want to read about here (although they are likely to want to ask you about such details). Also, the longer a business plan, the easier it is to repeat information. When repetition is appropriate, at least change the verbiage.

Tables and Graphics:

- Never pass up an opportunity to insert some great visuals such as models and tables. They are a welcome sight to most readers and can easily be worth more than a thousand words!
- Overall, pie charts have their place; tables are almost always beneficial; on average, bar charts are the least helpful.

Grammar and Miscellaneous Details

- Most investors very quickly notice grammar and spelling errors. This presents an image of incompetence and sloppiness. Consider asking other skilled individuals unfamiliar with a Bplan to read it.
- Use active voice in your writing.
- Develop structure and hierarchy to your plan. Use first, second, and possibly third order headings with frequency.
- Intersperse into your written presentation a series of bullet statements, tables, and models wherever possible. Try to have some variation from the typical narrative on every page. Double space between paragraphs.
- Use endnotes to reference your source information.
- Font type should be something common like Times Roman style and probably 12 point.
- Margins are to be at least 1 inch.

TABLE 22.2 Product Matrix for a New Physician Office Rapid Diagnostic Test

	New Diagnostic	Rapid Strep Test	Conventional Laboratory
Source of diagnosis	Saliva	Throat swab	Blood work
Wait time	10 to 15 minutes	10 to 15 minutes	2 to 3 days
Cost to produce	$18	$2	None
Price sold to doctors	$45	$3	Outsourced
Insurance reimbursement to doctors	$85	$17	Labs reimbursed

TABLE 22.3 Competitor Matrix for New TeleMedicine Dermatology Service

	TeleMedicine Dermatology	Conventional Dermatologist	DermLink MD	Spot Exam
Years in industry	Start-up	Decades	5 years	3 years
Service medium	Mobile	Face-to-face	Internet	Mobile
Actual consultation	Yes	Yes	Yes	No
Consultation timeframe	24 hours	Average 6 weeks	48 hours	24 hours
Consultation type	Acne only	Varies	Follow-up	Mole categorization
Price	$59	$78 to $139	$99	$4.99

The suggested outline above includes the multiple sections that go into making up a plan and it has been tried and tested many times. However, there are several things, such as the nature of the business, that can alter the outline. For example, if a venture is working on a new drug application with long FDA approvals to obtain, developing an extensive marketing program would not be appropriate. Consequently, flexibility is important but the completeness of the outline presented is to help the writer understand all the components that prospective stakeholders are often used to seeing and may inquire about.

PRESENTING THE WRITTEN BUSINESS PLAN

Having worked through the building of the content of your business plan, we need to explicitly address the presentation aspects of the plan—first the written presentation followed by a section on oral presentations. With the context of today's entrepreneur and investor, expectations can be quite varied. If one was pursuing a new start-up 20 years ago and needed funding, there were venture capitalists on the equity side and banks on the loan side. These are two very distinct types of financing, and the two rarely, if ever, compete for the same investments. We knew very little about business angels back then other than that they existed in the woodwork of communities. Today we still have venture capitalists and business angels, but each group seems to be becoming more diverse. The venture capital market seems to be emerging with a limited number of very strong players and many smaller players focused on various niches. In the business angel market, there are those who are still largely hidden in the woodwork of communities. However, there are also numerous groups of angel networks, and for example, may have monthly meetings to hear pitches and to pool their investments. Much more recently, we have crowdfunding emerging as a funding source for smaller amounts of capital for start-up ventures.

Along with the diversity of the today's investment community comes significant variation in the way that investors get their information delivered. The traditional way is the written business plan which is the ticket that gets you through the door to discuss your concept with a venture capitalist. The written business plan was the first screen, and entrepreneurs could rarely get to first base with a venture capitalist unless they cleared the hurdle with a quality concept and written plan that generated further intrigue and interest. With today's investment community, such preferences still exist but the expectations are much more diverse. Some prospective investors now want to read an executive summary or slide deck first; others want to hear a shorter oral pitch and then seek to engage a written plan if they are interested in moving their interest to a deeper level. In short, investor expectations vary widely. Entrepreneurs must be ready to jump in and provide prospective investors whatever they request or need. We will now address some of the modes and types of presentations, first written and then oral.

Types of Written Business Plans

Unless specified otherwise, when someone refers to or asks for a written business plan, they are usually referring to the *standard business plan* that typically consist of 20 to 30 pages, making up the main document plus appendices. Such written plans generally are able to offer enough depth that the reader can get familiar with the venture concept and how it is approaching the commercialization process. If the main part of the business plan exceeds 30 pages, most readers will become bogged down and lose interest. For internal planning purposes, some entrepreneurs will continue to expand the business plan and use it as an internal working document. Such documents are referred to here as the *internal business plan* and can reach 60 to 100 pages in length.

Shorter business plans are also used with some frequency in the marketplace. We address two here. The *dehydrated business plan* usually runs from 5 to 10 pages and, as the name suggests, it is a scaled-down version of the standard plan. Essentially, such a document covers the key points of the business plan by bringing particular attention to those issues that represent the heart of the business concept. Even with the dehydrated business plan, remember that you are telling a story of the origins of the business concept; why the founder(s) is the right individual to take this concept forward and the projected path of the venture's development. Such features are attractive in luring prospective stakeholders to the venture.

The final written form addressed here is the *executive summary*. It is the business plan in miniature and is usually 1 to 2 pages in length; sometimes as a stand-alone document it can run to 3 pages. The executive summary sets the tone by seeking to capture the pertinent points of the whole plan in a brief synopsis. Stated differently, the executive summary should be an honest and captivating overview that sells the highlights of your vision and objectives for the venture capitalist to garner further interest. The goal is to entice the reader to come seeking additional information. Remember that with both of these shorter versions the point is to use these as a means to invite the reader to something more, such as the standard business plan or engaging the entrepreneur directly.

Readability and Physical Layout

Most entrepreneurs want prospective investors to read the standard business plan if they have one. However, if readability problems with the business plan exist, prospective investors are likely to abandon the read and move away from further inquiry. Far too often a failure to read is because the business plan is put together in a way that makes it a challenging read. I strongly suggest that the business plan be put together in a way that can accommodate a 10-, 30-, or 60-minute plus read. Specifically, I suggest the following:

- Use the company name, logo, and mantra to help tell your venture story. These are similar tools that help a reader more quickly comprehend your business concept. Can someone get a good idea of what your venture is about by just looking at the name, logo, and mantra?
- Make the section titles talk. If everything was deleted except for the name, logo, mantra, and section titles, how

much could they tell you about the venture? Would they by themselves invite further inquiry?

- Structure the sections using multi-level headings. Take main headings like industry examination, market examination, competitive advantage, etc., and beneath them use subheadings. This helps the reader greatly by communicating the structure and overall direction of the business plan and what is being addressed.
- Leave a reasonable amount of "white" space on each page. The norm is single spaced text with one blank line between paragraphs.
- Each page should look different. Try not to have pages with just straight text in traditional paragraphs. A possible means of breaking up a page includes bullet statement subsections, tables and charts, and meaningful pictures that help tell your story. Meaningful charts and tables can be worth thousands of words; they can also help condense the length of the plan. Most readers would rather read a great summary table than 2 to 3 pages of typed detail. Your reader will appreciate you for it.
- Beware of repetition! With a document that encompasses as much material as a business plan does with multiple cross-linkages, it is easy to repeat oneself. Where it is appropriate to discuss something that has been discussed earlier, say it differently. Also, get someone with fresh eyes to read your business plan and help with things like this.
- Eliminate all grammatical errors. Like it or not, with just a few grammatical errors, most readers start making inferences about the capabilities of the person writing the plan. It is always a good practice to get someone with good writing and grammar skills to make the necessary corrections.

Accommodating Different "Reads"

As mentioned earlier, potential stakeholders have multiple preferences for how they like to become familiar with a new business concept (executive summary, dehydrated or standard business plans, slide decks, oral presentations, etc.). Now let's assume we have a group of potential stakeholders, all of whom have chosen the standard business plan to first become familiar with the business concept. There will be a very significant variance in the time and approach they take to reading it. As the author of your business plan, you need to be aware of these different reads. Some will read the executive summary and then leaf through the rest of the plan in a matter of a few minutes. At the other extreme will be those who give it a very solid read taking 60 to 90 minutes. In between there are those who will read little more than the section headings, bulleted statements and tables, and then perhaps supplement it with reading the sections they consider to be their most important section(s). To make things harder, most readers have their unique preferences about what they consider to be the most important sections! As a writer of your business

plan, it serves you well to keep the reading style of these various readers in mind and seek to write the plan in a way that accommodates multiple types of reads.

ORALLY COMMUNICATING YOUR BUSINESS PLAN

While the focus of this chapter is primarily on the written business plan, they usually go hand-in-hand with the oral presentation. While there are numerous materials dedicated to making effective oral presentations that are certainly worthy of further study, I will address a few central perspectives specific to business plans to keep in mind for the oral presentation.

Oral Presentation Length and Content

Just as prospective stakeholders have varying preferences on the length of the written business plan, they also have a specific length of time for the oral presentation. Some situations will call for a 1-minute presentation; another will call for a 5-minute presentation; yet another may allow 15 or even as long as 20 minutes. Again, nothing is set in concrete and rarely does the entrepreneur get to choose. So you have to be ready to adapt. This brings up the central point of any oral presentation: The goal is to give your audience a meaningful snapshot of your venture and how it addresses an important customer pain, key advantages you have moving forward, and what is in it for prospective investors. Entrepreneurs should *not* try to communicate everything they know about their concept, even if it is a longer presentation (like 20 minutes). Instead, with energy and passion, deliver the most important points that accurately reflect the venture. Think about it in terms of saying enough to bait some interesting questions that will lead to deeper interactions. More in-depth communications commonly come during the question and answer time and particularly within one-on-one conversations.

Preparing slides for a presentation is also very important. First, here are the four most common complaints that I hear about for business plan presentations.

1. The business concept is NOT understood.
2. Too technology-focused.
3. Too much industry and technology jargon.
4. No clear story; the flow is lost.

With these failures far too common in the presentation of business concepts, let me make the following suggestions:

1. Get the story right.
2. Bring solid energy and confidence to the presentation.
3. Always remember what is in it for your audience.

4. Plan for approximately one slide about every 45 seconds.
5. Use simple pictures and models where possible. Use variation from slide to slide.
6. No more than 15 to 20 words per slide.
7. Font size, no less than 28 point.
8. Use contrast—usually dark text on a light background.
9. Be well-dressed and neat.

Elevator Pitch

The elevator pitch is the most important part of the oral presentation. First, never assume that you have your audience's attention. If you miss them with your elevator pitch, in all likelihood, they are gone for the entire presentation. Second, develop a pitch that gets to the heart of the customer pain and the product that you deliver. Here are six different mechanisms around which elevator pitches can be developed:

1. Question—directed straight at the audience to get them involved.
2. A factoid—a striking or little known fact.
3. A physical object or demonstration.
4. An anecdote—a quick human interest story.
5. A quotation—an endorsement from a notable figure.
6. An analogy—a striking comparison.

CONCLUSION

A business plan is a wonderful tool that facilitates the communication process regarding the projected direction of the new venture and what it plans to accomplish. Business plans are written with the intent of helping to inform prospective investors and other stakeholders of the opportunities that lie ahead for the proposed venture and how it plans to achieve attractive outcomes. Business plans also serve as a valuable tool for helping the entrepreneurs to carve out a strategic plan and to better think through how all the different pieces of this business puzzle fit together in the venture going forward. The better the strategy of a venture is understood by the entrepreneurs in the context of competition and emerging technologies, the more prepared they will be in leading the venture onward towards a successful outcome.

Biotechnology Product Development

Therapeutic Drug Development and Human Clinical Trials

Donald R. Kirsch, PhD

Chief Scientific Officer, Cambria Pharmaceuticals, Cambridge, Massachusetts

The 1950s can be considered to be the start of the modern drug discovery era. Although a number of effective medicines were available for clinical use at the end of World War II, most of these were traditional medicines that had been discovered long ago and the vast majority of the medicines that had been discovered in the nineteenth and the first half of the twentieth centuries were basically found by pure chance. Only two medicines discovered during the late nineteenth and first half of the twentieth centuries could be said to have resulted from a pure directed effort to find a new therapy: the discoveries of arsphenamine (Salvarsan) by Ehrlich, the first effective treatment for syphilis [1], and streptomycin by Waksman, the first effective treatment for tuberculosis [2]. In both of these cases the inventors set out with the specific goal to find a new treatment for a specific disease and were successful.

Each of these directed discoveries provided invaluable discovery strategies that were adopted by the drug development industry. The lesson from streptomycin was that although substances with medicinal properties are very rare, medicines, or chemical compounds that could be modified and then turned into medicines, could be found through methodical screening approaches. The lesson from Salvarsan was that a drug could be created through the application of biological assays to guide chemical analog synthesis efforts to identify compounds with therapeutic value.

SMALL MOLECULE DRUGS

Small molecule drugs are either synthetic chemicals or chemical metabolites produced by plants or microorganisms. (In some cases these metabolites need to be chemically modified to produce a clinically effective therapeutic.) Synthetic chemicals are custom designed to be drugs, or in rare cases, chemicals that turn out to have drug properties by accident. The clinical utility of naturally occurring small molecule drugs is probably almost certainly due to chance since these compounds are not made by the plant or microorganism with the intended purpose of being drugs. In other words, the foxglove plant does not synthesize digitalis in order to treat heart failure. Rather, these naturally occurring metabolites are exploited by humans and repurposed for therapeutic use.

The contemporary approach to small molecule drug discovery was born out of, and is an amalgam of, the above century old research strategies. There is now a strong general consensus regarding the standard steps and phases of the drug discovery process (Figure 23.1) [3,4]. However, there is no standardized method for drug discovery and every novel drug is discovered in its own unique way. The consensus steps presented below should be taken simply as a broad experience-based, general guide to the drug discovery process.

Small Molecule Target Identification and Validation

The ultimate success or failure of any drug discovery project is fundamentally dependent upon the correct selection of the drug target for the chosen disease. As will be discussed in greater detail below, the drug discovery project will fail if the selected target is not in a pathway driving the underlying basis of the disease, or if the selected target affects other metabolic processes in the body that negatively affects viability (side-effects). The methods currently available to identify and validate effective drug targets are limited and imprecise as is the knowledge of the underlying molecular etiology of many important diseases. These shortcomings are a major factor driving the high failure rate in drug discovery. However, patients need medicines, and biopharmaceutical companies need new products, and therefore the drug discovery enterprise carries on.

Perhaps the single most important guiding concept in contemporary pharmacology is Paul Ehrlich's receptor theory which states that all drugs work by binding to a specific

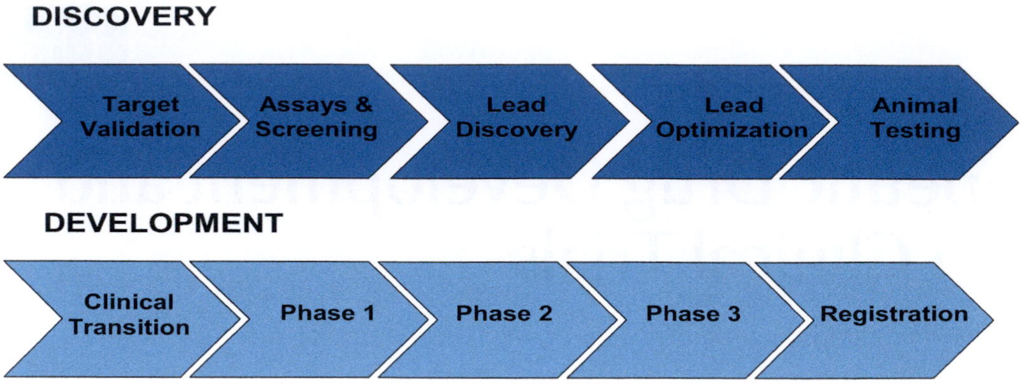

DISCOVERY

DEVELOPMENT

FIGURE 23.1 Drug discovery (therapeutic discovery and preclinical testing) and development (human clinical testing). Standard phases of drug discovery and development. Development processes, encompass the preclinical and clinical studies whose results will be used in regulatory submissions (to the FDA in the United States).

chemical component or receptor within the cell and that drugs act by modifying the activity of the receptor. Receptors are most commonly: (1) Enzymes which are proteins that speed up reactions within the organism; (2) Cellular switches that are actually called receptors because in many cases they were identified as drug targets before their biological cellular functions became known; and (3) Signaling pathway elements that act downstream from receptors (see Figure 23.2). While traditional drugs were discovered through serendipity, the field has changed so that instead of finding a drug by good fortune and then determining how it acts, receptor targets are now selected based on fundamental scientific principles and drugs are then sought that will act on the chosen receptor target.

All diseases have an underlying cause or molecular mechanism that produces the disease called the disease molecular etiology. This idea can probably be most easily understood for infectious diseases, for instance, the molecular etiology for tuberculosis is infection by the pathogenic bacterium *Mycobacterium tuberculosis*. The bacterium produces damage to the body and leads to the symptoms of the disease. Eliminate the bacterial pathogen and you cure the disease (of course you still need to identify a molecular target within the bacterium that will kill the bacteria without harming the patient). Other disease classes can be similarly understood. Heart disease can be caused by arrhythmia, a condition in which the natural heart beat or rhythm is disturbed, leading to a weakening of the action of the heart. The rhythm of the heartbeat is produced through the interaction of a number of receptors and ion channels (cell membrane proteins that allow inorganic ions such as sodium, potassium, or calcium to enter or leave the cell) within the heart. Drugs that act on these controllers of the heart rhythm can restore the heartbeat back to normal. Similarly, high-serum cholesterol can lead to heart disease, so drugs that block the synthesis of cholesterol within the body lower cholesterol levels and thus lower the probability of heart disease.

Since everything that follows depends on the correct selection of the target, much effort is put into providing confidence that the target has been correctly chosen. This is the process called target validation. Target validation is unfortunately far from a precise endeavor. One overarching problem is that for many diseases the underlying molecular etiology is not known with precision and, not surprisingly, these are the diseases for which new therapies are most desperately needed. The strategies used to validate hypotheses regarding disease etiology are far from definitive because of their inability to precisely model the disease in question (Figure 23.3). For such diseases there commonly are a set of competing unproven hypotheses regarding what causes the disease. While the drug developer could initiate a basic research program to identify with certainty the cause of the disease, this is a long and drawn out process with an uncertain outcome. Therefore, drug developers will most commonly make a highly educated guess as to which of the competing hypotheses is correct, knowing that successful development of a drug will be one means to provide confirmation of the underlying hypothesis.

As an example, many scientists working on Alzheimer's disease think that Alzheimer's could best be treated by targeting a protein called beta-amyloid protein [5]. Others think the best strategy would be to target a different protein called tau [6]. Perhaps one group is correct and the other wrong. Maybe they are both right and the disease is caused by multiple protein dysfunctions or that some cases of the disease are caused by the dysfunction of beta-amyloid protein and other cases are caused by the dysfunction of tau. Another possibility is that both groups are wrong and these protein dysfunctions are actually a result of the disease and that the actual cause is something upstream from beta-amyloid and tau. However, patients and their families (not to mention pharmaceutical corporate management) do not want to wait to find out. They want scientists to work on the development of a treatment despite the risk of failure. Thus the drug developer moves forward while research groups

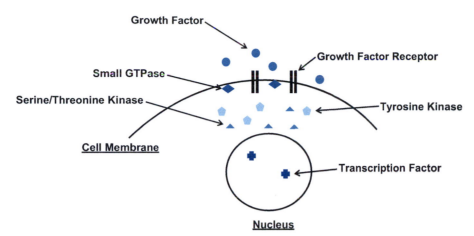

FIGURE 23.2 Drug targeting example. Growth factors are produced by specialized cells to induce the growth and division of target cells, acting through growth factor receptors present on the surface of the cell and spanning the cell membrane. These growth factor receptors, in response to the presence of growth factors, transfer the growth signal into the interior of the cell. The interior of the cell has a variety of components mediating cell growth and division including, in this example, a number of classic enzymes—tyrosine kinases, serine/threonine kinases, and small GTPases. When activated by signaling cascades, transcription factors enter the cell nucleus where they bind to specific DNA sequences and regulate genes that control cell growth and cell division.

Gene Knockout ≠ Inhibited Protein

Cell Culture ≠ Mouse

Disease Model ≠ Disease

Mouse ≠ Human

Human ≠ Human

FIGURE 23.3 Five sources of error that can produce discordance between studies to validate a drug target and the effects of a drug acting on that target in a clinical trial. See the text for details.

are competing with each other working on beta-amyloid or tau, depending on their best guess.

Once a disease etiology is selected, one still needs to select a drug target to counter the suspected cause of the disease. If you think that beta-amyloid causes Alzheimer's disease, you next have to come up with an approach to block the destructive actions of beta-amyloid and have good underlying evidence supporting the validity of the approach. Such evidence is commonly accumulated from multiple sources and approaches. One strategy is to start with an existing biochemical reagent that acts on the target in a nonselective fashion and test the reagent in a way that subtracts out the *nonspecific* actions of the chemical to try to predict the activity of a *selective* drug. However, often such reagents do not exist.

Another approach is to utilize standard molecular biology techniques. These techniques make it possible to up- or down-modulate a potential protein drug target in cells via reagents that up- or down-regulate or even knockout (eliminate) the gene that encodes it. The premise is that simply making more of the protein mimics a drug that stimulates the activity of the protein and making less of the protein mimics a drug that inhibits the activity of the protein.

A confounding issue is that many proteins have scaffolding functions in addition to their primary activity as a receptor or enzyme. Proteins commonly appear in complexes with multiple other proteins. Changing the level of a protein can have effects on all the proteins in the complex. Drugs however only affect the enzyme or receptor activity while molecular biology techniques affect both the enzyme or receptor activity and any scaffolding activity.

Additional limitations include the fact that testing in cells (*in vitro*) only approximates a portion of what goes on in an intact animal (*in vivo*). Alternately, one can use molecular biology techniques to produce gene knockouts or knockins in laboratory mice. This is where the gene encoding the target of interest can be disrupted (knockout) in the genome of a laboratory mouse, or a hyperactive version of the gene can be added (knockin) into a mouse genome. Characterization of the resulting mouse strain will reveal a number of important things about the target. For one, if the target has an essential function, the resulting knockout mouse strain will be dead or have some clear biological defect. Thus the drug developer will be warned away from inhibiting a target that could produce toxic consequences. The knockout/knockin can also be introduced into a mouse disease model to determine whether the genetic modification modifies the course of the disease. Finding that such a genetic change modifies the disease is highly encouraging, although not conclusive because a medicine is given only after the disease is diagnosed. In contrast, the gene knockout or knockin is present from the moment of conception and certainly precedes the onset of disease symptoms in the animal model. Therefore one might be validating a target that could only work if the drug was given prior to disease onset, something which is unlikely to happen clinically.

Target Identification and Validation—Areas of Uncertainty

Disease animal models are most commonly used to evaluate the effects of a potential therapeutic. However disease animal models are imperfect representations of the actual disease because mice are not people and there are biochemical, metabolic, and genetic differences between species. This is a particular concern for diseases of the elderly. For instance, current life expectancy at birth in the United States is approximately 78 years. Mice in contrast can live about a year in the wild and about 2 to 3 years in a highly protected laboratory environment. Since many diseases of the elderly are thought to be at least in part the result of long-term subtle toxic environmental exposures, mice arguably do not make a good model for such diseases. Even patients with a specific disease are not identical. As a result, patients do not respond in the same way even to well-established drugs. Clinical studies have shown that 10 to 30 percent of patients will not respond to a selected antihypertensive ACE inhibitor, 15 to 25 percent of heart failure patients will not respond to a selected beta blocker, 20 to 50 percent of patients will not respond to a specific SSRI antidepressant, etc. Thus, even for well-established therapies the physician will often empirically try different members of a drug class on their patient until they find one that works for them.

Given these limitations, on average only 30 percent of target validation projects are successful, meaning that the tested target appears to provide benefit in treating the disease. A target identification and validation study would typically take a year and cost $500,000 to $1 million to complete in an industrial laboratory (see Figure 23.4). If the target is not validated, this is a sunk cost and the research team proceeds to test the next candidate target. However, an even worse outcome is the incorrect validation of the drug target. In this case, work goes forward with mounting costs for a project that is ultimately doomed to failure. (Study costs, timing, and success rates in this and all succeeding sections were established by combining information taken from the following references: Brown and Superti-Furgam [7]; Drews [8]; Koppal [9]; Nwaka and Ridley [3]; and Reichert [10].)

Assay Development and High Throughput Screening

Once a therapeutic target is validated, the next step is to identify chemical compounds that act on the target in the desired way. This requires a screening assay, a biological or biochemical test that can clearly distinguish between active compounds that produce the desired effect, and inactive compounds that do not interact with the target. The screening assay must have the following characteristics:

1. The assay must be relatively inexpensive since a few hundred thousand compounds are commonly tested in a

Drug Discovery Phases and Metrics

Exploratory		
	Target Validation	Assays & Screening
Activity	Target ID, characterization	Assay development, HTS implementation
Duration	6-12 months	6-12 months
Success Rate	30%	65%
FTE/cost	1-2 FTE	2-3 FTE

Hit-to-Lead		
	Lead Discovery	Lead Optimization
Activity	Counterscreens, confirm hits, test analogs	SAR, *in vivo* testing, exploratory ADME, 2 series; 1 lead each
Duration	12-15 months	12-24 months
Success Rate	65%	55%
FTE/cost	3-5 FTE	8-12 FTE

Preclinical Studies		
	Animal Testing	Preclinical Transition
Activity	In vivo efficacy, animal ADMET	Process chemistry, scale up, formulation, GLP ADMET, IND
Duration	12 months	12 months
Success Rate		55%
FTE/cost	~$500,000	~$5.0 million

FIGURE 23.4 A summary of drug discovery phases with associated costs, staffing, durations, and historical success rates. See text for additional details and references.

typical screening campaign. (See below for a discussion of the selection of compounds for screening.) If each assay, fully loaded for reagents, labor, laboratory automation, and overhead, costs 10 cents per assay, expenses for the screening campaign alone will be about $20,000 not counting expenditures for assay design and validation. As a general rule of thumb, the per assay cost needs to be under $1 so that the screening campaign will cost no more than $200,000 to $300,000.

2. The assay must also be highly sensitive. At this point in the project the investigator is looking for a chemical lead, not a finished drug. One must expect that the crude chemical lead will have low potency that will be improved by subsequent chemical synthesis. Only a sensitive assay can detect such crude, weak leads.

3. The assay must be selective for the activity of interest. All biological assays are subject to artifacts and identify compounds that are not real hits. If such artifacts are both rare and anticipated ahead of time they can be easily weeded out through subsequent experimentation. If, however, they are common and confused with real hits the entire enterprise will fail.

Assay Development and High-Throughput Screening—Screen Implementation

Screening can commence once the assay is designed and validated. The question at this point is what samples and how many of them to screen. Because chemical optimization of a lead compound is a long and expensive process, it makes sense to start with a good lead that will hopefully limit the number of chemical iterations needed to produce the clinical lead compound. The assembly of chemical files for screening is a much-debated process. In the mid-1990s chemists at Ciba-Geigy, now part of Novartis, calculated the number of possible drug-type compounds that could in theory exist, estimating that there are 3×10^{62} such compounds [11].

Such a large number cannot be handled in practice. Therefore only a tiny subset of all possible compounds will actually be screened. During the 1990s a "more is better" philosophy took hold. Each of the established large pharmaceutical companies had a screening collection of around 50,000 to 200,000 compounds that had been prepared through their chemical synthesis efforts during the first 150 or so years of their existence. These collections came into being because it was standard practice to retain an aliquot for future screening every time a compound was synthesized at these companies. The 1990s was an era of intense mergers and acquisitions within the biopharmaceutical industry, and as a result many companies were in possession of the combined screening collections from multiple predecessors. American Home Products (later renamed Wyeth) had the chemical collections of Wyeth, Ayerst, Cyanamid/Lederle, and AH Robbins. SmithKline Beecham had collections from Beecham, Smith Kline, and the French, Richard and Company. Glaxo Welcome had the combined collections of Glaxo Laboratories and Burroughs Wellcome. Pharmacia had the combined historical collections of Searle, Upjohn, and Pharmacia. Bristol-Myers Squibb had the combined collections of Bristol-Myers and Squibb. Thus many hundreds of thousands of compounds became available for screening.

To address this perceived limitation, a number of combinatorial chemistry start-up companies were established during the same period. The goal of these companies was to make small-size samples of a large number of different chemical compounds for screening. The companies exploited laboratory robots and simple chemical reactions that could be performed with a wide range of starting materials in a combinatorial fashion. For example, a reaction of ten starting compounds of type "A" with ten starting compounds of type "B" in all possible combinations could rapidly yield 100 new compounds for screening. Such companies quickly built up collections of 100,000 or more new compounds for screening.

Unfortunately, the results from the "more is better" approach did not meet expectations. All companies came to roughly the same conclusion following their analysis of the output from multiple screening campaigns:

1. The types of compounds from the combinatorial chemistry companies were constrained by the necessity to run simple reactions in a massively parallel fashion. As a result of this constraint, the output compounds were most often not drug-like, did not result in good screening hits and was not worth the effort involved to screen the collections.

2. A subset of compounds from both the historical libraries and combinatorial collections were found to be active in a wide variety of assays. These compounds were named "frequent hitters" and their performance was inconsistent with the expectation that screening hits would selectively hit targets like a key fitting into a lock. After extensive follow-up research it was determined that such frequent hitter compounds were artifacts and produced activity because of chemical properties that would not make them useful drugs.

3. Other compounds were consistently inactive over an extremely wide range of targets suggesting that they lacked drug-like properties and were probably not worth screening.

4. Many active compounds were dropped following chemistry review because they lacked good opportunities for further chemical modifications.

This raised the question that if there was no opportunity for follow-up, why were these compounds being screened in the first place? The above observations led to a rationalization of the compounds being screened. Today screening campaigns are typically conducted using smaller rationally assembled chemical libraries, and a campaign including 50,000 to 200,000 rationally selected compounds is generally considered to be a reasonable test of a good volume of chemical space.

Assay development, validation, and implementation typically in aggregate takes about a year and costs $1 million or more in a large biopharmaceutical company. The overall success rate for this research phase is about 65 percent (see Figure 23.4). Failures principally come in two areas. First, it can be maddeningly difficult to develop assays for some biological processes, especially when the assay needs to meet the difficult combined criteria of low cost, robustness, ease and speed of operation, high selectivity, and freedom from artifact. Some screening assays are never successfully completed. Second, for reasons that are not completely understood, not all targets are equally "druggable," a term meaning that the target activity can be modified by the action of a drug or drug-like chemical. The only way to know with some confidence that your target is druggable is to test a compound file and see whether any bona fide actives are recovered. There have been many instances when I designed a screen, tested several hundred thousand of compounds, and found no active compounds.

Lead Discovery

Hopefully, at the end of the screening campaign the drug developer has a hit list—all the compounds that were active in the screen along with their chemical structures. What should a reasonable hit list look like? The first question is "what is the hit rate?" It is the percent of the tested compounds that showed activity. If one is looking for a treatment for an incurable disease, I think it is reasonable to expect that compounds with therapeutic potential will be rare, few, and far between. I have seen cases where investigators report that a few percent of the tested compounds are active. I think this is unreasonable. If such potential treatments were so common—a few per hundred random compounds—it stands to reason that they would have been found previously through pure serendipity and the disease would have been cured.

I believe that most screeners would say that a reasonable hit rate would be no higher than 0.1 percent. I find that a hit rate of 0.01 percent is very workable, producing about 20 actives from a screen of 200,000 samples. These actives are then characterized biologically and chemically to produce leads for the chemical optimization process. Artifacts are removed in so far as possible via biological secondary assays and the potency and efficacy of the true hits are determined. Potency indicates how low a concentration of a compound is needed to produce the desired effect, and efficacy means how strong a biological response can ultimately be produced by the compound. In general, it is best to focus work on high potency and efficacy actives since these compounds provide a starting point that is closer to the ultimately desired drug.

Chemical analysis will demonstrate whether similar chemical types are recovered repeatedly or whether all the actives are chemically unrelated. Finding similar compounds repeatedly is generally a good sign that the screen ran well since it would be reasonable to expect that certain chemical structural types will be best able to hit the target of interest. Chemical compounds that are structurally related to the actives are then purchased and tested to crudely identify which chemical features are needed to produce activity. It is a bad sign if the hit compound is active but all related compounds are inactive. This result suggests that it will be very difficult to find chemical analogs with improved activity. Similarly, it is a bad sign if virtually all analogs are active. Drugs fit into their site of action like a key into a lock. As a result, some analogs should work and others should be inactive. If everything works, it suggests that the hit is working indiscriminately, possibly because of its chemical reactive properties rather than because of its selective action on a target.

All the above information is used to select two to three actives as leads for further work. In many cases the biologists' favorite hits will be different from the chemists' favorite hits. This is because each group looks at the results through the lens of their own scientific discipline and training. Biologists look at the actives for high potency, efficacy and activity in a variety of relevant biological assays

coupled with validation in multiple models with appropriate selectivity and low toxicity. Chemists look at the actives for chemical novelty, drug-like character, ease of chemical synthesis, and opportunities to chemically elaborate the active compound. In addition, chemical intuition is important. The very best medicinal chemists who have repeatedly discovered useful drugs will have intuitive feelings regarding which actives can eventually turn into drugs. Such feelings cannot be rationally described, but they are important and will contribute to project success. The bottom line is that biologists and chemists have different, *but equally valid* perspectives on the drug-discovery process. Successful projects incorporate the perspectives from both disciplines.

Lead discovery typically takes over a year, at this point employing expanded staff and at an average cost of over $1.5 to $2 million. The success rate is on average 65 percent (see Figure 23.4). Failure is typically caused by poor leads or in some cases no leads. Poor leads have weak biological activity suggesting that it will require extreme effort to bring the lead to a point where it will have clinically relevant activity. Poor leads can also be chemically intractable with difficult multistep syntheses and poor potential for analog design. A decision to move forward commits to a lead optimization stage with significantly increased expenses and a longer timeframe.

Lead Optimization

Once a lead is selected the next step in the process is optimization. With a preliminary knowledge established regarding which chemical features are needed to carry the desired biological activity, it is common to now refer to the lead as a "scaffold." The concept is that while the basic form of the drug has been identified, this basic form, or scaffold, will now be decorated with chemical substituents to produce the final drug molecule. Analogs are made and then tested in multiple biological systems—initially in the test tube and later in cells and laboratory animals. Obviously, analogs will be tested for improved potency and efficacy against the target because highly potent and efficacious compounds can be dosed at low levels reducing the potential for side-effects. Testing is also conducted for selectivity to insure that the compound acts on the target of interest and not on similar proteins. Commonly, assays for the most closely related enzymes or receptors are established and run as counterscreens looking for inactivity or low potency.

However, drugs must act in the body of a living organism and not just in a test tube (*in vitro*). In traditional drug discoveries, compounds were tested in animals at the very earliest phases of the project. Thus, there would be early assurance that not only did the compound hit the target of interest, but that it was also pharmacologically well-behaved in animals. In current practice however, evaluation in animals is deferred until much later stages of development—arguably a major weakness of the current drug-discovery model.

In fact, in recent times some drug developers have continued to believe that postponing animal testing was completely wrong-headed. Probably the most famous of these critics was Dr. Paul Janssen, founder of Janssen Pharmaceuticals. Dr. Janssen's record of productivity speaks for itself [12,13]. Janssen and the scientists at Janssen Pharmaceuticals discovered more than 80 new medicines and four of Janssen's medicines are on the World Health Organization list of essential medicines—an absolute world record. Prior to his retirement, Janssen Pharmaceuticals was screening well over 10,000 chemical compounds annually directly in a group of animal-based assays.

The current discovery model defers animal testing largely because *in vitro* testing is less expensive, quicker, and higher throughput. However, it is recognized that it will not be effective to simply optimize compounds for effects on the target because issues of whether the drug will work in a living organism are crucial for the ultimate success of the project.

There are five types of pharmacological properties that characterize how a drug behaves in the body. This set of pharmacological properties is referred to as the drug's ADMET, an acronym standing for Absorption, Distribution, Metabolism, Elimination, and Toxicity. *In vitro*, test tube-based assays, are available to roughly measure each of these properties and such assays are currently employed during the lead optimization at early stages in place of animal testing [14,15].

Drug Absorption and Distribution

Oral activity is desired for most drugs since patients prefer taking a pill to an injection, suppository, or other alternate means of administration. Oral activity requires that the drug is able to survive the acidic environment of the stomach and that it can be absorbed from the digestive tract. Digestive-tract absorption is modeled using a system based on Caco-2 cells, cells derived from the lining of the digestive tract. Compounds that pass a monolayer will commonly, but not always, absorbed through the digestive tract.

Once in the body, various drugs will distribute differently, and where the drug goes is a crucial determinant of efficacy. For example, any drug that works on a neurological disease must enter the brain. However, there is an obstacle called the blood-brain barrier that keeps most compounds out of the brain. This barrier is believed to have evolved so that pharmacologically active substances in the foods we eat will be unable to enter our brains after a meal and disrupt neurological processes. The barrier is very effective although imperfect. For example, caffeine, present in many beverages, is able to enter the brain and disrupt sleep. The existence of this barrier is an important issue for drug

developers and much work has gone into the development of test tube models for the blood-brain barrier. Similarly, much work has also gone into producing drugs with appropriate brain distribution profiles.

As an example, histamine receptors in cells of the nasopharynx control the release of cellular metabolites that produce allergy symptoms—stuffiness and runny noses. Antihistamines block these receptors and produce good relief for allergy sufferers, but with one major problem—histamine receptors are also in the brain and antihistamines interact with these receptors causing drowsiness (sleepiness). The earliest antihistamines, for example diphenhydramine (Benadryl), penetrate well into the brain and cause sleepiness as a major undesired side-effect. Diphenhydramine in addition to being effective in relieving allergy symptoms is unfortunately a potent sedative and, although it was originally developed to treat allergy symptoms, it is now commonly used in over-the-counter sleep agents like Tylenol PM. In this case, pharmacologists wanted to block the brain penetration of the antihistamines to produce a superior nonsedating side-effect-free allergy pill. Terfenadine (Seldane) was an early antihistamine compound that was unable to enter the brain and was marketed as the first nonsedating allergy medication [16]. However, the structural changes that blocked brain penetration also enabled the drug to block an ion channel in the heart called the hERG channel. This effect was first discovered only after the drug was on the market and used in a larger population of people. Blocking the hERG channel can produce a heart arrhythmia called QT interval prolongation which in some cases causes a potentially fatal heart arrhythmia called "Torsades de pointes." The FDA later banned the drug and required its removal from the market. Subsequent drug development goals became more complex: to block the histamine receptor, to block brain penetration, and to not block the hERG channel. Further work led to the development of loratadine (Claritin), which is currently available as a safe, nonsedating allergy medication, advertised as "Claritin clear" because it leaves you nonsedated and clear-headed [17].

Drug Metabolism

The next property that needs to be considered in lead optimization is metabolism. There are well-established test tube-based assays to measure metabolism. Most drugs are metabolized (broken down) by liver enzymes called cytochromes P450. The liver eliminates toxic compounds in the diet and this activity allows us to safely eat many things that would otherwise be poisonous. However, these liver enzymes become a problem if they break down useful medicines too quickly. You can begin to understand how susceptible a drug is to these liver enzymes by examining the dosing information on the label. A drug that must be taken four times a day is most likely broken down quickly by these enzymes while a once-a-day medicine is probably broken down much more slowly. Patients prefer once-a-day dosing, but that can be difficult to achieve while maintaining a variety of other beneficial properties in a medicine. If it were easy, of course all drugs would be dosed once-a-day.

As an extreme example of a drug metabolism issue, cardiac patients will take a tiny pill by placing it under his or her tongue. The drug in this example is nitroglycerin, which is given to treat angina pectoris, pain in the chest that results because of insufficient blood flow through blood vessels within the heart. Nitroglycerin dilates or expands these vessels allowing more blood to flow through and thus relieves the pain. But, why not just swallow the pill instead of sticking it under your tongue? Nitroglycerin is very rapidly broken down by liver enzymes. Materials absorbed from the stomach go directly to the liver and nitroglycerin that is absorbed from the stomach is destroyed immediately and never makes it to the heart. In contrast, drugs placed under the tongue rapidly diffuse through the mucous membranes in the mouth, enter capillaries and the venous circulation, and can then go directly to the heart without first entering the liver and be metabolized. Thus nitroglycerin is effective when placed under the tongue but is ineffective when swallowed [18].

In current practice, chemists prepare analogs of the lead compound and each lead is tested for activity against the target; potency and efficacy and, using the above described *in vitro* assays, for desirable pharmacological properties; oral absorption, distribution to the diseased tissue/organs, and resistance to rapid metabolism. The overall goal is to synthesize at least one compound that can be moved forward into clinical trials. This stage of research employs a greatly expanded staff of about 8 to 12 scientists working in all disciplines. The greatest staff expansion is in the area of chemistry, with typically 4 to 8 chemists synthesizing compounds full-time. On average, and depending on the number of synthetic steps involved and the difficulty of the chemistry, each chemist can synthesize about two custom compounds per week. The synthesis of 1500 or more custom compounds would typically be needed to produce a clinical candidate and thus would take about 2 years with a cost on the order of $4 to $8 million. Historically the success rate for lead optimization has been about 55 percent (see Figure 23.4).

Clinical Candidate Compound Selection and Characterization in Animal Disease Models

The selection of a clinical candidate compound is not an exact science. Therapeutic products are not designed to meet a certain specification; rather they just need to incorporate a combination of properties that allows them to be both safe and effective. A truck will be designed to carry a certain load, carry a certain number of people, or pull a trailer of a certain weight. A computer will be designed to have a certain amount of memory or to operate specific software programs. In contrast, there is really no clear design specification for a new first-in-class medicine. The new medicine should treat the target disease, but beyond that it is not a matter of hitting a design specification but rather to provide some measurable clinical benefit for patients without burdensome side-effects. The exact nature of that benefit is not predesigned but determined in practice. In other words, the exact benefit is not known or predicted with any confidence going into the clinical trials, but rather is defined as a result of the clinical trials.

An almost imponderable question at any particular point is whether additional chemical synthesis will yield a superior compound or whether it is the right point to halt chemical efforts and move into the clinic. This is a question for hot debate among members of the project team. There is always the possibility that the next compound made will be superior to what is in hand. When do you stop? Commercial issues must be addressed as part of this debate. For instance, drugs need to be patent-protected, enabling companies to maintain exclusivity in the market for a period of time to insure profitability. The patent life clock begins to tick once patents are filed. Expanding development time in analog synthesis decreases profits by compressing the time on the market prior to the introduction of the generic version of the drug. Alternatively, delaying patent filing could provide the opportunity for a competitor to beat you to the patent office. There are also tactical issues. The research team typically is dissolved once the clinical candidate is called. What if a problem is identified during the next step, the clinical transition studies? Who will address the problem if the team has been disbanded and the members are off on a new set of projects? In many companies this last problem is often addressed by having the team identify a backup compound in addition to the clinical candidate, which will be in hand should the clinical candidate stumble.

Lastly, since costs will escalate at the next steps in the process, the team will carefully characterize the clinical candidate in multiple animal disease models before deciding to move it on into clinical transition studies. You want to be as sure as possible that your molecule merits the resources that will be needed for clinical testing. The strategic goal is if you are going to fail, and most projects do, fail as soon as possible before too much time and too many resources are wasted on a project that will not go forward. A failure at late stage is a disaster for all involved and is to be avoided whenever possible. Research teams therefore constantly try to design and implement what are commonly called killer experiments—studies that would provide a yes/no answer on whether to move the project forward.

LARGE MOLECULE DRUGS

Target Identification and Validation

Large molecule drugs are in a separate category from small molecule drugs, which include inorganic and organic polymers (such as proteins) and biochemicals (such as polysaccharides, nucleic acids, and proteins). Large molecule drugs are most commonly proteins already present in humans and animals that have evolved to carry out a specific function. That exact same function is utilized in the desired therapeutic application of the protein. So, while the small molecule drug developer looks outside the body for his or her drug, the large molecule drug developer looks within the body. Once a protein of interest is identified and its therapeutic activity validated, the goal is to manufacture it in quantity for therapeutic use, sometimes with, but commonly without, modification. Large molecule drugs largely fall into four categories: (1) hormones and other replacement proteins, (2) cytokines (signaling molecules employed by the immune system), (3) vaccines, and (4) antibodies.

Hormones

Insulin is the founding member of the large molecule hormone drug group, used to treat type 1 diabetics who are unable to synthesize insulin. Historically, it was extremely fortunate that insulin from animals, specifically cows and pigs, worked well in humans. Pancreas from these species was available in quantity from slaughterhouses to serve as source material for the preparation of therapeutic insulin. In more recent times true human insulin, made by recombinant DNA methods, is instead given to diabetic patients. Other commonly used replacement therapies include recombinant factor VIII (Recombinate, Kogenate) and factor IX (Benefix), both used to treat hemophiliacs who as the result of genetic mutations are unable to make these proteins and erythropoietin, a hormone that stimulates the production and survival of blood cells. Patients with end-stage renal disease produce little erythropoietin and must be given the hormone as a replacement therapy. Also, patients undergoing cancer chemotherapy commonly become anemic and such patients can better tolerate their chemotherapy when treated with erythropoietin. Relative to small molecule drugs, target identification and validation for these replacement-type proteins is much more straightforward. If it is clear that a missing protein is causing the disease, it obviously makes sense to treat the disease by replacing the protein [19,20].

Cytokines

Cytokines are employed therapeutically mainly because of their ability to modulate the immune system. The modulation could be "stimulating" to treat an infection, or "inhibitory" to treat autoimmune diseases in which the patient's own immune system is inappropriately attacking their body. Examples include human interferon alpha, used to treat hepatitis B and C (viral infections); human interferon beta, used to treat multiple sclerosis (an autoimmune disease); and modified interleukin-II to treat thrombocytopenia (another autoimmune disease). In terms of target identification and validation, when a disease course is known to be driven by the activity of the immune system, the therapeutic goal is to pair a known modifier of the immune system activity with the disease of interest, which is almost always determined via animal model testing [19,20].

Vaccines

Humans have two immune systems—innate immunity and adaptive immunity. The innate immune system defends the host from infections by pathogens in a nonspecific manner. This innate system recognizes pathogens in a generic way, sensing biochemical features of the pathogen that differ from the host. This immune system responds by producing generally toxic substances and as a result will harm the host as well as the pathogen. The innate system is ancient and ubiquitous and appears across the biosphere in plants and insects as well as in animals. The toxic effect of the innate system response is particularly easy to see in plants, where it is common to see an entire limb of a fungus-infected plant wither and die. The innate system sacrifices the limb to save the plant. This evolutionarily ancient defense strategy is the only immune system found in most organisms including plants, fungi, insects, primitive multicellular organisms, and some vertebrate animals. A second system, called adaptive immunity, is believed to have first appeared in jawed vertebrates (vertebrate species without a jaw such as the lamprey eel). Adaptive immunity provides jawed vertebrates with the ability to specifically recognize and remember each pathogen, generating a selective antibody response to a pathogen that can be rapidly mounted later in time if the pathogen is encountered again. The system is adaptive because although the organism is naïve to the first attack and responds slowly and weakly, a rapid robust response will be mounted to subsequent attacks by the same pathogen. Also, because the response is selective, collateral damage to the host is minimized. Vaccination is basically a method to prime the adaptive immune system to prepare it for attack by a pathogen that had never previously been encountered.

The traditional vaccine strategy is to prepare a pathogen in an inactivated form, one that is unable to produce the disease, and to then introduce the inactivated pathogen into the patient. Inactivation can be produced via chemical treatment (the Salk polio vaccine is a classic example) or via the isolation of a mutant form of the pathogen that has attenuated virulence (the Sabin live polio vaccine is a good example of an attenuated vaccine). However with the advent of gene cloning it has been possible to produce protein subunit vaccines. Subunit vaccines are made by producing viral pathogen surface proteins via recombinant DNA techniques and then utilizing the resulting proteins as a vaccine. An example of a protein subunit vaccine is the Hepatitis B virus in which viral surface proteins are produced by recombinant methods in yeast and then employed to formulate the vaccine protein [19,20].

Therapeutic Antibodies

Antibodies are the primary effector agents of the adaptive immune system. The adaptive immune system is activated by a pathogen and, after a lag, begins to make new antibodies directed against the structural proteins from which the pathogen is constructed. These antibodies physically bind to the pathogen. Antibodies are also very selective. They will bind to the proteins of a specific pathogen and commonly, not to a closely related pathogen. Importantly, antibodies normally do not bind to proteins which are part of the host's own cells. Once bound, the antibodies direct destructive components of the immune system to eliminate the pathogen, and once the disease resolves, memory cells are retained within the immune system to rapidly make this group of antibodies if, and when, the same pathogen strikes again. This is the underlying mechanism by which vaccines work.

The immune system has extremely broad capabilities. It is estimated that humans are capable of generating about 10 billion different antibodies, each able to bind to a distinct feature of a foreign protein. Thousands of new antibodies are produced when a pathogen infects an organism. This made it impossible to purify a specific antibody from this mixture for close study and as a result only the most general antibody characteristics were known. Prior to 1975, the only system through which large quantities of pure antibody could be obtained was from a rare cancer called multiple myeloma. In multiple myeloma, a single antibody-producing cell becomes cancerous and proliferates in the bone marrow. As the cancer grows it secretes huge quantities of the single specific antibody made by the cell. In many cases, so much antibody is produced that it spills out into the urine of the patient. In the mid-nineteenth century, urine-secreted proteins in this disease were called Bence-Jones proteins by physicians who were not yet aware of the nature of the spilled material. As a result, the entire field had to depend on these rare freaks of nature for their investigations. Most limiting was the fact that since multiple myeloma cancers occur at random, there is no way to know what the antibody produced in the disease binds to. As a result, if one has the key but not the lock into which it fits: not a good situation through which to figure out how antibodies work or, for that matter, to turn them into therapeutics. This situation dramatically changed in the late twentieth century through the work of Georges Köhler and César Milstein. Milstein developed a technique called the monoclonal antibody method through which pure individual antibodies directed against any protein of interest could be produced in quantity and studied in detail. Köhler and Milstein were awarded the Nobel Prize for Physiology or Medicine in 1984 for this work [21].

Scientists began to think about therapeutic applications for antibodies once it became technically possible to produce quantities of specific antibodies with a desired set of selected characteristics. Like any new idea, this concept was initially met with some negativity within the industry. Since antibodies are proteins, they would thus have to be administered via injection and possibly multiple times a day, a distinct disadvantage relative to traditional small molecule orally active drugs. Secondly, antibodies are extremely costly to produce when compared with traditional small molecule drugs, potentially reducing profits. Thirdly, manufacturing plants that produce therapeutic proteins are expensive to build and thus require substantial capital investment, another discouraging feature of the approach.

However, with time, the industry began to appreciate the positive features of therapeutic antibodies. Antibodies are hard to make, but they are also hard to copy, discouraging generic manufacturers from taking the market after patent expiration. It could also be possible to enter therapeutic areas where no pharmaceutical options existed and thus where no competing oral alternative was available. Lastly, antibodies can be very long lived in the body. For example, antibodies of the IgG class have *in vivo* half lives in the 7- to 23-day range and thus while antibody dosing is via injection, the injections can be infrequent, on the order of once a week, making the medicine more convenient and desirable to the patient.

With protein hormones and cytokines the objective is to replace or augment a naturally occurring protein. In contrast, antibodies are developed to inhibit and diminish the activity of a naturally occurring protein. While it can be clear when an important protein is missing and needs to be replaced, for example in the case of insulin, determining the therapeutic value of inhibiting a protein is much less straightforward. In a sense, this type of target identification closely resembles the target identification for small molecule drugs. As for small molecules, a candidate target is identified based on the scientific literature. The target is validated in cell culture and animals though the use of gene knockout methodology or some preliminarily-generated antibodies. If the idea proves out, work commences to identify the clinical candidate antibody [22].

Structure Optimization and Identification of a Clinical Candidate

Structure optimization follows two distinct courses for large molecule drugs. In the case of hormones and cytokines, where the goal is to replace or augment a naturally occurring protein, the objective is to precisely mimic and administer the natural protein. Therefore no optimization is required. In contrast, therapeutic antibody development strategically resembles small molecule discovery in that a number of desired features must be built into the clinical candidate antibody. The first goal is to find an antibody that binds the target with high efficacy and selectivity. This starting antibody will commonly be a mouse antibody as a consequence of the monoclonal antibody technology employed to identify the antibody of interest. One cannot develop treatments based on mouse antibodies because the patient will recognize the mouse antibody as a foreign protein and mount an immunological attack against it. This problem is overcome by "humanizing" the antibody, basically converting the mouse antibody into the human equivalent. More recently, methods have been developed that make it possible to start with a human rather than a mouse antibody. The next step is to consider the efficacy of the antibody—its ability to block the target. Binding to the target is determined by the Fab (fragment, antigen-binding) region of the antibody—the portion that binds to the antigen. In some cases, however, efficacy is determined by the Fc region (fragment, constant; the nonbinding portion) of the antibody and variants of this region are made and tested to optimize efficacy. Lastly, the half-life of the antibody will determine how frequently it needs to be administered, and structural variants are made and tested to optimize the half-life and thus optimize the dosing schedule.

Similar to small molecule drugs, making a change in an antibody that beneficially changes one characteristic can concomitantly affect other features negatively. Thus the final clinical candidate molecule can end up being a compromise of the desired target features. Lastly, antibodies are made in cells, not factories. Thus, a major consideration in selecting the clinical candidate is the development of a cellular production system that can be employed to make the antibody in an economically viable process for eventual commercialization.

CLINICAL TRANSITION STUDIES—INVESTIGATIONAL NEW DRUG APPROVAL

The goal of clinical transition studies is to demonstrate the safety of the drug before it is first dosed in humans. From this step forward, every experiment and study that is carried out will be reviewed by regulatory authorities (in the United States, by the Food and Drug Administration [FDA]). Review of drugs by the FDA is a relatively recent development. The law regulating the safety of new drugs, the Food, Drug and Cosmetic Act of 1938, established the functioning of the FDA as we now know it. Most every country has their own regulatory agency that reviews and approves human therapeutics, and many of their requirements for approval are similar.

The FDA currently has over 9000 employees and an annual budget of over $1.25 billion. The FDA Center for Drug Evaluation and Research (CDER) oversees the research, development, manufacture, and marketing of synthetic small molecule drugs. Since 2003, CDER has also been responsible for the regulation of biologic therapeutic products. CDER's involvement starts with the Phase 1 clinical study via their approval of a manufacturer's Investigational New Drug Application (IND). The IND application consists of the results from a highly defined set of studies designed to demonstrate the safety of new pharmaceutical agents and the consistency of the manufacturing process through which they will be produced. The core set of experiments conducted to support the submission of an IND dossier is commonly called the clinical transition studies.

A battery of specific studies is required to be included in the IND application. Although all scientists are trained to carry out experiments in a carefully designed and executed fashion and to record their observations with high precision, studies intended for submission to a regulatory agency are in addition subject to a system of management controls called Good Laboratory Practice (GLP). GLP was instituted as a standard meant to ensure the quality, integrity, and reliability of safety data following cases of safety and efficacy testing fraud by pharmaceutical and industrial manufacturers. Good Manufacturing Practice (GMP) is a similar parallel system for studies of manufacturing processes and analytical testing of active ingredients.

Regulatory authorities have established a set of requirements that drugs need to meet prior to entering clinical use, but have avoided providing a defined checklist of experiments, instead issuing general guidance notes for the required studies. Despite this, the required studies can easily be described via a checklist (for example, see below) [19,20].

Acute toxicity—The drug is administered to a laboratory animal, usually a rodent, in increasing doses and the animal is observed for toxic effects following each dose. The dose range is large; from very low doses to the highest well-tolerated level called the "no toxic effect level" and beyond to higher doses that produce obvious toxicity. At the end of the experiment the animals are sacrificed and autopsied to search for any effects the drug may have had on the internal organs.

Test for QT interval prolongation—It is well known that some pharmaceutical targets (human biochemical or metabolic functions) can be very difficult to inhibit while others are easier to inhibit, and some targets are so susceptible that they are sometimes unintentionally inhibited by drugs designed to act elsewhere. One of these easy-to-hit targets is the cardiac hERG channel, an ion channel involved in regulating the rhythmic action of the heart. Inhibition of the hERG channel causes prolongation of QT interval in the heart rhythm which can lead to a potentially fatal heart arrhythmia called Torsades de pointes. Drugs from many different therapeutic classes, including several tricyclic antidepressants, antipsychotic drugs (thioridazine and droperidol), antihistamines (astemizole and terfenadine), and certain antimalarial drugs (halofantrine), will inhibit the hERG channel. hERG-channel inhibition therefore needs to be measured by what is by now standard *in vitro* testing prior to the initiation of clinical trials [23].

Genotoxicity—Cancer is caused by gene mutations which can either be inherited or produced during the course of life by exposure to certain viruses, radiation, or mutagenic chemicals. It is therefore crucial to avoid producing drugs that have any mutagenic activity, as such drugs could be carcinogenic. Bruce Ames, one of the scientists responsible for our current understanding of the mutagenic nature of carcinogenesis, developed a straightforward bacterial-based test, named the Ames Test in his honor, to detect mutagenic activity and thus carcinogenic potential in a chemical compound. The FDA requires Ames testing as part of the IND application as well as related tests based on rodent cells for chromosomal abnormalities and chromosomal damage [24].

Chronic toxicology—The acute toxicity study described above looks for immediate damage produced by a drug. There are also concerns that toxicity can occur, even with low doses of a drug, when the drug is dosed repeatedly over time. This concern is addressed by chronic toxicology studies. Three or more drug doses are administered over a period of time: a dose known to be toxic from the acute toxicity study, a therapeutic dose, and an intermediary dose. This test is carried out using two species: a rodent, usually rats, and a nonrodent, usually dogs although monkeys and pigs are used in certain circumstances. The duration of the chronic toxicity trial must match the intended clinical use. A 2-week trial is adequate for a compound like an antibiotic that will only be given for a few days. Studies of 6 months of more in duration are required for drugs that will be given chronically, such as high blood pressure medications. Such studies can obviously be extraordinarily expensive because they are conducted over a long period of time, require a large number of animals (100 rats and 20 dogs would be typical for a long-term study), plus the chronic dosing consumes large amounts of drug test article which must be prepared in a costly fashion to meet FDA standards.

Costs are high to manufacture drug substance used in studies for a FDA submission because they must be prepared under GMP guidelines. The synthetic process must be clearly defined and described in detail and followed precisely from batch to batch. Analytical procedures must be developed and validated to insure quality control of the manufactured drug. The purity of the test article must be determined and any impurities present must be defined, characterized, and consistent from batch to batch. Also drugs are not just given straight up, but are dosed in a formulation that optimizes the delivery of the drug. The formulation must be optimized and defined at this point and remain set for all further studies. Studies for the IND regulatory submission are carried out in specialized GLP/GMP laboratories operated with close regulatory oversight.

While the cost for a minimal clinical transition study could be as low as $1-2 million, it would be prudent to budget at least $5 million for a clinical transition study on a specific compound. Costs can be significantly higher if long-term chronic studies are needed or if tests need to be modified and repeated. Historically the success rate for projects going through clinical transition is about 55 percent. It is clearly very hard to design a drug that is both effective and extremely safe (see Figure 23.4).

CLINICAL TRIALS

Phase 1

Clinical investigations of a new drug candidate start with a group of studies commonly called Phase 1 testing. A series of ethical considerations are involved in the design of all clinical studies since human subjects could potentially be put at risk:

1. **Social value**—The contemplated study should bring value to society, for example, by improving human health or advancing scientific knowledge.
2. **Scientific validity**—The clinical trial should be conducted in a scientifically rigorous way and with clear objectives so that the resulting data can be interpreted in a meaningful fashion.
3. **Fair subject selection**—The subjects for the trial should be selected based on pure scientific criteria and not because they are privileged or vulnerable.
4. **Informed consent**—The subjects should be well informed about the trial and consent to participate without coercion.
5. **Favorable risk/benefit ratio**—The risk/benefit ratio for the trial should be analyzed and must be favorable for the study to be conducted.
6. **Independent review**—An independent, disinterested group of qualified individuals must review the proposed trial to identify any possible conflict of interest issues.
7. **Respect for human subjects**—As the trial goes on, subjects must be informed without prejudice of any new developments, negative or positive, and any resulting decisions made by the subjects must be honored.

Phase 1 trials involve healthy volunteers, not patients, with the primary aim to assess the safety of the new drug and these volunteers are financially compensated for their participation in a manner consistent with the above ethical

Drug Development Phases and Metrics

	Phase 1	Phase 2	Phase 3	Registration
	1a/1b	2a/2b		
Activity	First in man, safety, tolerability, PK	Dose range, safety/efficacy profile, proof of concept	Large safety efficacy trial	
Size	20-80 subjects	300 patients	1000-3000 patients	
Duration	6 months	12-24 months	24-48 months	
Success Rate	70%	50%	65%	95%
Cost	$8000/subject	$10,000/patient	$6,000/patient	

FIGURE 23.5 Summary of drug development phases with associated costs, durations, and historical success rates. See text for additional details and references.

considerations. The Phase 1 study will also produce data on the pharmacokinetics of the drug (absorption, distribution, metabolism, and elimination) and its pharmacodynamic properties (biochemical and physiological effects on the body). These studies are conducted under what is called an "open label" format—everyone is aware of what drugs and doses are being given. There are commonly two components to the Phase 1 trial. First a rising dose study in which increasingly higher doses of the drug are administered to determine how much drug can be given without producing deleterious effects. This is followed by a multidose study in which one or more selected doses is administered repeatedly over time to determine the long-term effects of the drug. Such studies commonly involve 20 to 80 subjects and take about 6 months to complete. The cost for such a study is $3 million or more with an overall historical success rate of 70 percent (see Figure 23.5).

This high success rate of Phase 1 studies is a tribute to the effectiveness of clinical transition testing in demonstrating the safety of a drug which is then, in the majority of cases, confirmed in human testing. Even when safety is not confirmed, there is little chance for harm because of the slow and cautious design of the initial human tests. However, like anything in life mistakes do occur: *Errare humanum est*— to err is human. TGN1412 was a therapeutic antibody-type drug developed by TeGenero Immuno Therapeutics as a potential treatment for B cell chronic lymphocytic leukemia (B-CLL) and rheumatoid arthritis. Phase 1 clinical studies of TGN1412 were initiated in March 2006, conducted by Parexel, an independent clinical trials unit at Northwick Park and St. Mark's Hospital in London. Six volunteers were treated with the drug at a dose of 0.1 milligrams per kilogram, 500 times lower than the dose shown to be safe in animals. All six subjects became extremely ill shortly after treatment and were hospitalized, with at least four of the men suffering from multiple organ dysfunction. All of the men were reported to have experienced cytokine-release

syndrome resulting in angiodema, a rapid swelling of the skin and underlying tissue. Treating physicians said the men had suffered from a cytokine storm and that the men's white blood cells had almost completely vanished. It has been suggested that the men may never recover fully and suffer long-term disruption to their immune systems [25].

The reason why TGN1412 was safe in animals and yet highly toxic in humans may never be determined. In a preliminary report the Medicines and Healthcare Products Regulatory Agency (MHRA), the group that oversees clinical trials in the UK, found no deficiencies in TeGenero's preclinical work, no failure of disclosure, record keeping, or processes, and stated that TeGenero's actions did not contribute to the serious adverse events. TeGenero Immuno Therapeutics has, however, entered into insolvency as a result of these events.

Phase 2

The aim of Phase 2 clinical trials is to test the safety and, in a preliminary fashion, the effectiveness, of a therapeutic candidate compound in patients with the targeted disease. Phase 2 design most commonly includes a control group that is not given the drug and instead receives a placebo. In many illnesses, especially those in which the measurement of disease severity is difficult to quantify, the placebo can show substantial effects. For example, it is clear from many trials in clinical depression that simply entering into a trial and being repeatedly seen and counseled by a physician will produce significant therapeutic effects. These effects must be subtracted out to determine whether the test drug shows efficacy in its own right. Patients are carefully randomized into the control and drug groups to insure that average disease severity is the same in the two groups. If, for example, healthier patients were mistakenly placed in the drug group the study might lead to the false conclusion that an inactive drug was effective. A related common practice is to blind the trial, that is not to inform patients as to whether they are receiving the drug or placebo. In many cases the physician may also not be informed as to whether the test agent or placebo is being administered. This design is called a double-blinded trial. Data from the Phase 2 trial are used to select a dose regimen (amount, frequency, and duration) for expanded, and hopefully conclusive, studies in a larger group of patients in Phase 3.

Because Phase 2 trials have dual and sequential goals, they are commonly divided into two subtrials: Phase 2a and Phase 2b. Phase 2a concentrates on safety and dosing while Phase 2b is an extension of 2a with an increased focus on efficacy. The number of patients in a Phase 2 study can range from 50 to 500 and 1 to 2 years or more depending on the study design. A cost in the $3 to $4 million range would be typical for an academically led study, with industrial studies typically costing much, much more. The historical success rate for Phase 2 studies has been on the order of 50 percent (see Figure 23.5).

Phase 3

The goal of the Phase 3 trial is to unambiguously show whether or not a new compound is effective in treating the target disease. These trials are termed pivotal in the industry because they will make or break the success of the drug. The design of the Phase 3 trial combines scientific and financial considerations. If a drug is highly effective, only a relatively small number of patients may be needed to show a statistically significant positive effect. For example, if every patient who does not take the drug quickly dies and every patient taking the drug survives you do not have to be a professional statistician to conclude that only a small number of patients will be needed to produce a convincing data set. However, a larger number of patients will be needed if the effect of the drug is small. For example, patients with amyotrophic lateral sclerosis (ALS or Lou Gehrig's disease) typically live 3 to 5 years postdiagnosis. Riluzole (Rilutek), the only drug clinically approved for the treatment of ALS, extends life on average by 2 to 3 months. The Phase 3 study to register riluzole included more than 1200 patients who were treated for almost 2 years, a study size which was needed to convincingly demonstrate in a statistically significant fashion that the drug produced this small positive effect [26].

While from a scientific perspective it is critical to insure that the Phase 3 study is adequately powered, financial considerations will influence the design of the trial toward the minimum size that effectively meets the desired goal. A consideration that is intimately tied to statistical power is how drug effectiveness will be determined, commonly called "outcome measures." As in Phase 2 trials, this is especially important in cases where there is subjectivity in assessing effectiveness. For example, in neuropsychiatric

diseases, effectiveness is determined by the patient's verbal disclosure of his or her symptoms and the simple act of including a patient in a trial can be therapeutic. A clinical effect that can be measured with a simple blood test, like cholesterol level, will obviously produce clearer and less subjective results. Variation in patient response to a drug is another confounding issue that impacts the power of a clinical trial. Even well-established FDA approved drugs can vary in their effectiveness in different patients. In extreme cases 70 percent of patients will not respond to a drug that is highly efficacious in 30 percent of patients. Since patient response cannot be predicted ahead of time (although new personalized medicine studies are attempting to address this), the size of the Phase 3 trial may have to be increased to provide statistically significant results in a patient population that includes large numbers of nonresponders.

The Pfizer drug torcetrapib is an excellent example of the intersection of science and finance in clinical trials [27]. Torcetrapib inhibits the enzyme cholesteryl ester transfer protein (CETP). Inhibition of CETP would be expected to raise levels of the so called "good" high-density lipoprotein cholesterol (HDL), which would make torcetrapib a highly desirable therapeutic agent for lowering the risk of cardiovascular disease. In 2004, Pfizer initiated their Phase 3 ILLUMINATE trial to demonstrate the clinical efficacy of torcetrapib. However, in December 2006, and after investing $800 million, Pfizer learned that torcetrapib actually *raised* the risk of death and cardiovascular disease and therefore development of torcetrapib was halted. What happened?

Early-stage clinical trials of torcetrapib showed that the drug elevated blood pressure in treated patients. Pfizer experts said that a modest effect on raising blood pressure would be of minor importance relative to the HDL-stimulating effect of the drug and argued that costly Phase 3 trials should be initiated. The Pfizer commercial group also contributed to the decision-making process as Pfizer was anticipating the expiration of the atorvastatin (Lipitor) patent in 2011 with the concomitant loss of greater than $10 billion per year in revenue. Torcetrapib seemed to be just what the doctor, in this case the accountant, ordered with a prediction of $10 billion in good year sales. It was estimated that FDA approval could be in hand by 2011 if the Phase 3 trial was started in 2004. We can now see the process was rushed for commercial reasons. Roche is now developing its own CETP inhibitor dalcetrapib and Merck has a similar compound called anacetrapib. Neither dalcetrapib nor anacetrapib raise blood pressure showing that torcetrapib's hypertensive activity was neither a class nor mechanistic effect of inhibiting CETP. Roche initiated a 15,600-patient trial with their compound in 2008 and Merck a 30,000-patient trial in 2011. It turns out that torcetrapib, but neither of the other two drugs, increases aldosterone levels, leading to elevated blood pressure. (Increasing aldosterone is definitely not a good thing; in fact, drugs such as spironolactone were developed to act as aldosterone-antagonist diuretics for use in the treatment of hypertension.) With the wisdom of hindsight, Pfizer should have invested more time up front to synthesize a torcetrapib analog lacking hypertensive activity. This course might have been taken in the absence of commercial pressures on the project; but commercial pressures are a fundamental reality in the pharmaceutical industry.

In general, and including issues such as trial design, defining outcome measures, identifying performance sites, and recruiting patients, Phase 3 trials can be 3 to 5 years in duration and cost $50 to $100 million or more. Historically, approximately 65 percent of Phase 3 trials have been successful (see Figure 23.5). A new drug application (NDA) is submitted to the FDA following the successful completion of the Phase 3 trial.

NDA Approval and Postlaunch Surveillance

In recent years the FDA has approved 15 to 20 drugs annually. This is a significant decline from the late 1990s when typically 30 new drugs were approved each year. This decline has occurred despite dramatic increases in research and development spending during this period. A recent paper proposed "Eroom's Law" (Moore's law spelled backwards), which states that the number of new drugs approved per billion U.S. dollars spent on R&D is halved roughly every 9 years, falling around 80-fold in inflation-adjusted terms since 1950 [28]. The reason(s) for the decline in research productivity are not known with certainty, but obviously raises great concern regarding the long-term prospects for the pharmaceutical industry. Fortunately, once a drug achieves statistically significant efficacy in treating a disease, the FDA will approve the drug for sale approximately 95 percent of the time.

Following NDA approval, the drug goes on sale and will then be used for the first time to treat extremely large numbers of patients. The manufacturer is required to collect safety data on the product while it is on the market and to periodically analyze these data to look for any indication of a safety issue that was not revealed in the Phase 3 trial. It is estimated that up to 20 percent of new drugs will be recalled from the market as a result of safety issues only identified after the drug is used to treat very large numbers of patients.

A classic example of such a recall is terfenadine, marketed by Hoechst Marion Roussel (now Aventis) under the trade name Seldane as the first nonsedating antihistamine. Terfenadine was approved for marketing in the United States in 1985. By 1990 it had been prescribed for over 100 million patients worldwide and it was becoming clear that terfenadine was causing cardiac toxicity in some patients as the result of hERG inhibition. While terfenadine is not overtly hERG-inhibiting at therapeutic doses, the drug will accumulate to high toxic levels if dosed in combination with other drugs such as erythromycin and ketoconazole, drugs that inhibit the cytochrome P450 enzyme CYP3A4 that metabolizes terfenadine. Even more concerning and more difficult to control, one of the ingredients of grapefruit juice also inhibits the same enzyme. In June 1990 the FDA issued a risk report on terfenidine and 2 months later required the manufacturer to send a letter to all physicians alerting them to the problem. A black box warning describing the problem was added to the package insert in July 1992. (A black box warning indicates that medical studies have shown that the drug carries a significant risk of serious or even life-threatening adverse effects and is the strongest caution that is issued by the FDA.) Terfenadine was removed from the United States market by the manufacturer in late 1997 [29].

Areas of Uncertainty

It is difficult to think of any first-in-class pharmaceutical that was discovered using exactly the path described above. And, no two first-in-class compounds have been discovered in exactly the same way. The process described above is an amalgam of good practices, but each discovery is unique, with each drug campaign diverging from the above path in various ways. Ivermectin (Mectizan) was discovered using an animal-disease model primary screen of a group of fewer than 100 test samples, and the initial screening active compound possessed almost ideal ADME properties [30]. Initial clinical testing of imipramine was in schizophrenic patients. When the drug failed, it was empirically dosed in patients suffering from major depression where it showed activity [31]. Lovastatin (Mevacor) was indentified following the screening of only a few hundred samples [32]. Only 60 analogs were made in chemical optimization of captopril (Capoten) [33]. The lead upon which the antibiotic aztreonam (Azactam) was based on was virtually devoid of antibacterial activity [34]. Ezetimibe (Zetia) came from a research program to identify cholesterol-lowering acetyl-coenzyme A acetyltransferase (ACAT) inhibitors. Ezetimibe, however, lacks ACAT inhibitory activity and instead inhibits the NPC1L1 cholesterol transporter [35]. Sildenafil (Viagra) was developed to treat hypertension and then angina. The drug came to be used as a treatment for erectile dysfunction only because of side-effects that were noted during a failed angina clinical trial [36].

Secondly, there is rarely, if ever, organizational consensus regarding the future clinical value of a therapeutic under development. It is never clear that a drug will truly be beneficial until the very end of the development process or perhaps even until the drug is introduced into clinical use. Figure 23.6 provides a list of highly successful compounds that were almost cancelled during the development process. The list contains many now-recognized blockbuster drugs including cimetidine (Tagamet), the first billion dollar a

- **Welcome**
  - Acyclovir (Zovirax)
  - Azidothymidine (Retrovir)
  - Bupropion (Wellbutrin)
- **Park Davis/Warner Lambert**
  - Gabapentin (Neurontin)
  - Atorvastatin (Lipitor)
  - Troglitazone (Rezulin)
  - Fosphenytoin (Cerebyx)
  - Pregabalin (Lyrica)
- **ICI Pharmaceuticals**
  - Propranolol (Inderal)
- **SmithKline Beecham**
  - Cimetidine (Tagamet)
- **Squibb**
  - Captopril (Capoten)
- **Merck**
  - Lovastatin (Mevacor)

FIGURE 23.6 Drugs almost cancelled during development.

year selling blockbuster drug, and atorvastatin (Lipitor), the best-selling drug of all time with annual sales of over $14 billion per year [37].

SUMMARY

There is no one "correct" way to discover a new drug. Instead, drug developers have a "tool kit" of strategies and methods they can choose from among which, when properly deployed and exploited, will on occasion lead to the discovery of a new medicine. What constitutes a valuable new clinical therapeutic is commonly recognized only in hindsight. Thus, there is neither a clear path to drug discovery nor a marker to show that you have gotten there. Not surprisingly, drug discovery is highly inefficient, with less than 2 percent of project compounds moving from conception to regulatory approval, and frighteningly expensive, with costs of over $1 billion commonly estimated for the discovery of a new drug.

REFERENCES

[1] Bosch F, Rosich L. Pharmacology 2008;82:171.
[2] Sakula A. Br J Dis Chest 1988;82:23.
[3] Nwaka S, Ridley RG. Nat Rev Drug Discov 2003;2:919.
[4] Federsel H. Nat Rev Drug Discov 2003;2:654.
[5] Tanzi RE, Bertram L. Cellule 2005;120:545.
[6] Gotz J. Brain Res Rev 2001;35:266.
[7] Brown D, Superti-Furgam G. DDT 2003;8:1067.
[8] Drews J. Science 2000;287:1960.
[9] Koppal T. Drug Discov Development 2004;7:24.
[10] Reichert JM. Nat Rev Drug Discov 2003;2:695.
[11] Bohacek RS, McMartin C, Guida WC. Med Res Rev 1996;16:3.
[12] Black J. J Med Chem 2005;48:1687.
[13] Stanley TH, Egan TD, Van Aken H. Anesth Analg 2008;106:451.
[14] Kerns EH, Di L. Curr Opin Chem Biol 2003;7:402.
[15] Di L, Kerns EH. Curr Top Med Chem 2002;2:87.
[16] Slater JW, Zechnich AD, Haxby DG. Drugs 1999;57:31.
[17] Brown AM. Cell Calcium 2004;35:543.
[18] Hardman JG, Limbird LE, Gilman AG, editors. Goodman and Gilman's Pharmacological Basis of Therapeutics. 10th ed. McGraw-Hill; 2001.
[19] Ng R. Drugs From Discovery to Approval. 2nd ed. Wiley-Blackwell; 2009.
[20] Rang HP, editor. Drug Discovery and Development—Technology in Transition. Elsevier; 2006.
[21] Nissim A, Chernajovsky Y. Handbook Exper Pharmacol 2008;181:3.
[22] Reichert JM, Rosebsweug CJ, Faden LB, Dewitz MC. Nat Biotechnol 2005;23:1073.
[23] Hammond TG, Pollard CE. Toxicol Appl Pharmacol 2005;207 (Suppl. 2):446.
[24] McCann J, Ames BN. PNAS Proc Nat Academy Sci 1976;73:950.
[25] Hansel TT, et al. Nat Rev Drug Discov 2010;9:325.
[26] Miller RG, Mitchell JD, Lton M, Moore DH. ALS Other Motor Neuron Disease 2003;4:191.
[27] News and Analysis. Nat Rev Drug Discov 2011;10:163.
[28] Scannell JW, Blackley A, Boldon H, Warrington B. Nat Rev Drug Discov 2012;11:191.
[29] Alfaro CL. Psychopharmacol Bull 2001;35:80.
[30] Omura S, Crump A. Nat Rev Microbiol 2004;2:984.
[31] Fangmann P, Assion H, Juckel G, Gonzalez CA, Lopez-Munoz F. J Clin Psychopharm J Psychopharmacol 2008;28:1.
[32] Vagelos PR. Science 1991;252:1080.
[33] Ondetti MA, Rubin B, Cushman DW. Science 1977;196:441 (1077).
[34] Sykes RB, Bonner DP, Bush K, Georgopapadakou NH, Wells JS. J Antimicro Bial Chemotherapy 1981;8(Suppl. E):1.
[35] Betters JL, Yu L. Clin Pharm Acol Therapeutics 2010;87:117.
[36] Ghofrani HA, Osterloh IH, Grimminger F. Nat Rev Drug Discov 2006;5:689.
[37] Cuatrecasas J. J Clin Invest 2006;116:2837.

Chapter 24

Development and Commercialization of *In Vitro* Diagnostics: Applications for Companion Diagnostics

John F. Beeler, PhD

Director, Theranostics and Business Development bioMerieux, Cambridge, Massachusetts

The field of clinical diagnostics plays an increasingly important role in today's medical evaluations, clinical decision-making, and disease management (Figure 24.1). Among the group of products offering applications to this field are the *in vivo* and *in vitro* diagnostic tests. *In vivo* diagnostics include those radiology imaging tests performed directly on a patient such as ultrasound scanning, magnetic resonance imaging (MRI), and positron emission tomography (PET). In contrast, *in vitro* diagnostics refer to those tests that process biological samples taken directly from the patient (i.e., salvia, blood, urine, feces, etc.) and are analyzed outside the body to detect and quantify the presence of a specific biological marker. These specific markers or analytes include pathogens, circulating proteins, and electrolytes, as well as genomic alterations including gene mutations, chromosomal copy number variations, and messenger RNA transcripts.

The external measurement of a specific biological marker from a clinical sample via an *in vitro* diagnostic assay can be achieved by one of two distinct forms of commercial products including the laboratory-developed test (LDT) or an *in vitro* diagnostic device (IVD). Both LDTs and IVDs are used to analyze human samples outside the body but have significant differences in how both these products are developed, regulated, and commercialized, each having their own specific advantages and disadvantages (Table 24.1). The differences in their development, regulatory, and commercial characteristics can have a profound impact on development timelines, market adoption, and commercial success. For example, LDTs, also known as "Homebrews," are *in vitro* diagnostic assays developed and validated by individual testing labs for use in that facility only and subject to regulations of the Clinical Laboratory Improvement Act (CLIA). In contrast, IVDs are developed by device manufacturers for global distribution and subject to review by regulatory authorities such as the Food and Drug Administration (FDA). More specifically, the Federal Code of Regulations [21CFR.809.3], defines *in vivo* diagnostic devices as "those reagents, instruments, and systems intended for use in diagnosis of disease or other conditions, including a determination of the state of health, in order to cure, mitigate, treat, or prevent disease or its sequelae. Such products are intended for use in the collection, preparation, and examination of specimens taken from the human body." [1] From a regulatory perspective, an IVD therefore refers collectively to the device or kit which is a composite of all the components of the assay including reagents, ancillary buffers, and software working together on a compatible platform or instrument. For the purposes of this article, the focus will be on development of IVDs as opposed to an LDT *in vitro* diagnostic product.

The test results an IVD delivers, provides vital information that assist healthcare providers determine a course of action. Although accounting for only 2 percent of overall healthcare spending, clinical diagnostic products can influence 70 percent of medical decisions, illustrating their dominant role in determining healthcare outcomes ranging from risk assessment to monitoring disease progression [2]. The utility of these diagnostic products to provide actionable information is evident by the more than 6.8 billion IVD tests performed each year from a menu representing over 4000 products available for clinical use [3]. IVDs encompass a diverse range of technologies including clinical chemistry panels, microbiology cultures, immunoassays, and molecular applications including polymerase chain reaction- (PCR) based assays and *in situ* hybridization (ISH) techniques. IVD products assess a wide range of analytes from measuring the concentration of vital electrolytes (i.e. sodium,

Diagnostic Application of IVDs

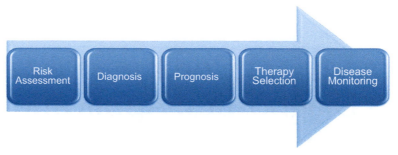

FIGURE 24.1   The application of *in vitro* diagnostics in the delivery of healthcare.

TABLE 24.1 Comparison of *In Vitro* Diagnostics (IVD) and Laboratory-Developed Tests (LDT)

Requirements	IVDs	LDTs
Marketing Authorization	FDA/Section 520 FD&C Act	CMS/CLIA Standards
Time to Develop	Long (12-24 months)	Short (4-6 months)
Subject to Quality Systems • Design Controls • Manufacturing Controls • Complaint Handling	Yes	No
Establish Clinical Validation prior to marketing	Yes	No
FDA guidance for use as a companion diagnostic	Yes	No
Global Reach/Distribution	Yes	No

potassium, magnesium, calcium, etc.) and other vital serum components (glucose, lipids, cholesterol) to detecting specific biomarkers such as procalcitonin (PCT), prostate-specific antigen (PSA), and troponin as well as specific genetic alterations such as mutations (BRAF, EGFR, KRAS), amplifications (HER2/neu), translocations (EML4-ALK), and polymorphisms (HLA-B*5701).

Together, these diagnostic products contribute to a global diagnostic market valued at approximately $45 billion and projected to grow at approximately 7 percent annually reaching a market size of $64.6 bilion in 2017 [4]. The fastest growing segment of the *in vitro* diagnostic market is the application of molecular diagnostics which is estimated to grow 12 percent annually through 2017. Much of the growth of molecular diagnostics to date can be attributed to infectious disease applications where testing for HIV resistance and identification of pathogens including hepatitis, cytomegalovirus, herpes respiratory syncytial virus, and human papilloma virus (HPV) dominate the market.

BRINGING IVD PRODUCTS TO MARKET

Traditionally, an assay is developed as an IVD only when the biomarker it detects has been well-characterized on the academic level, documented through a robust series of publications illustrating its clinical application, and demonstrating the need for a standardized and reproducible detection method [5].

The typical development process of an IVD assay, from its initial design through validation, is a lengthy and tedious process as illustrated in Figure 24.2. The development process of the IVD is focused on demonstrating that the assay's analytical performance reflects the capability of detecting the analyte in an accurate and reproducible manner as well as the clinical performance of the assay. Development timelines for IVD products are partially impacted by their inherent regulatory requirements and the need to fulfill data expectations. The regulatory requirements for the IVD are market-dependent and can vary substantially on where the product is to be registered.

In Europe, there is an absence of a formal regulatory review or approval process by a competent health authority for bringing an IVD product to market. Access to the European market is guided by the IVD Directive 98/79/CE (CE stands for Conformité Européene, or European Conformity) which currently stipulates self-certification for the diagnostic assay. Under this directive, the IVD manufacturer submits a technical file on the product along with information on their quality manufacturing (QM) system to a nationally accredited group. The accredited group performs an assessment of the IVD resulting in a conformity mark (CE mark) necessary for sales and distribution to the member states of the European Economic Area (EEA) and the European Free Trade Association. CE marking encompasses 32 member states including Switzerland and Turkey which has established mutual recognition agreements with the EEA. However it should be noted that the current IVD directive is under review and is anticipated to shift to a risk-based classification scheme that will dictate the new requirements needed to be established prior to an IVD coming to market

IVD Development

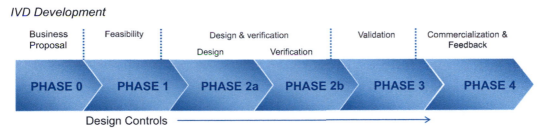

FIGURE 24.2   The *in vitro* diagnostic development process.

[6]. It is anticipated that the level of risk a device poses to a patient will determine the involvement of the notified body on the conformity assessment including requirements for QM systems and premarket review of the technical file.

In the United States, the FDA is responsible for administering regulatory oversight including premarket activities such as risk classification, review of marketing applications, as well as surveillance of IVD postmarket performance. Specifically, the Office of *In Vitro* Diagnostics and Radiological Health (OIR) within the Center for Devices and Radiological Health (CDRH) is responsible for administering the federal law pertaining to IVDs and assuring their safe and effective performance. The sponsor of the IVD to be marketed is required to submit a premarket submission to OIR and receive marketing authorization prior to commercializing the product. To facilitate development of IVD products, the CDRH periodically publishes guidance documents to address innovative approaches and the changing diagnostic landscape. Developers of IVDs are encouraged to check the CDHR's website for new guidance documents that may provide insights into relevant applications [7].

510(k) versus PMA

The FDA considers IVDs as medical devices subject to the premarket controls as defined in the Federal Food, Drug and Cosmetic (FD&C) Act and contained in the procedural regulations outlined in Title 21 Code of Federal Regulations Part 800-1200 (Table 24.2).

The level of control required to establish safe and effective use of the device is dictated by the FDA's risk-based classification system established for IVD products and categorizes IVD products as Class I, II, or III devices with Class III devices designated as high-risk devices (Figure 24.3). This classification system outlines the compliance requirements that will guide the development of the IVD product and whether the subsequent regulatory pathway will require a premarket notification (510(k)) or submission of a premarket approval (PMA) application for marketing authorization. The perceived level of risk is a reflection of the intended use of the IVD and there are examples where the FDA has approved assays detecting the same analyte under different regulatory pathways depending on how the assay was being employed. For example, the bioMerieux VIDAS

TABLE 24.2 Control Guidelines for *In Vitro* Diagnostics

General Controls	Special Controls
• Registering manufacturers and distributers	• Special labeling requirements
• Listing of device with the FDA	• Mandatory performance standards
• Manufacturing the device in accordance with Good Manufacturing Practices	• Postmarket surveillance
• Labeling devices in accordance with labeling regulations in 21 CFR Part 801 or 809	• FDA medical device specific guidance
• Submission of premarket notification [510(k)] prior to marketing device	**Special Controls For Class III Devices**
	• Full report demonstrating the device is safe and effective (ie clinical trial)

total PSA (TPSA) assay, which is indicated as an aid in the detection of prostate cancer, was approved by the FDA under the PMA pathway due to the perceived high level of risk to the patient for subsequent follow-up and treatment. In contrast, the NADiA® ProsVue™ PSA assay which is indicated for use as a prognostic marker in conjunction with clinical evaluation as an aid in identifying those patients at reduced risk for the recurrence of prostate cancer and monitoring the recurrence of prostate cancer is perceived as a lower level of risk to patients who had already been treated and therefore received clearance under the 510(k) pathway. The majority of IVDs reviewed by the FDA are cleared as 510(k) products. In 2012, the FDA approved 3,091 products under the 510(k) process while 39 products received original PMA approvals [8].

To facilitate a review of an IVD product, Congress passed the Food and Drug Administration Safety and Improvement Act (FDASIA) which provided the FDA with the authority to collect user fees on applications for medical devices which included IVD products. First enacted in 2002, the Medical Device User Fee Act (MDUFA) provides funding

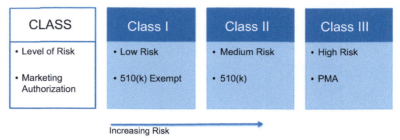

FIGURE 24.3 FDA *in vitro* diagnostic device classification.

to the FDA to support the staff of trained reviewers. The rates implemented for 2014 include a user fee of $258,520 for PMA applications and $5,170 for 510(k) notifications [9]. Reduced fees for small businesses are available.

The marketing application process for an IVD is intended to provide sufficient information verifying the product has been validated to ensure it is safe and effective for its intended use. In some cases, Class I products with low risk may be exempt from premarket submissions. For IVDs with low to moderate risk, the 510(k) submission process requires a sponsor to demonstrate that the product is substantially equivalent to a preexisting or predicate device already cleared by the FDA for the same intended use. Establishing substantial equivalence requires the submission of basic data requirements to provide the FDA with a reasonable assurance the product is safe and effective. In addition to demonstrating general controls are in place, the submission of preclinical data on the analytical performance of the assay illustrating accuracy, precision, limit of detection, linearity, and cross-reactivity is also required. While 510(k) filings do not generally require performing a clinical trial, the need to include clinical data varies on the assay being evaluated and its intended use. If the FDA determines substantial equivalence has been demonstrated to either a reference method (i.e. gold standard) or a predicate device for the same intended use, the IVD will be cleared for marketing. Other options available to the FDA include requesting additional information or determining the assay is not substantially equivalent (NSE). If the issuance of a NSE is the result of the lack of a predicate device, the sponsor has the option to seek approval of the device via a *de novo* 510(k) pathway or by submitting a PMA application. In 2010, the average time to clear a 510(k) device by the FDA was reported to be approximately 5 months (153 days) with approximately 73 percent of 510(k)s reviewed determined to be substantially equivalent and cleared for marketing.

IVDs designated as high-risk devices (i.e. Class III) are required to submit a PMA application to OIR. These include assays that are used to diagnose a life-threatening disease (i.e., PSA) and assays utilized as companion diagnostics and used to determine a course of treatment (THxID-BRAF). In contrast to a 510(k) application, a PMA filing does not seek to establish substantial equivalence to a preexisting product.

While a PMA application will include preclinical data on its analytical performance similar to that included for a 510(k) filing, PMA filings are required to include a more comprehensive demonstration of its safe and effective use. Therefore, a sponsor submitting a PMA application is required to perform a clinical trial and generate clinical data illustrating the test performs according to its intended use, using the designated samples (i.e., blood, tissue, sputum, urine etc....) from a defined patient population. The testing is required to be performed in a setting representative of where it is intended to be sold (i.e., clinical reference lab, physician lab office, etc.). Although prospective studies are encouraged, retrospective analysis of banked samples have been used to support an application's intended use (TheraScreen-KRAS). In addition to the submission of preclinical and clinical data, PMA applications are also required to include information on design control and manufacturing of the IVD product. Sponsors of PMA applications are subject to inspections prior to approval to assure adherence to Quality System Regulations (QSR) and implementation of Good Manufacturing Practices (GMP) to ensure IVDs are safe and effective. A key feature to mitigate regulatory risk is the availability to sponsors to engage feedback from the agency via the Pre-Investigational Device (pre-IDE) meeting. This mechanism allows sponsors to seek advice and clarification from the FDA on such matters pertaining to intended use of the assay, clinical protocol design, validation procedures, and other parameters required for approval. Although not binding on the FDA's part, pre-IDE meetings can provide valuable information and guidance on the FDA's expectations. In 2009, the average number of days between filing of a PMA application and receipt of the MDUFA decision (approval or nonapproval) was approximately 15 months (464 days) with approximately 68 percent of PMAs accepted for filing receiving regulatory approval.

SUCCESSFUL ADOPTION OF IVDS

In addition to obtaining the necessary regulatory clearance or approval to market an IVD product, there are several other market barriers that need to be addressed to drive a widespread adoption of an IVD and assure a product's commercial success. In addition to demonstrating robust and reproducible analytical performance, an assay must also demonstrate its validation in a clinical setting and confirm its intended use. While several of these requirements are generated to support regulatory authorization, other market barriers must be addressed postapproval. A key driver in the adoption of an IVD assay into routine clinical testing is demonstrating its clinical utility in which the assay must deliver clinically actionable data capable of influencing medical decisions [10]. Faruki and Lai-Goldman have presented intriguing data supporting the acceleration of test acceptance for several IVDs once clinical utility is definitively established. The "early development" period that precedes the establishment of clinical utility was reported to last up to 5 years and is characterized by performing clinical studies to support the incorporation of the assay into clinical practice guidelines. Finally, data must be generated illustrating the health economic benefits of a particular assay which is critical in establishing and obtaining maximum reimbursement and aiding in the adoption of the assay by test providers. Demonstrating these four parameters of analytical performance, clinical validation, clinical utility, and economic benefits are essential for achieving success in the market.

REIMBURSEMENT OF IVD PRODUCTS

In the United States, the reimbursement for clinical diagnostics is dictated by the Clinical Laboratory Fee Schedule, managed by the Centers for Medicare and Medicaid Services (CMS). Prior to 2013, reimbursement prices were established by collating the number of steps in an assay via Common Procedural Terminology (CPT) codes that were "stacked" to arrive at a final cost that a lab could submit for reimbursement of a particular assay. Beginning in 2013, reimbursement rates for many molecular-based assays transitioned from stacked codes to test-specific codes with finalization of payment determination for analyte specific assays effective as of January, 2014. The impact of these new rates on IVD developers is that the IVD kit must be sold at a fraction of the total reimbursement cost to the service provider to ensure profitability of the lab performing the assay. As a result, there is a significant challenge to the IVD developer to obtain pricing that is reflective of the value the IVD delivers.

In European markets, while mandatory CE marking under the IVD Directive 98/79/CE requirements facilitates access of diagnostic tests across the European Union, the use of the assay is dependent on a favorable health technology assessment outcome necessary to obtain reimbursement. The European market is characterized as a heterogeneous region in terms of these assessment and reimbursement approaches with every country having its own distinct requirements. As a result, potential differences arise across members of the European Union and developers of IVDs often lack information on the appropriate pathways required for technology assessment to secure reimbursement and thus drive adoption and utilization of their tests. In contrast to the evaluation mechanisms

in place for therapeutics in which many countries put drugs through a well-defined appraisal process on the national level, diagnostics are typically reviewed at the local level. This local approach to technology assessment and reimbursement of IVDs compared with national-level reviews for most drugs can result in substantial delays to reimbursement of a diagnostic product and hence its availability. For example, although Herceptin was approved in France in 2000, funding for Her2 testing was not approved until 2007 [11].

APPLICATION OF AN IVD AS A COMPANION DIAGNOSTIC

A growing area of interest is the application *of IVDs* to guide therapeutic selection. The pharmaceutical industry has been experiencing a paradigm shift in its drug development process, migrating away from its traditional "blockbuster" model in which every patient is treated with the same therapeutic for a particular condition, in favor of adopting a "targeted" approach in which therapeutics are directed to discreet populations based on the use of a patient's molecular information. Driving this adoption are the technological advances in proteomic, genomic, and gene sequencing applications which have the potential to identify patients more likely to benefit from this and enable personalized treatment options. As a consequence, there is an increasing number of therapeutics whose use is being guided by a diagnostic assay thus giving rise to the field of companion diagnostics. The codevelopment of a diagnostic paired with a therapeutic represents an innovative growth opportunity for IVD products.

While the pairing of an IVD product to guide the use of a therapeutic was first illustrated in 1998 with the approval of Genentech's Herceptin® and Dako's HercepTest™, the majority of companion diagnostic products have been approved by the FDA only recently (see Table 24.3).

In addition to Herceptin®, ten other therapeutics have been approved with a corresponding companion diagnostic with six occurring since January, 2012, demonstrating the growing trend of integrating diagnostics into the drug-development pathway. Although the vast majority of products codeveloped to date have focused on oncology applications, there are increasing trends of drug-diagnostic codevelopment approaches in other therapeutic areas as well. The codevelopment of a therapeutic along with it companion diagnostic and its ability to segment patients who are eligible to receive increasingly expensive therapeutics is providing attractive growth opportunities for IVD products. Sales of companion diagnostics are anticipated to have a compound adjusted growth rate (CAGR) of 29.2 percent between 2012 and 2018 and achieving sales of $897 million by 2018 [12]. When used as a companion diagnostic, IVDs carry a strong value proposition as it is anticipated that their ability to select optimal responders and spare other patients from ineffective and costly or even unsafe treatments will

TABLE 24.3 The Listing of Currently Available FDA-Approved Companion Diagnostic Device

Companion Diagnostic	Paired Therapeutic(s)	Analyte Measured	Target Tissue	Technology Platform	Original Approval
DAKO HERCEPTEST	Herceptin (trastuzumab) Perjeta (pertuzumab)	HER2 overexpression	Breast Gastric	IHC	10-27-98
HER2 FISH PharmDx Kit	Herceptin (trastuzumab) Perjeta (pertuzumab)	HER2 gene amplification	Breast Gastric	ISH	05-03-05
INFORM HER2 Dual ISH Cocktail	Herceptin (trastuzumab)	HER2 gene amplification	Breast	ISH	06-14-11
HER2 CISH PhrmDx Kit	Herceptin (trastuzumab)	HER2 gene amplification	Breast	ISH	11-30-11
BOND Oracle HER2 IHC	Herceptin (trastuzumab)	HER2 overexpression	Breast	IHC	04-18-12
SPOT-LIGHT HER2 CISH	Herceptin (trastuzumab)	HER2 gene amplification	Breast	ISH	07-01-08
PATHWAY HER2 (Clone cb11)	Herceptin (trastuzumab)	HER2 overexpression	Breast	IHC	11-28-00
PATHVYSION HER-2DNA Probe Kit	Herceptin (trastuzumab)	HER2 gene amplification	Breast	ISH	12-11-98
DAKO EGFR PharmDx Kit	Erbitux (cetuximab) Vectibix (panitumumab)	EGFR overexpression	Colon	IHC	02-12-04
c-KIT PharmDx	Gleevec (imatinib)	c-KIT overexpression	GIST	IHC	02-12-04
Therascreen KRAS RGQ PCR Kit	Erbitux (cetuximab)	KRAS mutations	Colon	PCR	07-06-12
Ferriscan RZ-MRI Analysis System	Erbitux (cetuximab)	Iron concentration	Liver	MRI	01-23-13
VYSIS ALK Break Apart FISH	Xalkori (crizotinib)	ALK translocation	Lung	ISH	08-26-11
COBAS 4800 BRAF V600 Mutation Test	Zelboraf (vemurafenib)	BRAF mutations	Melanoma	PCR	08-17-11
COBAS EGFR Mutation Test	Tarceva (erlotinib)	EGFR mutations	Lung	PCR	05-14-13
THxID BRAF	Mekinist (trametenib) Tafinlar (dabrafenib)	BRAF mutations	Melanoma	PCR	05-29-13
Therascreen EGFR RGQ PCR kit	Gilotrif (afatinib)	EGFR mutations	Lung	PCR	07-12-13

IHC: Immunohistochemical; ISH: *in situ* hybridization; PCR: Polymerase Chain Reaction; MRI: Manetic resonance Imaging; GIST: Gastrstromal Intestinal Tumors.
Source: http://WWW.fda.gov/MedicalDevices/ProductsandMedicalProcedures/InVitriDiagnostics/ucm301431.html

TABLE 24.4 Therapeutic Benefits from Companion Diagnostic Products

- Improves efficacy
- Reduces toxicity; Patients spared exposure to ineffective medicines
- Drug development timeliness shortened
- Lower drug development costs
- Regulatory risk mitigated
- Faster therapeutic adoption
- Improved pharmacoeconomics

provide numerous benefits (see Table 24.4). However, because of the significant costs associated with developing and validating companion diagnostics assays and the need for access to samples with well-annotated clinical outcomes data, it is envisioned that these requirements will necessitate the need for increased partnerships between IVD and therapeutic developers.

FORGING DIAGNOSTIC AND THERAPEUTIC PARTNERSHIPS FOR COMPANION DIAGNOSTIC APPLICATIONS

Developing a diagnostic assay to select patients most likely to benefit in parallel with the therapeutic requires exquisite planning and execution to align these two unique and complex development pathways (Figure 24.4). Furthermore, the FDA has asserted that any corresponding diagnostic assay that supports the safe and effective use of a therapeutic must be an FDA-approved assay [13]. This additional regulatory requirement therefore must be achieved prior to the therapeutic being approved for commercialization.

Although developers of therapeutics that require a companion diagnostic product have the option of developing their own companion diagnostic device, many lack the core competency required for the development of a diagnostic.

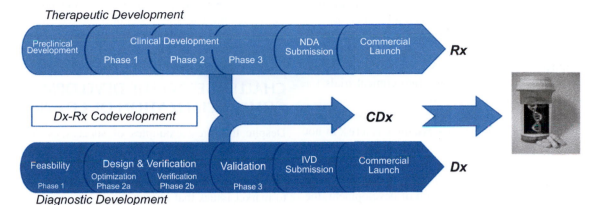

FIGURE 24.4   Bridging the development of a therapeutic and diagnostic.

The alternative approach is to partner with an IVD developer to provide the accompanying diagnostic product. In turn, developers of IVDs, particularly those with experience navigating the global regulatory requirements and having worldwide sales and marketing capabilities, offer a global solution. Those capable of placing the companion diagnostic wherever the pharmaceutical partner intends to sell its targeted therapies would appear to be the partners of choice for pharmaceutical developers.

This new paradigm of codevelopment creates significant opportunities for developers of IVDs and provides them with the opportunity to participate in this emerging field of personalized medicine. IVD developers will see their assays establish a new standard of care and segment the market into optimal responders and spare those who would not benefit from a particular therapeutic. It also affords IVD developers an opportunity to bring innovative technologies to the market as those with efficient technology platforms capable of providing comprehensive information from minimal amounts of material that will reap significant benefits.

However, the codevelopment process may be viewed as disruptive by both the pharmaceutical and diagnostic industry compared to the way they have traditionally operated and developed their respective products. Aligning the development of an IVD and therapeutic presents a unique set of the challenges that will need to be addressed. The pharmaceutical partner needs to be assured of the feasibility of the approach while the diagnostic developer needs to be properly incentivized to maintain engagement and provide these innovative diagnostic products. For example, pharmaceutical companies have traditionally controlled all aspects of the development and marketing of their therapeutic products. Those who have been brought into the development cycle have usually been compensated on a fee-for-service schedule, such as contract manufacturing organizations, clinical research organizations, and marketing and communication firms. In contrast, companion diagnostic codevelopment programs require

pharmaceutical companies to partner with a diagnostic provider and be dependent on their diagnostic product for the therapeutic to reach the market. Integrating a diagnostic assay into the drug development process may be characterized as adding complexity as well as higher development costs and increasing risks of delays to clinical development timelines.

For the IVD developer, adjusting currently planned R&D activities to accommodate a new companion diagnostic opportunity is challenging. In accepting a previously unplanned project, there is a need to reallocate existing projects and resources and reassign manpower. Typically, timelines required by the pharmaceutical partner presents a logistical challenge to have an assay available to support registration studies. Unless already available for use, the IVD will need to be developed prior to the start of the clinical studies that are designed to employ a patient stratification/selection strategy. In essence, the process of integrating a diagnostic into the drug development process requires joining two very unique and complex development programs run by two vastly different companies with significantly different development timelines for their respective products. Therefore, understanding the IVD development requirements is critical to aligning the development timelines of the paired products and incorporating the IVD assay into the development path for eventual simultaneous approval of the therapeutic and its companion diagnostic product.

INTEGRATING AN IVD INTO THE DRUG DEVELOPMENT PATHWAY AS A COMPANION DIAGNOSTIC

Companion Diagnostic Development Requirements

Companion diagnostics, like all IVDs, are considered medical devices and are subject to the premarket controls as defined in the Federal Food, Drug and Cosmetic (FD&C)

Act. Essentially all companion diagnostic products listed in Table 24.3 have typically been classified as high-risk, Class III devices, subject to a PMA application for marketing authorization in the United States. Therefore when used as companion diagnostics, IVDs have a high level of regulatory requirements to achieve which in turn has implications on development timelines of the IVD product and when it can be available to be incorporated into clinical trials for validation as a companion diagnostic.

When used as a companion diagnostic, unless initiated early in the drug development process, there is a risk of not having the IVD available at the start of pivotal clinical trials for patient selection and thus impacting delays to the development timelines of the therapeutic. Prior to integrating the assay into its clinical validation phase of development, the IVD will have had to complete its analytical validation in which the performance of the assay has been optimized and the design and specification of the assay have been verified. Essentially, an IVD product would have to complete Phase 2A and 2B, design and verification, at which time the assay design is considered "frozen" and can now move onto clinical validation or Phase 3 of development. It is not until the conclusion of design and verification, which can take up to 2 years to complete, that a prototype version of the IVD assay can be manufactured and utilized as an investigation use only (IOU) assay for validation in a clinical setting.

For the execution of clinical validation (Phase 3), it is envisioned that the therapeutic product and corresponding companion diagnostic will be developed simultaneously and the clinical performance and utility of the IUO assay will be demonstrated using data from the clinical development program of the paired therapeutic product. Ideally, the clinical data is generated prospectively by stratifying patients for inclusion into a clinical trial for treatment with the paired therapeutic and the clinical utility established when patient outcome data is correlated with the results of the companion diagnostic-selected patient population. However, there have been cases when the data is validated retrospectively as was the case for Qiagen's Therascreen KRAS assay.

If an IUO assay is not available to meet the therapeutic timelines, an alternative option to alleviate the time requirement challenges posed by IVD development is the laboratory-developed test (LDT). In contrast to IVDs which are developed with strict adherence to design controls and quality system regulations, LDT can be developed and validated by individual testing labs in as little as 6 months for use in that facility only. LDT assays have the advantage of bypassing the rigorous development requirements associated with an IVD and therefore represent the least impact on timelines for initiating clinical trial testing. However, the regulatory requirements for LDTs when used as companion diagnostics have not yet been addressed by the FDA. From a commercial perspective, LDTs are geographically limited and confined for use in the lab for which they were developed which could be a future barrier to access and have commercial implications on the therapeutic. Alternatively, the LDT could be subsequently bridged to the IVD, but this requires the meticulous banking of samples and retrospective testing to demonstrate high concordance between the two assays once the IVD is available.

CHALLENGES TO THE DEVELOPMENT AND COMMERCIALIZATION OF CDx PRODUCTS

Despite the latest examples of success as demonstrated by the recently approved companion diagnostic products (Table 24.3), challenges remain on several fronts including logistical applications, regulatory requirements and access to market issues that impact the adoption and commercial success of IVD products when used as companion diagnostics. Identifying strategies to overcome these challenges are critical for the future success of IVDs when used as these innovative products.

Logistical Challenges

All of the companion products approved to date have been for assays that detect a single analyte. For example the Therascreen EGFR RGQ PCR kit detects mutation in the EGFR gene in Non-Small Cell Lung Cancer (NSCLC) samples and is indicated for the use of Gilotrif in patients with EGFR mutation positive NSCLC. In contrast, the VYSIS ALK Break Apart FISH assay detects translocations in the ALK gene and is indicated for the use of Zelboraf in ALK-EML4 positive patients. However, as the therapeutic options for a single tumor type increases so too does the need to obtain comprehensive information from a clinical sample. Due to the limited material obtained from a clinical biopsy, it is unrealistic to expect reflex testing covering multiple assays will be feasible to profile a tumor sample to arrive at a clinical decision endpoint. How testing of a clinical sample will get prioritized when there are multiple choices remains to be seen but the need to develop IVD products that have multiplexing capabilities is clearly evident. The challenges to validate this multiplex approach when used with multiple drugs and the difficulties and limitations associated with validating biomarkers that are in low prevalence cannot be overstated.

Regulatory Challenges

Although the paired products are dependent on each other's regulatory approval for market access, there is a universal absence of structure allowing for the simultaneous submission and review of the paired products as one regulatory file. For example, a pre-market approval (PMA) submission is reviewed by the FDA's Center of Diagnostics and Radiological Health (CDRH) while in contrast, a new drug application (NDA) for a therapeutic is submitted and reviewed by a completely separate entity of the FDA, either the Center for Drug Evaluation and Research (CDER) or the Center for Biological Evaluation and Research (CBER). This lack of regulatory harmonization is evident across major markets including the European Union, where IVD Directive 98/79/CE (CE stands for Conformité Européene, or European Conformity) stipulates self-certification for the diagnostic assay while therapeutics are submitted to the European Medical Agency (EMA) for review by the Committee for Human Medicinal Products (CHMP). In Japan, a process for the simultaneous review of therapeutic-diagnostic (Rx-Dx) pairs is still lacking, and in emerging markets such as China, a process for CDx development is still being defined. Establishing a uniform process for simultaneous review and approval will create a more efficient system and help to mitigate risks in these codevelopment programs.

Commercial Challenges

The development of an IVD by device manufactures must represent a compelling investment opportunity. Device manufacturers invest significant resources in bringing an IVD to market including R&D, clinical trials, and regulatory compliance. The traditional IVD business model has been built on the concept that low margins can be offset with high-volume tests. However, recent companion diagnostics assays have tended to be niche indications representing "orphan-like" diagnostic opportunities. For example, the annual number of metastatic colorectal cancer cases and metastatic melanoma cases in the United States are approximately 50,000 and 10,000, respectively. Even the total number of annual cases of advanced/metatstatic NSCLC eligible for ALK-EML4 screening is less than 100,000 cases [14].

Although low volume can typically be offset by higher pricing (i.e. orphan therapeutics), IVD products tend to be prohibited from this approach and are challenged to obtain value-based pricing In addition to the challenges of niche market opportunities, low pricing and lags in reimbursement, IVDs are confronted with another set of challenges in the market place in the form of "home brews" or LDTs. Many reference and academic labs develop and offer their own tests in the absence of IVDs. However, once an IVD kit is regulatory approved, there is little compelling reason for labs to convert to the available kit, thus presenting the IVD developer with a competitive market beginning at launch of the IVD. The presence of competing LDTs, coupled with low volume, low pricing, and potential delays in reimbursement, present significant challenges to the traditional IVD business model. Coupled with the costs associated with IVD development, there is a risk in attaining a viable business model and therefore it is imperative to address these challenges and find solutions that incentivize the IVD developer to participate in this emerging field.

Solutions to these economic challenges can be addressed through creative partnerships between diagnostic and pharmaceutical developers and by reforming the current reimbursement system. To compensate for the typically modest volumes and pricing and to establish a viable IVD business model, requiring the therapeutic partner to fund assay-development costs is justified in light of the value the diagnostic developer brings to the codevelopment program. In addition, incentivizing the diagnostic developer with success fees or milestone payments for significant events such as regulatory approvals, launch in key markets or demonstrating a significant impact on sales should also be considered in regard to the value the Dx creates for it's paired therapeutic. To compensate for lags in reimbursement, creative strategies should be considered so that testing does not become a barrier for access to the therapeutic. There have already been some examples illustrating the feasibility of this approach in which the therapeutic developer either provides funding or directly pays for the test to be performed. Examples include the funding by AstraZeneca for EGFR mutation testing in the UK for Iressa and Merck KGaA supporting KRAS testing in Spain for Erbitux [11].

Although these are attractive short-term approaches, reimbursement reform will be needed to drive future innovation in the field of companion diagnostics. Reforming the current reimbursement system for diagnostics is one possibility to accommodate the innovation that is being delivered. Another consideration is to assess the coupling of the diagnostic and therapeutic as one true product in which the cost of the assay is bundled with the cost of the therapeutic and the pharmaceutical provider assumes responsibility for covering the cost of the diagnostic. The reality is that the therapeutic is deriving the bulk of the economic benefit and failure to recognize the value that the diagnostic component delivers is a risk to future investment in this area and a challenge to IVD developers to participate in this emerging application of personalized medicine.

FUTURE APPLICATIONS FOR IVD PRODUCTS

Aside from companion diagnostics, other future growth opportunities for IVDs are currently in the development stage and can be found on several fronts. These include an increased focus on full automation, point-of-care (POC) testing, and developing more efficient and sensitive diagnostic applications to drive personalized medicine initiatives. The latter being driven by technological advances to extract molecular information from patient samples for a more patient-specific diagnosis based on genetic information. These technologies include digital PCR, next-generation sequencing approaches, and single molecule arrays (SIMOA). Clinical segments that will spur investment in these innovative approaches include infectious disease testing, oncology, cardiovascular disease, and neurological conditions. However, uncertainty on both the reimbursement and regulatory landscape could impact the progress of developing IVDs for these innovative applications.

SUMMARY

IVD products are an integral component to the delivery of an optimal healthcare system. A growing application of IVD products are their use as companion diagnostics to select patients who are most likely to derive benefit from a corresponding therapeutic. Implementing companion diagnostics has reached a "tipping point" in which we have been able to witness a growing number of new chemical entities coming to market with their safe and effective use dependent on an IVD product. IVD manufacturers with their regulatory expertise and global sales and marketing capabilities can be ideal partners for pharmaceutical companies requiring diagnostic assays to guide therapeutic selection. However, despite the initial excitement, significant challenges remain to these partnerships that underscore the traditional IVD business model. Value capture remains a major challenge going forward, together with regulatory uncertainty and operational issues between codevelopment partners. These challenges remain to be addressed that allow the field to advance and deliver the benefits to patients that need it the most.

REFERENCES

[1] 21 C.F.R.Part 809.
[2] Aspinall MG. Hamermesh RG. Realizing the Promise of Personalized Medicine Harvard Business Review; October 2007:85(10):108–17.
[3] *http://advameddx.org/download/files/InfographicWeb.pdf.*
[4] Based on 2012 Market Statistics from Frost and Sullivan.
[5] Baker M. New-wave diagnostics Nature Biotechnology; August 2006: 24(8):931–938.
[6] Stynen D. Revision of Europe's IVD Directive 98/79/EC www.ivdtechnology.com/print/2412.
[7] *http://www.fda.gov/regulatoryinformation/guidances/.*
[8] U.S. Food and Drug Administration/Improvements in Device Review November, 2012.
[9] U.S. Food and Drug Administration. http://www.fda.gov/MedicalDevices/DeviceRegulationandGuidance/Overview/MDUFAIII/ucm313673.htm.
[10] Faruki H, Lai-Goldman M. Application of a Pharamcogenetic test Adoption Model to Six Oncology Biomarkers Personalized Med 2010;7(4):441–50.
[11] Miller I, Ashon-Chess J, Spolders H, Fert V, Ferrara J, Kroll W, Aska J, Larcier P, Terry P, Bruinvels A, Huriez A. Market Access challenges in the EU for high medical value diagnostic tests Personalized Med 2011;8(2):137–48.
[12] Based on 2013 Market Statistics from Roots Analysis.
[13] *In Vitro* Companion Diagnostic Devices: Guidance for the Industry and Food and Drug Administration Staff Issued April 25th, 2013.
[14] Howlader N, Noone AM, Krapcho M, et al. (eds). SEER Cancer Statistics Review, 1975-2010, National Cancer Institute. Bethesda, MD, http://seer.cancer.gov/csr/1975_2010/ based on November 2012 SEER data submission, posted to the SEER web site, April 2013.

Chapter 25

Regulatory Approval and Compliances for Biotechnology Products

Norman W. Baylor, PhD

President & CEO, Biologics Consulting Group, Inc., Alexandria, Virginia

National regulatory authorities (NRAs) regulate pharmaceutical products to enable patient access to high-quality, safe, and effective products, and restrict access to those products that are unsafe or have limited clinical use. When appropriately implemented, regulation ensures a public health benefit and the safety of patients, healthcare workers, and the broader community. Before new technologies can be used, they must be assessed and approved by authorized regulatory agencies. Detailed safety review during research and development stages, regulatory approval, and legal registration are necessary stages of product development. These regulatory processes ensure that products are safe and effective.

Biomedical products must be reviewed and approved or licensed by the NRA of the country in which they will be marketed and distributed. These authorities evaluate whether a product is safe for widespread use and whether manufacturers can consistently produce high-quality products. Among the issues regulatory authorities consider are:

- Whether the design for clinical testing is safe enough to warrant human participation.
- Whether there is sufficient data to ascertain risks and benefits.
- Whether the benefits from any given product outweigh the risks that may be associated with its use.
- Whether data collected in one country can be applied to the use of a product in another country.

After a product is approved, licensed, and marketed, it must be monitored throughout its lifecycle to ensure that its benefit continues to match expectations of safety and effectiveness. National and regional regulatory authorities—including the U.S. Food and Drug Administration (FDA), Health Canada, the European Medicines Agency (EMA), as well as other national regulatory authorities throughout the world oversee and manage the regulatory review and approval process. The approval process for biomedical products is similar in most countries; however, there are some aspects that differ based on specific laws and regulations in each country. In all countries, information submitted to regulatory authorities regarding the quality, safety, and efficacy of drugs is similar; however, the review process for clinical trials and marketing authorization applications may differ. The primary focus of this chapter will cover the U.S. FDA approval process. For specific information about the regulatory approval route in other countries it is best to seek guidance from the specific national regulatory authority (NRA) in those countries or from external experts familiar with those processes.

Regulatory reviews of products designed for use in the developing world present unique challenges. To reflect local priorities and health conditions, a regulatory review ideally is managed by the government or regional authority of the people for which the product has been designed. Challenges arise when regulatory authorities in developing countries do not have the skills and/or resources to manage the review. As additional products are developed for low-income countries, the strain on the resources of developing country NRAs may become even greater. The FDA and other regulatory authorities may provide assistance to these NRAs in an attempt to ultimately support product access to those who need them most. Some mechanisms, such as the EMA's Article 58 and the World Health Organization Prequalification Program, help assure safety and efficacy of products designed exclusively for the developing world [1].

Regulatory procedures impact all stages of biomedical product development. Therefore, it is critical that developers of biomedical products (drugs, biologics, devices, *in vitro* diagnostics, or some combination) possess the knowledge and awareness of the regulatory challenges and opportunities to expedite the development of safe and effective products in a cost-effective manner. The pathway from discovery to marketing of a new biomedical product can be long, complex, and costly. A clear understanding of the FDA regulatory process, regulations, and policies is essential when developing an effective product lifecycle management strategy, seeking product approval, and assuring that products are marketed in compliance with federal requirements. In order to minimize the risks and costs involved in the biomedical product development process, it is imperative that clear planning is done during the early stages of product development, with regular assessment of chemistry, manufacturing, and control (CMC), and nonclinical and clinical data as it is generated. The aim of this chapter is to provide an overview of the FDA regulatory product approval process and discuss considerations for successfully developing a regulatory strategy that leads to product marketing authorization from national regulatory authorities.

HISTORY OF THE FDA

The FDA is responsible for ensuring the safety of an array of consumer products. The FDA is part of the executive branch of the U.S. federal government located in the Department of Health and Human Services. The U.S. Department of Agriculture Bureau of Chemistry was the predecessor of the FDA. Prior to 1902 the manufacture of vaccines, antitoxins, and other biologicals was unregulated by the federal government. In response to the tragic deaths of 14 children due to contaminated diphtheria antitoxin, Congress enacted the Biologics Control Act of 1902 which gave the federal government the authority to grant premarket approval for every biological drug and for the process and facility producing such drugs [2]. This legislation contained the initial concepts for the regulation of biologics. In 1906 Congress passed the Federal Food and Drugs Act, to address increasing consumer concern about the safety of foods and drugs in the United States. The FDA was one of the first agencies established by the U.S. government dedicated to consumer protections [3]. In 1927 the regulatory functions of the Bureau of Chemistry were reorganized to become the Food, Drug, and Insecticide Administration, which in 1930 changed its name to the Food and Drug Administration. In 1938 the FDA was overhauled with the passage of the Pure Food, Drug, and Cosmetics Act.

The oversight of medical devices was the responsibility of the U.S. Post Office Department and the Federal Trade Commission to a limited extent prior to 1938 and came under the authority of the FDA after 1938. Although premarket approval did not apply to devices, the Pure Food, Drug, and Cosmetics Act equated them to drugs for regulatory purposes [4]. With the proliferation of medical technology, and an increasing rise in the development of various types of medical devices, Congress considered passing laws for the regulation for devices which would be comparable to the 1962 Drug Amendments Act. This legislation failed and the Secretary of the Department of Health, Education, and Welfare commissioned the Study Group on Medical Devices which

recommended in 1970 that medical devices be classified according to their comparative risk and regulated accordingly. In the early 1970s, a government report documented thousands of injuries resulting from medical devices [5]. Soon after, the Dalkon Shield intrauterine device was withdrawn from the market after more than 200 second trimester septic abortions and 11 maternal deaths occurred. In response to these adverse events Congress enacted the 1976 Medical Device Amendments to enhance the FDA's ability to establish the safety and effectiveness of medical devices.

Additional refinements to the function, organization, and authority of the FDA continue as new public health threats and issues emerge. There are several different departments within the FDA that handle issues such as drug development, food safety, cosmetics, blood products, medical devices, vaccines, veterinary medicine, and radiation-emitting products. Under current law, every medical product is classifiable as a drug, device, biologic, or combination product. The classification of the product determines the particular review and approval processes the FDA may use in accessing the safety and efficacy of the product for human use. In addition to evaluating new products before they are released onto the market to determine their safety and effectiveness, the FDA also periodically inspects existing products and the facilities in which they are manufactured, and evaluates labeling, advertising, and other claims made about the products for which it regulates.

The U.S. FDA's organization includes, among other units, the Office of the Commissioner and four directorates (Medical Products and Tobacco, Foods, Global Regulatory Operations, and Policy) overseeing the core functions of the agency (Figure 25.1). The Office of Medical Products and Tobacco provides high-level coordination and leadership across the Center for Drug Evaluation and Research (CDER), the Center for Biologics Evaluation and Research (CBER), the Center for Devices and Radiological Health (CDRH), and the Center for Tobacco Products (CTP).

The agency responsible for the regulation of biological products previously resided under the National Institutes of Health. This authority was transferred to the FDA in 1972. Currently, both CBER and CDER are responsible for regulating therapeutic biological products, including premarket review and oversight.

CBER regulates biological products for human use under applicable federal laws, including the Public Health Service Act (PHS Act) and the Federal Food, Drug, and Cosmetic Act (FD&C Act). (See Table 25.1.)

Products regulated in CBER include blood and blood products, vaccines, allergenics, cell and tissue-based products, gene therapy products, and therapeutic proteins derived from plants, animals, humans, or microorganisms. New biologics are required to go through a premarket approval process similar to that for drugs. However, the Public Health Service Act provides that marketing approval for a biologic shall be obtained through the submission and approval of a Biologics License

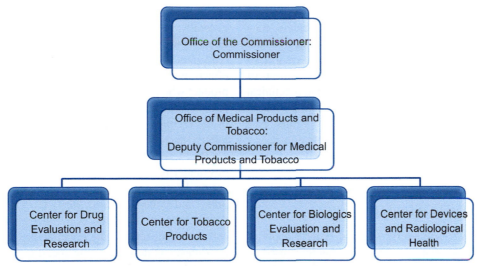

FIGURE 25.1   The organization chart of the U.S. FDA.

TABLE 25.1 Acts and Regulations Pertinent to the Development and Licensure of Biomedical Products

Congressional Acts
Public Health Service Act (42 USC 262-63) Section 351
Food, Drug & Cosmetic Act (21 USC 301-392)
Food and Drug Administration Modernization Act, 1997
Food and Drug Administration Amendments Act, 2007
Title 21 Code of Federal Regulations (CFR)
Subchapter A—General
21 CFR 58 Good Laboratory Practices
21 CFR 56 Institutional Review Boards
21 CFR 50 Protection of Human Subjects
Subchapter C: Drugs: General
21 CFR 201
21 CFR 210-211 Good Manufacturing Practices
Subchapter D: Drugs for Human Use
21 CFR 314.126 Adequate and well-controlled trials
21 CFR 312 Investigational New Drug Application
Subchapter F: Biologics
21 CFR 600-680 Biological Product Standards
Subchapter Devices
21 CFR 807

Application (BLA). CBER also regulates medical devices related to licensed blood and cellular products under the FD&C Act's Medical Device Amendments of 1976 [6]. Moreover, the medical devices regulated by CBER are intimately associated with the blood collection and processing procedures as well as the cellular therapies regulated by CBER.

CDER regulates over-the-counter and prescription drugs, including biological therapeutics and generic drugs. CDER has different requirements for the three main types of drug products: new drugs, generic drugs, and over-the-counter drugs. The FD&C Act requires a sponsor to submit a new drug application (NDA) for the FDA's evaluation to market a drug. The biological therapeutics regulated by CDER require the submission of a BLA and include monoclonal

antibodies for *in vivo* use designed as targeted therapies in cancer and other diseases; proteins intended for therapeutic use, including cytokines (interferons) and enzymes (e.g., thrombolytics); immunomodulators (nonvaccine and nonallergenic products) intended to treat disease by inhibiting or modifying a preexisting immune response; and growth factors intended to mobilize, stimulate, decrease, or otherwise alter the production of hematopoietic cells *in vivo*.

CDRH regulates all medical devices under the FD&C Act, inclusive of radiation-related devices, that are not assigned categorically or specifically to CBER. The FDA has divided devices into three classes to identify the level of regulatory control applicable to them. The highest category is Class III and includes those devices for which premarket approval is required to determine the safety and effectiveness of the device. There are two primary pathways by which the FDA permits medical devices to be marketed: premarket clearance by means of a 510(k) notification, or premarket authorization by means of a premarket application (PMA) or product development protocol (PDP). *In vitro* diagnostic products are medical devices as defined in section 210(h) of the Federal Food, Drug, and Cosmetic Act, and may also be biological products subject to Section 351 of the Public Health Service Act. Like other medical devices, IVDs are subject to premarket and postmarket controls. IVDs are also subject to the Clinical Laboratory Improvement Amendments (CLIA '88) of 1988.

Product types continue to merge as a result of technological advances and blur the historical lines of separation between the FDA's medical product centers, i.e., CBER, CDER, and CDRH. Combination products are therapeutic and diagnostic products that combine drugs, devices, and/or biological products. A combination product is classified, assigned to a specific center within the FDA, and may be regulated as a drug, device, or biologic depending upon its primary mode of action as determined by the FDA. Because combination products involve components that would normally be regulated under different types of regulatory authorities, and frequently by different FDA centers, they raise challenging regulatory, policy, and review management challenges. Differences in regulatory pathways for each component can impact the regulatory processes for all aspects of product development and management, including preclinical testing, clinical investigation, marketing applications, manufacturing and quality control, adverse event reporting, promotion and advertising, and postapproval modifications.

REGULATIONS RELATED TO BIOMEDICAL PRODUCT DEVELOPMENT

A single set of basic regulatory approval criteria apply to biomedical products regardless of the technology used to produce them. The current legal authority for the regulation of biologics derives primarily from Section 351 of the PHS Act and from certain sections of the U.S. Food, Drug, and Cosmetic Act [7,8]. The statutes of the PHS Act are implemented through regulations codified in Title 21 of the Code of Federal Regulations, parts 600 through 680 which contains regulations specifically applicable to biologics. The PHS Act requires individuals or companies who manufacture biologics for introduction into interstate commerce to hold a license for these products. FDA issues these licenses. In addition, because biologics meet the legal definition of a drug under the FD&C Act, manufacturers must comply with the drug Current Good Manufacturing Practices (CGMPs) regulations (parts 210 and 211). Regulations applicable to biomedical products are summarized in Table 25.1. These regulations include the minimum requirements for the manufacturing of biologics, drug, devices, and combinations thereof, as well as the requirements for performing clinical trials.

The FDA periodically publishes various guidelines and guidance documents to assist developers of new biomedical products in regard to the manufacture and clinical evaluation of these products. In addition, international guidelines developed and published by the International Conference on Harmonization (ICH) have been adopted by the FDA. Guidance documents do not have the force of law, but are intended to provide useful and timely recommendations and represent the agencies' current thinking on particular topics. These documents are particularly useful in rapidly progressing areas of science and for specifying a degree of detail beyond what is included in the regulations.

To understand how the FDA regulates biomedical products, it is important to understand some of the more pertinent operational definitions contained in the statutes and regulations. Section 351 of the PHS Act defines a biological product as any virus, therapeutic serum, toxin, antitoxin, vaccine, blood, blood component or derivative, allergenic product, or analogous product applicable to the prevention, treatment, or cure of diseases or conditions of human beings [9]. Biological products, in contrast to chemically synthesized small molecules, which can be thoroughly characterized, are generally derived from living material, are complex in structure, and usually cannot be fully characterized.

Safety is defined as the relative freedom from harmful effects to individuals affected directly or indirectly by a product when prudently administered, taking into consideration the character of the product in relation to the condition of the recipient at the time. Thus, the property of safety is relative and cannot be ensured in an absolute sense.

Purity is defined as the relative freedom from extraneous matter regardless of whether it is harmful to the recipient or deleterious to the product. Usually, the concepts of purity and safety coincide; purity most often relates to freedom from such materials as pyrogens, adventitious agents, and chemicals used in the manufacture of the product.

Potency is defined as the specific ability or capacity of the product, as indicated by appropriate laboratory tests or by adequately controlled clinical data obtained through the administration of the product in the manner intended, to effect a given result. Potency, as thus defined, is equivalent to the concept that the product must be able to perform as claimed, and, if possible, this must correspond with some measurable effect in the recipient or correlate with some quantitative laboratory finding.

Standards mean specifications and procedures applicable to an establishment or to the manufacture or the release of products that are designed to ensure the continued safety, purity, and potency of biological products. The word standard is also used with a secondary meaning, usually in the sense of a reference preparation, such as a bacterial or viral antigen that can be used in evaluating potency or, in some cases, safety and purity.

The regulations regarding biological products, in addition, define effectiveness as the reasonable expectation that, in a significant proportion of the target population, pharmacologic or other effects of the biological product, when administered under adequate directions for use and warnings against unsafe use, will serve a clinically significant function in the diagnosis, cure, mitigation, treatment, or prevention of disease in humans.

Current good manufacturing practices define a quality system that manufacturers use as they build quality into their products. The regulations outline the minimum manufacturing, quality control, and quality assurance requirements for the preparation of a drug or biological product for commercial distribution. For example, approved products developed and produced according to CGMPs are safe, properly identified, of the correct strength, pure, and of high quality.

CURRENT REGULATORY PATHWAYS

The regulatory pathways for evaluation and approval of biomedical products are outlined in Table 25.2.

The regulatory requirements for biomedical products cover both the premarketing phase, consisting of the

TABLE 25.2 Current US FDA Regulatory Pathways

Biologic products
IND—Investigational new drug application
BLA—Biologics license application
Drugs
IND—Investigational new drug application
NDA—New drug application
Medical devices
510(k)
IDE—Investigational device exemption
PMA—Premarket application
21 CFR 812
21 CFR 814

TABLE 25.3 Product Development Phases

Discovery/basic research—(pre-IND)
Process and analytical development (pre- and post-IND)
Process— Development and optimization
Manufacturing consistency
Assays—Development and specifications
Identity, purity, potency
Stability indicating
Drug substance (bulk substance) and drug product characterization
Product development phases
Preclinical animal studies (pre-IND)
Proof-of-concept
Toxicology
Safety pharmacology
IND submission
Clinical trials
Phase 0, 1, 2, and 3
Product approval/licensure
Postmarket studies (phase 4)

investigational and licensing phases, and the postmarketing phase. These requirements can be found in the Investigational New Drug (IND) or the Investigational Device Exemption (IDE) regulations [10]. The first step, prior to evaluating a new product in human clinical trials, is the preclinical phase. The FDA requires that certain animal tests be conducted before humans are exposed to a new molecular entity. The objectives of early *in vivo* testing are to demonstrate the safety of the proposed product. For example, tests should prove that the compound is not toxic at the doses that would most likely be effective in humans. The results of these tests are used to support the IND application that is filed with the FDA. Sponsors are encouraged to request a pre-IND (or pre-IDE) meeting with the FDA to discuss preclinical studies, clinical study design, and data requirements that may need to be agreed upon prior to the initiation of human clinical studies.

TRANSLATIONAL DEVELOPMENT

The industry's goals are to develop a commercially viable product and make a meaningful contribution to available therapeutic options while satisfying a myriad of regulatory requirements. The introduction of new biomedical products typically involves a long and expensive process that may begin with a relatively simple initial discovery but includes an extended period of development, which addresses formulation and manufacturing, preclinical evaluation, safety, efficacy, and commercial potential. Table 25.3 includes a list of the phases in product development from discovery through postlicensure.

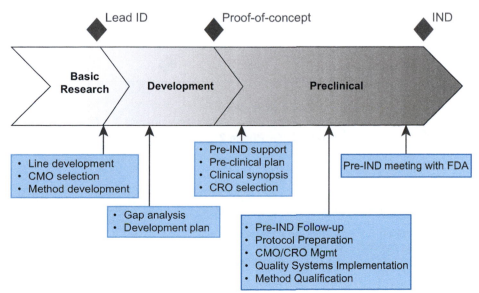

FIGURE 25.2   Impact of the regulatory process on key early development milestones.

In order to understand the timeframe required for a product to become commercially available, one must understand how the product development stages are intertwined with the stages of the regulatory process.

Translational development involves the process of transitioning from the basic research and discovery phase to a regulated product development phase beginning with the preclinical stage (Figure 25.2).

The research and discovery phase may be empirical and based on trial and error and occurs in an unregulated environment; whereas, the impact of regulatory affairs on clinical development is significant and expands the IND phases through licensure and beyond. Although there is no FDA regulatory oversight in the basic research and discovery phase as described at the beginning of this chapter, each of the product development stages beginning with the preclinical stage is impacted by the regulatory process. (Figure 25.3).

Failure to understand and appreciate the regulatory impact for future product development can result in significant delays when attempting to transition a product from the research lab to the clinic. A discovery process that is focused on the development of a drug for one purpose may lead to its use in another, unanticipated, disease indication. Once a potential candidate drug is identified, it must be evaluated in the structured highly regulated environment as previously described.

Once product development enters the regulated environment there are challenges that must be overcome. Preclinical studies must be done under good laboratory practices (GLP); chemistry, manufacturing, and control procedures must be done under current good manufacturing practices (cGMP); and clinical studies must be done under good clinical practices (GCP). It is highly recommended that a gap analysis of all development areas be done as part of a product development plan (PDP). Comprehensive product development planning should be based on a clear understanding of the FDA regulations and expectations. This includes effective communication with the FDA to assure concurrence with the development plan. The execution of the PDP should be overseen by a project management expert. Product development requires a team effort and success is highly dependent on support from upper management and availability of appropriate resources. Product development regulatory goals should include:

- Developing a reproducible process that can yield a consistent product and that can be manufactured under cGMPs.
- Developing analytical procedures that can reliably measure product parameters that are stability indicating, and can demonstrate product comparability following changes to manufacturing, facilities, or equipment.
- Develop animal models that can demonstrate proof-of-concept and safety.
- Demonstrate safety and efficacy in clinical trials.

Once appropriate preclinical studies are completed, the FDA requires that sponsors of regulated products first obtain preliminary permission for conducting clinical trials in humans. The clinical development of a new drug in the United States usually begins with a sponsor approaching the FDA for permission to conduct a clinical study with an investigational product through submission of an IND application form. Clinical trials in support of a PMA may be conducted only after the FDA has issued an IDE. In the application, the sponsor (1) describes the composition, source, and method of manufacture of the product and the methods used in testing its safety, purity, and potency;

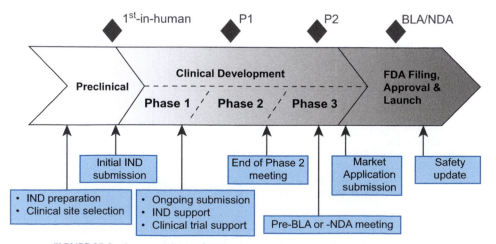

Regulatory Affairs Impact
Key Clinical Development Milestones

FIGURE 25.3 Impact of the regulatory process on key clinical development milestones.

(2) provides a summary of all laboratory and preclinical animal testing; and (3) provides a description of the proposed clinical study and the names and qualifications of each clinical investigator. The FDA has a maximum of 30 days to review the original IND application and determine whether study participants will be exposed to any unacceptable risks. As part of the IND process, each clinical investigator files information describing his or her qualifications for performing clinical trials, details of the proposed study, and assurance that a number of conditions specified by the regulations will be met. A signed informed consent must be obtained from each study participant [11]. Approval for the study must be obtained in advance from a local institutional review board. Once the FDA is satisfied with the documentation, the Phase 1 clinical trial can begin. If the documentation is inadequate, the FDA can place the IND on clinical hold [11].

HUMAN CLINICAL TESTING PHASES

Only licensed or approved biomedical products may be shipped from one state to another; however, during the premarketing phase, interstate shipment of products for investigational use is allowed under the law and regulations [11]. There are generally three separate phases (Phase 1, 2, and 3) in the clinical evaluation of experimental biomedical products at the premarketing stage.

These phases may overlap, and the clinical testing may be highly iterative because multiple Phase 1 or 2 trials may be performed as new data are obtained. The respective responsibilities of the regulatory authority, i.e., the FDA and the sponsor are also outlined in Figure 25.4. One should note that the FDA is not responsible for completing

the appropriate studies in support of the safety and efficacy of the product. This is the sole responsibility of the sponsor.

In a Phase 1 trial, generally, 20 to 100 volunteers are enrolled, which is primarily focused on an assessment of the safety of the product. During this stage, low doses of the product are administered to healthy volunteers who are closely supervised. During the Phase 2 trials, the drug is administered to 100 to 300 volunteers with the intent to determine the drug's effective dose, the method of delivery, and the dosing interval, as well as to reconfirm product safety.

Pre-IND meetings with the FDA are particularly important for new sponsors and for products that incorporate novel features. Other meetings with the FDA are also encouraged at critical points throughout the IND review, including "end-of-Phase 2" meetings. The purpose of an end-of-Phase 2 meeting is to assess the adequacy of the Phase 2 safety and effectiveness data that support advancement to Phase 3, to evaluate the Phase 3 plan and draft protocols, and to identify any additional information necessary to support a marketing application for the uses under investigation. The end-of-Phase 2 meeting is generally held before major commitments of effort and resources to specific Phase 3 studies are made.

A Phase 3 trial may involve anywhere from 1000 or more volunteers across multiple study sites and is considered the pivotal efficacy trial. These studies are used to demonstrate further safety and effectiveness and to determine the best dosage. As far as efficacy evaluation, efficacy is demonstrated ideally in randomized, double-blind, well-controlled trials. The endpoints will be product specific. Additional controlled safety studies are often requested when the numbers of subjects included in the efficacy studies are deemed insufficient to provide adequate safety data. The studies

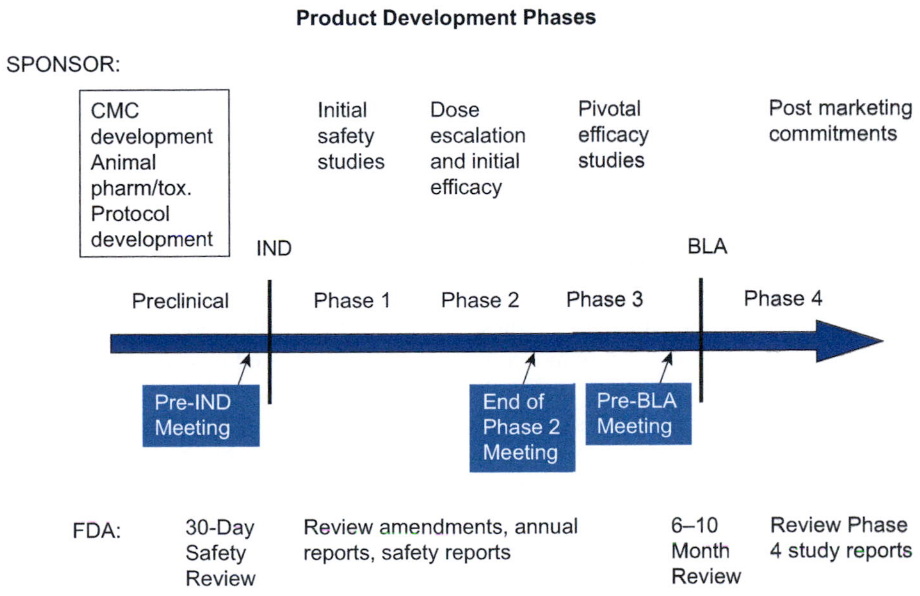

FIGURE 25.4 Product development phases.

need to be designed in such a way that statistical methods may be applied to their evaluation. Safety studies may be unblinded if the number of injections, route of administration, or schedule differs between groups, in particular when infants and young children are involved. Phase 3 trials are the final step before seeking FDA approval.

BIOLOGICS LICENSE APPLICATION (BLA)

Biological products require FDA approval through a biologics license application (BLA) as opposed to new molecular entities, which are approved through a new drug application (NDA) or new devices which are approved through the 510(k) procedures or premarket applications (PMA). Types of products requiring a BLA include vaccines, blood and blood byproducts, some types of monoclonal antibodies, and tissue and cellular products. Once all three phases of the clinical trials are complete, the sponsoring company analyzes all of the data. If the findings demonstrate that the investigational product is both safe and effective for its intended use, the company may file a BLA with the FDA requesting approval to market and distribute the product commercially. FDA experts review all the information included in the BLA to determine if the data demonstrates that the product is safe and effective enough to be approved. Following rigorous review, the FDA can either (1) approve the BLA, (2) send the company a "complete response " letter requesting more information or studies before approval can be granted, or (3) deny approval.

The review of a BLA usually includes an evaluation by an advisory committee which is an independent, external panel of FDA-appointed experts who consider data presented by company representatives and FDA reviewers. The advisory committee then votes on whether the data support the safety and effectiveness of the product in order for the FDA to consider approval of the BLA, and under what conditions. The FDA is not required to follow the recommendations of the advisory committees, but often does.

Prior to the submission of a BLA, a pre-BLA meeting with the agency is strongly encouraged to discuss the sponsor's product developmental plan. The FDA has determined that delays associated with the initial review of a BLA may be reduced by exchanges of information about a proposed marketing application [12]. The primary purpose of a pre-BLA meeting is to discuss any major unresolved issues, to identify those studies that the sponsor is relying on as adequate and well-controlled to establish the product's effectiveness, to identify the status of ongoing studies, to acquaint FDA reviewers with the general information to be submitted in the BLA (including technical information), to review methods used in the statistical analysis of the data, and to discuss the best approach for the presentation and formatting of data in the application.

The BLA should contain details of the manufacturing facility and equipment as well as data derived from nonclinical laboratory and clinical studies that demonstrate that the manufactured product meets prescribed requirements for safety, purity, and potency. Information should be submitted in the BLA that confirms that there is compliance with standards addressing requirements for:

- Organization and personnel.
- Buildings and facilities.
- Equipment.
- Control of components, containers, and closures.
- Production and process controls.
- Packaging and labeling controls.
- Holding and distribution.
- Laboratory controls.
- Records to be maintained.

Furthermore, a full description of manufacturing methods; data establishing stability of the product through the dating period; sample(s) representative of the product for introduction or delivery for introduction into interstate commerce; summaries of test results performed on the lot(s) represented by the submitted sample(s); specimens of the labels, enclosures, and containers; and the address of each location involved in the manufacture of the biological product should be included in the BLA. The manufacturing facility must also be inspection-ready at the time the BLA is submitted. If the information provided meets FDA requirements, the application is approved and a license is issued allowing the firm to market the product. Issuance of a biologics license is the final determination that the product, the manufacturing process, and facilities meet applicable requirements to ensure the continued safety, purity, and potency of the product.

Regulatory oversight continues after licensure. Phase 4 studies are required to assess the safety of the product in larger populations. Additionally, any changes to the manufacturing process or change in therapeutic indications must be reported to the FDA for approval in the form of a BLA supplement.

SUMMARY

Development of biomedical products is an expensive and lengthy process that requires significant advanced planning. Regulatory procedures impact all stages of the biomedical product development process. In order to successfully develop a marketable product it is critical that developers are not only aware of, but have an understanding of regulatory obligations and opportunities. Moreover, clear regulatory planning during the early stages of product development is essential to develop a focused regulatory strategy that can be presented to the regulatory authorities.

REFERENCES

[1] Global Health Technologies Coalition. Regulatory Processes for New Technologies. http://www.ghtcoalition.org/regulatory-pathways.php February 2014. Retrieved.

[2] Kondratas RA. Death Helped Write the Biologics Law. FDA Consumer 1982;16:23–5.

[3] Regulatory Information. "Other Laws Affecting FDA." Legislation. http://www.fda.gov/regulatoryinformation/legislation/default.htm. March 2013. Retrieved.

[4] FDA website: http://www.fda.gov/aboutFDA/whatwedo/history/origin/ucm055137.htm. Retrieved March 2013a.

[5] Maisel WH. Medical Device Regulation: An Introduction for the Practicing Physician. Annals of Internal Medicine 2004;140:296–302.

[6] FDA website: http://www.fda.gov/biologicsbloodvaccines/developmentapprovalprocess/510kprocess/default.htm. Retrieved February 2013b.

[7] Federal Food, Drug and Cosmetic Act. 21 United States Code, Sec 321.

[8] Public Health Service Act. (1944). Chap. 373, Title III, Sec.351, 58: Stat. 702, 42 United States Code, Sec.262.

[9] Code of Federal Regulations. (2012a). Title 21, Part 600.3(h). Definitions. Washington, D.C. Office of the Federal Register, National Archives and Records Administration.

[10] Code of Federal Regulations. (2012b). Title 21, Part 312 and Part 800, 2012b. Definitions. Washington, D.C. Office of the Federal Register, National Archives and Records Administration.

[11] Code of Federal Regulations. (2013c). Title 21, Part 312. Definitions. Washington, D.C. Office of the Federal Register, National Archives and Records Administration.

[12] U.S. Food and Drug Administration. "FINDINGS: Issues and Communication: Independent Evaluation of FDA's First Cycle Review Performance—Final Report. http://www.fda.gov/ForIndustry/UserFees/PrescriptionDrugUserFee/ucm127153.htm. April 2013. Retrieved.

Chapter 26

The Biomanufacturing of Biotechnology Products

John Conner, MS*, Don Wuchterl**, Maria Lopez***, Bill Minshall, MS†, Rabi Prusti, PhD††, Dave Boclair†††, Jay Peterson‡ and Chris Allen, MS‡‡

*Vice President Manufacturing Science and Technology, Cytovance Biologics, Inc., Oklahoma City, Oklahoma, **Senior Vice President Operations, Cytovance Biologics Inc., Oklahoma City, Oklahoma, ***Vice President Quality Systems, Cytovance Biologics Inc., Oklahoma City, Oklahoma, †Senior Vice President Regulatory Affairs, Cytovance Biologics Inc., Oklahoma City, Oklahoma, ††Executive Director Quality Control, Cytovance Biologics Inc., Oklahoma City, Oklahoma, †††Manager Manufacturing Downstream Operations, Cytovance Biologics Inc., Oklahoma City, Oklahoma, ‡Manager Manufacturing Upstream Operations, Cytovance Biologics Inc., Oklahoma City, Oklahoma, ‡‡Senior Manager Facilities and Engineering, Cytovance Biologics Inc., Oklahoma City, Oklahoma

What is biologics manufacturing? How is it different from small molecule pharmaceutical manufacturing? Biologics manufacturing, or biomanufacturing for short, is a complex process that produces a product largely derived from discoveries using recombinant DNA technology to develop processes and analytics to manufacture biotherapeutic products. These recombinant products were developed from several platforms such as whole *multicellular* systems encompassing transgenic plants, animals and *unicellular* microbials (bacteria and yeast), and insect and mammalian cell cultures. The discovery and "proof-of-concept" from the research bench is transferred to a process and analytical group that will use science and engineering as well as regulatory experience to scale-up the product efficiently with sufficient product yield to support the clinical program and a quality product expressing the quality attributes of the product as well as profile any product-associated impurities. The process for different biologic platforms are complex and unlike traditional chemical synthesis the biologic product resulting from a living system is not as an exact science as chemistry.

The long-existing paradigm for biologics was "the process is the product" and any variation in the process could impart a change in the product's safety and efficacy. Although today's raw materials, process and analytics are better defined and allow a lot more flexibility in the design and development of the process. Changes in the process or materials could severely alter the product's safety and characteristics, thus one may end up with a product with a different profile. Changes in the manufacturing process can alter the "impurity profile" of a biologic, thus imparting changes in the product's purity which can have an adverse effect on safety. It has been demonstrated that endogenous adventitious viruses may result from processing changes or the extension of the production process. Therefore, end of production processes and genotypic studies on the cell line have been required to understand the implications of changes in the production process that can affect the product's quality attributes, impurity profiles that could impact the safety of the therapeutic. Today's biologic manufacturing facilities incorporate analytical and process development capabilities to develop and test the scale-up of the process to deliver sufficient productivity of a quality product. The development will support a Phase 1 clinical study focusing on safety and efficacy of the product. If the product can demonstrate safety and efficacy, the product with regulatory agency and business-positive feedback will continue the manufacturing of the biologics until reaching final approval and licensing.

THE HISTORY OF BIOTECHNOLOGY AND BIOMANUFACTURING

Biotechnology is technology based on biology. It utilizes the biology of living systems and their genetic manipulations of these systems and processes to develop technologies and products that help improve the lives and health of individuals worldwide. These biological processes of microorganisms have been used for thousands of years to make food products from fermentation, such as bread, beer, wine, pickles and cheese—these processes are still used today. Modern biotechnology provides discoveries of recombinant DNA technology to discover and develop therapeutic biologics. The following is a chronological history of significance to the field of biotechnology and biomanufacturing (http://www.bio.org/articles/history-biotechnology?page):

500 B.C.—In China, the first antibiotic, moldy soybean curds, is put to use to treat boils.

A.D. 100—The first insecticide is produced in China from powdered chrysanthemums.

1761—English surgeon Edward Jenner pioneers vaccination, inoculating a child with a viral smallpox vaccine.

1870—Breeders crossbreed cotton, developing hundreds of varieties with superior qualities.

1870—The first experimental corn hybrid is produced in a laboratory.

1911—American pathologist Peyton Rous discovers the first cancer-causing virus.

1928—Scottish scientist Alexander Fleming discovers penicillin.

1933—Hybrid corn is commercialized.

1942—Penicillin is mass produced in microbes for the first time.

1950s—The first synthetic antibiotic is created.

1951—Artificial insemination of livestock is accomplished using frozen semen.

1958—DNA is made in a test tube for the first time.

1978—Recombinant human insulin is produced for the first time.

1979—Human growth hormone is synthesized for the first time.

1980—Smallpox is globally eradicated following a 20-year mass vaccination effort.

1980—The U.S. Supreme Court approves the principle of patenting organisms, which allows the Exxon Oil Company to patent an oil-eating microorganism.

1981—Scientists at Ohio University produce the first transgenic animals by transferring genes from other animals into mice.

1982—The first recombinant DNA vaccine for livestock is developed.

1982—The first biotech drug, human insulin produced in genetically modified bacteria, is approved by the FDA. Genentech and Eli Lilly developed the product.

1985—Genetic markers are found for kidney disease and cystic fibrosis.

1986—The first recombinant vaccine for humans, a vaccine for hepatitis B, is approved.

1986—Interferon becomes the first anticancer drug produced through biotech.

1988—The first pest-resistant corn, Bt corn, is produced.

1990—The first successful gene therapy is performed on a 4-year-old girl suffering from an immune disorder.

1992—The FDA approves bovine somatotropin (BST) for increased milk production in dairy cows.

1993—The FDA approves Betaseron®, the first of several biotech products that have had a major impact on multiple sclerosis treatment.

1994—The first breast cancer gene is discovered.

1994—The Americas are certified polio-free by the International Commission for the Certification of Polio Eradication.

1995—Gene therapy, immune-system modulation, and recombinantly produced antibodies enter the clinic in the war against cancer.

1996—A gene associated with Parkinson's disease is discovered.

1996—The first genetically engineered crop is commercialized.

1997—A sheep named Dolly in Scotland becomes the first animal cloned from an adult cell.

1998—The FDA approves Herceptin®, a pharmacogenomic breast cancer drug for patients whose cancer overexpresses the HER2 receptor.

1999—A diagnostic test allows for the quick identification of Bovine Spongicorm Encephalopathy (BSE, also known as "mad cow" disease) and Creutzfeldt-Jakob Disease (CJD).

2000—Kenya field-tests its first biotech crop, a virus-resistant sweet potato.

2001—The FDA approves Gleevec® (imatinib), a gene-targeted drug for patients with chronic myeloid leukemia. Gleevec is the first gene-targeted drug to receive FDA approval.

2002—The EPA approves the first transgenic rootworm-resistant corn.

2002—The banteng, an endangered species, is cloned for the first time.

2003—China grants the world's first regulatory approval of the gene therapy product, Gendicine (Shenzhen SiBiono GenTech), which delivers the p53 gene as a therapy for squamous cell head and neck cancer.

2003—The Human Genome Project completes sequencing of the human genome.

2004—The United Nations Food and Agriculture Organization endorses biotech crops, stating biotechnology is a complementary tool to traditional farming methods that can help poor farmers and consumers in developing nations.

2004—The FDA approves the first antiangiogenic drug for cancer, Avastin®.

2005—The Energy Policy Act is passed and signed into law, authorizing numerous incentives for bioethanol development.

2006—The FDA approves the recombinant vaccine Gardasil®, the first vaccine developed against human papillomavirus (HPV), an infection implicated in cervical and throat cancers, and the first preventative cancer vaccine.

2006—The U.S. Department of Agriculture grants Dow AgroSciences the first regulatory approval for a plant-made vaccine.

2007—The FDA approves the H5N1 vaccine, the first vaccine approved for avian flu.

2009—Global biotech crop acreage reaches 330 million acres.

2009—The FDA approves the first genetically engineered animal for production of a recombinant form of human antithrombin.

A TYPICAL BIOMANUFACTURING PROCESS

Figures 26.1 to 26.2 show typical biomanufacturing processes for upstream processes, and regulatory milestones from preclinical, clinical, BLA, and NDA submissions.

A Typical Biologic Product Development Diagram and Regulatory Milestones from Preclinical, Clinical, BLA, and NDA Submission

There are various regulatory opinions in the United States, European, Japanese pharmaceutical industries, and other countries that regulate biologics. It is quite confusing and overlaps in opinions and redundancies. In order to bring together these regulatory authorities, the International Conference on Harmonization of Technical Requirements for Registration of Pharmaceuticals for Human Use (ICH) was formed in 1990. This organization brings together these regulatory authorities to discuss scientific and technical aspects of drug registration. Since 1990 the increase in drug development has grown globally and at an incredible pace. ICH has harmonized regulatory guidance documents to help biopharmaceutical entities to register and develop safe, quality, and effective drugs. There are guidances covering quality, safety and efficacy guidelines. Below is a list of ICH guidances that are relevant to the manufacture of a common biologic, a "therapeutic protein" known as a monoclonal antibody (mAb). The following slides lists the pertinent ICH guidance document for a mAb biomanufacturing process and the diagram illustrates the typical biomanufacturing process flow for a mAb. (See Figures 26.3A and B.)

Biotechnology products are derived from manipulation of various cells and their subsequent products these engineered cell systems produce. These biologic products are produced from various biomanufacturing platforms. One platform produces therapeutic proteins such as monoclonal antibodies, cytokines, fusion proteins, and a number of therapeutic and process enzymes. There are also vaccines, whole cell, and gene therapy products being developed and biomanufactured.

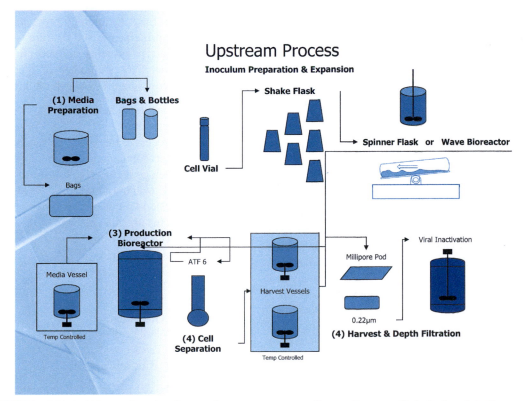

FIGURE 26.1   A Typical biomanufacturing diagram of an upstream process. (*Source: Cytovance Biologics Inc., John Conner, 2013.*)

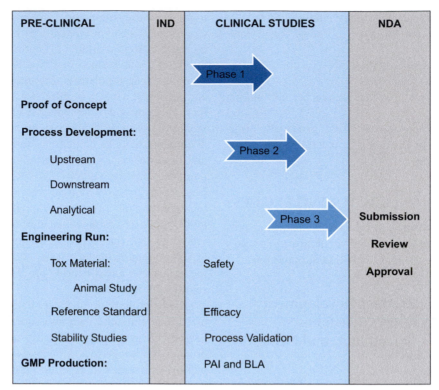

FIGURE 26.2 A typical biologic product development diagram and regulatory milestones from a preclinical, clinical, BLA, and NDA submission. (*Source: Cytovance Biologics Inc., John Conner, 2013.*)

A biologic therapeutic product, also known as a biologic, is a therapeutic product developed to treat a variety of diseases. This biologic product can be a monoclonal antibody, a vaccine, a tissue, or various proteins such as cytokines, enzymes, fusion proteins, whole cells, and viral and nonviral gene therapies. Biologic products are derived from living systems that may or may not be altered. Recombinant DNA technology has produced many biological products and has allowed research an avenue to discover many more. The paradigm for biologics "the process is the product" still is viable today. Biologics are also known as large molecules (nucleic acid and protein platforms). It is generally known that a therapeutic biologic is a product derived from or part of a cell or tissue. While the term biologic is used more often when the medical product consists of a cellular or tissue

There are several classes of biologic products. Some are naturally occurring biologics such as whole blood and blood components, organ and tissue transplantations, vaccines and recently stem cell therapy. Those therapeutic biologics that are derived via recombinant DNA technology have developed a large number of therapeutics and have replaced older naturally derived drugs with recombinant DNA technology such as "insulin" that was originally derived up until the 1980s from insulin extracted from cattle and pig pancreas (When comparing non-recombinant insulin, there are only three amino acid differences between cattle and human insulin. There are also only one amino acid difference between human and pig

insulin). Today, most insulin is biomanufactured via recombinant DNA technology or "genetic engineering."

Recombinant DNA technology products are wide ranging and include proteins derived that are monoclonal antibodies, signaling-type proteins, and receptor-type proteins.

In general here are a number of types of biologics derived from recombinant DNA technology:

- Article I. Monoclonal antibodies
- Article II. Cytokines
- Article III. Process or intermediates used in manufacturing
- Article IV. Recombinant proteins
- Article V. Therapeutic vaccines
- Article VI. Growth hormones
- Article VII. Blood production-stimulating proteins
- Article VIII. Insulin and analogs
- Article IX. Therapeutic enzymes
- Article X. Fusion proteins
- Article XI. Therapeutic peptides
- Article XII. Therapeutic oligos
- Article XIII. Vaccines
- Article XIV. Gene therapy
- Article XV. Whole cells
- Article XVI. Tissues
- Article XVII. Biosimilars

A biologic can be defined as a large complex molecule produced from or extracted from a biological or living system.

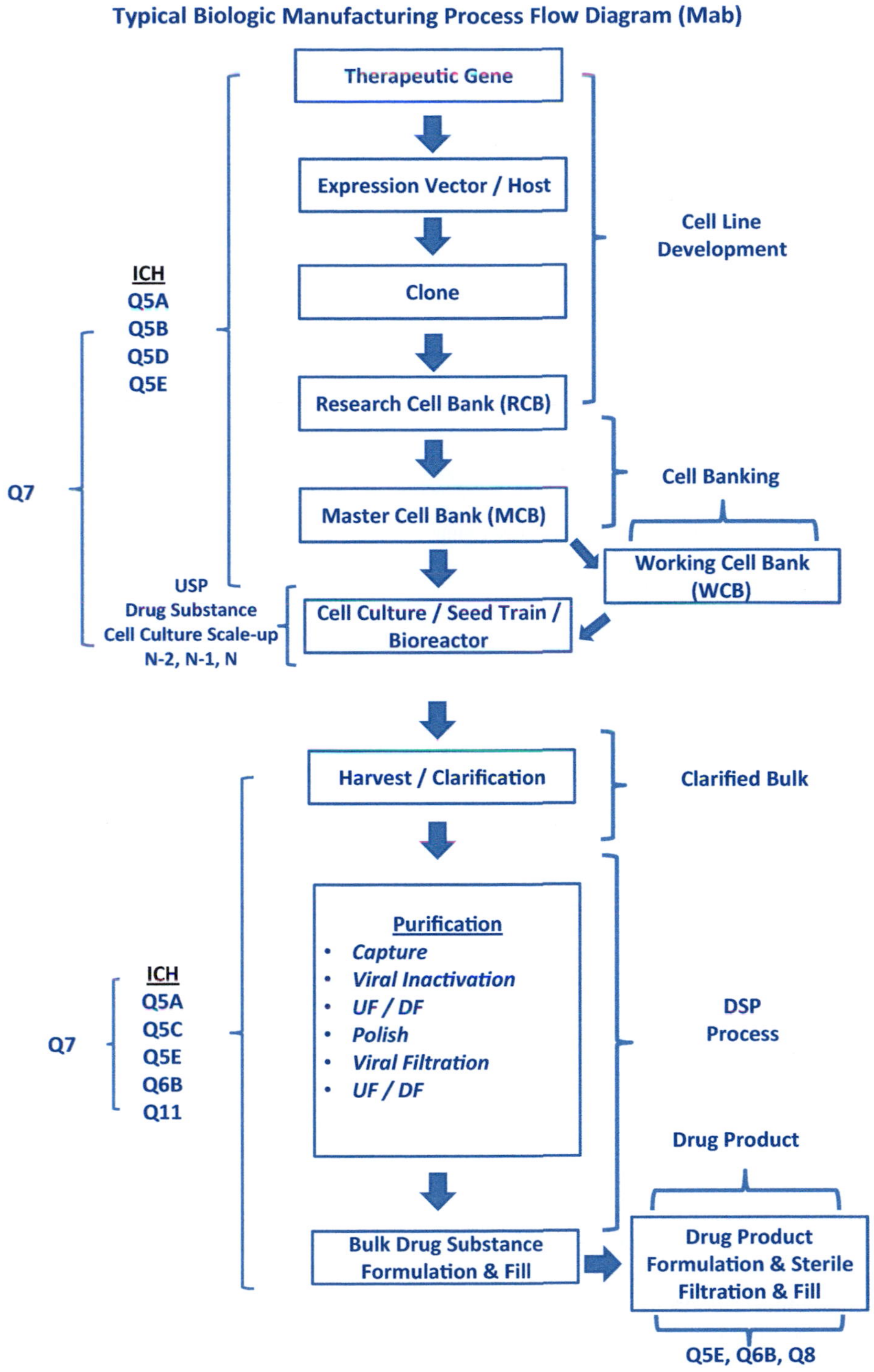

Typical Biologic Manufacturing Process Flow Diagram (Mab)

FIGURE 26.3 A typical biologic manufacturing process flow diagram with appropriate ICH guidance per steps. *(Source: Cytovance Biologics Inc., John Conner, 2013.)*

The biomanufacturing process, process controls as well as the complete physiochemical and biological testing all together characterize the biologic product. For example, in regards to the biomanufacturing process, a biologic can be derived from biotechnology or it may be prepared using more conventional methods as is the case for blood- or plasma-derived products and a number of vaccines. In regards to the nature of a biologic's active substance, it may consist entirely of microorganisms or mammalian cells, nucleic acids (DNA or RNA), be a protein (antibody, cytokine, enzyme, protein-like, etc.) all originating from either a microbial, animal, human, or plant sources.

TABLE 26.1 A Variety of Biologics

Designation	Name	Indication	Technology	Mechanism of Action
Abatacept	Orencia	Rheumatoid arthritis	Immunoglobin CTLA-4 fusion protein	T-cell deactivation
Adalimumab	Humira	Rheumatoid arthritis, ankylosing spondylitis, psoriatic arthritis, psoriasis, Crohn's disease	Monoclonal antibody	TNF antagonist
Alefacept	Amevive	Chronic plaque psoriasis	Immunoglobin G1 fusion protein	Incompletely characterized
Erythropoietin	Epogen	Anemia arising from cancer chemotherapy, chronic renal failure, etc.	Recombinant protein	Stimulation of red blood cell production
Etanercept	Enbrel	Rheumatoid arthritis, ankylosing spondylitis, psoriatic arthritis, psoriasis	Recombinant human TNF-receptor fusion protein	TNF antagonist
Infliximab	Remicade	Rheumatoid arthritis, ankylosing spondylitis, psoriatic arthritis, psoriasis, Crohn's disease	Monoclonal antibody	TNF antagonist
Trastuzumab	Herceptin	Breast cancer	Humanized monoclonal antibody	HER2/neu (erbB2) antagonist
Ustekinumab	Stelara	Psoriasis	Humanized monoclonal antibody	IL-12 and IL-23 antagonist
Denileukin	Ontak	Cutaneous T-cell	Diphtheria toxin	Interleukin-2
Diftitox		Lymphoma (CTCL)	Engineered protein combining Interleukin-2 and Diphtheria toxin	Receptor binder

(**Source:** *http://en.wikipedia.org/wiki/Monoclonal_antibody_therapy#FDA_approved_therapeutic_antibodies*.)

A biologics mode of action may describe a biologic platform such as an immunotherapeutic, gene therapy or a cellular therapeutic. (See Table 26.1.)

BIOSIMILARS

What is a biosimilar? How is it different than a generic? Generic is the designation for (off-patent) small-molecule drugs that are exactly identical to the properties and the process to manufacture is the same and reproducible. In essence, chemically synthesized drugs are pretty much: add component A + B = C (product) almost all of the time. Biosimilars are much more complex and larger molecules can be influenced by the manufacturing process. Because of the biologics complexity, biosimilar manufacturers cannot guarantee that their biosimilar is exactly identical to the original manufacturer's version, but rather it is similar to the original biologic. The biosimilar manufacturer's manufacturing process may be slightly different. This may produce significantly different effects which may impact product quality, have no effect, or in some cases elicit additional quality attributes—now you have a biobetter, thus requiring

clinical development. A disadvantage of the biosimilar developer is that in developing the innovator's process to produce the biosimilar, the innovator's starting material, i.e., the recombinant cell line or clone, is not available to the developer unlike generics where raw materials and process chemicals are known or can be derived. Finally, the impurity profiles may impart a variety of similar impurities or degradation products that may elicit harmful side-effects.

Thus, biosimilar manufacturers produce products that are slightly different than the innovator's and cannot guarantee that their biosimilar is as safe and effective as the innovator's product. So, unlike generics, biosimilars were not authorized in the United States or the European Union through the procedures that allowed generic approvals. So as a result, to date all biosimilar drugs have targeted well-known approved and coming off patent biologic drugs. The regulatory agencies have required biosimilar therapeutics to undergo a very detailed comparability review and testing. In 2012, the United States Federal Drug Agency (U.S. FDA) published a guidance as part of the "Patient Protection and Affordable Care Act of 2010" part of the Public Health Service Act (PHS Act) which was created to provide an approval pathway known as the Biologics Price Competition and Innovation Act (BPCI Act). This approach or law allows for a potential approval of biological products that can demonstrate "biosimilar" properties that are "very similar" to the original biologic or one that "closely resembles" the FDA-licensed biological product.

The European regulatory authority (EMA) has provided an approach and coined their biosimilar as "similar biological medicinal products." Their document guides biosimilar companies in the manufacture and approval of these complex biologics to demonstrate comprehensive comparability of the biosimilar to the innovator's product. The European Medicines Agency (EMA) accomplished this well before the FDA. Thus, the EU has been further ahead of the United States in biosimilars with the EMA approving the first biosimilar "Omnitrope" in 2006. In June 2010, a biosimilar copy of Amgen's Neupogen was approved and since then a total of 12 biosimilars have been approved between 2006 and 2012. In July 2013, two monoclonal antibody (mAb) biosimilars (Remsima-Celltrion and Inflectra-Hospira) were approved by the EMA. These mAbs were very similar to the innovator molecule known as Remicade (infliximab) originally approved in 1999 for rheumatoid arthritis, Crohn's disease, ulcerative colitis, psoriatic arthritis, and psoriasis. All of these diseases are classified as autoimmune diseases.

Therefore, a biosimilar product is similar to a biologic reference or innovator product, has the same mechanism of action for the intended use, preapproved label use, has the same route of administration, dose formulation, and has similar potency or strength as the reference or innovator product. The biosimilar also should show no clinical differences between the biosimilar and the innovator product in terms of the safety, purity, and potency.

Therefore, the regulatory theme for the manufacture and approval is midway between testing and comparability for a new therapeutic biologic and more than the testing of a generic drug. Comprehensive comparability is the key! Below is a list of classes of biologics that are in the current biologic development or have been approved:

- Epoetins
- Filgrastims
- Insulins
- Growth hormones
- Monoclonal antibodies
- Low-molecular weight heparins
- Beta interferons

Key Phases of Biologics Development

The biologic product to be developed and manufactured starts with the discovery and proof-of-concept studies characterizing the product as well as defining the actual molecule and its mode of action. The study and knowledge of the molecule's characteristics will be important in designing cell culture and bioreactor parameters in order to scale-up and produce a sufficient yield of product to satisfy early experiments and analytical development. This crude product will also be used for early clarification, downstream process development, and formulation studies. During the discovery phase *in vitro* and *in vivo* (small animal) studies will be performed. Once the product proof-of-concept is achieved, a decision to move forward with process development and the eventual investigational new drug (IND) finally is agreed upon. In today's drug development world, the next step is to secure funding to continue developing the therapeutic. This usually involves forming a company and securing funding from private sources, venture capital or government grants. Most of these companies don't have sufficient funding to build development, manufacturing and quality laboratories nor the time it takes to build this infrastructure. These companies partner with Contract Manufacturing Organizations (CMOs) to help develop and manufacture the drug as well as offer Quality and Regulatory support.

DISCOVERY

Target identification of a therapeutic biologic molecule involves choosing a disease with an unmet need or an improvement of a current therapeutic, and usually the group or person may have a personal or scientific interest in studying and developing a drug candidate. These biologic drugs are usually discovered in academic and biotech research labs. Once a molecule is chosen, the biochemical mechanism and other biological characteristics are tested for their interaction with the drug or disease target. There are thousands of biologic molecules studied and they go through a very arduous process to profile and characterize the molecule and its potential drug or disease target. Proof-of-concept *in vitro* and *in vivo* (small animals such as rodents) must be validated before any drug can move from discovery and into a clinical development program. Once a promising therapeutic candidate or several leading candidates are validated, the company or group will set up and budget a preclinical development program.

PROCESS DEVELOPMENT

All biologic products transition from bench scale research and proof-of-concept to the next stage of product development called process and analytical development. The therapeutic protein candidate's characteristics, purification strategies, analytical methods for in-process and final product characterization, and any stability data are supplied to the process and analytical development groups. This is typically called the technology transfer or "tech transfer." The tech transfer is the most important phase of product development as it is the hand-off to the scale-up team (process and analytical development—PD and AD respectfully), manufacturing science and technology (MST), manufacturing and quality assurance (QA), and quality control (QC) teams. A thorough understanding of the product's characteristics and the process at bench scale is necessary in order to facilitate the transfer of all of the critical parameters.

Once the tech transfer is initiated from the client, the upstream process development (USP), or cell culture group, embarks on accessing the media and cell culture conditions relative to the correct identification (ID) of the cell line, the growth and viability of the cell line is robust, and the productivity of the cell line's product (therapeutic protein) titer (yield) is adequate to scale-up. Once, the cell line and growth conditions are confirmed, the PD group will make a development cell bank from the research cell bank (RCB) and will use this to develop a scale-up process and optimize the media and supplements used in the cell culture. The USP development will also make material to be used in the downstream process development (DSP) which is the purification and formulation development group. This group will also work on the postharvest clarification (removal of the cells and other large molecules as well as some large protein and DNA aggregates) prior to the first chromatography or purification steps. The first steps post clarification is usually a capture- or affinity-binding step. In essence the therapeutic protein is bound to a chromatographic resin's (example Protein A mAbSelect Sure™ from General Electric (GE) packed in a column allowing for impurities to flow through the column. The bound therapeutic protein (TP) is then pulled off or eluted from the resin and collected for the purification steps which takes the TP through various chromatographic column steps to remove impurities and aggregates such as host cell proteins (HCP) and host DNA. All of these chromatographic purification and polishing steps are designed based on the protein properties and characteristics described during the discovery bench scale or preclinical phase of the product development. The DSP also will include viral clearance studies to reduce the risk of viral contaminants. Several resins or filters significantly reduce viral load or give "x amount of Log reduction of virus." The DSP team also develops the formulation steps for bulk drug substance (BDS) and the final formulation of the drug product (DP) and excipients (other materials in the formulation that impart a property such as providing stability to the DP). During the DSP process, the development and optimization of the DSP team will provide the analytical development team process/product material to work on designing, confirming, qualifying, or validating analytical methods needed for in-process and release testing.

As the process development phase of the product development proceeds the manufacturing science and technology group will work with the PD and AD teams to capture and work on the tech transfer from the development groups into the manufacturing and quality groups.

CLINICAL MANUFACTURING
Preclinical Trials

In the preclinical phase the product is further characterized. The biologic molecule's phenotypic, genotypic, and biochemical profiles must be determined. Attributes and parameters useful in determining its strengths and weaknesses such as shape, amino acid sequence, isoelectric point (PI), drug candidates mechanism of action, its potential bioactivity or availability, and any possible toxicity issues are some of the characterizations that will need to be studied or elucidated. These will be the building blocks of information that will be transferred to other groups responsible for process and analytical development.

How are we going to manufacture the novel therapeutic biologic? During this phase a process is developed to scale-up the process to manufacture a quality product that can be used in a Phase 1 clinical trial. Typically a master cell bank (MCB) will be produced from a research cell bank (RCB) or a pre-MCB. A working cell bank (WCB) may be produced from a MCB that has been fully tested for bio-safety and has also been fully characterized. If a WCB is produced it to will be tested as the MCB was tested for bio-safety and characterized as defined per the Q7 ICH Guidance. These cells will be used in PD DEMO (demonstration) runs and the data from the PD work will be transferred (tech transfer) to manufacturing. Concurrently analytical development will be working on developing and qualifying in-process and release analytics which will then be transferred into quality control (QC).

Manufacturing scientists and engineers will then take the process and design a scale-up plan and tech transfer into manufacturing. The first run will be a non-GMP engineering run that will lead to a GMP run. Typically the engineering run is a process dress rehearsal for the Good Manufacturing Practice (GMP) run. This run will manufacture products for:

- Toxicology-primate study
- Viral clearance/validation
- Reference standard
- Stability studies
- Storage
- Shipping
- Container closure DBS and DP
- Analytical development (ex bioassays)
- Other analytical methods work
  - Compendial
  - Method qualification/validation work

The GMP run will be prepared by reviewing the engineering run outcome based on the process review, in-process data, and final testing of the product. The engineering run will be deemed successful and ready for GMP production if there are no major process or testing issues and the product has met all of its quality parameters allowing for the release of the drug substance and if the drug product is formulated to pass all of the acceptance criteria which would allow for the product to be released. The documents would be revised and updated from the engineering run redlined batch records. The final production records would be reviewed and approved for GMP production. The GMP run would provide material to support the following needed for IND filing and the start of the Phase 1 clinical trial:

- Clinical Trial Material
- Stability
- Reference standard
- End-of-production (EOP) cell bank
- Genetic stability

The GMP clinical trial material is held in quarantine at the biomanufacturing site and when it passes all of the release testing and document review, the GMP lot will be released to the in-house clinical distribution group for clinical studies once the IND is approved. The clinical trials are usually managed by the in-house clinical group or outsourced to companies like Almac, Quintiles, or Covance.

Another important part of the preclinical phase of the product development is drug formulation and drug delivery. How are we going to present this drug to the patient's biologic system? Formulation, delivery, and container/closure development must be studied at this early stage. If you cannot develop a stable formulation matrix and do not know the delivery path, the drug candidate development will be delayed or stopped. Formulation and the product's delivery parameter development is a critical element that must be developed and understood. The key is stability (biosafety and product maintains its quality attributes) of the drug candidate's formulation, safety as determined initially by biosafety testing of the bulk, and final product. It must also be noted that this formulation and drug delivery system may be revised during the development of the product.

Once formulated, several other important studies are important to develop and understand the formulated biologic drug. Pharmacokinetic (PK) studies look at absorption, drug distribution, metabolism of the drug, and the excretion or elimination of the biologic drug. Why is this important? PK data from animal toxicity (TOX) studies (product produced from non-GMP scale-up or engineering run) will be used to compare to the eventual early-phase studies. These preclinical TOX studies are typically dosing studies (acute and chronic dosing that help determine the specific dose and range in the animal TOX and first in the human Phase I clinical study). Other toxicity studies look at carcinogenic, mutagenic, and reproductive toxicity. This should give an idea of the potential degree of safety and efficacy of the formulated drug candidate as well as a foundation to support the process development, analytical

development, and the investigational new drug (IND) application filing. Once filed and approved, the preclinical and discovery information will help support the clinical development of the biologic drug. *Note:* all of the proposed preclinical toxicity studies are actual guidances from various regulatory agencies.

In order to understand and support the product characteristics and quality attributes and support preclinical and clinical in-process and release testing bioanalytical testing must be developed in the preclinical phase of the biologics development. Thus the analytical development group will support methods for cell culture, fermentation, assay to determine titers or process yields as well as bioassays, and other assays to elicit the identity, potency, purity, and safety of the product (e.g., in monoclonal antibodies [mAbs]) to use size exclusion chromatography (SEC) to determine the percent of purity by evaluating the amount of aggregation and other product impurities. It is important to understand the impurity profile of the product and the final formulated product.

CLINICAL TRIALS

Clinical studies are grouped according to their objective into three types or phases (Phase 1, 2, and 3). How does biomanufacturing activities correlate to the different phases of a clinical trial leading up to the commercialization of a biologic product? Manufacturing of the therapeutic biologic will continue through the prelinical and clinical phase of the trial to supply the clinic with the trial product to the patients enrolled in the clinical study, stability programs, additional reference standards, additional process optimization studies, and additional studies as needed to support investigations.

Phase 1 Clinical Development

Thirty days after a "biotech" company has filed its IND, it may begin a small-scale Phase 1 clinical trial to demonstrate human pharmacology and safety. Phase 1 parameters such as pharmacokinetic (PK) and tolerance in healthy recruited volunteers will be studied. These studies include acute and chronic dosing studies including initial single-dose, a dose escalation, and repeated-dose studies.

Phase 2 Clinical Development

Phase 2 clinical studies are small-scale trials to continue to evaluate the safety and PK of the biologic and also to evaluate the efficacy and possible side-effects in a small set of patients (commonly 100 to 200). Typical Phase 2 objectives are:

- Safety
- Efficacy
- Risk assessment
- Process review
- Raw materials

- Analaytical methods
- BDS container closure
- DP container closure
- Storage
- Shipping
- Phase 2b (Phase 2a and b review and requirements to move to Phase 3)

Phase 3 Clinical Development

Phase 3 studies are large-scale clinical trials for continued safety and efficacy in a larger patient population. While Phase 3 studies are in progress, there are several interim analyses available to show continued safety and efficacy. During this phase the final process is determined and "locked down." A gap analysis of the process to support process validation is conducted and any gaps or risks are addressed. Process validation commences, and if all goes well the company will commence manufacturing of the three registration or conformance lots prior to the filing of a Biologics License Application (BLA) or a New Drug Application (NDA). Typical Phase 3 objectives are:

- Safety
- Efficacy
- Risk assessment
- Lock down process
- Process and analytical gap analysis (FMEA)
- Process validation
- Minimum 3 conformance or registration lots
- BLA submission
- PAI facility and quality assessment inspection
- BLA approval
- Secondary labeling and packaging-approval
- Inventory build

Phase 4 Marketing

Prepare for Commercial Launch and Commercial Manufacturing

Once a BLA and NDA have been approved, the biotech company will be seeking to launch the released drug product in the approved market. The inventory to launch may be the three conformance lots or other released lots manufactured in anticipation of an approved license to manufacture, distribute, and market the new drug.

GOOD MANUFACTURING PRACTICES

Requirements

Biologics manufacturing requires the use of good manufacturing practices (GMP) or current good manufacturing practices (cGMP) to ensure that adequate history is maintained for each product run. As the product

manufacturing process is developed and defined and as it matures from the lab bench development through Phases 1, 2, and 3, the regulatory expectation is that appropriate GMP be applied to help ensure subject safety. This is especially critical at Phase 1 where the clinical trial focus is safety and efficacy.

In order to support clinical trial drugs, manufacturers are expected to implement manufacturing controls that reflect product and manufacturing considerations, evolving process and product knowledge, and manufacturing experience. As the process becomes better-defined, critical control points are identified, and experience in the process increases, increased GMP documentation must be implemented and maintained. This means that information that is gained from the lab development bench scale all the way through Phase 3 trials must be translated into compliant GMP documents that house product production history.

Code of Federal Regulations and European Regulations

The United States Food and Drug Administration (FDA) and the European Union provide regulations for the manufacture of drug products. These are the laws that biologics manufacturers are required to follow.

The FDA regulations are defined in 21 CFR 210, "Current Good Manufacturing Practice in Manufacturing, Processing, Packaging, or Holding of Drugs; General" and 21CFR211, "Current Good Manufacturing Practices for Finished Pharmaceuticals." EU regulations are defined in the EudraLex, Volume 4, "EU Guidelines to Good Manufacturing Practice Medicinal Products for Human and Veterinary Use."

Additionally, the United States publishes guidance documents that provide the agencies current thinking on topics. These guidance documents provide valuable details into how the agencies expect manufacturers to show compliance to the regulations. The most used guidance documents can be found at http://www.fda.gov/Drugs/GuidanceCompli-anceRegulatoryInformation/Guidances/ucm065005.htm. Here is a list of the ICH Guidances specifically related to Quality and Manufacturing of Biologics:

FDA Guidance for Industry—Q7A Good Manufacturing Practice Guidance for Active Pharmaceutical Ingredients, August 2001
FDA Guidance for Industry—Q8 (R2) Pharmaceutical Development
FDA Guidance for Industry—Q9 Quality Risk Management
FDA Guidance for Industry—Q10 Pharmaceutical Quality System
FDA Guidance for Industry—Q11 Development and Manufacture of Drug Substances

FDA Guidance for Industry—Sterile Drug Products Produced by Aseptic Processing—Current Good Manufacturing Practices

FDA Guidance for Industry—CGMP for Phase 1 Investigational Drugs

FDA Guidance for Industry—Investigating Out-of-Specification (OOS) Test Results for Pharmaceutical Production

FDA Guidance for Industry—Process Validation: General Principles and Practices

EU Guidelines to Good Manufacturing Practice—Annex 1, Manufacture of Sterile Medicinal Products

EU Guidelines to Good Manufacturing Practice—Annex 12, Investigational Medicinal Products.

Oversight and Compliance

Regulatory compliance in biologics manufacturing requires that the implemented quality unit and system be robust enough to support product production throughout its clinical phase maturation.

The quality unit is expected to be independent of the operations/manufacturing unit and that it fulfills both the quality assurance and quality control responsibilities. Their roles and responsibilities should be defined and documented. Critical roles of the quality unit are the review and approval of all quality-related documents; disposition of raw materials, intermediates, packaging, labeling materials, and the final product; conduct internal and supplier audits; review completed batch production and laboratory control records before determining disposition; approve changes that could potentially affect the intermediate and final product; and ensure the complete investigation and resolution into deviations and complaints.

In biologics manufacturing, especially with Phase 1 material, not all critical parameters, control points, and at times raw material may all be defined or identified. Knowing this and knowing that the process will continue to grow through its clinical phases, oversight from the quality unit must ensure that the manufacturing process adheres to the foundational components of GMPs. These foundational components are those that ensure full support of the product production and are maintained within the quality system. All components of the quality system are controlled through written and approved policies and procedures.

Documentation

Change control—A system established to evaluate all changes that could affect the production and control of the product.

Personnel—A system for maintaining and evaluating personnel qualifications and training for job-related functions

Building and facilities—Systems that provide evidence of the adequacy of the facility. These systems include at minimum, design, qualification, calibration, cleaning, maintenance, and monitoring.

Laboratory control records—Systems that ensure records include complete data derived from all tests conducted to ensure compliance with established specification and standards.

Batch records and specifications—A system that ensures that documents related to the manufacture of intermediates and product be prepared, reviewed, approved, and distributed according to written procedures.

Materials management—A system for the receipt, identification, quarantine, storage, handling, sampling, testing, and disposition of material.

Production and process controls—A system for the control of critical steps such as weight and measurement; time limits; in-process sample testing; and contamination control.

FACILITY REQUIREMENTS

The facility and the utility requirements are the fundamental backbone of the process flow and production effectiveness. In facility design, it is important to consider the regulatory nature of the industry and seeking some in-depth knowledge of the requirements will pay big dividends in the long run. Let's briefly look at a few of these systems and their importance to the overall health of the business platform. (See Figures 26.4A and B.)

Air-Handling Equipment

Large volumes of air are required to properly satisfy the international standards for clean room air. This is an area where many people may underestimate their current and future needs. This can be a costly upfront mistake and can further restrict a company's ability to grow additional revenue streams. Industry air flow standards are dictated by international standards. Air flows dictate cleanroom classifications. Current classifications and room air changes per hour are found in Table 26.2.

These clean air room classifications must be considered as they dictate the allowable operations in each area. Due to the large volumes of air flows, building chilling capacity must be a strategic part of the facility design as well.

Process Water (Purified Water [PW] and Water for Injection [WFI])

Another crucial element in the success of your production processes is the demand and need for ultra-pure water, which cannot be overstated. Purified water is to be used for

(A)

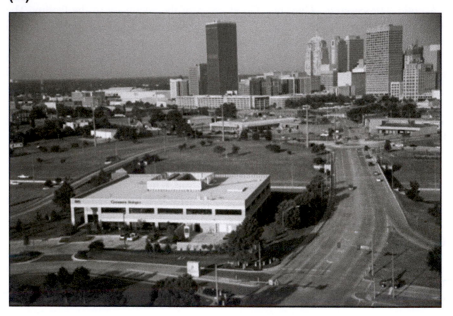

(B)

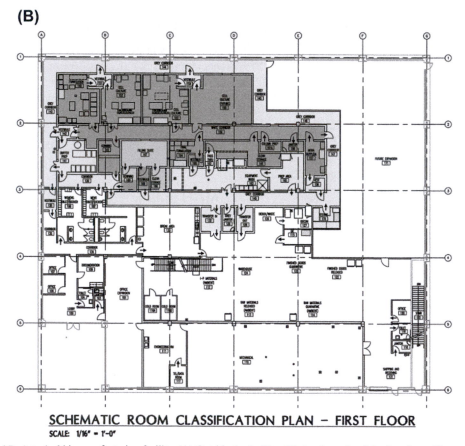

SCHEMATIC ROOM CLASSIFICATION PLAN – FIRST FLOOR
SCALE: 1/16" = 1'-0"

FIGURE 26.4 A and B. A typical biomanufacturing facility. (A) Outside the facility. (B) A schematic of the first floor. *(Source: Cytovance Biologics Inc., 2013.)*

TABLE 26.2 International Air Flow Standards for Cleanrooms: Current Classifications and Room Air Changes

FS Cleanroom Class	ISO Equivalent Class	Air Change Rate (per hour)
1	ISO 3	360–540
10	ISO 4	300–540
100	ISO 5	240–480
1,000	ISO 6	150–240
10,000	ISO 7	60–90
100,000	ISO 8	5–48

Source: IEST. *http://www.iest.org/Standards-RPs/ISO-Standards/ISO-14644-Standards.*

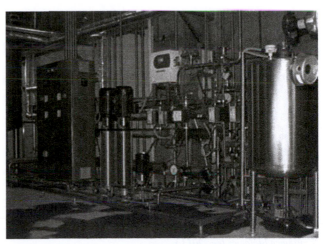

FIGURE 26.6   Typical water for injection system. *(Source: Water Sciences.* http://www.watersciences.biz/Purified_Water_Generation_Plant.html.*)*

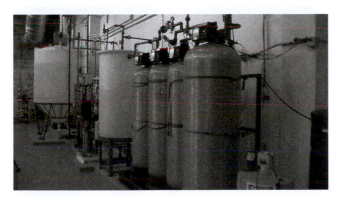

FIGURE 26.5 A typical purified water system. *(Source: Cytovance Biologics Inc., 2013.)*

the production of USP products. Purified water and sterile purified water may be obtained by any suitable process (see Figure 26.5). Water for injection is water purified by distillation or reverse osmosis (see Figure 26.6). As cost is an important factor in the implementation of these systems, at a minimum, a healthy Reverse Osmosis Deionized water (RO/DI) or distillation system should be utilized. Attention should be given to the design and installation of this critical system. Details such as storage, sanitization, number of water loops (ambient and hot), and the number of water drops need to be carefully planned in advance. In addition, the maintenance of the purified water systems is the most important element of continuously producing USP-acceptable water to support the facility's biological manufacturing processes.

Building Automation and Alarm Systems (BAS)

Proper building automation and alarming is paramount to effective and efficient operations. Clients and auditors will want to see if you have control of critical facility and

process-related parameters such as differential pressures, temperatures, humidity, pressure, flows, and more. There are many off-the-shelf systems that provide control and capture of important and useful information. Skillful use of automation and alarms can quickly pay dividends in facility utility costs. In addition, these automation software packages provide tools for trending, tracking, and troubleshooting various production-related applications. Building automation and alarm systems is an essential part of a current good manufacturing practices enterprise.

Additional Facility Requirements

In addition to the above referenced critical systems, there are many areas of consideration when designing or operating a compliant good manufacturing facility and organization. Topics noteworthy of additional study are included, but not limited to: cleanliness, validation and commissioning, process-material personnel and air flows, cold storage, dry storage, emergency procedures, safety, security, pest control, environmental monitoring, preventive maintenance and calibrations, and all possible redundancies that may be required to support utility and processes.

THE BIOMANUFACTURING TEAM—THEIR TYPICAL ROLES AND RESPONSIBILITIES IN A BIOLOGICS MANUFACTURING FACILITY

Manufacturing-related Functions

Manufacturing-related positions typically make up the majority of positions in a biologics manufacturing facility. These can be classified as positions that directly interact with the manufacturing process. Typical functions include

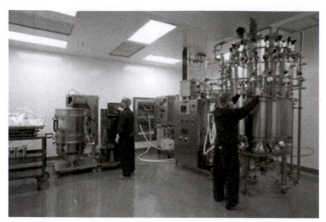

FIGURE 26.7   Upstream manufacturing: bioreactor operations. *(Source: Cytovance Biologics Inc., 2013.)*

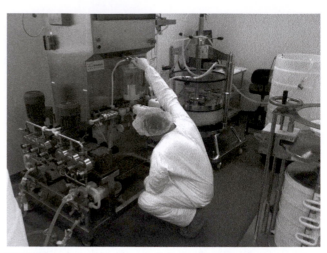

FIGURE 26.8   Downstream manufacturing: chromatography operations. *(Source: Cytovance Biologics Inc., 2013.)*

upstream manufacturing, downstream manufacturing (purification), fill/finish operations, a manufacturing support team, and a manufacturing technical support function.

Upstream Manufacturing

Upstream manufacturing responsibilities routinely include operations related to cell expansion steps starting with a single vial of frozen cells and growing these exponentially into larger and larger systems eventually reaching your large-scale terminal reactor where the targeted protein is expressed. These operations require highly skilled specialists trained in microbiological processes, Good Manufacturing Practices (GMPs), fermenter and bioreactor systems, automation systems, and in-process analysis instruments. While not always required, typical employees will have a bachelor's degree in biology, microbiology, or a similar science. (See Figure 26.7.)

Downstream Manufacturing

Downstream manufacturing, or commonly referred to as purification, is focused on the capture and isolation of a targeted molecule and the removal of impurities. This is accomplished through several different processes to include filtration, column chromatography, and tangential flow filtration (TFF). These operations also require highly skilled specialists trained in chemical properties, chromatography, TFF, filtration systems, Good Manufacturing Practices (GMPs), automation systems, and in-process analysis instruments. Typical employees will have a bachelor's degree in chemistry, chemical engineering, biology, or a similar science. (See Figure 26.8.)

Production Support

The production support function is commonly utilized in biologics manufacturing facilities. While these functions can be performed by the upstream and downstream

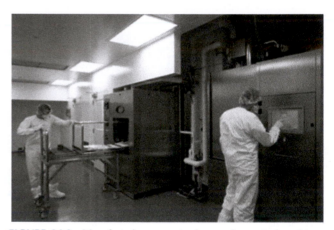

FIGURE 26.9   Manufacturing support: glass washer, autoclave (steam sterilizer), and prep area. *(Source: Cytovance Biologics Inc., 2013.)*

functions, the amount of coordination and activity in these areas would usually warrant a separate team. These functions perform a variety of supporting tasks to include: media and buffer preparation, equipment and component preparation, chemical dispensing, equipment and environmental cleaning, and some in-process testing. Associates on this team are trained in the use of glass washers, autoclaves, solution prep equipment, and Good Manufacturing Practices (GMPs). Typical employees will have a bachelor's degree in science or engineering. (See Figure 26.9.)

Fill/Finish Operations

The fill/finish team is a specialized function within the manufacturing team dedicated to the manufacture of the drug product. A drug product refers to the final formulated product in its delivery container. In most cases for biologic products, these will be traditional glass vials. Other systems include prefilled syringes or intravenous (IV) bags. As these steps in the process are the last manufacturing

(A)

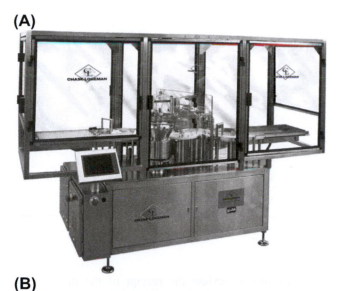

(B)

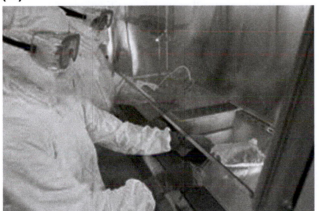

FIGURE 26.10 (A) Fill/finish operations: Chase Logeman automated vial fill machine. (*Source: Cytovance Biologics Inc. and Chase Logeman, 2013.*) (B) Fill/Finish Operations. (*Source: Cytovance Biologics Inc., 2013.*)

steps, they must be performed in highly contained environments. Typically these areas will be the cleanest areas in the facility with the highest levels of control. (See Figure 26.10A and B.)

Manufacturing Technical Support (MTS)

The MTS function provides scientific support to the manufacturing team. Their roles include tech transfer activities from the process development group, new equipment identification and qualification, on the floor support for complex process steps, troubleshooting complex process related issues, and support technical investigations. Skilled specialists and engineers on this team are familiar with the scientific principles related to one or more areas of a traditional process. They are also skilled and knowledgeable on the process equipment utilized throughout the process train. Specialists on this team will typically have many years of relevant experience as well

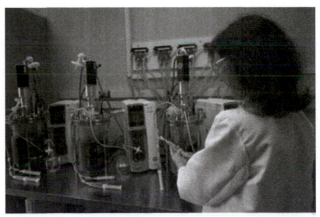

FIGURE 26.11 Manufacturing technical support. (*Source: Cytovance Biologics Inc., 2013.*)

as bachelor's level degrees in a scientific discipline (many have advanced degrees). (See Figure 26.11).

Quality Assurance

One of the most important functions in a biologics manufacturing facility is the quality unit. As this is a heavily regulated industry, a robust internal quality system is required to ensure adherence to all regulations as well as patient safety. Quality assurance provides a fully independent look at all documentation, production areas, and supply chain functions to ensure compliance. Quality is responsible for ensuring all raw materials, procedures, and areas are released for production. They will also perform reviews of all documentation, quality control samples, and final release specifications before approving a batch for release. Typically the quality unit will be the second largest function in the facility behind the manufacturing staff. Specialists on this team will typically have bachelor's degrees in a scientific discipline.

Quality Control

The quality control unit is responsible for performing testing on raw materials, in-process and final product testing, and environmental monitoring activities in a biologics facility. Analysts on this team will typically have bachelor's or master's degrees in chemistry, biology, microbiology, or engineering. (See Figure 26.12).

Facilities and Engineering

The facilities and engineering teams oversee all of the key systems required to keep the manufacturing plant operational. This includes base building systems, process equipment, utilities, building automation, and heating, ventilation, and air conditioning (HVAC). They also perform routine and nonroutine maintenance activities on the aforementioned systems. These teams are staffed with skilled

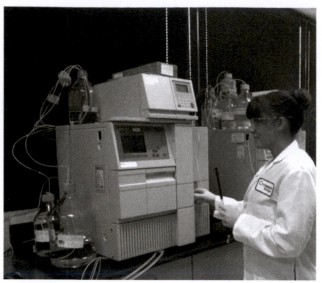

FIGURE 26.12 A quality control laboratory. *(Source: Cytovance Biologics Inc., 2013.)*

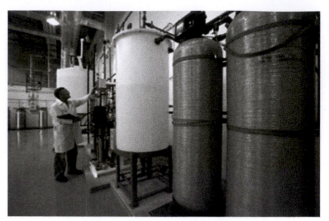

FIGURE 26.13 Facilities and engineering. *(Source: Cytovance Biologics Inc. 2013.)*

trade's people, plant and process engineers, and calibration (metrology) professionals. (See Figure 26.13.)

Supply Chain

The supply chain function is responsible for the procurement, warehousing, delivery, and management of all materials used in the process. This includes all shipping and receiving activities for raw materials as well as finished products.

MATERIAL MANAGEMENT

Materials utilized in the production of biological manufacturing is required to be controlled through documented systems that ensure adequate controls beginning from vendor selection through receipt, inspection, and release for use.

All raw materials should be acquired from a reputable source that has been audited and approved by quality assurance. The raw materials should be animal-component free. An audit of all product contact materials should be performed and animal-component free statements acquired from the manufacturer. All materials should have manufacturer specifications and certificates-of-acceptance (COAs) when received. Material specifications are required to be established for all materials utilized in the manufacture of the product. These specifications should include COAs, certificates-of-sterility, and requirements for any testing and release of the material. The specifications will be used by manufacturing and the supply chain or purchasing department to acquire the appropriate material for GMP manufacturing. Once the material is ordered, the receiving department will use the purchase order and the material

specifications to review the receipt of the material and ensure that it meets all material specifications.

It is important that the quality system that governs material management include controls to determine sampling requirements and quantities required per the vendor lot. These requirements can be found in the United States and the EU regulations and guidance documents. Raw material sampling and testing is required for all phases of clinical trials and the expectation is that a robust sampling program be implemented prior to commercialization of the product.

Raw material specifications will spell out the incoming sampling for ID testing and the storage conditions, and will require a COA from the vendor. All raw materials should be sampled and tested per the material specifications. The impact of a raw material that is not ID tested or any quality attribute could have a significant impact in the production of the product or its release. Not vetting the raw material ID or quality will impact Phase 2 and 3 clinical trials. Any issues during these late phase trials could have a significant setback to the development of the drug product. (See Figures 26.14 and 26.15.)

BIOLOGICS DRUG SUBSTANCE MANUFACTURING

An example of a typical biologics manufacturing process is shown in Figure 26.16.

Upstream Biologics Manufacturing

Cell Banking

Biotechnology requires the creation of a cell that has the capabilities to produce the monoclonal antibodies (mAbs) or proteins desired for use. These cells are created by transfecting the required genes with a marker into a host cell. Once this transfection has been completed, cells that exhibit the traits of the marker that was introduced are isolated and

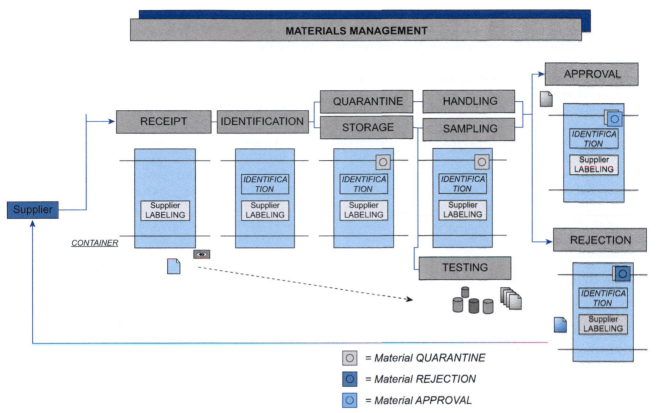

FIGURE 26.14   Materials management flow chart. *(Source:* http://2.bp.blogspot.com/-HLm1RlaWsN8/UArpSsteZII/AAAAAAAABJk/xLZIA9oulow/
s1600/MATERIAL+MANAGEMENT.JPG.*)*

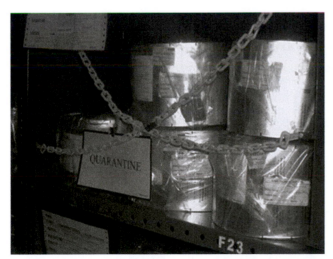

FIGURE 26.15   Materials quarantine. *(Source: Essential Medicines and Health Products Information Portal: A World Health Organization resource.)*

cloned. These clones are then frozen in small quantities and therefore producing a research cell bank (RCB). RCBs are evaluated for production capabilities and normally one RCB will be selected to move forward with testing and/or production.

Once a specific RCB has been selected, a two-tiered cell banking system is utilized (see Figure 20.17A and B). The first tier is referred to as a master cell bank (MCB). This cell bank is manufactured from the selected research cell bank. One vial of the RCB is thawed and expanded until a required number of cells are available for the creation of the cell bank. These cells are then aliquoted into small-volume cryopreservation vessels and frozen using DMSO (5 to 10 percent) at less than −130°C. These conditions limit the cellular activity which allows for long-term storage. Once produced, the MCB is tested for cell growth, cell viability, characterization, sterility, and various other tests as deemed necessary.

Once the MCB has been tested, the second tier or working cell bank (WCB) is initiated. One vial of the MCB is thawed and expanded until the required number of cells are available. These cells are again aliquoted into cryopreservation vessels for storage in DMSO (5 to 10 percent) at less than −130°C. Each WCB that is produced undergoes testing (cell growth, cell viability, characterization, sterility, etc.) before using further manufacturing processes.

Production of the targeted substance (mAb or protein) begins by preparing the inoculum to be used in the production bioreactor. This inoculum begins by thawing a vial of the tested working cell bank. The WCB culture is suspended in a specialized growth medium within a shake flask. The culture is then maintained in a monitored incubator that controls temperature, CO_2 concentration, and shaking rate. As the initial culture grows, it proceeds through scale-up increasing the volume of the shake flasks. This allows the inoculum volume to increase with each step. The scale-up process might use any number of vessels that allow for increasing the inoculum volume.

Once the inoculum culture has reached a sufficient cell density and volume, it is used to inoculate the production bioreactor. Bioreactors allow for the control of various conditions, including pH, dissolved oxygen (DO), gas flow, and temperature. The controlled conditions allow for the creation of an ideal environment for the cell culture to produce the targeted substance.

Bioreactors

There are two main types of bioreactors: multiple-use (stainless steel) or single-use bioreactors (disposable).

Multiple-use bioreactors are made of stainless steel and currently are the predominant version of bioreactors used in production settings. Multi-use bioreactors generally require a large capital investment for purchase and installation. They also require validated processes for cleaning, and sterilization increases cost and time

of maintenance and a skilled staff for operation. For this reason, in smaller-volume operations, disposable bioreactors are being used increasingly. (See Figures 26.18 and 26.19)

Disposable bioreactors utilize a disposable sterilized cell chamber in which the cell culture is maintained. This cell chamber minimizes the risks of cross-contamination as it is only used for one growth operation. The use of disposable bioreactors decreases the amount of validation, cleaning, sterilization, and maintenance needed per bioreactor run. For this reason, disposable bioreactors runs are able to be scheduled closer together allowing for an increase in plant production.

After the bioreactor has been inoculated there are three main types of bioreactor processes that are used: batch, continuous, and fed-batch. Batch bioreactor processes consist of filling the bioreactor with medium and inoculum and operating the bioreactor without additions of nutrients or medium until the growth profile is finished. Continuous bioreactor processes continually feed nutrients and medium into the bioreactor while also continually harvesting material from the bioreactor. Being as material is continuously being harvested, these processes can result in larger amounts of harvested material and longer bioreactor campaigns. Unfortunately, the longer bioreactor campaigns greatly increase the chance for contamination.

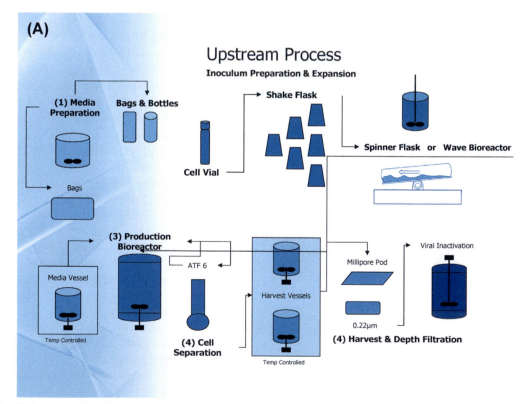

FIGURE 26.16   Biologics manufacturing process. (A) Upstream process, (B) Downstream processes and (C) Fill finish processes. (*Source: Cytovance Biologics Inc. John Conner 2013.*)

(B)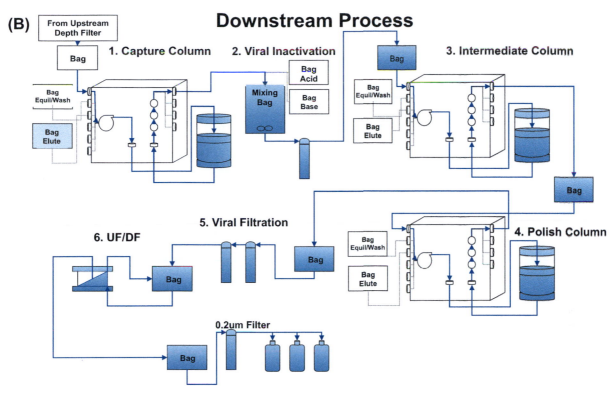

FIGURE 26.16B

(C)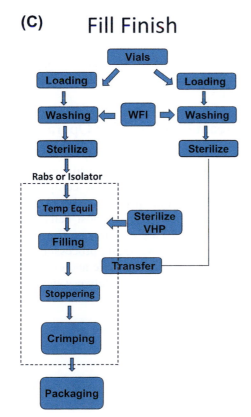

FIGURE 26.16C

Fed-batch bioreactor processes are the most common bioreactor processes used. This process starts with a lower starting volume and feeds nutrients and medium on a set schedule without a contentious removal of harvest material. Once the process has finished, the material is harvested for downstream processing.

Microbial Upstream Operations

Microbial fermentation involves the growth of a specific microorganism that has been programed to produce a specific protein. An example of a host organism used for this purpose is *Escherichia coli*. Production of the target substance begins with the thawing of the microbial cell bank. This cell bank is resuspended in growth medium and incubated within an incubator/shaker that controls the temperature and agitation rate of the culture. The culture is incubated to allow growth to the proper optical density for inoculation of the production fermenter. The production fermenter is designed to control parameters including dissolved oxygen, pH, temperature, and gas flows. This control allows for an optimized environment to be created for the growth of the microorganism. The fermentation process usually utilizes a fed-batch process which allows for feeding of additional specialized medium and supplements designed to support growth of the microorganism. (Figure 26.20)

(A) **(B)**

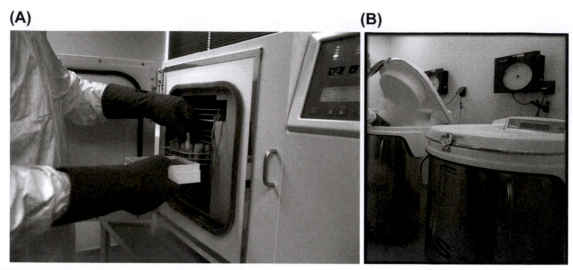

FIGURE 26.17   A and B. (A) Manufacturing cell bank production. (B) Cryopreservation and cryostorage. *(Source: Cytovance Biologics Inc., 2013.)*

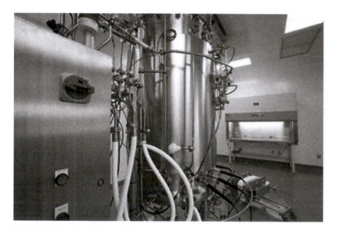

FIGURE 26.18   Mammalian upstream bioreactor operations. *(Source: Cytovance Biologics Inc., 2013.)*

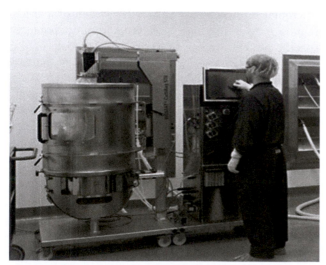

FIGURE 26.19   Mammalian upstream single-use bioreactor (SUB) operations. *(Source: Cytovance Biologics Inc., 2013.)*

Once the fermentation process is completed (approximately 48 hours) the microorganisms are harvested by centrifugation. This is important as the targeted substances are intracellular (inside the host cell). The centrifugation step allows for the removal of the growth medium. Being as the targeted substance is intracellular, the host cells must be disrupted to allow the extraction of the product. A common practice to accomplish this is the use of a high-pressure homogenizer. Once the targeted substance has been released for the cell, the resulting lysate must be centrifuged. This last centrifugation step results in the separation of the inclusion bodies from the remaining cell debris (a result of the homogenization process). The isolated inclusion bodies may then be frozen and stored before further downstream purification.

Downstream Bioprocessing Operations

Downstream processing, as it applies to biomanufacturing, refers to the separation, purification, and modification of macromolecules from complex biological feedstocks. Most commonly the feedstock is a cell suspension containing billions of "host cells" that synthesized the macromolecule of interest. The ultimate goal of a pharmaceutical downstream processing operation is to prepare a drug product for safe and effective delivery into humans or animals. The delivery method is a primary focus of fill/finish operations and can be parenteral, oral, or topical.

Pharmaceutical macromolecules are used in a vast array of applications including:

1. Cancer therapy
2. Enzyme replacement for enzyme-deficiency syndromes
3. Immune system suppression for autoimmune disorders
4. Elimination of infectious agents

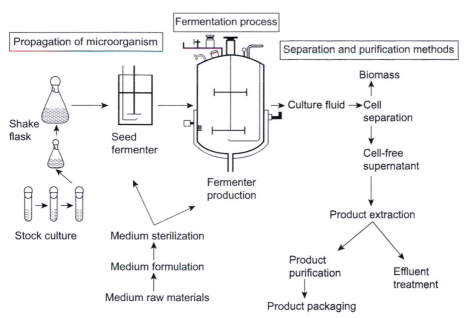

FIGURE 26.20   Microbial fermentation operations. *(Source: Intech.* http://www.intechopen.com/books/biomass-now-sustainable-growth-and-use/continuous-agave-juice-fermentation-for-producing-bioethanol.*)*

5. Anemia
6. Diabetes
7. Gene therapy

Downstream processing has undergone drastic advances in the last 30 years as new strategies have emerged to increase throughput, purity, and process yield. The recent technology advances in downstream processing have driven operating margins upward and have broken down costly barriers to entry into the biologics market. Start-up companies who are mindful of the recent cost-saving and process-optimization technologies in downstream processing are now more able than ever to bring life-saving biologic therapies to market, often tapping into the expertise of contract manufacturers and clinical research firms. Furthermore, regulatory agencies around the globe have established robust guidelines to ensure the new strategies being implemented in downstream processing keep the safety of the patient as a top priority. Due to the close proximity of downstream process operations to the final drug product, patient safety considerations are absolutely critical.

Downstream Process Flow

A downstream unit operation, a single step in the downstream process, can be categorized into a mechanical separation, chemical separation, or dual mechanical/chemical separation step. In other words, the molecule of interest is separated from the remaining impurities mechanically, by its dimensional (size, shape) characteristics, or chemically, by its biochemical (electrical charge, interaction with other macromolecules, oiliness) properties. Several downstream processing techniques apply both mechanical

and chemical separations simultaneously, and can be highly selective for the molecule of interest. Product separation and purification is accomplished through a series of process steps including, but not limited to: filtration, chromatography, precipitation, and centrifugation. As a general rule of thumb, product purity increases and volume decreases through each unit operation of the downstream process (see Figure 26.21).

In addition to the separation and purification of the target drug molecule, downstream processes modify the drug molecule and its environment. These modifications can be minor or extensive, depending on the ability of the expression system to produce the molecule. Some examples of product modification in downstream processing include:

1. Complete reconstruction of the product in solution (protein refolding).
2. Increasing the concentration of product in solution.
3. Attaching synthetic molecules to the product to enhance immune response or product stability.
4. Splitting of the product into multiple subunits.
5. Adding excipients (salts, amino acids, detergents, emulsifiers) to enhance product stability.

Harvest and Clarification

Downstream processing begins with the separation of large insoluble contaminants from the feedstock or "harvest" solution, usually whole cells and cell debris. This mechanical separation process is referred to as clarification. For expression systems in which the molecule of interest is secreted out of the cell into the surrounding solution (mammalian cell culture) and a relatively low density of cell debris is present, depth filtration is a common clarification technique. Depth filtration is a 3-D filter matrix that serves to remove the bulk of large particulates from the feedstock, analogous to a sand bank at the foot of a river. Water and very small particles pass through the sand while large debris cannot.

The advantage of depth filtration is low equipment cost and seamless transfer from bench scale to production scale. Several varieties of depth filters are readily available with some acting as both mechanical and chemical separators that bind charged contaminants from the host cell such as DNA and proteins (see Figures 26.22A and B).

Certain feedstocks with a high density of cell debris (microbial fermentation broth) require a primary clarification with a centrifuge prior to, or in lieu of, depth filtration. In contrast to traditional laboratory centrifuges that require multiple batches to process large volumes, continuous flow centrifuges mechanically separate the product from the feedstock in a single batch, taking advantage of density differences between liquids and solids. The feedstock is split into two or more portions: product stream(s) and a waste stream. The waste stream is discarded and the product stream(s) captured for further downstream processing. (See Figure 26.23.)

After the large insoluble particulates have been removed via depth filtration and/or continuous flow centrifugation, the harvest solution is passed through a fine filter that ensures all living cells are removed. This final filtration step ensures further downstream processing steps are protected from unwanted contaminants and debris.

Chromatography

Chromatography is a general term that refers to the separation of molecules that exist together in a solution. Chromatography is the primary tool used in downstream processing, enabling biologics manufacturers to separate

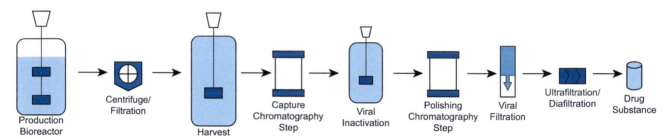

FIGURE 26.21 Typical downstream processing flow of a monoclonal antibody (mAb). The arrows represent the flow of the antibody product between unit operations. Each unit operation mechanically or chemically separates the antibody from host cell contaminants. *(Source: Figure modified from: Ahmed, I., B. Kaspar, and U. Sharma. (February 2012). "Biosimilars: Impact of Biologics Product Life Cycle and European Experience on the Regulatory Trajectory in the United States." Clinical Therapeutics.)*

(A)   **(B)**

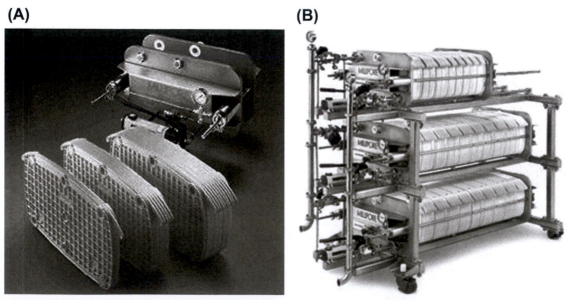

FIGURE 26.22 A and B. Typical depth filtration used in cell culture harvest clarification. Example of a small (A) and large (B) production-scale disposable depth filtration system. These units are Millipore Millistak+®POD disposable depth filters manufactured by EMD Millipore. *(Source: www.millipore.com.)*

a product molecule from thousands of others in solution. Column chromatography is by far the most common form of chromatography in biomanufacturing, in which a liquid "mobile phase" containing the molecule of interest passes through a solid "stationary phase." Columns are essentially hollow tubes made of glass, plastic, or steel with nets on both ends that contain the stationary phase within the column. A pump system with an array of monitoring

devices pushes the mobile phase through the column and directs the product stream away from the waste stream. Based on the scale of the operation, columns can vary in size from 1 centimeter in diameter to 200 centimeters in diameter and greater. Regardless of size, the principle of column chromatography remains the same. (See Figures 26.24A and B.)

The stationary phase, commonly referred to as chromatography resin or media, contains immobilized chemicals called "ligands" and can operate in different ways depending on the downstream process operation. The ligands can bind to the product molecule, allowing other unwanted molecules to pass through the column and be discarded. This strategy is referred to as "bind-and-elute" chromatography. The exact opposite occurs in "flow through" chromatography, in which the product molecule passes through the column and is captured while impurities bind to the ligands. Lastly, all molecules pass through the column in size-exclusion chromatography, with separation being achieved because molecules travel at different speeds through the column. (See Figure 26.25.)

Only a small portion of a chromatography column is actually ligand, with most of the column volume consisting of a polymer that holds the ligands upright and typically does not interact with macromolecules in solution. The polymer backbone is a highly porous spherical bead in column chromatography, or in a 3-D matrix in the case of membrane chromatography. In both cases the goal is to maximize the exposure of ligands to the surrounding solution so that chromatographic separation can occur. (See Figure 26.26.)

Column packing refers to the various strategies used to optimally place chromatography media within a column tube. A delicate balance exists with packing a column with

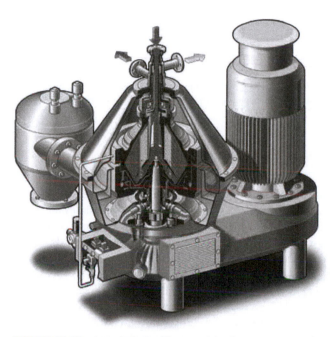

FIGURE 26.23 A typical centrifuge used in downstream operations to separate product from feedstock. A specialized centrifuge from GEA/Westfalia for the separation of a feedstock into low-density liquid, high-density liquid, and solid components. *(Source: GEA Westfalia Separator Group.* www.westfalia-separator.com.*)*

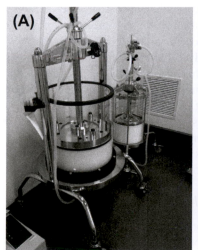
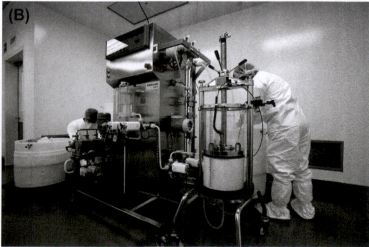

FIGURE 26.24 A and B. (A) Typical Chromatography columns packed with various chromatography resins. (B) Downstream purification Technician using a Chromatography Skid connected to buffer and chromatography column to purify protein therapeutics. Note the white resin matrix used to separate the macromolecules in solution. *(Source: Cytovance Biologics Inc., 2013.)*

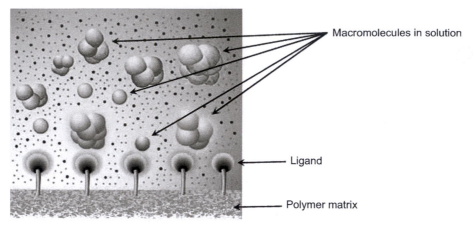

FIGURE 26.25   Chromatography Resin in Action: Highly magnified artist's model of a chromatography resin in action. Blue and green macromolecules do not interact with the ligands, while the orange and red macromolecules are bound to the ligands. *(Source: http://microsite.sartorius.com/sartobind-phenyl/hic.html.)*

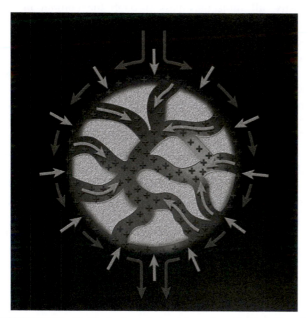

FIGURE 26.26   Positively charged chromatography resin bead. Note the porous nature of the bead, with channels throughout to allow access to the surrounding solution. Light gray arrows represent macromolecules that pass through the interior of the bead, while dark gray arrows represent macromolecules that are excluded from the resin bead. Plus signs (+) represent ligands affixed to the polymer matrix. *(Source: Pall Corporation. www.pall.com.)*

media: chromatography. Media should be installed into a column tube to ensure it remains stationary (hence the "stationary phase"), but does not become damaged or compressed to the extent that ligands cannot be accessed by the molecules in solution. A variety of strategies exist to pack columns and the appropriate method should be selected based on the resin's properties and the type of column hardware used in the manufacturing facility. In recent years, automated column packing methods (GE AxiChrom) have been developed to improve the reproducibility and robustness of column chromatography unit operations.

Capture Chromatography

The capture chromatography step is the first chromatography step of a downstream process and is the "workhorse" of the entire process. Imagine a gold prospector on an average day in the field who pans for several hours, ending up with a few small gold flakes at the end of the day. Hundreds of pounds of silt, water, and microscopic gold dust pass through the pan for every visible gold flake. Even the visible gold flakes are compounded with other metal impurities. The gold gathered is not the final product yet, but the prospector is much closer to the end result than he or she was several hours ago. Capture chromatography follows the same principle as gold panning; a relatively small loss of product yields huge dividends with at least a 100-fold increase in purity. Capture chromatography is typically the most efficient downstream process step.

Capture chromatography usually involves the use of an affinity ligand, a molecule that strongly attracts the product's macromolecule. A common affinity ligand is Protein A, a naturally occurring bacterial protein that "locks on" to human antibodies. Protein A-based resins are widely used in biomanufacturing to separate monoclonal antibody products from mammalian host-cell impurities. For nonantibody products, most chromatography resins can be used as the initial capture step. Fine tuning is often required to capture nonantibody products from a feedstock solution, and precise conditions must exist to bind the macromolecule product and allow others to pass through.

Polishing Chromatography

Polishing chromatography is the general term that refers to additional chromatography unit operations after the capture step. Polishing chromatography further enhances the purity of the target macromolecule to greater than 95 percent, in preparation for delivery of the drug to the patient. If applied

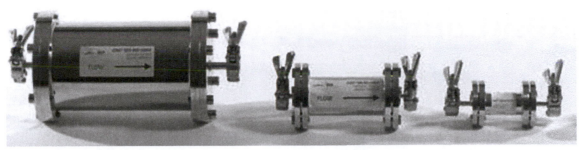

FIGURE 26.27   A membrane chromatography column. The steel cylinder contains a 3-D matrix with bound ligands rather than spherical beads. (Family of CIM® Monolithic Columns from BIA Separations.) *(Source: BIA Separations.* http://www.biaseparations.com.*)*

to the gold panning analogy, polishing chromatography is the metallurgist that transforms the dull gold flakes into pure 24K gold bars. Hundreds of resin types for polishing chromatography are available in varying bead sizes, ligand types, and polymer matrices. The vast diversity of biological macromolecules is a reflection of the numerous types of polishing chromatography resins and strategies which contract manufacturers can expect to work with.

Membrane Chromatography

Membrane chromatography is an alternative to traditional column chromatography, as ligands are attached to a 3-D matrix rather than a spherical bead. Membrane chromatography exists in most of the same ligand types as traditional resin. The use of membrane chromatography is advantageous for some downstream processes as higher flow rates through the chromatography matrix can be achieved as compared to most traditional resin types, and capital costs are lower without the need for expensive column hardware. However, membrane chromatography can be cumbersome to use at commercial production scales, where the material costs of the membranes can outweigh the capital cost savings of opting out of column chromatography.

A small subset of membrane chromatography systems combines the flow rate advantages of membrane chromatography with the reusability of traditional column chromatography (see Figure 26.27). BIA Separations has developed a membrane chromatography column for production use. The steel cylinder contains a 3-D matrix with bound ligands rather than spherical beads.

Buffer Preparation

While choosing the proper stationary phase is critical to a downstream processing operation, selecting the right mobile phase is equally as important. The salt solutions passed through chromatography media that establish the proper mobile phase conditions are called buffers. A great deal of attention is directed at buffer preparation to ensure the chemical components meet rigorous regulatory standards for pharmaceutical use and the buffers are prepared

correctly. A buffer that does not meet the requirements for its downstream unit operation can mean the difference between the product macromolecule binding to the resin or being discarded to waste. Advances in disposable technology are particularly applicable to the buffer preparation process. A capital cost to store large volumes of buffer solutions in stainless steel tanks is not feasible for most biomanufacturers, so disposable plastic bags are preferred.

Tangential Flow Filtration

Tangential flow filtration (TFF) is a technique widely adopted in downstream processing and is similar in principle to dialysis. Tangential flow filtration is used to remove the buffer surrounding the macromolecule product and add another buffer to the product that is more suitable for the next process step. The pores in a tangential flow filter are small enough that the drug product does not pass through— it moves parallel to the filter surface. Impurities, salts, and water pass through the filter and are discarded. TFF can be utilized as a preparative step between chromatography steps or to formulate the product of interest with the optimal salts and excipients. The exact formulation delivered by a TFF system varies greatly from product-to-product. Salts, amino acids, sugars, and surfactants are common additives. (See Figure 26.28A and B.)

Viral Reduction Techniques

Several mammalian expression systems contain viruses that are intentionally present to manufacture the drug macromolecule. Foreign viruses can also contaminate the cell culture and can be difficult to detect. To protect patients from harmful viral agents, downstream processes have built-in safeguards to eliminate viral contamination, known as "viral clearance."

The primary viral clearance operation in most downstream processes is known as viral filtration. Many types of viral filters are available, they are all highly specialized filters with precise pore sizes that allow the product molecule to pass through but trap viruses. The challenge with viral filtration is some viruses, especially parvoviruses, are

(A)   **(B)**

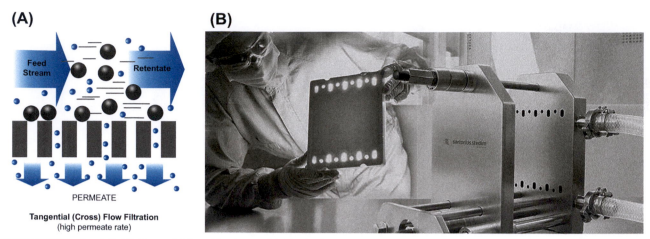

Feed
Stream   Retentate

PERMEATE

Tangential (Cross) Flow Filtration
(high permeate rate)

FIGURE 26.28   A and B. (A) Tangential flow filtration model. The feed stream containing the product molecule, travels in parallel to the filter surface. Only impurities such as salts and smaller molecules pass through the filter. (*Source:* Spectrum Labs. *www.spectrumlabs.c.*) (B) An example of a production-scale tangential flow filtration system. The stainless steel plates on the right are used to hold the tangential flow filters (held by the technician) in place. (*Source: Sartorius. www.sartorius.com.*)

incredibly small and similar in size to product molecules. The precision to which these filters are made is critical for patient safety. To ensure the filter performs properly, an air test is performed to detect microscopic leaks that could have allowed a virus through.

Viruses are often susceptible to acid and detergents, while many biologic drugs are not as sensitive. Acid treatment is a common tactic for viral reduction in a monoclonal antibody downstream process, while detergent treatment is sometimes used to reduce viral contamination for enzyme products. Chromatography often doubles as a viral clearance tool. Electrically charged chromatography resins are particularly effective at removing viral contaminants as the ligands attract viruses like a magnet.

Bulk Filtration and Fill

Bulk fill is the final step in the downstream process after the product has been formulated appropriately. A sterile filter is used to ensure any potential contaminants that may have been inadvertently introduced into the product are removed. Downstream processing specialists that perform a bulk fill operation must be highly trained and are monitored for contaminants throughout the process. Once the formulated drug product passes through the filter, it is delivered into sterile containers that are stored in highly controlled areas.

Equipment Cleaning

All equipment that has direct contact with products in downstream processing must be vigorously cleaned between uses to remove soilants that remain bound to the equipment surface. The cleaning agents used are either acidic or alkaline, often contain detergents, and can be

heated to increase cleaning potency. Applications with difficult-to-clean soilants or applications using large equipment often necessitate automated clean-in-place systems that distribute cleaning solutions to the equipment surfaces. Whether automated clean-in-place or manual cleaning is performed, all cleaning solution residues must be rinsed away with medical-grade water before using the equipment again. Highly sensitive analytical assays, such as the total organic carbon (TOC) assay, are industry standard for the detection of residual soilants and cleaning agents. (See Figure 26.29.)

Drug Product Manufacturing

For biological drug products, having a stability and robust final product formulation buffer is critical to the drug product manufacturing process. Developing a drug product formulation involves the characterization of a drug's physical, chemical, and biological properties in order to identify those ingredients that can be used in the drug manufacturing process to aid in the processing, storage, and handling of the drug product. Evaluating the drug substance under a variety of stress conditions such as freeze/thaw, temperature, and shear stress to identify mechanisms of degradation is extremely important.

Formulation studies should consider such factors as particle size, polymorphism, pH, and solubility that can influence the bioavailability and the activity of a drug. The drug in combination with inactive additives must ensure that the quality of drug is consistent in each dosage unit throughout the manufacture, storage, and handling to the point of use. It is essential that these initial studies be conducted using drug samples of known purity. The presence of impurities can lead to erroneous conclusions. Stability testing during each stage of drug development is a critical

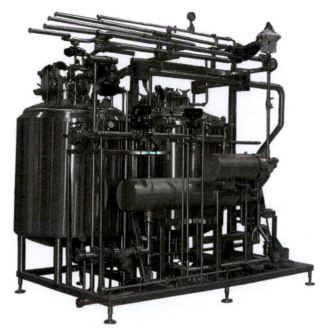

FIGURE 26.29 A typical clean-in-place system used to clean upstream and downstream process equipment. The tanks in the background are used to mix and heat up the cleaning solutions before delivery of the cleaning solutions to the downstream process equipment through a network of piping. (*Source: Turn-Key Modular Systems.* http://www.tkmodular.com/StandardProducts/CIPSystems.aspx.)

facet to ensuring product quality. Drug stability testing is important during preclinical testing and clinical trials to establish an accurate assessment of the product being evaluated. Stability data is required at each of the various stages of development to demonstrate and document the product's stability profile. A product's stability must be assessed with regard to its formulation; the influence of its pharmaceutical ingredients; the influence of the container and closure; the manufacturing and processing conditions; packaging components; storage conditions; anticipated conditions of shipping, temperature, light, and humidity; and the anticipated duration and conditions of pharmacy shelf-life and patient use. Holding process bulk intermediates or product components for long periods before processing into finished drug products can also affect the stability of both the intermediate component and the finished product. Therefore, in-process stability testing, including testing of intermediate components, is essential. The following harmonized guidelines provide an outline of the regulatory requirements for drug substance and drug product stability testing to aid in formulation development:

1. Stability testing of new drug substances and products.
2. Quality of biotechnological products: stability testing of biotechnology/biological.
3. Drug products.
4. Photo-stability testing of new drug substances and products.
5. Stability testing of new dosage forms.

A drug's kinetic and shelf-life stability profile is the extent to which a product remains within specification limits through its period of storage and use while maintaining the same properties and characteristics that it possessed at the time of manufacture. Stability studies should address several key drug stability concerns:

1. Active ingredients retain their chemical integrity within the specified limits.
2. Drug physical properties are retained.
3. Sterility and/or container integrity is maintained.
4. Potency/therapeutic effect of the drug remain unchanged.
5. No increase in toxicity occurs.

Drug products should be subjected to long-term stability studies under the conditions of transport and storage expected during product distribution. In conducting these studies, the different climate zones to which the product may be subjected must be evaluated for expected variances in conditions of temperature and humidity. A drug product may encounter more than a single zone of temperature and humidity variations during its production and shelf-life. In general, long-term testing of new drug entities should be conducted at $25°C \pm 2°C$ and at a relative humidity of 60 percent $\pm$ 5 percent.

There are many agents and ingredients that can be used to prepare the final formulation buffer of a drug substance to enhance the stability profile of the drug. These ingredients may be used to achieve the desired physical and chemical characteristics of the product or to enhance the stability of the drug substance, particularly against hydrolysis and oxidation. In each instance, the added agent or ingredient must be compatible with and must not detract from the stability or potency of the drug substance.

Hydrolysis is the most important cause of drug decomposition primarily because of the number of active agents that are susceptible to the hydrolytic process. Hydrolysis is a process in which drug molecules interact with water molecules to yield breakdown byproducts. There are several approaches to the stabilization of drugs subject to hydrolysis. The most obvious is the reduction or elimination of water from the system. In some liquid drug products, water can be replaced or reduced in the formulation through the use of glycerin, propylene glycol, and alcohol. In certain injectable products, anhydrous vegetable oils may be used as the drug's solvent to reduce the chance of hydrolytic decomposition. Decomposition by hydrolysis may also be prevented in other liquid drug formulations by suspending them in a nonaqueous vehicle. For certain unstable active agents, when an aqueous preparation is desired, the drug may be supplied in a dry form for reconstitution by adding a specified volume of purified water just before dispensing to a patient. Refrigeration is generally required for most drugs subject to hydrolysis. In addition to temperature, pH is also a factor that affects the stability of a drug prone to hydrolytic decomposition. Drug stability can frequently be improved though the use of buffering agents between pH 5 and pH 6.

Oxidation is another destructive process that produces instability in drug products. Oxidation is the loss of electrons from an atom or a molecule. Each electron lost is accepted by some other molecule, reducing the recipient. Oxidation frequently involves free chemical radicals, which are molecules containing one or more unpaired electrons such as oxygen and free hydroxyl. These radicals tend to take electrons from other chemicals, thereby oxidizing the donor. Oxidation of a drug substance is most likely to occur when it is not kept dry in the presence of oxygen, when it is exposed to light, or combined with other chemical agents. Oxidation of a chemical in a drug substance is usually accompanied by an alteration in the color of that drug and may also result in precipitation or a change in odor. The oxidative process can be controlled with the use of antioxidants that react with one or more compounds in the drug to prevent the oxidation progress. Antioxidants act by providing electrons and hydrogen atoms that are accepted more readily by the free radicals rather than those present in the drug. Among those most frequently used in aqueous preparations are sodium sulfite, sodium bisulfite, sodium metabisulfite, hypophosphorous acid, and ascorbic acid. The FDA labeling regulations require a warning about possible allergic-type reactions, including anaphylaxis, in the package insert for prescription drugs that contain sulfites in the final dosage form.

Because oxygen can adversely affect their stability, certain drugs require an oxygen-free atmosphere during processing and storage. Oxygen is present in the airspace within the storage container or may be dissolved in the liquid vehicle. Oxygen-sensitive drugs must be prepared in the dry state and packaged in sealed containers with the air replaced by an inert gas such as nitrogen. Light can also act as a catalyst to oxidation reactions by transferring energy to drug molecules making them more reactive. As a precaution against light-induced oxidation, sensitive drugs must be packaged in light-resistant or opaque containers. Because most drug degradations proceed more rapidly as the temperature increases, it is also advisable to store oxidizable drugs under refrigerated temperatures. Another factor that can affect the stability of an oxidizable drug in solution is the pH of the formulation buffer. Each drug must be maintained in solution at the pH most favorable to its stability. This varies from preparation-to-preparation and must be determined on an individual basis for the drug.

Formulated drug substances and drug products are stored in container closure systems for extended periods of time. For biological drugs, container closures typically include plastic bags/containers, bottles, vials, and syringes. The containers are typically made from glass or plastic. It is important to determine that there are no interactions between the drug and the container. When a plastic container is used, tests should be conducted to determine if any of the ingredients become adsorbed by the plastic or whether any plasticizers, lubricants, pigments, or stabilizers leach out of the plastic into the drug. The adhesives for the container label need to be tested to ensure they do not leach through the plastic container into the drug. Trace metals originating from the chemical in the drug, solvent, container, or stopper may also be a source of concern in preparing stable solutions of oxidizable drugs.

Freezing and thawing of bulk protein solutions are common practices in bulk intermediate, drug substance, and drug-product manufacturing. Freezing-induced aggregation and denaturation caused by cryopreservation or a pH shift due to crystallization of buffer components can lead to a significant loss in biological activity of the drug. Formulation development and analysis of the impact of freezing on proteins are a significant part of optimizing biological drug storage systems involving cryoprotectants, stabilizing excipients, freezing process parameters, and cryocontainers. Cryoprotectants function by lowering the glass transition temperature of a solution. The cryoprotectant prevents freezing, and the solution maintains some flexibility during the freezing process. Some cryoprotectants also function by forming hydrogen bonds with biological molecules displacing water molecules. Hydrogen bonding in aqueous solutions is important for proper protein and DNA function. As the cryoprotectant replaces the water molecules, the biological material retains its native physiological structure and function. Conventional cryoprotectants, such as glycerol and dimethyl sulfoxide (DMSO), have been used to reduce ice formation in biological material stored in liquid nitrogen. For some biological material, mixtures of cryoprotectants have less toxicity and are more effective than single-agent cryoprotectants. Cryoprotectant mixtures have also been used for vitrification (solidification without crystal ice formation). Vitrification has important applications in preserving embryos, biological tissues, and organs for transplantation.

Similar to cryoprotectants, lyoprotectants are molecules that protect material during lyophilization. Lyoprotectants are typically polyhydroxy compounds such as sugars (mono-, di-, and polysaccharides), polyalcohols, and their derivatives. Lyophilization is frequently used for biological drugs to increase the shelf-life of products, such as vaccines and other injectables that are subject to hydrolysis degradation. By removing the water from the material and sealing the material in a vial, the material can be easily stored, shipped, and later reconstituted to its original form for injection. The development of freeze-dried formulations involves selecting a suitable lyoprotectant that stabilizes the drug within a defined amorphous matrix and control key drug process parameters: freeze concentration, solution-phase concentration, product appearance, minimizing reactive products, increasing the surface area, and decreasing vapor pressure of solvents. During the lyophilization process, the freezing phases are the most critical. Amorphous materials do not have a eutectic point but instead have a critical temperature typically between −50°C and −80°C, below which the product must be maintained to prevent melt-back or the collapse of the biological material during the lyophilization primary and secondary drying steps.

During the primary freeze-drying phase, the pressure is lowered to the range of a few millibars and the temperature controlled based on the molecule's latent heat of sublimation. It is important to cool the material below its triple point, the lowest temperature at which the solid and liquid phases of the material can coexist. During this initial drying phase, approximately 95 percent of the water in the form of ice is removed from the product by sublimation. This phase is typically a slow process to avoid altering the molecular structure of the biological material. During this phase, pressure is controlled through the application of partial vacuum. The vacuum speeds up the sublimation during the drying process.

The secondary drying phase removes the remaining unfrozen water molecules from the primary phase. This part of the freeze-drying process is governed by the material's adsorption isotherms. In this phase, the temperature is raised higher than in the primary drying phase, and can even be above 0°C to break any physicochemical interactions that have formed between the water molecules and the frozen material. Usually the pressure is also lowered in this stage, typically in the range of microbars or fractions of a Pascal, to encourage desorption. After the freeze-drying process is complete, the vacuum is broken with an inert gas, such as nitrogen, before the container is sealed. At the end of the lyophilization process, the final residual water content in the drug product is typically around 1 to 4 percent.

The lyophilization process includes the transfer of aseptically filled product in partially sealed containers. To prevent contamination of a partially closed sterile product, an aseptic process must be designed to minimize exposure of sterile articles to the potential contamination hazards of the manufacturing operation. Limiting the duration of exposure of sterile product components, providing the highest possible environmental control, optimizing process flow, and designing equipment to prevent the introduction of lower-quality air into the Class 100 (ISO 5) clean area are essential to achieving a high assurance of final product sterility. In an aseptic process, the drug product, container, and closure are first subjected to separate sterilization methods before being assembled. Because there is not a terminal sterilization process for biological drug products, it is critical that containers be filled and sealed in an extremely high-quality environment. Before the aseptic assembly of a final product, the individual parts of the final drug product are sterilized by separate processes: glass containers by dry heat; rubber closures by moist heat; and liquid dosage forms are subjected to filtration. Each of these manufacturing processes requires validation and control to eliminate the risk of product contamination. Both personnel and material flow must also be optimized to prevent unnecessary activities that could increase the potential for introducing contaminants to exposed product, container closures, or the surrounding environment. The number of personnel in an aseptic processing room should be minimized. The flow of personnel should be designed to limit the frequency of entries and exits into and from an aseptic processing room. The number of transfers into the critical area of a cleanroom, or an isolator, must be minimized, and movement adjacent to the critical area should be restricted. Any intervention or stoppage during an aseptic process can increase the risk of contamination. The design of equipment used in aseptic processing should limit the number and complexity of aseptic interventions by personnel. Personnel interventions should be reduced by integrating an on-line weight check device that eliminates a repetitive manual activity within the critical area, sterilizing preassembled connections using sterilize-in-place (SIP) technology eliminating significant aseptic manipulations, and the use of automation technologies such as robotics to further reduce contamination risks to the product (See Figure 26.30 A and B.).

Product transfers should occur under appropriate cleanroom conditions. Carefully designed curtains, rigid plastic shields, and the use of isolator systems can be used to achieve segregation of the aseptic processing line. If stoppered vials exit an aseptic processing zone prior to capping, appropriate controls should be in place to safeguard the product until completion of the crimping step. Use of on-line detection devices to identify improperly seated stoppers provides additional sterility assurance. Aseptic processing operations must be validated using microbiological growth media fill process simulations. Media fill process simulations should incorporate risk factors that occur during normal product manufacturing such as exposure to product contact surfaces of equipment, container closure systems, critical environments, and process manipulations. Media fills should closely simulate aseptic manufacturing operations incorporating worst-case activities and conditions that may occur during aseptic operations.

MANUFACTURING SUPPORT FUNCTIONS

Quality Assurance (QA)

Good manufacturing practices require that all persons involved in manufacturing be responsible for quality and that the manufacturers implement an effective system for managing quality. This system should require that the quality unit be independent of the manufacturing unit and that the quality unit be involved in all quality-related matters.

(A)

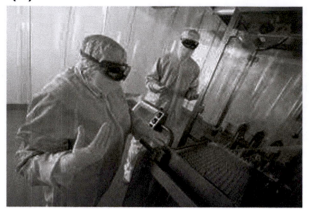

(B)

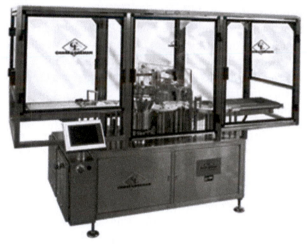

FIGURE 26.30 A and B. (A) Drug product manufacturing: formulation and final container fill finish. An example of a typical glass vial filling operations. (*Source*: Google Images.) (B) Cytovance biologics chase-Logeman Vial Fill Finish System. (*Source: Cytovance Biologics Inc. 2013.*)

Most manufacturers establish the quality unit by developing subteams that support the various manufacturing functions.

Incoming Quality Control/Quality Assurance (QC/QA)

This group performs functions related to assessment, testing, and disposition of materials that are designated to be utilized in the manufacture of intermediates and final products. They ensure proper storage, labeling, and segregation of materials is maintained and also document disposition of incoming material.

Operations Quality Assurance

This group performs functions throughout the actual manufacture of intermediates and final product. They are the independent "eyes" on the floor that provide quality oversight to the manufacturing activities. Their specific activities include but are not limited to verification of critical process steps, line releases, the audit of production areas, and perform in-process inspections.

Document Control

This group performs functions related to the control of all quality records. They ensure that revision history is maintained for documents, that processes for the distribution and reconciliation are maintained, and that change notifications are processed and maintained. Some of the types of quality records that are maintained are:

1. **Standard Operating Procedures (SOPs)**—Contains written instructions on how to perform manufacturing processes and support functions.
2. **Batch records**—Provides a record of actual executed manufacturing steps.
3. **Material specs**—Contains requirements for materials utilized in the manufacture of intermediates and final products.
4. **Training documents**—Provides objective evidence of personnel qualifications and completed training on required processes that are part of or support the manufacture of intermediates and final products.

Quality Assurance for Batch Disposition

This group performs an independent review of product batch records, associated investigations, and test results to verify that all production and testing requirements have been met and/or resolved before determining the final disposition. This group has the authority to determine whether a product will be accepted or rejected.

Quality Compliance

This group provides oversight to the entire quality system and manufacturing functions. They perform roles in quality management by ensuring that internal and external audits are conducted, establish and implement systems that govern quality system monitoring, and are the hosts to inspections and audits from regulatory agencies, customers, and clients.

Qualification/Validation

Good manufacturing practices require that manufacturers establish systems to ensure that their facilities, equipment, processes, test methods, and automated systems are adequate for the support of intermediate and final product manufacture. This system requires that critical product and process attributes be identified and measures implemented to control, test, and monitor these attributes. These systems require that documented qualifications and validations be executed and documented in order to provide evidence of suitability. These systems are driven and overseen by personnel not involved in the manufacture of product and are made up of personnel with engineering, facility, and quality backgrounds. These personnel perform multiple yet segregated roles in writing, executing, reviewing, and approving the documents that are utilized in qualifications and validations.

Facility and Equipment

When new facilities are built or reconfigured, building utilities (water, electrical, and HVAC) must be qualified to ensure that the facility can meet the requirements of the manufacturing process.

Process

As manufacturing processes are defined and critical parameters that include ranges and boundaries are established, objective evidence through validation protocols must be executed to ensure that the manufacturing process is robust and controlled at a level that can repeatedly produce the same product that meets the same specifications.

Analytical Methods

During the manufacture of intermediates and products, the verification of critical steps can be determined through sample testing. The test utilized must be qualified or validated. The qualification and/or validation of test methods ensure that the defined method can detect the required component or product ingredient. Depending on the test material, standard pharmacopoeia methods can be implemented or new methods can be developed. These methods must meet the requirements of analytical method validation and show specificity, accuracy, precision, detection limits, quantitation limits, linearity, range, and robustness.

Quality Control

Analytical Methods

Suitable analytical test methods are extremely critical components for establishing identity, quality, purity, and strength/potency of a drug product. The current good manufacturing practice regulations [21 CFR 211.194 (a)] require that test methods used for assessing compliance of pharmaceutical products with established specifications must meet proper standards of accuracy and reliability. All test methods are established as standard operating procedures (SOP) in the quality control (QC) laboratory. While it is not necessary to have analytical methods being qualified for testing process development (PD) demonstration run materials or scale-up engineering run material, all test methods need to be at least qualified for any GMP lot material during early stages of the drug development and manufacturing program. The need

and scope of analytical method qualification/validation should be defined under the master validation plan for the organization. This should be established in the form of an approved SOP.

It is necessary to perform qualification/validation of the test methods according to the International Conference on Harmonisation (ICH) Tripartite Guideline "Validation of Analytical Procedures: Text and Methodology, Q2 (R1)." Based on the ICH guideline, certain key parameters from the full assay validation program are addressed during the assay qualification. The analytical methods qualification/validation package should include (1) SOP, (2) assay qualification/validation protocol, (3) assay qualification/validation report, and (4) relevant analytical data. Method qualification and validation can be performed in a QC laboratory and/or analytical science laboratory (under R&D unit) of the organization. However, the release tests for the GMP manufactured products must be performed in the QC laboratory. Analytical method qualification/validation needs to be performed with qualified and calibrated instruments/equipment including the material storage units. While noncompendial test methods need to be qualified/validated based on ICH guidelines, according to the regulations [21 CFR 211.194 (a) (2)] all compendial methods as described in the United States Pharmacopeia (USP) and the National Formulary (NF) are not required to validate accuracy and reliability of these methods. These methods merely need to be verified for their suitability under actual conditions of use.

Quality Control Laboratory

The quality control laboratory is set up to support the manufacturing department for the production of drug substances and drug products. As defined in 21 CFR Part 211.22 the responsibility and authority of the quality control unit includes testing and approval (or rejection) of all components, drug product containers, closures, in-process materials, packaging material, labeling, and drug products. According to the regulations, a QC unit also has the responsibility for approving or rejecting all procedures or specifications impacting on the identity, strength, quality, and purity of the drug product. It also requires that the responsibilities and procedures applicable to the QC unit shall be in writing and such written procedures shall be followed.

A Description of In-Process and Release Tests Performed in a QC Laboratory for the Product Manufactory Process

The scope of this section is to provide a list of tests generally performed for protein-based drug manufacturing platforms. For nonprotein-based (biologics) drug development program testing, requirements can be different which are highly dependent on the nature and characteristics of the product. The production process of protein drugs (e.g., antibody and other proteins) is a two-stage process. The first stage is a growth and production phase which begins with different protein expression platforms like a mammalian expression system (e.g., Chinese hamster ovary [CHO] cell lines) or a microbial expression system (e.g., *E. coli*). The second stage is a downstream purification and formulation process. In general, the required in-process tests while manufacturing a product is defined by the product development phase of the project. All the specifications are developed and established during the process validation in order to define various process control steps. This activity is in turn guided by the process development activities of product development. Release tests for a drug substance (DS) and drug product (DP) are established based on the DS and DP in question in addition to certain regulatory guidelines, and the tests should demonstrate/establish identity, strength/potency, quality, and purity of a drug product. Several of the release test methods also serve as stability-indicating test methods during the required stability study program for DS and DP.

Microbiology (See Figure 26.31)

In-Process Tests For unprocessed bulk harvest common in-process tests are:

- Bioburden
- Mycoplasma detection with mycoplasmastasis
- *In vitro* assay for nonendogenous or adventitious viruses
- Detection of Mouse Minute Virus (MMV) DNA by quantitative polymerase chain reaction (qPCR),
- Transmission electron microscopy (TEM) of supernatant

Endotoxin testing is performed on the clarified bulk harvest.

Release Tests for Drug Substance

- Bioburden
- Endotoxin

Chemistry (See Figure 26.32)

In-Process Tests

- pH
- Conductivity
- Protein content by UV A280
- Titer analysis (e.g. Protein A-HPLC [high-performance liquid chromatography] for antibody, or enzyme-linked immunosorbent assay- [ELISA] based test method for other protein products)
- Sometimes size exclusion-HPLC (SE-HPLC), reverse-phase-HPLC (RP-HPLC), and sodium dodecyl sulfate

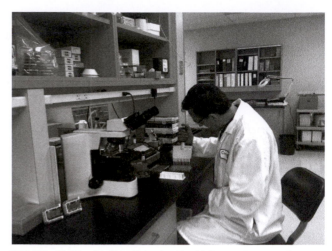

FIGURE 26.31   Quality Control Microbiology. (*Source: Cytovance Biologics Inc., 2013.*)

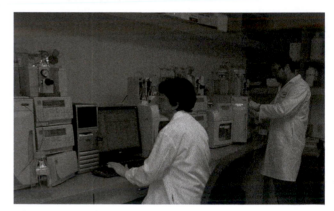

FIGURE 26.32   Quality control analytics. (*Source: Cytovance Biologics Inc., 2013.*)

polyacrylamide gel electrophoresis (SDS-PAGE) (reduced/nonreduced) methods are also used as in-process tests to monitor the efficiency of purification steps, state of aggregation of the product, and step-wise improvement in the product quality. Occasionally suitable potency or activity assay is also performed as an in-process test to monitor product quality as one moves through the manufacturing process. (See Table 26.3.)

Environmental Tests

For a compliant biomanufacturing facility, it is essential to develop a contamination control program. This program needs to address three basic tasks:

1. Control (minimization) of bioburden throughout the process of product manufacturing.
2. Control (minimization) of cross-over contamination of residuals from batch-to-batch production.

TABLE 26.3 Quality Control Release Tests for Drug Substance

Attribute	Drug Substance	Drug Product
Safety	Endotoxin	Endotoxin
Safety	Bioburden	Sterility
Impurities	Host cell protein (HCP)	N/A
Impurities	Residual DNA	N/A
Impurities	Tween 20 or Tween 80 or Triton X 100 or any other excipient (if added during formulation)	N/A
Impurities	Residual Protein A (if Protein A was used during purification process, e.g., for antibody product)	N/A
Quality	pH	pH
Quality	Osmolality	Osmolality
Quality	Appearance (color, visible particulate matter)	Appearance (color, visible particulate matter)
Quality	N/A	Subvisible particulate matter (10 µm, 25 µm), (2 µm, 5 µm, 8 µm for information only)
Quality	N/A	Volume in container
Quality	N/A	Container closure integrity
Strength/content	Protein concentration by A280 (or any other assay such as Bradford, BCA, etc.)	Protein concentration by A280 (or any other assay such as Bradford, BCA, etc.)
Purity	SE-HPLC	
Purity	SDS-PAGE (reduced and nonreduced), CE-SDS	SDS-PAGE (reduced and nonreduced), CE-SDS
Purity	RP-HPLC	RP-HPLC
Identity and charge heterogeneity	IEF, cIEF	IEF, cIEF
Identity and charge heterogeneity	CEX, CZE	CEX, CZE
Identity	Peptide map	Peptide map
Potency	Binding ELISA	Binding ELISA
Potency	Bioassay	Bioassay

Source: *Cytovance Biologics Inc., 2013.*

3. Control (minimization) of cross-over contamination of residuals from cleaning materials during the production period.

In order to achieve these goals it is critical to establish suitable laboratory test methods and operational practices. Appropriate gowning procedures, personnel monitoring, environmental monitoring (EM), air quality monitoring with settling plates, facility surface cleaning and disinfection monitoring, and purified water monitoring (by total organic carbon [TOC] analysis) are key programs that need to be established in the form of SOPs and implemented for a compliant biomanufacturing facility which is engaged in the production of quality drug products. (See Figure 26.33A and B.)

CONTRACT (CMO) VERSUS IN-HOUSE MANUFACTURING

Traditionally in the pharmaceutical industry the paradigm was to build small molecule manufacturing facilities that could manufacture large quantities of product reproducibly. These plants had enormous amounts of stainless steel and required a large facility footprint as well as a large workforce. With the discovery of therapeutic biologics or (large molecules), biopharmaceutical and biomanufacturing facilities were both newly constructed and others were converted into biomanufacturing facilities. These early in-house facilities were expensive to construct and at times retrofits were not right for the technology or difficult to

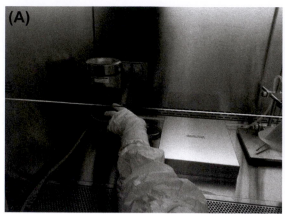
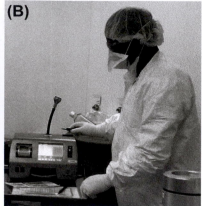

FIGURE 26.33 A and B. (A) Environmental Monitoring (EM) Technician setting up test equipment to monitor viable air particles (microbials) during processing. (B) the EM Technician setting up a Particle Counter to monitor particles in the air of the production suite. Quality control environmental microbiology/environmental monitoring. *(Source: Cytovance Biologics Inc., 2013).*

scale and reproduce. Thus many companies outsourced development and manufacturing of their biologic products to contract development organizations (CDOs) or contract manufacturing organizations (CMOs) or contract development and manufacturing organizations (CDMOs). Most CMO facilities were designed to have a scaled process to support preclinical through Phases 1, 2, and 3 and some that could support the commercial launch of complex biologic products.

Academic facilities, small biotech companies, medium seasoned biotech companies, large biopharmaceutical companies, and virtual companies have varying abilities to financially support and build a facility for multiple biologic platforms in-house. Most CMOs have already built manufacturing capabilities to produce and purify biologic drugs at a certain scale to accommodate their scale or "niche" market. These capabilities are large capital expenditures such as stainless steel bioreactors, fermentors, mixing tanks, water systems, chromatography skids, chromatography columnsclean roomsms, QC labs, EM Labs, process development labs as well as Quality systems. The advantage of a CMO facility is that it is ready for manufacturing the developed product. Although, today there are a variety of disposable options in the small-scale manufacture of biologics which would allow a small company to consider biomanufacturing in-house. There are single-use bioreactors (SUBs) that range from a 25 liter to a 2000 liter scale as well as single-use mixing units (SUMs) in the same scale. Some biotech companies are using disposables to perform small-scale studies to support some preclinical or pilot-scale work and then transfer the process and further scale-up to a CMO. This allows the biotech company more control and hands on during early-process development.

A major disadvantage for the in-house model is the capital outlay for an in-house facility. In terms of time

and equipment, an in-house facility would be very costly in respect to supporting in-house expertise to manage the design, fabrication, installation and qualification of the facility, process, and support equipment. There are other considerations such as cleaning and maintenance of all product contact surfaces such as bioreactors and mixing tanks. These require studies and validation of the cleaning processes. Samples would have to be taken and tested creating additional in-house expertise, time, and resources and this would be contingent on suite availability to develop and manufacture the product. Whereas outsourcing these activities to a contract manufacturing organization (CMO) would shorten the timeline significantly because the CMO would already have the expertise, process, and facility equipment in place to support the development and manufacturing activities. Other aspects that need to be considered is the support for biomanufacturing with QA and QC groups that are necessary for the GMP documentation, in-process testing, and release testing. The Chemistry, Manufacturing and Control (CMC) section of a company's investigational new drug (IND) could be completed by the CMO and would be support for the biotech company as one of the CMO's regulatory offerings.

The availability of reliable and functional disposable equipment at small scales such as SUBs and SUMs mentioned previously might be reasonable for some small companies that may have a modular (factory-built panels delivered and assembled on-site with a factory-impervious finish) or stick-built (onsite piece-by-piece construction such as framing, sheet rock, and epoxy-type finishes) facility with proper cleaning and HVAC (that can deliver a classified or controlled environment) to bring in a SUB or SUM. The disposables or single use equipment offers quick installation, flexibility and no cleaning validation as compared to it's stainless steel bioreactor, buffer tanks and mixer predecessors. However, a company would still have to invest in clean rooms and infrastructure to support biologic GMP production. At the end of the day it would be more cost and time line effective to enlist a CMO to carry the "heavy lifting" of the drug development process. As a result, many biotechnology and biopharmaceutical companies are more commonly outsourcing some or all of their biomanufacturing needs. Outsourcing allows a company to remain focused on the crucial components in-house while taking advantage of a CMO to supply their resources for process development, analytical development, manufacturing, quality and regulatory support. Utilizing a CMO for outsourcing can help reduce or eliminate the need to build, manage, and maintain a facility, or it allows a company time to grow until it can justify a permanent facility.

SUMMARY

The incredible amount of recent biologic therapeutic discoveries has led to an increased need for scientific and engineering knowledge available to characterize and biomanufacture these large and complex molecules. In this chapter we have followed what role biomanufacturing has in the development of a biotherapeutic product. We have followed the biologic product's development from "proof-of-concept," examined the history of these large molecules, and developed a knowledge-base that we would use in developing a scaled process that would be tech-transferred into manufacturing. Within this chapter we also discussed key partners in the biomanufacturing process such as raw material suppliers, outsource testing vendors, as well as key support teams such as facilities, engineering, process development, quality assurance, quality control, environmental monitoring, manufacturing, and manufacturing science and technology teams required to fully develop and manufacture a biologic that can meet all of the critical safety, quality, and regulatory parameters.

It is essential that the biomanufacturing process be able to deliver and demonstrate a safe therapeutic drug at each step of the clinical trial, be economically able to reproducibly manufacture sufficient inventory with a stable shelf-life, and to successfully traverse the regulatory and efficacy hurdles in order to obtain regulatory approval. In biomanufacturing "the process is the product" is an old paradigm, but it is still relevant in the development and manufacture of a biotherapeutic.

The Later-Stage Biotechnology Company

Chapter 27

Company Growth Stages and the Value of Corporate Culture

Craig Shimasaki, PhD, MBA

President & CEO, Moleculera Labs and BioSource Consulting, Oklahoma City, Oklahoma

All companies transition through growth stages along their pathway to commercialization and maturity. This transition is a real process that subtly occurs over time. There are discrete growth stages of every company and during these stages there are certain characteristics of successful companies that distinguish these stages. Also, it is during these transition phases a company successfully or unsuccessfully moves to the next stage. Knowing and understanding this transition process, and the factors that influence it, will help the leader affect the culture and guide the company through each growth stage in a positive way. Successful transition is also influenced by the leadership's ability to implement appropriate process changes. For instance, the procedures and policies that work for 5 employees do not work optimally for a company of 50 employees, or for 500 employees. In addition, the leaders are also risk managers of the company and they must effectively manage the changing risks of a growing and transitioning company. As this transition takes place there is a corporate culture that is established, and it evolves from simply the core values of the founders to the sum total of the core values of the majority of the new hires.

In this chapter we will cover a variety of topics related to the growth, transition, and management of a company over time. These topics include an overview of the developing company transition stages and the changes that management must make, the corporate culture and core values of the company, the risks that must be managed by the leadership, and the potential impact of the continual hiring of new employees. As companies transition through these different development stages, they are accompanied with changes in communication methods, processes for making corporate decisions, and the level at which certain decisions are made. Being aware of company development stages is vital because problems can occur when an entrepreneurial company transitions into the next development stage but their leaders do not. As an organization makes a transition, the leader must also make a transition,

particularly in their management and communication style if they hope to effectively lead their company to accomplishing their goals. The purpose of this chapter is to help the entrepreneur be more effective in managing a highly dynamic scientific business that is dependent on working effectively with knowledgeable and highly motivated individuals.

As a company accomplishes each successive objective toward creating a valuable product or service, it adds staff, expands activities, establishes corporate relationships, and their business practices evolve. Changes and adjustments also occur in the process of how a company makes decisions at all levels. A company that is comprised of 10,000 employees in 5 geographic locations that manufactures and markets products in locations worldwide, makes decisions differently than a start-up organization with a handful of employees and one product in development. The optimal methods and decision-making processes for an early-stage company does not necessarily work well for a mature company and vice versa.

In the early stages of corporate development, the leadership of the organization is usually comprised of one individual. As it grows, leadership responsibilities are shared with other key individuals. As the company continues to grow, leadership responsibilities expand to a greater number of key managers and employees. Throughout this chapter, the term "leadership" may refer to one or more individuals, yet it always will reference the individuals empowered with the responsibility and authority to make final decisions.

CORPORATE DEVELOPMENT AND TRANSITION STAGES

The development stages of an organization are outlined below, and these represent a continuum which all organizations transition through as they grow. Every organization is dynamic. By recognizing these transition stages and understanding the characteristics of different corporate development stages, the entrepreneur leader can improve their leadership ability to effectively manage their organization for long-term success. It is not necessary to understand everything about each corporate development stage, it is only important to recognize *when* it occurs and *what* changes and adjustments to make so that your organization can keep forward momentum and increase in strength as you move toward your corporate goals. (See Table 27.1.)

All companies eventually transition through each of these corporate development stages whereas the time spent at each stage will vary by company. The following section contains a discussion of the characteristics of each development stage along with some of the likely key activities. Each of the key activities may differ for each organization and it will be based upon the type of product and the biotechnology sector in which the company operates. Also, I describe some aspects of the leader's management style during these phases.

THE START-UP PHASE

For those who are founders, the start-up phase is an exciting experience, and yet at times it can seem frightening because it feels as if you are staring at a vast unknown. When establishing a new company, there is excitement, anticipation, and expectation of the future. There is a sense of newness. In reality, the start-up phase is the most fragile growth stage of the company and many do not proceed past this stage for a multitude of reasons. A good analogy to the start-up phase is that of the first pioneer settlers who colonized and established the providences in America. They had no roadmap or best practices to guide them, and yet the opportunity was unlimited. However, success was dependent upon the creative ideas and inherent ability of the founders to create and build something of great value.

Start-Up Phase Key Activities

In all start-ups there is usually one or more founders, and occasionally a very small team of individuals who may be working part-time or operating in a consulting capacity at the newly formed company. If the technology is owned by a research or academic institution, key activities will be to negotiate and secure the license, secure or file patents, set up the proper corporate structure, and formalize agreements between the company and the founders, including issuing stock and creating a business plan. In addition to these corporate activities there will be a multitude of product-development activities to move the product forward to milestones and raise start-up or seed capital.

During this stage, the biotech entrepreneur will be accomplishing or overseeing almost everything. There will

TABLE 27.1 Corporate Development Stages and Focuses

Corporate Development Stages		Key Management Focuses	Work Environment Characterization
Start-Up Phase	Establishment	Proper corporate structure, license agreement, key consultants, product development milestones, creating a business plan, raising start-up capital	Newness, excitement
Development Phase	Early	Investors and future funding, outside collaborators and contract organizations, meeting product-development milestones, hiring key employees	Anticipation, discovery
	Middle	Major funding, hiring employees, significant product-development milestones, developing market strategy	Expansion, gaining strength, milestone successes, growth
	Late	Additional funding, additional employees, key management, regulatory milestones, prototypes and clinical trials, product launch	Navigating challenges, critical decisions
Expansion Phase	Early	Corporate partnerships, expanding market and channels, reimbursement	Market entry and success
	Late	Additional management, additional market applications, developing new products, and expanding applications of existing products	Growing market share
Decline Phase	Decline	Dealing with competitor products, internal and external challenges, decreasing sales revenue	Internal and external issues, employee concerns

be a myriad of activities and all of them will be important, and all must somehow get done. While trying to get the company properly established, the entrepreneur may already have a full-time job which means working long hours, nights, and weekends. The biotech entrepreneur quickly learns that regardless of what their expertise is, they must adapt and become a jack-of-all trades.

Start-Up Phase Management and Decision-Making

During this stage the entrepreneur leader will be shaping the future and the direction in which the organization will be headed. Because the entrepreneur will be the only individual with the completeness of the vision for the organization and the product, he or she will be leading the organization with a "command-and-control" management style at this phase. "Command-and-control" simply refers to the fact that all decisions are being made by one individual who then directs the work of others and evaluates the outcomes. This individual then makes decisions about these outcomes as to their appropriateness, compared to what is required to reach their ultimate goals. This management style can also be called the "entrepreneurial" management style. During the start-up stage this style of management is essential because the team members are counting on the leader to communicate the company's direction and objectives and to tell them what success looks like. This style of management is not the same as micromanaging tasks, but all tasks must be directed toward making incremental advancements toward the desired outcome.

An inappropriate connotation of the "command-and-control" management style is that of a military boot camp where a demanding leader is ordering recruits around. Whereas, this management style is interactive, information- and opinion-gathering, yet the ultimate decisions are still made by the leader who is aligning each decision to result in the progressive movement toward their envisioned goals. During this time all team members will be depending on the leader for direction and to make quality decisions. Therefore, the leader cannot be tentative or be someone who vacillates in their decisions. The leader must know their goals and know how the team will achieve them, even if some of these goals are still being determined along the way. The absence of a strong visionary leader and/or poor strategy and poor execution will result in the demise of a start-up before it has a chance to transition to the next development stage.

THE DEVELOPMENT PHASE

Early-Development Phase

During this phase, an organization has made a significant transition from a start-up to a development-stage company. At this stage there are still only a handful of individuals

who are responsible for accomplishing the company goals. These individuals may be working part-time, operating in a consulting capacity, or there may occasionally be a full-time employee or two, depending on the funding situation. At this phase an initial funding event will have occurred and the company will have some capital to work with for advancing the product further along in development.

Early-Development Phase Key Activities

The company is most often operating as a virtual organization where most of the activities are contracted out to other organizations, including the laboratories of the original inventors. The major focus is on achieving critical product-development milestones using the early capital raised. Other activities include finding key employees and raising additional capital for the next stage of product development. Plans are being made for future regulatory goals and objectives, and refining the market strategy.

Early Development Phase Management and Decision-Making

The early-development phase requires a strong leader with a clear vision and a strategic plan because all activities are essential and need to be completed, and everything seems equally important. Still, without clear priorities, nothing will be completed in a timely manner. The leader must continually communicate the corporate plans and the product values to internal and external stakeholders. If the leader is unsure, unclear, or inconsistent in priorities, goals, and objectives, the company's growth becomes stunted and these limited resources are yielding limited value. At this stage the leader must still manage with a command-and-control style and ensure that company growth and progress moves in the right direction and that all activities are directed toward the correct goals, though, at this stage there should be team members who the leader can trust to share a portion of the leadership responsibilities. These individuals share the same vision as the entrepreneur, possess similar values, and understand and agree with the goals and objectives of the company and the product being developed. Consistency and persistence are the essential characteristics for companies at this early-development phase. Some organizations never make it past this stage because of unforeseen external or internal challenges, inability to raise capital, or lack of clear leadership. In order to move to the next phase, the company must persist in accomplishing what it set out to do, being resourceful, and often making some course corrections that improve the value of the developing product or improve its market interest.

Mid-Development Phase

During this phase, the organization continues to grow with steady and consistent progress being made toward its corporate- and product-development objectives. Major funding has been secured to advance product development to the next significant milestone, and greater value is being attributed to the organization. The employees are content with the organization and its future and they feel informed about the company and its progress, and enjoy their work. There is early public interest in the product being developed and the anticipation that it will meet some important need.

Mid-Development Phase Key Activities

The company has been building internal capabilities but it still outsources most activities, however more of these are being integrated and supported within the organization. Major funding has provided ample working capital for additional hires to expand internal functions. Product development progress has reached key milestones and the company is overcoming many challenges encountered during its growth and during product development. Preliminary meetings are occurring with potential partners and public relations is resulting in some recognition for the company.

Mid-Development Phase Management and Decision-Making

At this phase the leader must begin transitioning from managing through a command-and-control style to a delegate-and-inspect management style. If the leader does not adjust their management style during this transition stage they can become an impediment to the company and the product-development progress. Management-style transition is as much a change for the employees as it is for the leader who in the past made all the decisions. At this stage there should be other key management who have the leadership skills that can be trusted to make many of the decisions for a particular function, and they should be given that responsibility. This transition will not occur instantly, but gradually over time as the leader begins delegating more responsibility to other key management. The leader must still communicate a clear vision for the company, and must constantly convey, internally and externally, the company's development progress. In spite of this management style transition, employees must still believe that they can go to the leader for solutions to major problems if necessary, and be confident that the leader is approachable. The leader must create an expanding leadership team and operate in the company's unique strengths. They must not forget that one key strength is their quickness and agility in creatively responding to problems and external challenges.

Late-Development Phase

Because of the lengthy product-development process for all biotechnology products, many companies may spend a great deal of time in this development phase. This is also the stage where large amounts of capital are consumed as companies move through lengthy clinical trials and regulatory processes. By now the company has closed several large rounds of funding. And often at this stage the company encounters product-development challenges, product-testing issues, and possibly regulatory issues, which all must be overcome. During this phase there may be tensions developing as to the future of the company, or there may be questions about how the company will overcome these challenges.

Late-Development Phase Key Activities

Key activities include product and field testing, such as human or prototype testing, meeting with regulatory agencies, examining scale-up options, and partners. Other activities include sourcing and meeting with potential marketing partners or those interested in late-stage clinical trial development or as a potential acquirer of the company. The staff and personnel number is increasing and there usually is an additional layer of management added within the organization.

Late-Development Phase Management and Decision-Making

By this stage the leader must have made a complete transition to a delegate-and-inspect management style. By now the hired managers and employees have sufficient expertise and possess untapped capabilities which will be underutilized if the leader does not make the transition by this stage. Regarding management style, the leader should be focused on articulating the important and strategic business goals to the senior management and provide the team with measurable goals to evaluate progress. The management team should consist of seasoned individuals having vast experience, but all must support identical goals for the product, the market, and the organization. These individuals may include a Chief Scientific Officer (CSO), Chief Medical Officer (CMO), Chief Financial Officer (CFO), Business Development Executive, Regulatory executive, to name a few. If the company is relatively small then these individuals may not be that senior, but they often will cover these same functions. It is important that the leader has fully completed the management-style transition and be functioning effectively with the leadership team. If this has not occurred by now, managers and employees will experience growing frustration and a lack of challenge to themselves and their own career.

One obvious reason for the management style transition is that by now the individuals whom a leader manages usually possess more knowledge and understanding about a problem or situation than the leader will. Therefore, these individuals are the best ones to make certain decisions; this is true of all levels of employees. If the management style does not transition, employees become ineffective and usually find nonproductive activities to occupy their unused capacity, or most often, they will leave to find more challenging positions of employment. A leader who still directs task-oriented work will deprive capable employees of the opportunity to step-up and contribute at a greater responsibility level.

EXPANSION PHASE

Early-Expansion Phase

Organizations that reach this stage have successfully passed the hurdles of product development and have received regulatory approval for their new product (if required), and they are manufacturing their product and expanding the market for their product. Reaching this phase means there is tremendous potential for the company and staff is being added and capabilities are being expanded. By now, the company will have made some mistakes along the way, but none have been beyond repair and these are corrected quickly. Management must maintain a start-up mentality and not set up a bureaucracy that impedes the company's agility and its ability to respond quickly. Management's challenge will be that of balancing a standard process infrastructure but maintaining the flexibility and creativity that was a strength in their previous development stage.

Early-Expansion Phase Key Activities

At this stage the company's product is in the market and much activity is concentrated around executing the market strategy, managing market channels, manufacturing activities, and reimbursement challenges (for medical products). Companies now must execute their plan and monitor their external environment for changes that impact them and their products.

Early-Expansion Phase Management and Decision-Making

At this phase, the management style has become more similar to that of larger corporate entities, yet there still should be a relatively flat organization, meaning that there are very few layers of management. The company should still have the ability to make decisions in a way that takes advantage of a smaller company's strengths. Management focus should include training more leaders at new levels of the organization rather than just better managing tasks, as these new leaders can impact greater portions of the organization. The leadership and management are quite capable of handling development and growth needs but they still experience a few crises every now and then. Communication is vital within the organization and management should ensure that all employees feel they are informed about the progress of the company.

Late-Expansion Phase

The companies that reach this phase are successful in their own right. They have developed great capabilities and are efficient producers, manufacturers, and marketers of their products, and they are increasing their market share. Companies such as Amgen, Genentech, Biogen-IDEC, and Genzyme reside at this phase. Of course, each of these organizations have encountered challenges and many of their early employees may have moved on, some to start companies of their own. It is interesting to note that employees who were there in the early days remember a different company and they may believe that the company had become "institutionalized." No doubt a few "bureaucratic processes" may have been adopted, but enough individuals adhere to the importance of just getting the job done rather than creating additional processes. Some companies will have been acquired by now or merged with a larger organization.

Late-Expansion Phase Key Activities

The company is focused on market strategy, reimbursement (if medical products), manufacturing, improving quality, and new-product development. If the company is not acquired or the first product is not licensed to a marketing partner, there may be financing activities for securing mezzanine rounds of capital for expansion.

Late-Expansion Phase Management and Decision-Making

One key characteristic of successful companies at this corporate stage is clear and frequent communication from management to staff and employees. As organizational structures enlarge, communication channels tend to break down. When this occurs, corporate communications problems begin. The absence of information can cause employees to think and presume information that may or may not be true. Several things can help a successful transition through this stage. One activity is frequent and meaningful communications between the leader, the senior staff, and all levels of the organization about the goals, the plans, and the reasons for these choices. Employees need to know what is going on outside of their own discipline, which will help them work more knowledgeably. Management must be sure to communicate progress about all aspects of the business to employees, even if it changes frequently. The leadership must continue to share with employees the vision for the future and demonstrate that there is purpose and value in what they are doing.

DECLINE PHASE

This is not a planned stage of corporate development and it is one that must be avoided. Reaching this stage is not a milestone, but it means that either the company or its products have become irrelevant to the market or that their products are nearing the end of their life cycle. Finding a company at this stage can also mean that they have stopped innovating and relied on a single product for their growth. Arriving at this stage is much less frequent in the biotech industry, but it still happens if products become commodities and the company fails to continue product innovation and only focus on sales and marketing.

Decline Phase Management and Decision-Making

We will not elaborate much on this except that it is management's responsibility to lead and guide their organization through each corporate-development stage without reaching this one. Biotech companies are known for innovation and product leadership, and as such it would be unusual to find many biotech companies that reach this stage very often.

THE CEO'S ROLE IN THE TRANSITION OF LIFE STAGES

It is the responsibility of the leadership, particularly the CEO, to lead change and to guide their company and employees successfully through each development stage. The CEO must recognize each transition phase and respond by managing in an appropriate manner for that development stage. A command-and-control management style is optimal for a start-up company with one part-time administrative assistant, a scientist, and a technician. However, this management style will not be effective for 50 employees including a senior management team of a Chief Scientific Officer, Chief Financial Officer, Chief Medical Officer, and Business Development Executive. The CEO's management style must transition as the organization transitions, or the CEO may not be leading the company for long.

Sometimes the CEO does not know how to change, or they may have difficulty adapting to change and resort to managing as in the start-up stage rather than making a management-style transition. Often the CEO does not want to change. Encountering resistance to change is not uncommon when an entrepreneur who founded the start-up organization becomes CEO and then grows the company to the next level and receives a major round of funding. If the company has received venture capital, a VC partner will be on the company's board. The VC will have limited patience with a CEO that is resistant to change, but most often will give the entrepreneur CEO an opportunity to make changes. If the entrepreneur CEO cannot make appropriate changes, the VCs will replace the CEO and bring on a seasoned and experienced person that understands how to manage a growth company. Venture capitalists may be seen as only interested in their investment, but they also want the company to succeed or they will not have many future

investment opportunities themselves. Seasoned and experienced VCs can quickly recognize the signs of an unhealthy organization and will do what they can to correct the situation so that the organization can survive. Founding entrepreneurs know there are significant challenges to building a successful biotech company, but *they* should not be one of those challenges as it is counterproductive and can be prematurely fatal to the company.

MANAGEMENT SKILL SETS

The CEO is the *leader*, but the *leadership* includes all individuals given responsibility and authority for making decisions for the company. As the organization grows, the leadership will include others responsible for scientific, corporate, marketing, regulatory, and manufacturing functions. Unfortunately, not everyone who is given responsibility for a function carries great management skills. There are an abundance of helpful books available for improving management skills, and a young company should invest time and energy in training and equipping their managers and leaders. For brevity, the following is a list of characteristics that are important to be sure are present in all managers. If the leader does not possess these traits, the first thing they should do is work on improving their own management skills so they can help teach and instill them in others.

Five Qualities of Successful Managers

1. **They identify**—Successful managers have or acquire the ability to recognize the right people for the right positions based upon needs at that time.
2. **They lead and inspire**—The knowledge of how to inspire and motivate individuals to achieve their goals, objectives, and tasks and see the vision set before them.
3. **They teach**—The ability to teach and instruct individuals to accomplish the objectives that align with the vision the company has created
4. **They inspect**—The ability to appropriately monitor and inspect the progress and results from the efforts of these individuals and make necessary adjustments to continue progress towards those goals.
5. **They reward**—The understanding of the value of praise, appreciation, increased responsibility, incentives, and remuneration; a different mix is required for different individuals.

CORPORATE CULTURE AND CORE VALUES IN A BIOTECHNOLOGY COMPANY

Every company is unique in its culture, its employee mix, and the manner in which it conducts its business. One can say that each company has a personality all its own. Typically, the collective characteristics of a company are referred to as a corporate culture. A company's culture is tangible in that outsiders and customers can sense a real difference between one company's employees and those of another organization. For instance, one company may have a culture that is characterized by innovation, excitement, and collaboration, motivating employees to ignore the traditional work hours and do whatever is necessary to get a job done regardless of the time of day. Conversely, another company may have a minimalist culture with clock-watching employees, doing only what is required and only if it is written in their job description.

Your corporate culture will be a strength or a weakness. Every company encounters problems and challenges and it seems like biotechnology companies have more than their fair share of them. But the corporate culture of a company is a good predictor of their ability to overcome a crisis.

Example of the Tylenol Scare of 1982

In 1982, seven consumer deaths occurred when these individuals ingested tainted Tylenol Extra Strength capsules laced with cyanide. This crisis situation has been analyzed as a case study in business schools around the world as an example of how to successfully respond to crisis. Ortho McNeil's employees (a Johnson & Johnson company) responded according to their corporate culture of putting first the well-being and needs of the people they serve. It was quickly discovered that the Tylenol capsules were tampered with *after* they left the manufacturer, and the contamination was not the company's fault. However, Ortho McNeil executives made the decision to immediately recall 31 million bottles of Tylenol at a cost of over $100 million. To further protect the public, the company nationally advertised not to consume any products containing Tylenol. Most interesting is that this type of crisis management was not really "taught" to the Ortho McNeil employees, nor was it a rehearsed response. It was later recognized that these actions were based upon their organization's core values [1] established by their founder and this is what guided the employee's decision-making. Ortho McNeil possessed a company culture and core values that were an asset, but these values only became visible to the public as a result of this crisis. As a result, Ortho McNeil created many of the commonly used over-the-counter (OTC) product manufacturing safety measures. This crisis, which could have taken a company down, only helped demonstrate the core values of the company and their product's value.

Development of a Corporate Culture

For a biotechnology start-up, developing a corporate culture may not seem like a high priority compared to the need of finding money, hiring a team, and quickly making product-development progress. Yet, it is critical to pay attention to the development of a culture because at some point the company reaches a critical mass, and like concrete, the culture of the organization becomes set. A company may temporarily ignore the development of a corporate culture without much consequence, but at some point this will impact the ability to effectively accomplish objectives. One thing is certain, there will be a company culture whether it is by design or default. Every company's corporate culture is somehow different and there is no universal culture that is optimal for everyone. For instance, an organization operating in a highly ordered industry such as accounting may not be best suited to have a culture based upon creativity, but rather one of constancy; yet there are other beneficial qualities that are valuable to many. If a company has a fully developed culture that is counter-productive to progress, now is time to do something to change. Choose to purposefully create a culture that adds strength, rather than on that is divisive or detrimental to progress.

As previously discussed, all companies transition through distinct growth phases, and everything does not always work out exactly as planned. Internal and external changes and adjustments are inevitable as a company grows. Your corporate culture will be a help or a hindrance in overcoming these challenges in product development and organizational growth. Fortunately, most start-up biotechnology companies begin with an entrepreneurial culture that is energetic, creative, and persevering. When founding team members and management hold themselves to a defined set of core values, the organization operates in a consistent manner and the employees have confidence as to how problems and issues will be resolved.

Every Individual Defines the Corporate Culture and Core Values

An organization's strength is the sum total of all the individual strengths. Each employee makes decisions based upon their own knowledge and their core values. An employee with a core value of "mutual respect for others" does not think about how they may leave an unfinished task for another employee to complete. Someone with a core value of "acceptance of responsibility for ones actions" will readily admit a mistake rather than cover it up or blame someone else. These examples may seem minor by themselves, but add these up amongst 15, 150, or 1500 employees and this becomes the prevailing culture of the organization. Individuals who do not share the same company values arrive at different conclusions based upon the same information, and this causes internal conflicts which would have been disastrous for Ortho McNeal during their Tylenol crisis. The corporate culture does not always impact whether or not things get done, but rather *how* and *when* things get done.

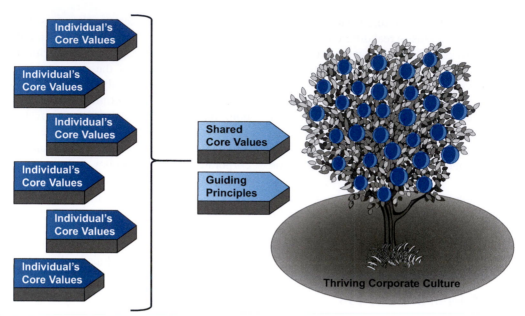

FIGURE 27.1   Developing a Corporate Culture.

For stability, organizations need foundational values that are clear and unwavering. Core values that are only framed and hung on a wall but do not penetrate into the hearts and minds of the leadership are eventually resisted or resented by all employees. The leadership must demonstrate in their daily activities that they operate and make decisions in accordance with their core values. Values that are demonstrated to apply to senior management will be reinforced, embraced, and even expected of all employees throughout the organization. A company without a driving set of core values is equivalent to a ship without a compass.

Core Value Examples

There are a multitude of core values that many great companies espouse and these values may be different for every company. The key is that an organization has core values that employees embrace and live by. Core values can be thought of as the seeds of an organization's future. The selection and incorporation of a particular set of core values will ultimately bear the fruit innate to those values. Just as a farmer planting orange trees would not expect to harvest tomatoes, likewise, the selection of certain core values predict the type of culture a company will yield as it matures. (See Figure 27.1.) Below are some examples of core values and guiding principles that may be embraced by a start-up company. Remember, these are not the only ones nor are they necessarily the ideal ones for every company, but they are examples of some that are associated with significance.

Corporate Core Value Examples

- **We are team players**—We help each other grow within and across departmental functions to be part of a greater purpose; it is not just a job.
- **We show mutual respect to everyone**—We value each other and it is exemplified by our behavior. We listen to each other, using tact and giving reasons why we do the things we do.
- **We value honesty and integrity**—We say what we mean and we do what we say, whether it is convenient or not.
- **We are accountable and responsible**—We take ownership for our actions, both right and wrong.
- **We have open communications**—Across all levels and functions of the company for internal and external information, both good and bad news.
- **We are focused**—We have defined plans and ideas that are prioritized to reach our goals. We have the discipline to say "no" when appropriate.
- **We are empowered**—We perform our tasks with creativity to reach our goals while developing new solutions to problems. We understand the value we contribute to the overall goal of the organization.

From these defined or simply understood core values a company will develop and adopt a mission statement. Mission statements are standard convention and it is rare that an organization does not have one. However, a company's underlying core values are even more important to an organization's future than its mission statement. A mission statement is an aspiration of the company, whereas core values are inherent within the company's employees. In order to fully establish a corporate culture, the core values must be translated into more tangible "guiding principles."

Guiding Principle Examples Based Upon Core Values

Core values must be translated into guiding principles which help individuals better understand how the organization desires its employee to make decisions and operate. A set of guiding principles can be defined or they can be just understood. Below are some examples of guiding principles that are based upon various core values.

- We are a diverse group of individuals with differing backgrounds who share the same core values and encourage each other and also remind each other if we don't live up to our own values.
- We value our partners and patients highly and are loyal to them and their needs. Our partners are our physicians, employees, vendors, and suppliers. Our patients are our mission.
- We are a relationship-oriented company. We will incorporate into all our business, market, and science endeavors a relationship orientation with our "partners" in achieving common goals that benefit each other. We will seek relationships with partners sharing common or mutually beneficial goals.
- We will differ from our competitors by incorporating innovation into all of our products. In addition, the products that we develop will not be an end in themselves but tools to improve healthcare in the broadest sense.
- Our profitable differences will be seen in our product innovation value discipline and not in the commoditization of products. Our product positioning will be "best-in-class" where there are competitors. This will be accomplished through our products themselves and the collateral services and programs provided that create more value to the customer than the product alone.
- When our products are launched, we will work to improve outcome measurements such that the true long-term benefit of our products will be understood.

The Impact of Core Values

If the leader esteems core values, so will the organization. Leaders will exemplify the core values that the company will espouse, such as in the Credo developed by Robert Wood Johnson in 1943 for the Johnson & Johnson Company. Core values can be thought of as a belief system and a set of non-negotiable behaviors that a group of individuals value. Having core values does not automatically guarantee business success, however they will provide the highest likelihood of

success. Once the company is successful, strong core values ensure the likelihood of sustaining that success. If your desire is to build an organization with lasting value, core values cannot be ignored. Possessing strong core values are beneficial not only in business but they apply to family life and relationships. A good book with simple truths about core values written by an ex-school teacher is titled *Life's Greatest Lessons: 20 Things that Matter* [2].

Select Partners and Service Providers Based Upon Common Core Values

The selection of critical suppliers and service providers should be evaluated similarly to the hiring of a senior or executive staff member of the organization. The same care, scrutiny, and examination of common goals should be evaluated prior to forming a relationship because as the organization begins to grow and make progress, the company will become interdependent on the quality and reliability of these external relationships. Since start-up organizations outsource many activities during early development, it is vital that these suppliers and service providers share similar core values. The last thing a growing biotech company needs is to experience problems such as the break-down of trust and confidence with critical partners. The 80/20 rule is true in external relationships, meaning that 80 percent of the company's time is spent working on 20 percent of the worst relationships. These are simply manifestations of inconsistencies in core values between the two parties. These incompatible relationships divert management attention away from building the business and reaching their goals.

The best time to evaluate a relationship is before it is consummated. When choosing a partner, service provider, or supplier, do not make choices based upon pricing alone. You must evaluate all aspects of the partnership including communication, strategic direction, corporate values, and their interest in a long-term synergy rather than just pricing a transaction. We all know that relationships will face difficulties at some time, but these challenges should be opportunities to alter a process, improve a communication channel, or modify a working relationship, rather than a suboptimal way of doing business. When substandard behavior becomes tolerated as the norm, working with these relationships become weary and burdensome. Great suppliers and service providers should be willing to concede short-term financial gain to work through issues if your interest is in a long-term relationship and you have a partnership orientation. Be sure to communicate a long-term partnership goal, and it will reduce the time spent on any one particular issue, and both parties can work toward equitable solutions. Also, do not neglect to give feedback to suppliers and service providers. Let them know how they are doing, and give them recognition for their effort.

GUIDANCE FOR HIRING TEAM MEMBERS

Before an organization can build a desired corporate culture, the company needs a hiring process that carefully identifies ideal members to add to your team. During growth phases a company must ensure their desired culture is maintained, or it will unknowingly transition to the least common denominator of the majority of new employees. Realize that a rapidly growing organization will hire the equivalent of its entire company many times over, until it reaches a critical mass. If a company indiscriminately hires individuals who do not share common company core values, divisions occur and new employees may be driven by motivations not shared by the majority of the company.

No biotechnology enterprise can successfully accomplish its goals without the help of a myriad of individuals and external resources. Seasoned entrepreneurs and executives all reach a point in their career where they recognize that their success is no longer determined by what they can do by themselves—but by what they can accomplish with and through the help of others. Building a successful biotech company requires an ever-expanding team. Therefore it is important to find the right mix of individuals with complementary expertise having the leadership characteristics necessary to establish and direct a growing organization to a common goal.

The careful selection of team members is important because: (1) these individuals provide the expertise required to reach your corporate and product development goals and (2) these individuals are evaluated by investors and they influence the likelihood of securing investment capital. Choose your team wisely, as their credentials, backgrounds, and experience are viewed as indicators of future success. For more information about a new interview and hiring process, who to hire first, compensation and benefits in the biotechnology industry, see "Chapter 11: Hiring a Biotech Dream Team" in *The Business of Bioscience: What Goes Into Making a Biotechnology Product* [3].

When considering someone for a full-time position, the company must first narrow the applicants down to a small group of "ideal candidates" for the position. Multiple candidates are screened and interviewed for this position in the hopes of finding the right person for the job. How do you determine who is the right person for the position? All companies know the importance of finding individuals who possess related experience for a position. However, there are two other characteristics that are rarely considered, but are equally as important as related experience. When interviewing individuals to find the ideal candidates at least three characteristics should be examined for fitness: (1) having related experience; (2) having the ability to execute; and (3) possessing shared core values. The Venn diagram in Figure 27.2 depicts these characteristics as distinct but intersecting, showing their interdependence. The opacity indicates the ability to see these characteristics during a typical interview process.

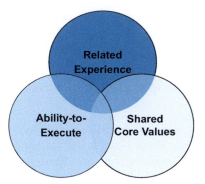

FIGURE 27.2 Ideal candidate characteristics.

Having Related Experience

When considering a candidate to hire, all companies look for related experience. Without question, related experience is vital to the position and it is the easiest quality to identify and evaluate, unfortunately all too often it is the only factor examined. Just because an individual has related experience this quality alone should not make them "an ideal candidate" for the job. Related experience should be only one of three required qualities examined before considering an individual as an ideal candidate for a position. Related experience qualifications include depth and breadth of experience, academic credentials, and the type of work experience and length of time in a position. These are all well-understood and easy to assess, therefore we will not elaborate on this quality much further.

Having the Ability to Execute

Having the ability to execute is a quality that characterizes "doing" rather than talking or thinking about something. Character qualities such as "finishing a job started," and "always coming through," are qualities that exemplify having the ability to execute. Individuals that lack this quality usually can talk the language but cannot complete or finish even the simplest of tasks. Those without this quality think they are making progress because they can talk the talk, but upon examination they come up empty-handed time and time again. These individuals are time-consumers for management because they divert attention from other work and require constant monitoring and maintenance to keep their project from being in jeopardy. The ability to execute is difficult to teach on the job and management certainly cannot help them complete all of their tasks. In most organizations, finding out if the new hire has the ability to execute is often realized several months after hiring.

Ideal candidates should have related experience *and* possess the ability to execute. Possessing the combination of these two qualities ensures that an individual can think of ideas, form a strategy, and execute a plan. Although the ability to execute quality is difficult to recognize; a good interview process will help identify individuals possessing these characteristics. The ability to execute *and* related experience are two important qualities that ensures a person is able to deliver what is needed in the position. However, having these two characteristics still does not constitute and ideal candidate for employment.

Having Shared Core Values

An individual who possesses relevant experience, the ability to execute, *and* shared core values makes an ideal candidate for a position. Without shared core values, two people cannot work together effectively for a sustained period of time nor can they work to their full potential. We previously elaborated on some core values, but core values are as diverse as people. They can include qualities such as "a good work ethic," "responsibility to get the job done," "honesty in all situations," "reliability," and "loyalty to the company."

Everyone possesses core values. No team can be effective without sharing some of the same core values—even street gang members, although their core values are negative ones. Interestingly, even negative core values unite individuals together. The most effective teams are comprised of individuals who share a maximum of common core values and influence each other to accept additional core values that are important to the rest of the team. Core values become our personal "well of conscience" from which we draw when we face difficult situations, problems, or crisis and we do not know what to do. To become an effective team, all individuals must draw from similar wells, especially when problems are encountered, as all responses need to be consistent with company values. This is how the Ortho McNeil team responded rapidly and in unity to the Tylenol tampering crisis. The most successful leaders are individuals with the ability to recognize good character qualities and great core values that match those that they espouse. Great companies learn to identify shared core values in people before they hire them.

RECOGNIZING WHEN TO LET SOME PEOPLE GO

One of the most difficult decisions for a leader is the decision to let an employee go. This can be more difficult if the employee was hired at the beginning and if they are a cofounder. Often these individuals are not unruly or contentious, they may simply be underperformers or difficult to work with and lack the skills needed to perform at that level. This situation can arise if an individual performs adequately during the company's early-development stage but later cannot contribute to the growing or changing needs of the organization. Occasionally these individuals were set-up for failure because they were given exaggerated senior level titles such as vice president or C-level positions just because they were cofounders or early hires.

Because the entrepreneurial leader has many pressing matters to deal with, personnel issues may be side-stepped because these are difficult to deal with or there is uncertainty about what to do. Entrepreneurs should not be afraid of making tough decisions. Once it becomes clear that an individual is not a good fit and ample effort has been made to deal with the situation to correct it, the situation must be handled swiftly and decisively. If the leader procrastinates in dealing with personnel problems, someone else must make up for that person's short comings or others must double-check their work because of the lack of confidence in their capabilities. If the problem is with an individual in a senior leadership position, you must weigh the significance of management time, damage to employee morale, and the likelihood of the individual's future contribution to the organization. Ask yourself, "would this individual, be a great asset for the organization as it continues to grow?" If the answer is clearly "no," then you are setting up the organization for extended and expanded problems by not dealing with this now.

Sometimes there can be good alternatives to this situation, but these depend on the type of problem and the inherent capabilities of the problem individual. If the problem stems from their abilities being misaligned with their job description, possibly they can be given alternate job responsibilities that are consistent with their skills. For instance, if the individual is a great strategic thinker but is a terrible manager, then consider a role as a nonmanaging member of the organization. If the individual is creative and provides ideas but cannot carry out or manage projects, then possibly a consultant role to the organization will work. However, if the problem stems from the individual's inability to work with others, a misalignment with the company's core values, or the absence of one or more of the three characteristics of an ideal candidate for the position, then termination is usually the only alternative.

Recognize that human relations (HR) issues should be documented throughout this correction process. Some of these activities include performance reviews, corrective actions with clear details about their performance and expectations, documentation of the problems and assistance in helping to remediate the problems, warnings that the lack of correction or improvement can result in termination. These and other solutions should have been tried prior to reaching a termination decision. Most states in the United States acknowledge what is called "at-will" employment, meaning there is an understanding that employees can be terminated "at-will" provided there is no discrimination against any member of a protected group of individuals, such as the aged, handicapped, minorities, and various others. In issues where termination is involved, it is always advisable to consult with an HR attorney or if the company has a shared-employer professional employer organization, they can provide guidance during this process.

If the leader ignores personnel problem issues, this diminishes the effectiveness of the organization and over time damages the trust with other employees, especially if this individual holds a key role in the senior management. Ultimately, these decisions should result in what is best for the organization rather than what is best for one individual. In rescue missions and stories of heroics "the good of the one outweighs the good of the many." However, in start-up and development-stage companies, the good of the one cannot outweigh the good of the many. It is not uncommon that in a rapidly growing biotechnology company, the responsibilities and the organization's needs surpass the capability of the founding CEO or other founding employees. Unfortunately, the "one" may even be the founding CEO. There are times when the founding CEO needs to depart for the good of the company. Sometimes this may be hostile but in the best of situations this should be a planned succession.

SUMMARY

Having the ability to recognize the different development stages of an organization is key for an entrepreneurial leader. All companies transition through these development stages, but the time spent within each stage is dependent upon the type of product being developed. At the start-up stage the leader will manage the team with what is called the "entrepreneurial" or "command-and-control" management style. This management style is characterized by centralized decision-making with strong controls. During the corporate development phase, as the experience level and number of employees increase, the leader must make a management style change. The leader must successfully transition to a "professional management style," or what is known as "delegate-and-inspect" management style. The professional management style is characterized by a delegation of decision-making responsibilities and formal control mechanisms. Unfortunately, some entrepreneurial leaders do not know how to change or may not want to change. Failure to make this management-style transition will become detrimental to the company and it will impact the future success of the organization.

A company's new hires are key to getting a strong start on product development and expanding your internal expertise. These individuals also have an impact on your ability to raise capital as a biotech start-up organization must have experienced and qualified individuals in all functions where the company professes expertise. In order to hire the best, develop an interview process that permits the examination of the three important qualities for an ideal candidate such as having related experience, having the ability to execute, and possessing shared core values. Make sure that you have a well thought-out strategy for hiring individuals at an appropriate level within the organization. As the company grows, be sure to address employee and personnel issues quickly, as these can quickly destroy a team's motivation and restrict a company's ability to make important product-development progress. Each member of the team will either be an asset or a detriment to progress, so it is critical to identify the best ones, and continually help them to become better managers and leaders.

REFERENCES

[1] Johnson & Johnson. "Our Credo Values." http://www.jnj.com/connect/about-jnj/jnj-credo/.

[2] Urban H. 4th ed. Life's Greatest Lessons: 20 Things that Matter. Fireside Books; 2003. 165.

[3] Shimasaki CD. Hiring a Biotech Dream Team. In: The Business of Bioscience: What Goes Into Making a Biotechnology Product. New York: Springer; 2009. Chapter 11.

Chapter 28

Biotechnology Business Development: The Art of the Deal

Jack M. Anthony* and Phil Haworth, PhD, JD**

*Founder and Principal, BioMentorz, Inc., Healdsburg, California, **Principal, Biomentorz, Inc. Redwood City, California*

In the biotechnology industry, the need for cash is constant. Very few, if any, biotech companies can raise enough capital to cover all the research, development, clinical, regulatory, and manufacturing costs through to commercialization. During the early days of the biotechnology industry, the need to find new sources of capital for later-stage human clinical trials opened a door for a new breed of individuals within the biotech industry who could integrate the skills of a salesperson, strategic planner, financial forecaster, telemarketer, paralegal, and effective science-friendly presenter, to name a few important traits. These are the traits and skills required by business development (BD) executives. These individuals who fulfill the function of the BD executive are typically assigned the responsibility to find and negotiate partnerships with large corporations such as pharmaceutical companies, to provide cash and help with later-stage product development, marketing, and commercialization of the biotechnology company's product. In a typical partnership, the biotech company may receive upfront payments, milestone payments, fee-for-service payments and, eventually, royalties on sales. In exchange, the pharmaceutical partner receives ownership or exclusive license and marketing rights to the biotechnology company's product. All companies within each of the different biotech sectors will greatly benefit from the business development activities described, however, we will mostly elaborate on biotherapeutic examples. The goal of this chapter is to offer insight into the business development function, understand how to organize your efforts, keep the momentum moving, and create an opportunity to reach a successful outcome. Keep in mind that successful deals can take at least 12 months to bring about, so early planning and preparing is essential.

The concept of "partnering" or "biotech collaborations" was born out of necessity. In 1978 Genentech, one of the first biotechnology companies, realized that upon being the first to clone the human insulin gene, it would take an enormous amount of cash to fund their program through the remaining phases and into the marketplace. At that time, big pharmaceutical companies "owned" the (animal) insulin market and they had capabilities and resources far beyond Genentech's. Early on, Genentech entered into discussions with a number of potential clients, and Eli Lilly, a major pharmaceutical company, licensed Genentech's technology and took it through the remaining development stages to commercialization as a product called Humulin®. The upfront payment and milestones from this deal resulted in needed cash to grow Genentech, and it also covered the previous expenditures for development of recombinant insulin, whereas subsequent royalties provided a cash-flow well into the future of the company. As a result, and out of necessity, the template for partnering of future biotechnology products to pharmaceutical companies was realized, and it became evident that business development was a key discipline to be mastered by all biotechnology companies.

Deloitte Recap showed that there may be another reason to partner: utilizing the embedded knowledge and resources of a large partner may give a biotech company an edge in successfully advancing a drug candidate because partnered compounds are three times more likely to reach the market than unpartnered compounds (Figure 28.1).

It is apparent that being proficient at conceiving and executing a business development plan and attracting a global or regional partner is an important strategic activity of any biotechnology company. The list of biotech/pharmaceutical company collaborations formed since the late 1970s includes just about every major pharmaceutical company and almost every biotech company. The total dollars ascribed to these deals are in the tens of billions, not to mention the capital received from acquisitions and downstream royalties from many of the deals. While venture capital and angel investors can take credit for funding the early efforts of a majority of biotech companies, the influx of cash from partnering deals with major pharmaceutical companies has funded much of the downstream activities and commercial successes.

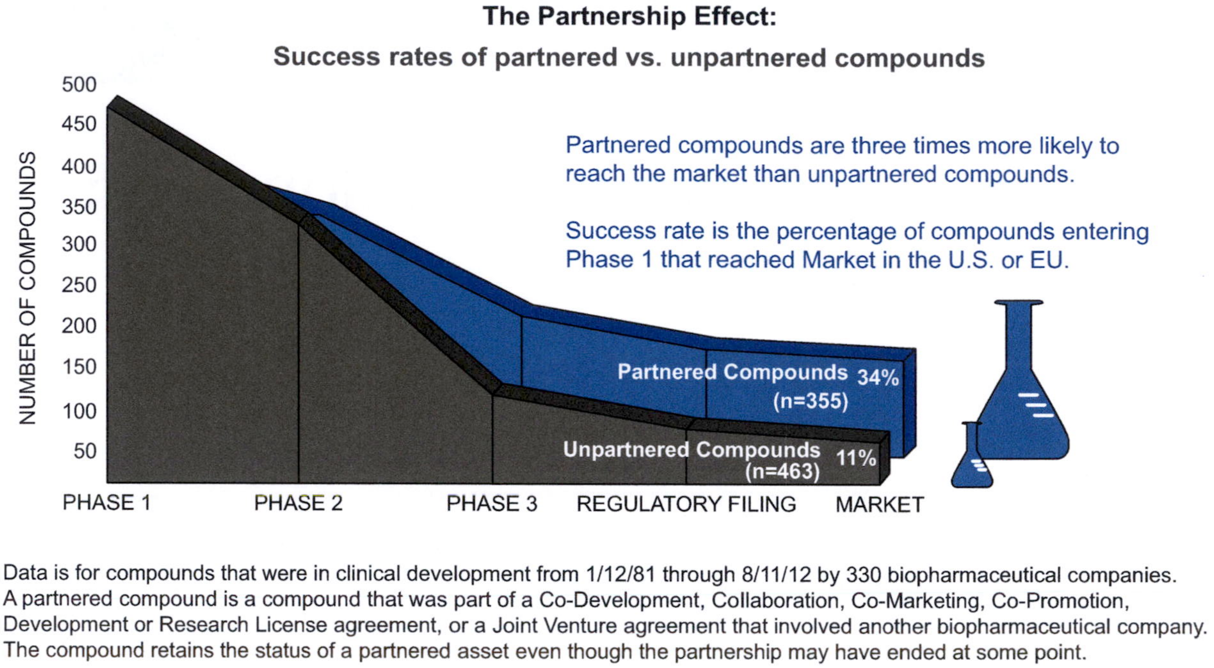

The Partnership Effect:

Success rates of partnered vs. unpartnered compounds

Partnered compounds are three times more likely to reach the market than unpartnered compounds.

Success rate is the percentage of compounds entering Phase 1 that reached Market in the U.S. or EU.

Partnered Compounds 34% (n=355)

Unpartnered Compounds 11% (n=463)

Data is for compounds that were in clinical development from 1/12/81 through 8/11/12 by 330 biopharmaceutical companies. A partnered compound is a compound that was part of a Co-Development, Collaboration, Co-Marketing, Co-Promotion, Development or Research License agreement, or a Joint Venture agreement that involved another biopharmaceutical company. The compound retains the status of a partnered asset even though the partnership may have ended at some point.

FIGURE 28.1   The effect of partnerships on success of compounds reaching the market. *(Source: Deloitte Recap.)*

BACKGROUND OF BIOTECHNOLOGY LICENSING AND PARTNERING DEALS

To get an idea of the magnitude and significance of these types of deals and partnerships between biotechnology and pharmaceutical companies, we look at the deals that were completed in the first half of 2012 and compare to the first half of 2013. According to Thomson Reuters, there were approximately 1234 deals completed with life science companies in the first half of 2013 that amounted to a total of $73.3 billion. The average deal dollar amount for the biotechnology company across all stages when licensed is approximately $300 million (Figure 28.2).

While the appetite for deals between biotechnology companies and large pharmaceutical and other institutional partners remains robust, the variables of a deal in terms of dollars, milestones, and staging has shifted somewhat. In our experience, and in discussions with potential partners, it suggests that negotiating upfront payments versus downstream milestones and even royalties has become more challenging as "buyers" are applying more pressure on the biotech company to produce and be successful. In short, biotechnology companies must demonstrate proof-of-relevance early in a product development program, do more with less, and be certain they are meeting changing market needs. It would be difficult to project where the biotech deal, financing, and partnership markets will be in the future based on past statistics, but following comparables available from a number of sources suggests some trends (Figures 28.3 and 28.4).

Every biotechnology company's survival is determined not only by its success in the laboratory and the clinic, but also by the number and/or size of the transactions it completes—whether they be licensing transactions, mergers, and acquisitions (M&A) transactions, or investment transactions (Table 28.1).

Without the occurrence of one or more of these events there will be limited clinical development pipelines and fewer therapeutic and medical device products reaching the marketplace. A key for the success and future growth of any biotechnology company is creating an environment for deal-making through business development (BD). While a talented start-up CEO usually fulfills the BD role in the early days, bringing onboard an experienced BD executive is essential for the company's long-term growth if funding is to keep pace with its own organic growth.

WHAT IS A BUSINESS DEVELOPMENT "DEAL?"

Before we proceed to describe the "art of the deal" let's pause and describe "what is a deal?" If you look up the word "deal" on Wikipedia, the first two descriptions are (i) a contract and (ii) the distribution of cards. In this context, both definitions can be considered correct. The deal, when completed, describes the exchange of goods or assets between two parties. The parties may be two companies or alternatively, the parties may be one company and a group of shareholders in which technology is sold or rented for present or future cash. The deal is a transaction in which, hopefully, both parties realize essential gain in the interest of their respective company. In our world, the deal includes all forms of licensing transactions, M&A, and the sale of equity to investors. If you are considering a career in this field, you will also need to

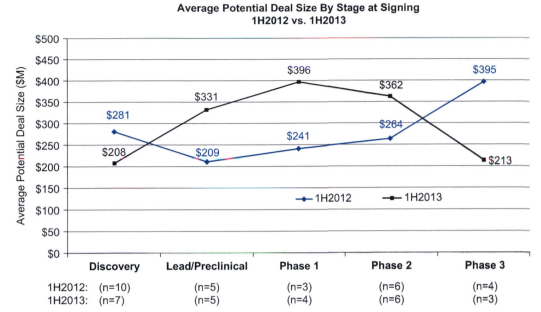

FIGURE 28.2   The average potential deal size for life science companies in the first half of 2012 and 2013 based upon the stage at signing. *(Source: Thomson Reuters.)*

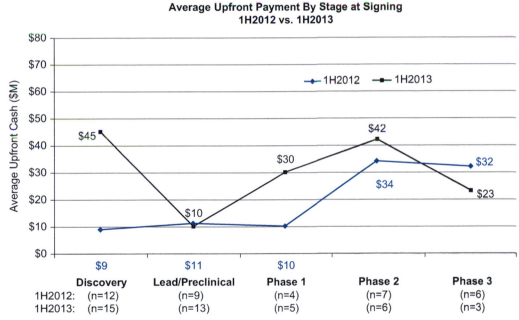

FIGURE 28.3   The average upfront payment to life sciences company by the stage of signing during the first half of 2012 and 2013. *(Source: Thomson Reuters)*

learn how to distribute the "cards" such that a contract works to your company's benefit while simultaneously providing value to your partner company.

Let us be clear at the outset that deal-making is a form of selling, however biotech deal-making differs from "sales" in one very important aspect. In traditional sales, a transaction can be completed by an individual salesperson skilled in the art of presenting product benefits and appropriate closing techniques, but in biotechnology, creating a deal requires the inclusion, cooperation, and coordination of a group of people across all company functions. The successful completion of a deal requires a choreographed performance involving scientists, clinicians, manufacturing experts, consultants, and other contributors. It can be a challenging job

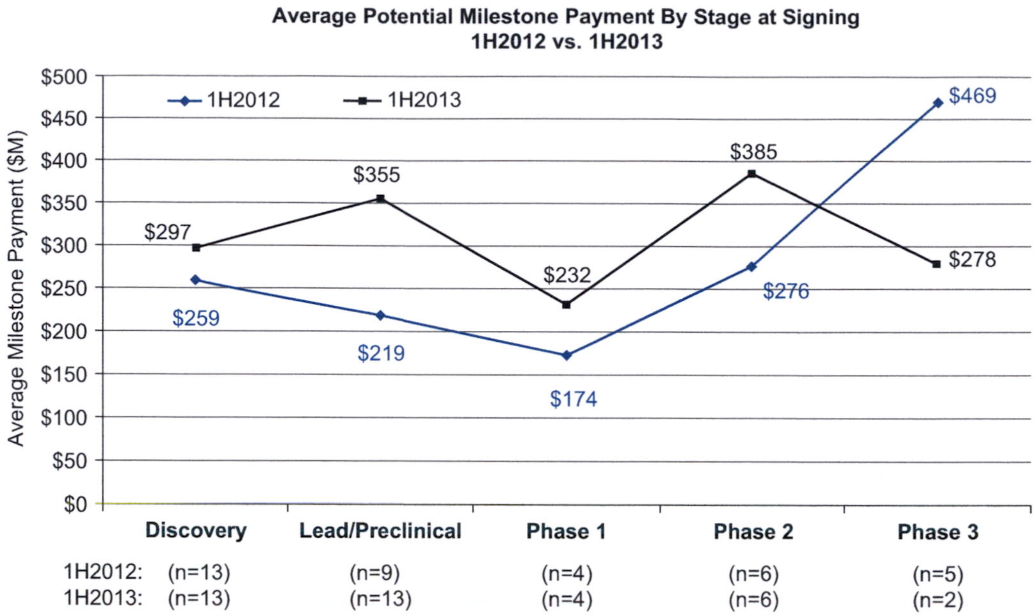

Average Potential Milestone Payment By Stage at Signing
1H2012 vs. 1H2013

| 1H2012: | (n=13) | (n=9) | (n=4) | (n=6) | (n=5) |
| 1H2013: | (n=13) | (n=13) | (n=4) | (n=6) | (n=2) |

FIGURE 28.4   The average potential milestone payments for life science companies by the stage of signing during the first half of 2012 and 2013. (*Source: Thomson Reuters.*)

to sell what are essentially "futures" on today's projects. The importance of doing deals is at least as crucial to the success of a biotechnology company as scientific excellence, translational biology, and clinical development. Talented, experienced, and smart business development people are essential to any successful biotech effort.

STARTING THE PROCESS

Before you start the "deal" process there are four questions that must be asked and answered by you and your company:

What is being Sold?

The first and most important step in any transactional process is to identify precisely what it is you wish to sell. Typically there are three broad categories of products for sale:

1. **The entire company and its vision.** For example, in May 2013, GlaxoSmithKline (GSK) acquired a Swiss genetic vaccine developer for $325 million.
2. **A specific technology with multiple potential applications.** For example, in June 2013, Pfizer partnered with CytomX, a South San Francisco company to access their antibody-drug conjugate technology for a $25 million upfront payment.
3. **A single product.** For example, in July 2013, Johnson & Johnson acquired a Phase 3 prostate cancer drug (ARN 509) from San Diego-based Aragon Pharmaceuticals for a reported $1 billion.

Reaching internal agreement on what your company is about to sell can be more difficult than you might expect. There is no magic formula for this process, but this must be worked out before you begin any transactional process. In general terms, it is best to pick an asset with clearly defined intellectual property (IP) protection and a clearly identifiable application and demand. Until you have defined what you have to sell it is difficult to identify those who might want to buy it, and it is impossible to calculate or agree upon what it might be worth. Even though your company may not have proven the product opportunity yet, you still must have a clear understanding of what the technology will lead to, the tools to get there, and a plan to get it done.

Why are You Selling It?

Next you need to agree on why you want to complete a transaction? The most obvious answers to this question are either: (1) you need the money and resources that a partner can bring to bear or; (2) you need the "validation"[a] that a partner would bring to your company. Any deal must have a purpose that is greater than simply a short-term cash payment. Often deals are transacted to access resources that in the long-term will generate more value for the company if you sell it now, than if you did not. In other words, if the

---

a. Validation has become a term of art often used by biotech people which has little to no substantive meaning. In essence, the term tries to capture the notion that if "someone important cares about what I am doing then what I am doing must be important." We can all understand the attractiveness of this idea but in truth in is just the lack of self-esteem.

TABLE 28.1 The Average Potential Milestone Payments for Life Science Companies by the Stage of Signing During the First Half of 2012 and 2013.

1H2013 Deal Trends: Licenses & JVs						
Licensor/ Seller	Licensee/ Buyer	Total Size	Upfront	Asset Description	Stage	Therapeutic
MacroGenics	Gilead	$1,115M	$30M	DART bispecific mAb programs against up to 4 undisclosed targets	Preclinical	Cancer
FORMA	Celgene	>$945	Undisclosed	Discovery of drugs targeting the protein homeostasis pathway	Discovery	Diversified
Lundbeck*	Otsuka	$825M	$150M	Expansion of 2011 CNS pipeline collaboration to include Lu AE58054 for Alzheimer's Disease	Phase II	Neurology
MorphoSys	Celgene	$818M	$92M cash $60M equity	MOR202, HuCAL antibody targeting CD38 for multiple myeloma	Phase I/IIa	Cancer
CytomX	Pfizer	> $635M	Undisclosed	Probody Platform to develop Probody-Drug Conjugates (PDCs)	Preclinical	Cancer
Chiasma	Roche	$595M	$65M	Oral octreotide oral for acromegaly and neuroendocrine tumors	Reformulation	Endocrine/
MorphoSys	GSK	$579M	$29M	MOR103 fully human HuCAL antibody for inflammatory diseases, including RA and MS	Phase I/II	Autoimmune/ Inflammatory
Edison Pharma	Dainippon	$545M	$35M	EPI-743 and EPI-589 redox factors and mitochondrial augmentors for CNS disorders in Japan	Phase III	Neurology
Seattle Genetics	Bayer	$520M	$20M	Uristatin-based antibody-drug conjugate (ADC) technology with antibodies to multiple cancer targets	Not Applicable	Cancer
Cytokinetics	Astellas	$490M	$16M	Skeletal muscle activators, including CK-2127107, for conditions associated with muscle weakness	Phase I	Neurology

(*Source: Thomson Reuters.*)

company's value or "pie" gets bigger with this transaction, your slice, or ownership, has more value than it did before the deal was signed. For example, it is very hard for a small biotechnology company to ultimately sell, distribute, and market a chronic-use cardiovascular drug without having hundreds of sales representatives calling upon general practitioners and cardiologists. So a deal with a large pharmaceutical company like Pfizer or AstraZeneca might be the best option for your drug and your company.

Alternatively, the real purpose of the deal might not be an immediate need. Sometimes another reason for doing a deal is to unload an asset that no longer fits with the company's skills, strategies, or resources and will be shelved without a new home. Whatever the reason, it is important to reach agreement on the deal rationale among the board of directors and the management team of the company. The deal process is long—9 months to 1 year if you are fortunate, but it could take twice that long. During that time you, the team, and/or the board may even lose sight of, or interest in, the transaction and the person tasked with completing it (you!). Without a clear rationale for why this deal is important to the company, frustration from the time and resources spent on the deal process may inevitably focus upon the BD executive tasked with this transaction.

Providing early clarity about why the deal should be done will also help the BD person to recognize when to abandon or substantially modify a proposed transaction. Unless you are simply doing transactions for the sake of doing transactions, it is entirely possible that the deal you have spent the last 12 months working on is no longer important either because the circumstances have changed or the proposed deal terms no longer meet the reason for doing the deal in the first place. Part of the BD executive's job is to know when to say "no" to a deal. Open, constant, and clear communications up and down the company chain-of-command are critical in the deal-making process. An astute BD executive understands this even if others do not. They understand that part of their job is to be in front of this type of discussion no matter which direction it takes.

At this point we should talk a little about negotiation theory and the concept of the "best alternative to a negotiated agreement" (BATNA), which is a concept introduced into common linguistics back the 1980s [1]. If you choose to say "no" to an offered deal, it is critical to understand and to be able to explain the consequences of that decision. In other words, what are your options if you don't take this deal? In negotiation theory, BATNA is the course of action available to a party if the negotiation fails and an agreement cannot be reached. In practice, most biotech companies find themselves without an alternative to negotiating an agreement, and they may not have any other good options available to them if they don't take the deal. In true adherence to negotiation theory [2] a party should not accept a deal worse than its BATNA. However, as is often the case, the only alternative to a negotiated agreement may be closing down the company because without the deal there may not be any more cash to operate. It is important to understand whether or not you have a BATNA. This is essential before starting any transaction [3] because having a BATNA makes a difference [4]. For example, let's say you have two products in development and you need to out-license one of these products in order to fund a Phase 3 human clinical trial for the second drug. Your alternative might be to go for an "IPO" to raise additional funds for the Phase 3 trial rather than to out-license one of your products. By telling your potential licensing partner you are working on filing for a public offering can only help your desired licensing discussion. Consequently, the BATNA to the licensing deal is an IPO. Unfortunately, in many of the situations experienced by small biotechnology companies, the alternative to not doing a deal or additional funding may be to close down the program or the company. While it is difficult to consider closing the company as the "best alternative," no one has ever published a thesis describing "no alternative to a negotiated agreement."

How Much is it Worth?

Assuming that at this point the team has agreed on what it is going to sell and why they want to sell it. Now comes the hard part. How much is it worth? This can be a very delicate discussion both internally and externally. The person charged with leading the deal process has to employ an unbiased, credible and acceptable valuation process. Otherwise placing a dollar-value on an asset is a futile exercise where only the true believers see the value. Needless to say the individuals on the other side of the transaction rarely consist of true believers, so a valuation that is acceptable internally must encompass a valuation that is credible externally.

There are basically two methods commonly utilized to value a precommercial-stage asset. The best method, but most difficult, is to use some form of discounted cash-flow model such as a net-present value (NPV) calculation or a Monte Carlo Analysis [5]. The difficulty in calculating these values does not lie in the mathematical component since it is possible to download tools on the Internet that will achieve that result [6]. The problem arises when an organization is unwilling or unable to effectively assess the risk, cost, and time associated with commercializing a particular asset. Accurate discounted cash-flow calculations can and do occur, but seldom in a small biotechnology company due mainly to the absence of the necessary objectivity.

A more realistic approach would be to base the valuation of your product on comparables for deals completed on similar products or assets. This method of evaluating comparables is a similar methodology to that used when determining home value in the real estate market. Searchable biotechnology deal databases can be accessed at a cost through organization such as Recap by Thomson Reuters (www.recap.com) or EvaluatePharma (www.evaluatepharma.com). Typically these databases can be searched on selectable criteria, for instance, "Phase I antibody for solid tumor oncology in Japan." The database will return a selection of transactions meeting these criteria which will include the name of the parties, the date and subject matter of the transaction, and (to greater or lesser extent) information on the deal terms. It is unlikely that the search will turn up a deal involving an asset that is identical to yours but there should be some that are close enough to provide a range of values related to licensing a Phase 1 Antibody to treat solid tumor cancers in Japan. The best part about this approach is that it is driven by objective external data that can be presented to everyone on both sides of the transaction. One last comment on valuation—the techniques that do not work are "I need $3 million for next year's budget—go get a deal," or "We spent $15 million on this program therefore it must be worth twice that…."

Who will Want to Buy it?

The fourth and final step in preparing your partnering campaign is to determine who may be likely to sign up to pay for your asset. In classical business school terms the Venn diagram methodology for selecting a corporate partner is a strategic modeling approach called the 3C elements of success. The 3C term was originally coined by Kenichi Ohmae, a business and corporate strategist (*http://www.kohmae.com/en/*) who referenced the three elements of success as: the customer, the competitors, and the corporation. In the context of biotechnology partnering and deals the 3Cs have evolved into: the cash, the competency, and the commitment. In short, this translates into: can they pay for it, can they develop it, and will they develop it. (See Figure 28.5.)

In a perfect world, one would begin a partnering campaign with a certainty about who has the competency and commitment to develop your drug. You would then limit your search to companies that have the necessary cash, competency, and commitment to such a deal. Alas, we do not live in a perfect world. One real problem with the commitment to any deal is often it may only last as long as the scientist or business executive remains employed at the acquiring company, and regrettably these individuals may not be there throughout the entire development cycle of a pharmaceutical product. Both authors of this chapter have been involved in licensing transactions that at the outset seemed like the perfect marriage between companies, only to see "Prince Charming" move to a different kingdom! So, to complete the analogy, while it is good to have a list of "princes" it is wise to kiss many frogs.

In an attempt to update the 3Cs approach to finding a partner we include some valuable nuggets to consider [7]. According to Sarah Shaw (*http://theentreprenettegazette.com/about/*), when deciding to bring on a partner there are ten questions you need to ask yourself and we selected the five most relevant to biotechnology deals. They are:

1. What are they contributing that we cannot?
2. What business tactics, systems, or connections are they bringing to the table that will benefit us?
3. Do they have integrity?
4. What makes them as committed as we are to the business?
5. Do they keep and honor their commitments?

If you can answer these questions in a positive manner you can feel good about your choice of partner. Ms. Shaw's Blog also generated some great interviews on this subject and we have included a few that seemed most on point for us:

"Till Death Do You Part"

How to find the best partner: *The right one may be more important than the right time. Bringing on a business partner is almost like getting married. Go into it with your eyes wide open and with much thought. Some benefits of a partner are the accountability, moral support, and complementary skills or personality traits. But you also have double incomes to cover, and the real potential for conflict and disagreement. So DO know each other well, identify who will do what, and have an exit strategy should it not work out.*

Jennifer Leake of Consultants Gold, Inc.

How to find the best partner: *Being in business is intimate and involves some of our most heartfelt dreams and aspirations. Choose your business partner with the care and consciousness as you'd choose a mate. Prerequisites: common goals, shared vision, the ability to resolve conflict, and a plan for what to do when conflict inevitably arises.*

Kim Wright of Cutting Edge Law

THE DEAL REQUIRES A PLAN

It is likely that every business development executive accepts the axiom, "it is better to be lucky than smart" but every experienced BD person also knows that in all likelihood getting a deal done will require something more than luck—a plan! A transaction is going to take time—12 months plus or minus. Without a plan, the transaction is going to be lost in a sea of a distraction and a pool of frustration. The plan will need to encompass every aspect of the deal process from identifying the company contacts to selecting the lawyer for the final contract negotiation. Below is a template of the plan, the first four steps of which should now be familiar to you:

1. What do you want to sell?
2. Why do you want to sell it?
3. What can you expect to get for it?
4. Who can you expect to buy it?

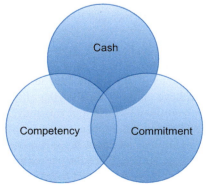

FIGURE 28.5 The "3Cs" of finding a partner.

The essential nature of these first four elements should be obvious by now and hopefully getting that far in the process has created a forum for developing the rest of the plan.

Who is Going to be Responsible for the Deal Process?

The process needs to have a leader and the likely candidates include the CEO, the CFO, the General Counsel (GC), or the head of BD. The authors of this chapter have a strong bias toward having the leader be the senior BD person, assuming they have the ability and the experience. In most instances the GC or CFO will approach a deal based upon their individual technical expertise, whether it be law or finance. While the expertise of a GC and/or CFO can be invaluable in the deal-making process, simply viewing the deal as a purely legal or financial document can be annoying to the other party. To be honest, most BD types just don't want to negotiate with the "lawyers" and the "accountants." While your CEO may have the necessary experience and knowledge to carry out the deal, they will almost certainly be too busy to be engaged in every element of the process. Most importantly, there can be a very real advantage in not having the final decision-maker in the room during key parts of the negotiation. There is a sound academic basis for using a phrase that is heard from every car salesperson in America, "*I need to take that to my manager.*" [8] It actually works in a negotiation. It works because it allows time for a more thoughtful response and it works because it tells the buyer they are pushing close to the limits of the deal.

Who is on the Deal Team?

Initially, everyone may want to play a role in the deal (this enthusiasm will decrease over time!) but it is essential to define and limit the core membership of the team. Recruitment to the team should be based partially on the skills and experience of individuals, but the BD person will also need to make some decisions based on an individual's personality. Who would you want to spend a rainy, grey weekend in a foreign country with? If the thought of this concerns you when you think about any particular individual, they may not be the best person to include on your deal team. Not everyone in your organization has the skill and temperament to do this work; so while your chief scientific officer (CSO) might be the best scientist on your team, he or she may not have the patience or time to schlep around after the BD guy. Pick your team wisely and keep them happy. Often, potential partners may be located in a country other than yours and for a number of months you may end up spending more time with these folks then your spouse and your children. Before the deal is over, you will know their favorite foods and music, their political views, and even

their religious beliefs. As the deal team leader, you need to recognize that in addition to working on this deal, your team members have a regular day job and you need to reward and encourage your team: a good meal in a fun restaurant (the Quinea in Mayfair!) goes a long way, take them to a sporting event in some new city (baseball at the "Big Egg" in Tokyo), or try the Pergamon Museum in Berlin. Make sure they have something to talk about with their colleagues upon their return. If this kind of expense doesn't work with your company policies you may have to pay it out of your own pocket—but that just binds the team to you more closely! The essential elements of any deal team will be BD, R&D (Clinical), and legal, although it is less likely that legal will be required on the traveling squad at least at the beginning stages of the process. Other occasional team members might include members from finance, commercial, manufacturing, and regulatory. It is important to recognize that some of the team may view the intended transaction as a threat to their jobs, therefore, the larger the size of the deal team the more likely it is to include the resistance. Managing that part of the deal team is a test of leadership skills. If you have time to read it, there is a great book that can help with these issues called *Thinking Fast and Slow* by Daniel Kahneman [9].

Establish the Role of Each Member of the Deal Team at the Outset

There are a number of serious conversations that will need to occur between you and your team members. Defining each team member's role in the deal process and making sure each member understands their role is vital. For instance, a scientist and or clinician will at some point start to speculate on data that has yet to be generated or yet to be shared with your potential partner. Any good scientist or clinician requires a healthy dose of introspective analysis and skepticism, or what one academic calls the "irony of abnegation" [10] which we interpret to mean, a technical person cannot define success without first exploring and explaining every source of failure. Although his approach is a legitimate asset in becoming a better scientist, this type of communication with your potential partner can turn your deal into a train wreck in minutes!

It is not that you must ask your scientist to lie, but merely to answer the question as it is posed and not as it might be interpreted. For example, the answer to the question, "do you have animal data showing efficacy" is "Yes, let me show you the data from our rat study." The answer *should not be* "We couldn't make it work in dogs so we did it in rats." The discussion about the failed dog experiment should and will occur later when the parties are in diligence, but on a first date there is no need to talk about your early tentative efforts. Potential partners need to first see value in the deal before they hear the concerns, otherwise you will never find a partner. Before each and every meeting, review with your team the goals and scope of the meeting/presentation and make sure they understand the limits of the subject matter to be discussed at any particular moment in time.

Keeping the CEO, the Board, and the Scientific Advisory Board (SAB) Updated

Even if the CEO is not on the deal team let us not pretend for a moment that they will not be involved in your deal. The amount of CEO involvement is directly proportional to the importance of the deal to the company. If the CEO has no interest in the deal you should probably think about working on something else. As we have previously discussed, not having the CEO involved in the day-to-day of a deal has its advantages. However while you may be running the deal, the CEO is still running the company. If you and the CEO are not in agreement at the outset, the situation is unlikely to improve over time. It is a good idea to remind yourself that the CEO directly answers to the shareholders and those shareholders are not part of the deal team and are mainly influenced by events outside of your company. So if the shareholders pressure the CEO, the CEO will pressure you.

Working with the CEO while still managing the deal process is a balancing act that all BD executives must accomplish. There are things that can help make this work:

- Make sure you and the CEO have regular face-to-face meetings in which you provide an accurate and honest update on the process.

- Make sure there are no surprises for the CEO; keep him or her up-to-date so he or she can inform the board effectively.
- Avoid making predictions and try never to quantify the possibility of getting the deal done.

We suggest that all the key players, the CEO, and the board get regular updates on the deal process. We prefer to use an Excel spreadsheet that can easily be modified and converted into PowerPoint in a moment's notice. Our sample "transaction tracker" template is included below (Figure 28.6).

Regardless of how you may choose to keep track of the deal process, tracking is an essential part of your function as the lead business development executive. The spreadsheet we suggest is self-explanatory in terms of the content. The most immediate benefits to this type of tracking are that you maintain a concise record of companies which have been contacted, the contact individual, and the time and manner in which you contacted them. You should also record the responses (both positive and negative) you receive to your proposed deal. You need to know who you have spoken to, who has yet to respond, who is interested, and also why others are not interested. This is an essential tool for describing to your board and CEO, what is, or is not, happening to your transaction. Without such a record your activities will be subject to misinterpretation and re-interpretation that becomes more and more difficult to manage.

Select and Manage the Point(s) of Contact in Each Target Company

The next step in the plan will be to work out who within each target company will be the initial point of contact for your

Business Development Tracking Spreadsheet								
Company Name	Priority	Contact Name	Contact Information	Non-Con sent	CDA	Confidential Meeting	Status & Next Steps	Comments
Apple Pharma	1	Joan Smith	j.smith@applepharm.com	3/13/2012	Declined			No longer active in this therapeutic area
Baker Therapeutics	1	Larry Brown	lab1@bakerThera.com	3/13/2012	5/17/2012	6/19/2012	Internal review August 25	
Charlie Co	2	Asish Patel	ashih.p@charlieco.com	4/8/2012	5/22/2012	6/19/2012	need to review commercial forecast prior to October Executive committee meeting	interested but may be a low bidder
Dog Therapeutics	1	Peter Kugel	peter.kugel@dogT.com	4/2/2012	Declined			Only looking for antibody drug against this target
Easy Pharma	2	Chie Wu	C.Wu@easypharm.com	2/19/2012	3/22/2012	5/19/2012		Too expensive for Easy Pharm
FOX AG	1	Bryan Jones	bryanj@foxag.com	2/19/2012	Declined			Only wants Phase 3 drugs

FIGURE 28.6   The business development tracking spreadsheet example.

proposition. Our advice on this point is to recruit as much help as you can to develop this list—it makes everyone feel involved and it actually helps. There are some fundamental questions that need to be answered such as how will the dialog begin and who will management it? Sometimes business development, sometimes R&D, and sometimes another person in your company will manage the initial contact. By working an inventory of individuals who have contact with any given target partner, you give your company the best opportunity to get a deal done. Also note that the best method of approach for one target company may not be the best method for the next company. Care must be taken that the first discussion with the target company is informational and casual so it would not result in a hard "no" which is memorialized in their database somewhere. A no can last for years, or at least until significant data erases them. Consequently, choosing the initial contact point at a target company can have significant impact on your licensing process. Regardless of how the first discussion begins, a thorough consideration about the message content and its potential impact should occur before any communication is made.

Develop a Script for your First Communication

The first communication between you and any potential partner is perhaps the most critical and most difficult to prepare. Later in this chapter we will describe the various pitch formats that the deal team will require in order to reach a successful conclusion. This first communication is little more than a written variation of the company's known "elevator pitch." There are no more than five things you should try to communicate in this first step:

1. The mission and purpose of your company.
2. What your technology is capable of achieving.
3. What you are trying to sell.
4. The stage of development of your asset.
5. How your asset will help this potential partner.

To do this effectively the initial pitch should be no more than 1 page of text or approximately 10 to 15 PowerPoint slides. All individuals involved in delivering a pitch to any potential partner should use the same documents. It is incumbent upon the deal team leader to make sure that everyone understands the key points of the message and to ensure that team members are willing and capable of delivering the key points with no, or limited, "editorial insights." Key team members all need to be singing the same music—that is to say that each member must deliver the same company message, not their personal message.

Prepare a Number of Presentations for your Deal Campaign

Although the partnering campaign will begin with a simple, short nonconfidential introduction such as described above, it requires much more than this to get the deal done. It is anticipated that you may need up to five different presentations in addition to the nonconfidential introduction. These presentations are intended to reveal increasing levels of details and confidentiality. In our experience, the process more or less follows the steps below, with the required presentations highlighted in bold:

1. Nonconfidential introduction
2. **Nonconfidential presentation (more information than the introduction but still not everything)**
3. Sign (first) confidential disclosure agreement (CDA)
4. **First confidential presentation (new data included)**
5. **Second confidential presentation (plans and progress)**
6. Sign second CDA (sometimes required)
7. **Intellectual property (IP) presentation**
8. **Commercial presentation that may include forecasts (if appropriate)**
9. Diligence

It is best to have these presentations prepared at the outset of the process, although they will need to be updated as time passes. Getting these presentations prepared will require help from various members of your deal team, some of whom are only partially involved at the outset of the process, notably IP, clinical, and commercial. There may be resistance to preparing these presentations months in advance of their actual requirement. However, one good reason for doing these in advance is that these presentations aid in understanding your IP or commercial strategy so you can steer early conversations in the right direction while simultaneously fulfilling one of the cardinal rules of doing deals—no surprises.

Start Planning for the Diligence Process

It may seem overly optimistic to think about the due diligence process at the beginning of the partnering campaign, but preparing the diligence documents early can positively impact the deal process in a number of ways. There are three main benefits to considering the due diligence process at this early stage. First, the team will be forced to confront the status of the documentation required to support the transaction including in-licensing documents, patent files, FDA correspondence, lab work, marketing data, competitive analysis, etc. If the gaps in this paper trail can be identified at this stage of the process there is time to remedy or correct the flaws. If the flaws cannot be corrected (and there are circumstances where this might occur) the understanding of these deficiencies can at least be factored into the partnering process and the valuation exercise. Second, it offers an excellent opportunity to "bond" the deal team. Running through the process of constructing the paper trail around a licensing candidate is a very egalitarian process. Every member of the team adds value. Perhaps more importantly, every member has the opportunity to learn of the contributions made by their teammates. It is not often that the chief medical officer (CMO) sits down and talks to the patent attorney! Generating a level of mutual respect among the members of your deal team will pay real dividends in terms of team morale and team performance later in the process. A third benefit to preparing the diligence documents early is that it can have significant positive impact on the actual deal itself. At some point a potential partner will want to access the diligence documents and if they are ready to go it sends the message that your company is competent and confident. It also suggests that they might not be the first or only party to begin diligence.

Determine Who will be on the Negotiation Team

The negotiation team is not the same group of people who make up the deal team. Typically the negotiation team is much smaller, comprising usually two or three members—we prefer the two-member team, one from business development and a transaction lawyer (many times an outside lawyer) who has been brought in when discussions get serious because often, a company's general counsel is not going to be a transaction lawyer. The relationship between the lead negotiator and the transaction lawyer is the key to a successful negotiation and both individuals need to develop a clear understanding of the other's roles. On occasion, the negotiation team may also include someone from finance or some technical discipline if the deal hinges on some creative financing structure or on some complex technical element. As with the deal team, there are advantages to the CEO not being on the negotiations team, yet the CEO has an essential role in the negotiation. Using the presence and absence of the CEO in a well-organized manner can be a key element in closing the deal. *In abstentia*, the CEO can be both a "good cop/bad cop"[b] that can influence deal discussions at critical points; but this type of role play has to be used sparingly otherwise eventually the other side will insist on negotiating directly with the CEO.

CLOSING THE DEAL

There will come a point in the discussions when some kind of financial proposal will be appropriate to make since one side or the other will insist upon it. Assuming that your party is selling the asset, we are great believers in retaining the power of the pen, meaning that the first proposal should come from you. Once this initial offer is presented, assuming it has some basis in commercial reality, both parties tend to treat it as a benchmark. We recommend discussing your opening bid in person (face-to-face or over the phone) before submitting the formal written offer as it limits surprises and saves embarrassing misunderstanding. Once you have discussed what your opening bid will be, your second decision becomes how you want to appear to the other party, i.e., a hard bargainer or moderate. Whichever you choose, the chances are that the other negotiator will respond in kind, so make sure you select a style with which you are comfortable because it is likely to be present throughout the negotiations. Your opening offer will be met, hopefully, with a counteroffer, and thus the negotiations begin. By the time the parties have exchanged two or three versions of the term sheet or contract, it should be apparent where the deal is heading and, with any good fortune, the terms and conditions agreed in those drafts will be consistent with the terms discussed in the deal preparation process.

If the terms don't meet your desired goals there are some difficult decisions to make, but first it is helpful to understand why. There can be a number of reasons, the most likely being a lack of leverage in the negotiation. The absence of an alternative buyer always limits leverage and the other side eventually knows they are the only party at the table. Your leverage in a negotiation can also be reduced by other circumstances, including your company's financial position or the failure of a related technology or product which can undermine the perceived value of your asset. It could be that the world around your asset has changed or perhaps the strengths of your program have been undermined or devalued by new information on IP or the discovery of another disease mechanism. Do you take the offered terms or walk away? It is much easier to accept less than optimal terms if there is a rational explanation for why a difficult decision still has to be made. There can be no universal answer to this question and each organization will need to carefully examine its BATNA and the original reasons for doing the deal. That is why those preparatory activities you conducted are so important to the deal process.

Negotiation is more of an art than a science, although negotiation works best if not improvised and the process is well-planned. Occasionally, negotiations can be simple; each side giving something up in return for something else—but in most biotech/pharma deals, power imbalances will frequently lead to win/lose negotiations. This is why we stress that at the outset you must agree on what it is you are prepared to sell and how much you might reasonably expect to get from it. The main message of this chapter is that a deal is not an event that occurs in isolation but a process based on preparation—the four issues we identified at the outset.

---

b. The good cop/bad cop analogy has evolved from a stereotypic style used in television shows and movies where it was routinely used as a psychological tactic in interrogation. The "bad cop" takes an aggressive, negative stance towards the subject, making blatant accusations, derogatory comments, threats, and in general creating antipathy between the subject and himself. This sets the stage for the "good cop'" to act sympathetically: appearing supportive, understanding, in general, showing sympathy for the subject. The good cop will also defend the subject from the bad cop. The subject may feel he can cooperate with the good cop out of trust or fear of the bad cop. He may then seek protection by and trust the good cop and provide the information the interrogators are seeking. These same techniques are used regularly in the context of a negotiation.

Mostly, negotiations fall into one of two styles; the win/ win where both sides believe in enlarging the pie before dividing it, or the distributive approach where the size of the pie is fixed and one side wins as the other loses. If you have a choice, although you may not, avoid the distributive approach. Often, the parties that adopt this method do not have interest in a relationship and inevitably these deals do not stand the test of time. We should point out that because the biotechnology/pharma world is relatively small it is very likely that you will know someone who has done a deal with the organization with which you are about to enter into negotiations. Talk with them on the phone and ask how the other side operates—it will help you prepare for the next steps. If you find out they don't have a track record of adopting the win/win approach you can adjust your style accordingly.

Regardless of the approach, we recommend that during the negotiation it is best to avoid adopting direct conflict as a strategy for completing the negotiation. If you are the smaller company it is unlikely this path will be tolerated for long by the larger party. Obviously avoidance of conflict is much easier to accomplish in a "win/win" strategy. If conflict does occur, the leader needs to refocus all parties on the mutual benefits of the deal, rather than the specific issue and then pursue an indirect approach to resolving the source of conflict. If conflict is unavoidable it needs to be managed in such a way as to not become personal. Your responsibility as the negotiation leader is to control any conflict that might arise and limit the amount of damage to the credibility of your side. Demonstrations of anger, no matter how much they are provoked, are usually not the best way to get your argument across. If there is a point at which the proposed position is unacceptable to you or is inconsistent with a previously agreed position, say "no"—at some point the other side needs to know that there are some things you cannot agree to.

If the discussion gets emotional, try to stop the discussion and refocus. There are a number of alternatives which can be used by themselves or together:

- Take a break (someone always needs to go to the restroom or get some fresh air).
- Break the tension by making a joke, but not at the expense of the protagonist.
- Table the subject for now and move on to a more resolvable topic.

Keeping the dialog moving forward can significantly change the dynamic in the room.

Most conflicts are based on one or more of the following traits: competitive personalities, misperceptions and bias, poor communication of the issues, and rigid commitments. The basic personalities cannot probably be changed although the flash points can be limited by careful scripting by your side. Unless the issue is truly to die for, rigid commitments should be avoided as they do not allow for concessions or discussion. You have two ears and one mouth and it is good to use them in that ratio. What we have observed is that negotiators who are willing to take time to probe more patiently (or indirectly) and listen more carefully are usually the most successful.

If you reach an acceptable end by narrowing the differences, you are now ready to close the deal. It is essential to close the deal as quickly as possible. The deal should never be assumed to be done until the contract agreement is signed. Sometimes there is a desire to "just sign the term sheet and announce that the deal is done." This comment reflects the fatigue and desperation associated with the deal process and should be avoided at all costs. In order to help close the deal quickly, create some context of a ticking clock, the end of the fiscal year will always have an impetus. Other common methods to resolve the few outstanding items is to split the difference, or some variation of this in which both parties agree to concede one position in exchange for another. In any negotiation you will need to make concessions if for no other reason than to allow the other party to feel they have gotten something out of the negotiation. Decide in advance what key concessions you will not make and what is really important to you.

At the end of the negotiation you will have won some points and lost some points. To get the deal approved you are going to have to match the points won and lost with the goals that were agreed upon at the outset of this process. If you have communicated effectively throughout this process and followed the rule of no surprises, the CEO and board are more likely to approve the final transaction. If you don't think the deal is good enough to sign, tell your CEO and board and let the board override you if they want. If you believe the deal is good but the CEO or board does not approve it, then somewhere along the way you have made a mistake in your process. Work out what that mistake was and don't make it again!

A SUMMARY OF THE DEAL DANCE

We refer to the process of bringing a deal to the table and closing it as a "dance." Like dancing, it can only be learned by practice, not out of a book or off a DVD. To give the readers a flavor (the secret sauce) of this dance we conclude with some, but by no means all, of the steps involved. And remember, great business development executives make up their own steps to fit the circumstances.

- **The role of business development is different in every company:** These can include in-licensing, out-licensing, alliance management, strategy development, fundraising, product development, and many others. Understand the true needs of your business and be careful not to be distracted or sidelined by other assignments such as: the annual report, setting up off-site meetings, attending too many industry meetings, and even being the interim finance officer. At the end of the day the core business development needs must be taken care of while all else is secondary.

- **Understand the environment into which you will be "selling:"** Understand what drives companies, people, competitors, suppliers, bankers, and the board. By understanding these players, it will help you plan a partnering campaign. Large pharmaceutical companies may seem bizarre to you. But they are not bizarre. They are just large, multinational, risk-adverse companies in a risky business trying to manage their portfolios for future growth. You must understand them and how each one thinks. Pharmaceutical companies review thousands of opportunities each year so you must take the initiative to present your opportunity in its most favorable light.

- **Think first:** BD is not a "ready, fire, aim" process. Thoughtful analysis, talking with contemporaries, and "reading between the lines" are all part of the preparation before you approach your targets. There is a huge amount of background information available to you. Take some time to review it.

- **Understand Big Pharma (or the inverse, Small Biotech):** If you have not walked in their shoes, you need to learn about the pressures and constraints they operate under. Take someone in that organization to lunch and listen.

- **Get your "elevator pitch" down cold:** If you cannot tell your story and have their interest in 30 seconds or less, you are in trouble. Don't use a computer or props; nothing but your golden voice. Practice it every day, in the car, to your partner, to the dog, to your co-workers. This elevator pitch will grow into an opening slide of your presentation and change over time. See it as the backbone of everything your company is. If you lack an elevator pitch you will be fighting an uphill battle going forward. In our Secret Sauce Seminar we are always unpleasantly surprised by the number of executives who cannot give a coherent pitch or answer obvious questions. Shame! And the elevator pitch doesn't just belong to business development. It should be part of every deal-associated person in your company.

- **Understand what you want to buy or sell:** If you don't, then the path is long and rough and you may never get to complete a deal.

- **Think through all of the materials you need to line up:** Collateral materials, slide decks, patent summaries, bibliographies, scientific champions, an internal survey of employees for industry contacts, and lots more.

- **Prepare multiple presentations:** The partnering meeting slide deck, the nonconfidential introduction deck, the confidential deck I and II (hold something back for another meeting), the podium deck, and the VC deck. Avoid background colors, too much animation, and slides that cannot be read from the back of the room for which you always apologize. Never distribute slides to the other side in anything other than a pdf format. The decks are YOURS. They should be the essence of clarity, conciseness, and simplicity!

- **Always review materials before sending:** Circumstances, data, and messages change. No excuses accepted! At the same time, avoid creating new decks for every request or there will be confusion and chaos.

- **We have a mantra about carefully listening to others: "You have two ears and one mouth…for a reason!"** If you have ever been exposed to a sales technique course you learn early to listen to your customer carefully. Use open-ended questions (indirect probes) and listen carefully to the answer. Use direct probes only when a yes-or-no answer is appropriate. The more you listen, the more you will uncover needs, concerns, and get direction on moving forward.

- **Partnering meetings:** You can spend a lifetime and a fortune going to these meetings. They are very helpful when introducing a company or a project or after a major inflection point. Go to meetings to inform, not to close. If you close too soon a big "no" may go into a database and stall future progress. Just keeping people informed is easier because if they see something they like, they will reach out to you. *At some point sitting in partnering booths is not appropriate,* meeting offline is. Your constant objective is to get to another meeting with them.

- **Bluebirds and frogs:** Even though you have your priority target list, sometimes serendipity works in your favor. *Open all your windows and sometimes a bluebird will fly in. Said another way, kiss all the frogs. There is a prince there somewhere.* With whom and why deals get done is not entirely predictable. It is a mistake not to allow serendipity to help.

- **Follow-up:** Like everything else in life, follow-up is critical. Keep doors open, respond to requests, summarize meetings, send new information, build your case, and get to another meeting.

- **Entertainment:** Lots of fun perhaps, but does it make a difference? Potential partners are pretty savvy. They are in a hunt, and a dinner won't distract them. Besides, your competition can always out-entertain you. Use entertainment judiciously with the right people and at the right time in the dance, and have a message to send. Be conscious of the message you want to send.

- **Term sheets:** Pretty standard formats. Creativity here is many times not appreciated. Mark everything draft. Never agree to a binding term sheet. If they want a deal, do the deal. Keep term sheet development low key with lots of back and forth. Keep the board informed. Move to approvals once all the cats are herded and key points are settled. Generally a term sheet is prepared by the seller.

- **Agreement draft:** Who writes? Emotional issue. Either side can write, but the power of the pen is real. Small companies can avoid large legal fees by letting the other team write. Yes, there will be some bias but that can work in the seller's favor. Set a timeframe for completion.

- **Negotiations:** Yes, you can take a workshop or just use common sense. Know your MUSTS versus your WANTS. Have a good, experienced transaction lawyer alongside you. Work out roles and responsibilities with your attorney before you sit down. Leave egos at the door.
- **Due diligence:** Use electronic data rooms. Answer direct questions—directly. If you don't have a data point or know an answer, just say so. No "hand-waving" please.
- **After the signing:** Have a nice social affair and a little gift token. Give good toasts. Enjoy.
- **Alliance management:** As important as all that has gone before, keeping a deal going is as important as getting it. BD should remain involved as they know the faces and the background. Do not distribute the entire contract to new players internally, only the grant, the governance clauses, and other key operating terms.

The future of every biotechnology company is really related to the filling of major unmet market needs with vital products and at a development cost that is rational. Strategies that focus on unmet needs linked to well-executed programs by experienced company leaders attract attention from pharmaceutical companies and result in deal funding that is, for the most part, nondilutive and can lead to portfolio expansion and/or future merger and acquisition activity. Business development executives who are intensely focused, understand their trade and can lead the process, possess the essential elements of biotech corporate success.

Why is this "Secret Sauce" so Important?

As an early senior executive of Genentech once remarked, the really great BD executives possess a "secret sauce" to make things happen when others might give up and walk away. The secret sauce of BD executives include the experience necessary to lead a company's internal team to success in completing a deal. What may appear to be a series of random events may be in actuality a very organized effort, over many months or years, to attract significant funding for company operations from partners.

Business development executives are partially born and partially made. The right temperament, style, sense of humor, ability to know when to press and when not to, the ability to read people, a sense of drama, etc. is probably ingrained into a personality from their early years. This can be described as the ability to know when to talk and when to listen, process information, ask direct probing questions or indirect probing questions, engage in light conversation, and look people in the eye when addressing them. It includes the ability to write and talk precisely, avoid the "ums" and "you knows" that one hears so often from the podium, and understanding about cultural sensitivity—these come from experience on the job and just plain common sense about your profession. Everyone can develop their own secret sauce. It's about style, timing, and momentum. Having a mentor or two somewhere along the way speeds the process. You will know you have it when the first time a potential partner says to you "Okay, sounds good, let's do this deal…"

REFERENCES

[1] Fisher R, Ury W. Getting to Yes. Penguin Books; 2011. pp. 1–170.
[2] Myerson RB. Nash Equilibrium and the History of Economic Theory. Nash Equilibrium and the History of Economic Theory. Journal of Economic Literature Retrieved 1 October 2012.
[3] Honeyman A, Schneider C. The Negotiators Fieldbook: Desktop Reference. American Bar Association 2006:200–300.
[4] Hawkins J, Steiner N. "The Nash Equilibrium Meets BATNA." *Gamed Theory Varied Uses in ADR*. Boston, MA: Harvard University Press; Retrieved 1 October 2012.
[5] Ulam SM, Eckhardt R. Stan Ulam, John von Neumann, and the Monte Carlo Method. Los Alamos Science 1987; (Special Issue (15)):131–7.
[6] Stewart JJ, Allison PN, Johnson RS. Putting a Price on Biotechnology. Nature Biotechnology September 2001;19:813–7.
[7] Shaw S. How to Find the Best Partner; March 9, 2011. www.adimpact.com/BySarahShaw.
[8] Desai PS, Purohit D. Let Me Talk to My Manager: Haggling in a Competitive Environment. Marketing Science; Spring 2004 March 2004;23(Issue 2):219.
[9] Kahneman D. Think Fast and Slow. Penguin; 2011.
[10] Pappas, H.J. "How to be a Good Scientist: The Irony of Abnegation." Kunkliga Tekniska Hogskolan School of Information and Communication Technology. Denmark.

Chapter 29

Biotech-Pharma Collaboration—A Strategic Tool: Case Study of Centocor

Lara V. Marks, D.Phil. (Oxon)

Senior Research Fellow, Department of Social Science, Health and Medicine, King's College, London, England

Today the estimated value of alliances signed between pharmaceutical companies and biotechnology companies is $160 billion per annum [1]. Underlying the vast sums being paid out for alliances is the fact that such collaboration is a lifeline for pharmaceutical companies scouting for new products to fill their dwindling portfolios in the face of expiring patents and rising generic competition. It is also vital to biotechnology companies seeking to raise funds for their research and development (R&D) and establishing a footprint on the market.

Since their inception, biotechnology companies have depended on partnerships for their survival and growth. This chapter looks at the pivotal role alliances played in the foundation and growth of Centocor, one of America's pioneering monoclonal antibody companies. Set up in 1979, 3 years after Genentech, the world's first dedicated biotechnology company, Centocor was among the first handful of biotechnology companies started in the 1970s. Within 5 years of its founding, Centocor had become a highly competitive and profitable diagnostics company based on monoclonal antibodies (mAbs). As this chapter shows, much of this success rested on the collaborations its founders secured with research institutes and larger healthcare companies. Through skillful networking, Centocor's executives secured the scientific and technological expertise, products, capital, and market distribution necessary to mature from a small start-up company to a major player in the global diagnostic market. In 1992, however, Centocor faced imminent collapse, brought on in part by its executives' decision to go it alone in the development and marketing of the company's first therapeutic. What saved the company from extinction and allowed it to subsequently succeed in therapeutics was a reversion to its strategy of collaboration [2].

THE BIRTH OF CENTOCOR

In May 1979, Hilary Koprowski, a Polish virologist, immunologist, and director of the Wistar Institute [3], entered a partnership with Michael Wall, a MIT-educated electrical engineer and founder of several electronics, computer, and biological start-up companies, to establish a new biotechnology company [4]. Calling the company Centocor, Koprowski and Wall aimed to create, develop, and market diagnostics and therapeutics based on mAbs. Monoclonal antibodies were new to the scientific and commercial world, having been devised by César Milstein and Georges Köhler at the Laboratory of Molecular Biology, Cambridge in 1975. Derived from natural antibodies (proteins produced by the immune system that are designed to attach to and inactivate foreign particles, or antigens) mAbs were produced as a result of the fusion of myeloma cells with antibodies taken from the spleen of previously immunized animals [5].

Providing for the first time a long-lasting and standardized form of antibodies that could be used for various medical applications, mAbs were quickly adopted by various academic and commercial laboratories globally. This included Koprowski and his team at the Wistar Institute. Using cells sent by Milstein, Koprowski, and his colleagues began to develop mAbs against the influenza virus and malignant cancer tumors [6]. Funded by government grants, this research formed the basis for patent applications in 1978. Granted in 1979 and 1980, these patents were the first-ever patents for mAbs [7]. In 1978, Koprowski offered to license the patents to Boehringer-Ingelheim for $500,000 annually over 10 years. The pharmaceutical company, however, had dragged out negotiations for 6 or 8 months before saying no on the basis that they saw no future for mAb products [8].

Frustrated by his experience with Boehringer-Ingelheim and other companies, Koprowski realized that the only way forward would be to establish a separate company. He decided to do this in partnership with Wall. At the time that Wall and Koprowski started discussing their plans for a company, Wall was getting itchy feet for a change of scenery, having just sold Flow Laboratories, a company he had set up to produce and sell cell cultures and related products. Wall had various business schemes in mind, including growing orchids. His idea of founding a company based on flowers, however, soon dissipated on talking to Koprowski. What captured Wall's attention was the fact that Koprowski believed he could have in hand a mAb diagnostic very quickly. This was named 19-9, a mAb developed at the Wistar Institute that Koprowski saw as having potential as a diagnostic for pancreatic cancer [9].

Setting up an office in downtown Philadelphia in May 1979, Wall started to build Centocor's executive team as the company chairman with scientific support from Koprowski and the Wistar Institute. One of the first to join the executive team was Ted Allen. Allen's background was ideal for Centocor as he had been a marketing manager at Corning Medical, a Boston-based division of Corning Glass Works. More importantly, he came from a company which had begun to establish a strong portfolio of diagnostic immunoassays. Such diagnostics were rapidly replacing the more traditional chemical-based tests that had dominated the diagnostics market since the 1940s [10].

With Allen on board, Centocor soon attracted the interest of another Corning employee who would prove pivotal in moving the company forward. This was Hubert Schoemaker, one of Allen's former Corning colleagues who had been instrumental in building up Corning's pioneering portfolio of diagnostics. Schoemaker was a biochemist by training and had completed a doctorate at MIT within a department at the cutting edge of biotechnology research. One of the factors determining Schoemaker's decision to join the Centocor start-up was his desire to find a way to improve people's lives. His inspiration came from the profound disabilities of his daughter, who was born with lissencephaly, a rare brain malformation causing severe mental disability and motor dysfunction. Schoemaker joined Centocor initially in an unofficial capacity, helping with research and planning while continuing to work at Corning. In early 1980, however, he began officially, taking

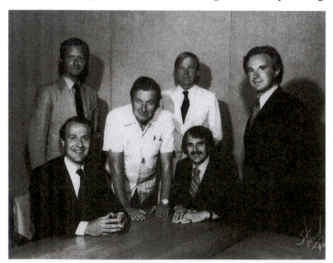

FIGURE 29.1 The earliest founders of Centocor. In the front, from left to right are: Schoemaker, Koproski, Zurawski, and Evnin. Behind from left to right are Allen and Wall. (Photo credit: *Anne Schoemaker.*)

over the position of chief executive officer in the wake of a sudden departure by Allen [11]. (See Figure 29.1.)

Within months of joining Centocor's team, Schoemaker had sourced another individual who soon became vital to the company's operation. This was Vincent Zurawski. He joined Centocor in August 1979 as the company's first Chief Scientific Officer. Zurawski came well-equipped for the post. A chemist by training, he had been a pioneer in mAb production at Harvard Medical School and Massachusetts General Hospital (MGH), where he had held a postdoctoral research fellowship.

THE COLLABORATIVE JOURNEY BEGINS

The founders decided to focus their resources initially on diagnostics, predicting $17 million in revenues by 1984, [12]. with therapeutics as their long-term goal. Diagnostics were easier to develop and could win regulatory approval more easily than therapeutics, thereby enabling faster revenue growth [13]. In addition to developing diagnostic products, they aimed to supply antibodies on contract to other companies for use in their proprietary diagnostic kits [14].

Entering the diagnostics sector was ambitious. The $2 billion diagnostics market was highly competitive, dominated at that time by healthcare giants like Abbott Laboratories, F. Hoffman-La Roche, and Warner Lambert who had developed tests that could only be analyzed through their own proprietary instruments. In 1979 two companies were already offering mAbs on a commercial basis: Sera Lab, a British company (with which César Milstein was involved) and Hybritech, a San Diego start-up founded in 1978 by Ivor Royston, a professor at the University of California San Diego and his research assistant Howard Birndorf. Both of these companies were marketing mAbs as reagents to researchers and exploring their use as diagnostics [15]. The competitive landscape, however, quickly changed. By 1983 over 150 companies, including large pharmaceutical companies, had mAb-based diagnostic programs, and 23 such diagnostics were being marketed and another 100 were in the pipeline [16].

From the start Wall and Koprowski saw collaboration as key to their business model. The very name "Centocor" was derived from the words "cento" which describes (in Latin) an old garment made of hundreds of patches of material or a literary or musical composition made up of parts of other works, and (2) "cor(e)" as in the center [17]. Centocor's collaborative philosophy was unusual for the time. In 1979 most start-up biotechnology companies were trying to do everything internally from the discovery process through development. Centocor's founders believed, however, that rather than depending solely on in-house research they should use internal skills to identify and fund prominent external researchers and laboratories working in areas the company wanted to develop and where there was an appropriate license for the technology [18]. As Wall told *Forbes* magazine in May 1985, "You can have a garage full of Ph.D.s working on a project and nine times out of ten some guy across the street is going to come up with the discovery that beats them all" [19].

Central to Centocor's policy of collaboration was Wall and Schoemaker's remarkable ability to network [20]. By being well-connected and plugged into the academic world, Wall and Schoemaker realized they stood a better chance of finding promising products at a relatively early stage when they were not unduly expensive [21]. As Schoemaker later recalled, "We realized it was a lot cheaper to roam academe and pay a royalty back for what we developed than start our own research facilities. Collaboration was the best way to be competitive" [20].

One of Centocor's strongest academic collaborations was with the Wistar Institute, fueled in part by Koprowski's connection with the company. In 1979 Centocor signed three licensing deals with the Institute for rights to four approved and pending patents for diagnostic and therapeutic purposes. Centocor paid $25,000 upfront and agreed to make royalty payments of 4 to 6 percent for any resulting products [23].

Centocor's alliance with the Wistar was helped by the fact that the latter had its own charter and board. This allowed greater flexibility for an academic-company collaboration than otherwise was normally possible in the late 1970s. Although the pioneering academic-company relationship between Centocor and the Wistar raised some concern about conflict of interest for one Wistar board member, this was soon overcome [24]. The relationship set an important precedent for the partnerships Centocor entered thereafter [25].

Centocor, like other biotechnology companies, was helped enormously by the passing of the Bayh-Dole Act in late 1980, which established for the first time uniform guidelines for the patenting and commercialization of government-funded academic research [26]. Between 1985 and 1990 Centocor's partnerships with research institutions grew from 15 to over 80 worldwide, many involving license and license-option agreements [27]. These collaborations were vital to Centocor's business, providing materials for some of its early products [28]. Crucially, it allowed the company to keep its costs to a minimum while increasing sales: between 1984 and 1990 Centocor's R&D budget remained at the same level while its sales increased fivefold [29].

In addition to partnering with research institutions to fill its product pipeline, Centocor pursued marketing alliances. Facing a highly competitive environment, Wall and Schoemaker realized they could strengthen the company's market position by having licensing agreements with companies that had well-established market positions and distribution channels. This would eliminate the time and expense of establishing Centocor's own distribution mechanism and facilitate faster entry to the market [30].

Centocor's team deliberately secured agreements with key diagnostic companies, whereby the companies would buy and sell Centocor's antibodies in completed test kits as well as separate antibodies to be used in their own proprietary machines [31]. All of Centocor's diagnostic tests were designed to be compatible with existing diagnostic systems that allowed for both the testing and analysis of results, such as those marketed by Abbott and Roche, and used by the majority of clinical laboratories [32]. This arrangement not only helped Centocor gain a broad market penetration, but allowed it to leverage its technical strength without threatening competitors [33]. As David Holveck, who headed up Centocor's diagnostics department from 1983, stated, "Because of the marketing strategy of networking with all of the major suppliers, we insulated ourselves from competition because we were the suppliers of the reagents, and they were looking for ways of adding tests to their instrumentation [34]. In 1983, 61 percent of Centocor's product sales were being sold by major distributors. Two years later this had increased to 74 percent [35]. (See Figure 29.2.)

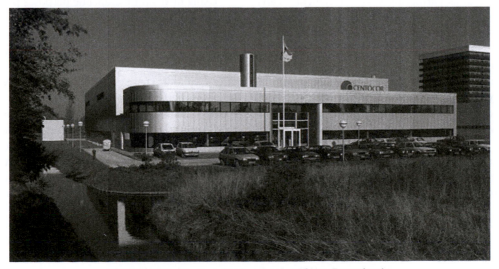

FIGURE 29.2   Centocor headquarters in Malvern, Pennsylvania.

An important catalyst in Centocor's early success was its swift winning of regulatory approval for two diagnostic tests: one for gastrointestinal cancer (using an antibody licensed from the Wistar) and the other for hepatitis B (developed by Zurawski and licensed from Massachusetts General Hospital). Both tests had reached the market by 1983. The approval of the hepatitis test was significant as it was the first mAb-based test approved for this disease by the FDA. Centocor's hepatitis B test was in high demand because from the early 1970s many countries, including the United States, required the screening of blood intended for blood transfusion. Some idea of how popular the test was can be seen from the fact that between April and December 1983 Centocor sold 600,000 of its hepatitis tests.

Between 1983 and 1986 Centocor introduced another three tests to the market: one for diagnosing ovarian cancer (licensed from the Dana Faber Cancer Institute), the first diagnostic tool available for the disease; a test for breast cancer (licensed from Scripps Clinic and Research Foundation); and another for colorectal cancer (licensed from the Wistar) [36]. All three tests are still used in clinical practice today. In addition to these diagnostics, Centocor also put into the market the first diagnostic test for multidrug resistance, a major problem for cancer patients. By 1990 Centocor had captured more than a quarter of the world's market for antibody-based tests for cancer [37].

Between 1979 and 1985 Centocor's team built up a profitable business with revenues of just under $50 million. It was highly lucrative because most of the bottom-line revenue came from royalties [38]. By 1987 Centocor was one of the very few monoclonal antibody companies with earnings [39].

FINANCE: "GRAB AS MANY COOKIES AS YOU CAN"

Just as fundamental as partnering was to Centocor's early success, was Wall and Schoemaker's ability to find capital. What helped this process was the fact that soon after setting up the company, Wall, using his previous reputation in the business world, persuaded Tony Evnin, a senior partner in Venrock Associates, a venture capital firm, to become one of the company's directors. This was important as Venrock had a history of investment in the diagnostics and therapeutic sector. Venrock subsequently became the first major investor in Centocor, providing $300,000. This would just be the start of raising funds. Between 1979 and 1981 Centocor raised approximately $7 million through private placement of its stocks [40]. The Centocor executives raised further cash from public offerings in 1983, 1986, 1990, and 1991, the last raising $100 million [41].

Wall and Schoemaker also secured funds through research and development (R&D) limited partnerships. First used by the Delorean Car Company in 1975, R&D

partnerships allowed companies to raise capital from private individual investors for specific research projects off the balance sheet, providing investors with tax benefits and potentially higher returns than equity investments [42]. In 1982, Genentech was the first biotechnology company to use the mechanism to develop human growth hormone and gamma interferon drugs [43]. Centocor was one of the most successful and aggressive users of R&D limited partnerships within the biotechnology industry, establishing at least four such partnerships between 1984 and 1987 [44].

Central to Centocor's fundraising was Schoemaker's philosophy that it should not be driven by the company's business plan. He believed that even if Centocor had a lot of money on the balance sheet, more money should be raised whenever the opportunity arose. As he explained, "In Centocor's early days, Bill Hambrecht of Hambrecht and Quist advised me: "When the cookie jar comes around, grab as many cookies as you can because you'll never know when it comes around again." He also advised me to discard all of the traditional business evaluations such as cash flow, price/earnings, etc. in deciding when and how much money to raise. He told me that each week he had five CEOs in his office who had insufficient capital and that he had never had a CEO come to him and tell him he had too much money" [45].

EXPANDING ITS MARKET POTENTIAL

While initially funneling resources into blood-based diagnostics, Wall and Schoemaker quickly looked for ways to expand into the therapeutics sector. Therapeutics posed greater uncertainties than diagnostics. Much of the commercial attention in the nascent biotechnology therapeutics industry was focused on using recombinant DNA technology for the production of drugs for which there were existing therapeutic models and markets [46]. Therapy based on mAbs was a novel idea and remained uncharted territory.

Using mAbs for therapeutic purposes presented considerable new challenges. Unlike the blood-based diagnostics that Centocor had heretofore been developing, which involved the deployment of mAbs in tests on blood removed from the human body, therapeutics required the administration of mAbs directly into the human body. mAb antibody drugs therefore posed greater safety concerns. Therapeutics also required far greater quantities of mAbs than needed for diagnostics, posing new manufacturing and quality-control challenges [47].

In order to gain experience in the therapeutic sector, Centocor devised a strategy to initially develop mAbs as contrast agents for diagnostic-imaging procedures. While not therapies in themselves, the use of mAbs as imaging agents tested the safety of mAbs for potential therapies and provided useful aids for the evaluation and therapeutic treatment of a patient. In 1985, Centocor established an *in vivo* diagnostic-imaging unit and began to develop three products directed towards imaging diseases such as cancer and conditions of the cardiovascular system. The market for mAb-imaging diagnostic products was expected to be between five and ten times larger than that of blood-based diagnostics [48]. Within the field of cancer alone, imaging diagnostics were expected in 1985 to grow by 200 percent each year, reaching $200 million by 1988. The market size for cardiac imaging was also projected to increase from $70 million to $130 million between 1985 and 1988 [49].

In their reports to investors, Centocor's executives predicted the company's imaging diagnostics would swiftly be on the market within a couple of years of their first testing [50]. What they hoped to do was capitalize on the mAbs it was already deploying in the development of its *in vitro* blood tests. To this end, early on the team looked into developing CA 19-9 as a tool for imaging gastrointestinal cancers and CA-125 for imaging ovarian cancer [51]. Progress, however, was slow and not as straightforward as anticipated. One of the problems was that while the mAbs proved good imaging agents, they took a long time to clear from the body which delayed the reading of the images and thus obtaining the diagnostic results [52].

Centocor's difficulties in utilizing mAbs for imaging diagnostics were not unique. Indeed, many other companies would struggle to reach the market with such products and their overall worldwide sales would remain small. In 1998, for example, the worldwide sales of diagnostic-imaging products using mAbs was worth $10 million. The sales revenue would grow over the coming years, but would continue to be small, estimated to be $15 million in revenue in 2005. Such figures were well below the projected figures Centocor and others had forecast back in the 1980s. Back in 1987 one financial analyst had forecast the annual sales for Centocor's cardiovascular imaging tests could reach between $300 million and $400 million [53].

Despite the slow progress, in August 1989 Centocor won European approval for its first imaging product called Myoscint®. Licensed originally from MGH, Myoscint® could locate and estimate the amount of dead heart tissue from a heart attack. The product was first marketed in France, Germany, Italy, Spain, and the United Kingdom and then in America from 1996 [54]. Overall the product did not take off in a significant way. By the time the product reached the market, other methods had appeared that proved less invasive for the patient and more accurate in terms of the data they provided. In the end Myoscint® proved more useful for detecting heart transplant rejection and myocarditis (inflammation of the heart muscle). It was used for these purposes off-label in Europe, where those performing heart transplants found it an invaluable tool [55].

THERAPEUTICS

While the experience with imaging diagnostics proved disappointing, it gave the Centocor team some expertise in the development of mAbs for use directly in humans. This was invaluable in going forward in the creation of mAb-based medicines. Importantly, it provided a starting point in terms of what was needed for the R&D for a therapeutic as well as learning the ropes for clinical trials and manufacturing. Going, forward with therapeutics, however, was by its nature a much bigger risk for the company. Nothing could fully prepare Centocor's executives, then more familiar with the business model for developing diagnostics, with what would be needed for the development of mAbs as drugs. Moreover, they had little to go on from the nascent biotechnology therapeutics industry. At the time, companies in this sector had more expertise in using the new recombinant DNA technique to develop drugs in disease areas for which there were already well-established treatment protocols and market systems. By contrast, few knew which disease areas mAbs could be successfully used therapeutically or which market they would be able to penetrate.

Early on, Wall and Schoemaker recognized that the time and cost required to bring therapeutic products to market exposed their newly emerging company to unacceptable financial risks, which could divert resources and hinder innovation. In order to minimize the risk and gain financial, scientific, and technical resources as well as credibility, they therefore devised a strategy to generate relationships with leading companies. By 1983, Centocor had established collaborations with two companies for this purpose: the American chemicals company FMC Corporation and the Swiss-based pharmaceutical company F. Hoffman-La Roche [56].

Centocor's alliance with FMC began in 1980 with FMC agreeing to contribute a total of $12.4 million. Split 50/50 and managed by a committee with a representative from each company, each partner had the option to purchase all of the other's interest in the joint venture [57]. One of the aims of the collaboration was to find a way to produce mAbs from cell-lines more closely resembling human antibodies. This was particularly important if Centocor was to gain leadership in the mAb therapeutics field. Most of the early mAbs developed from the time of Köhler and Milstein were derived from mouse cells. These mAbs had certain drawbacks: a short half-life, poor recognition by receptors in the human body, necessitating administration in high doses, and had greater potential to cause life-threatening allergic reactions and viral safety problems. For Centocor, human antibodies not only promised greater safety and efficacy for therapeutic products, but provided a competitive advantage in securing investment [58]. In 1986, Centocor gained exclusive rights to the human antibody technology developed through the venture. In return FMC received 1.35 million shares of Centocor's stock [59]. The only other biotechnology company that had managed to develop human antibodies by then was Cetus [60].

CENTOCOR GOES IT ALONE

In 1986, Wall and Schoemaker decided that while they would continue to develop therapeutic products through joint ventures, the profits generated from the highly successful blood test business and contract revenue from technology licensing, and selected product marketing arrangements could be used to build Centocor into a major pharmaceutical company. Their ambition was for the company to be as big as Merck, by the year 2000 [61]. Transforming Centocor into a globally integrated pharmaceutical company was not an unusual goal for the time. Other executives from leading biotechnology companies were pursuing the same vision with some success. In 1985 Genentech launched Protropin® to treat growth hormone deficiency in children. It was the first recombinant pharmaceutical product to be manufactured and marketed by a biotechnology company without the help of a partner [62].

By 1988, Centocor's research group had identified 30 new entities for possible drug development and had 12 Investigational New Drug Applications filed with the U.S. Food and Drug Administration (FDA), many of which were mAbs, and had clinically evaluated 10 products [63]. While many of Centocor's competitors at this time were focusing on deploying mAbs for cancer treatment and Centocor had its own cancer program [64], Centocor's preferred lead candidate was an antibody-targeting septic shock, a deadly disease usually acquired in hospitals and traditionally treated, ineffectively, with antibiotics. By 1986, Centocor had two human antibodies, one developed in-house through their collaboration with FMC, and one licensed in from the University of California San Diego, known as HA-1A [65].

At least a third of septic shock cases are caused by gram-negative bacteria, a class of bacteria that possesses a unique outer membrane that hinders cell penetration by antibiotics and other drugs. During the 1980s gram-negative sepsis was the third leading cause of death in the United States, with over 100,000 people dying from the condition each year, accounting for up to $10 billion in healthcare expenditures annually. Wall and Schoemaker believed that should Centocor develop a drug to combat a critical medical problem, they would have a major blockbuster. The estimated market for products to treat septic shock in 1990 was over $300 million [66].

In order to maximize the potential of HA-1A, trade-named Centoxin, Wall and Schoemaker, in part encouraged by their Wall Street advisors, decided that rather than selling the rights to the drug to another company they would develop and market Centoxin internally. This they believed would give them greater control over the product and larger revenues [67]. As Tony Evnin, one of Centocor's first investors and directors, explained, "At that point in time it seemed like such an important product and it was a product in a new area. We wanted the ability to keep it all

to ourselves. Perhaps we were a bit greedy, but it seemed like it was something that, by bringing in…additional talent [from the pharmaceutical industry], we could take on ourselves" [68] (Figure 29.3).

One of the reasons the Centocor executives decided to develop and market Centoxin internally was that it would help build the necessary infrastructure for becoming an integrated pharmaceutical company [69]. This, however, required major upscaling of the company's manufacturing capabilities and marketing which involved large sums of cash. At least $150 million was needed to get Centoxin to market. Between 1986 and 1992, Centocor went through nine different equity, debt, and off-balance sheet financings, netting more than $500 million. By 1992, $450 million had been spent on clinical trials, building a sales force of 275 people (200 in the United States and 75 in Europe), and building two new factories—one in Holland and one in the United States [70].

Heeding advice from Wall Street, the management team was also restructured to bring on board skills in pharmaceutical development, regulation, and marketing by the hiring of staff from large pharmaceutical companies. In December 1987, James Wavle, the former president of Parke-Davis,

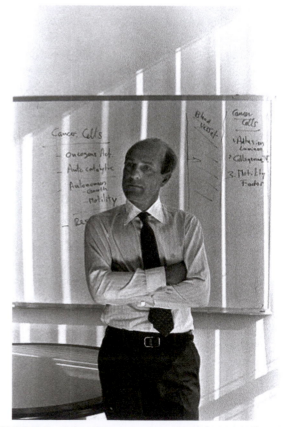

FIGURE 29.3 Hubert Schoemaker during his early years at Centocor. He was known for being able to convey very quickly a vision of the future as well as listening to those around him. Those who worked with him recall his overwhelming sense of optimism. (Photo credit: *Anne Schoemaker.*)

Warner-Lambert's pharmaceutical unit, became Centocor's president and chief operating officer. Working alongside Schoemaker, who retained his position as chief executive officer and replaced Wall as chairman, Wavle took on the responsibility for turning Centocor into a globally integrated pharmaceutical company [71]. The recruitment of pharmaceutical executives had a major impact on the culture within Centocor, bringing in new management styles, more aggressive marketing, and a higher cash burn [72].

Confidence was high that Centoxin would succeed. Such optimism was not unfounded. In February 1991, a leading American journal ran an article indicating Centoxin reduced gram-negative sepsis by 39 percent. For those who went into septic shock, the drug reduced mortality by 47 percent [73]. The same month the United States Army administered the drug to soldiers fighting in the first Gulf War [74]. A month later the European drug regulatory body approved Centoxin for the treatment of gram-negative sepsis. Six months later, in September 1991, a FDA panel advised approval of Centoxin to treat septic shock [75]. Centocor's sales were predicted to soon be in excess of $1 billion. On this basis, Schoemaker believed Centocor would have more than 50 percent of the share of the antibody pharmaceuticals market in Europe, the United States, and Japan by 2000 [76].

"CENTOCORPSE": CENTOCOR IN CRISIS

The good news, however, did not last. In late October 1991, an American federal court ruled that Centocor's patent for Centoxin infringed on one held by Xoma Corporation, a competitor biotechnology company based in California developing a similar drug for septic shock in partnership with the pharmaceutical company Pfizer Inc [77]. Centocor's executives were unsure how they should handle the matter. This was the first major case of litigation they had experienced. Initially Schoemaker wanted to settle, but Wavle persuade him to fight based on the belief that a settlement could result in cross-licensing and thereby a loss in revenues. The hope was Centocor might strike as lucky as the biotechnology company Amgen in its patent dispute with Genetics Institute [78]. In retrospect, Schoemaker believed the decision to fight Xoma was one his biggest strategic errors [79]. Losing the patent battle to Xoma, the litigation cost Centocor dearly in terms of time and money. It also publicly aired questions about the design of Centoxin's trials and the data analysis [80].

Adding to the company's woes, from late 1991, some medical practitioners began to question the potentially high price of Centoxin (between $3000 and $4000 for each patient) and the degree to which they could predict which patients would most benefit from the drug [81]. By early 1992, initial European sales of the drug were also far below expectations. More pessimistic news was to follow

when, on February 20, 1992, the FDA requested additional information about Centoxin. Triggering shock in the financial community, the tidings sent Centocor's shares tumbling 19 percent or $8.125 a share, closing at $33.125 a share. Only 2 weeks before, the stock had traded at $50 a share. The slide in Centocor's share represented a $675 million drop in its market value [82].

Despite the negative publicity, Schoemaker believed the problems could be resolved. Three months later, however, on a public holiday in April, he received a telephone call at home from David Kessler, head of the FDA, indicating Centoxin would not be approved because of insufficient evidence to establish its efficacy and the necessity of more trials before it could be reconsidered for approval [83]. For Schoemaker, usually a great optimist, this news was "the worst thing that could have happened." The devastation was great for everyone in the company [84].

Hitting media headlines on April 15, 1992, the news stunned investors. Nicknamed "Centocorpse" by Wall Street, Centocor's stock dropped 41 percent in 1 day [85]. In the week that followed, disgruntled investors filed six lawsuits against Centocor's executives alleging violation of federal securities laws and called for damages [86]. Shareholders had seen $1.5 billion of Centocor's market capitalization disappear, its stock rate having fallen from a high of $60 to just $6 [87]. Sensitive to the calamities of one of its leading companies, the biotechnology industry suffered its own financial aftershock [88].

COLLABORATION—A MEANS OF RESCUE

The FDA's decision had not killed Centoxin, but Centocor desperately needed time and money to save the drug, develop its other products, and survive. With the future of the company at stake, Schoemaker and Wall immediately crafted a rescue strategy. To stop the company's cash burn they rapidly laid off hundreds of people, primarily the sales representatives hired for Centoxin's launch. Within a short period the company's employee base had shrunk by a quarter. The company's management team was also reshuffled: Wavle and other recent recruits from the pharmaceutical industry departed.

Crucial to the company's financial survival was also Schoemaker and Wall's reversion to collaboration. The income generated from the diagnostics division, which was bringing in millions of dollars, was insufficient to keep the company afloat and they could not rely on the investment community with the fall in Centocor's stock [89]. Within days of the FDA's announcement Wall and Schoemaker plunged into a frenzy of partnership and fundraising efforts with a number of pharmaceutical companies, including SmithKline Beecham and Eli Lilly [90]. Schoemaker's dynamism and optimism were major factors in driving this forward [91].

What Wall and Schoemaker had on their side were some other promising products in Centocor's pipeline plus the fact that half the industry wanted to obtain Centoxin despite its problems. J.P Garnier, who headed SmithKline Beecham at the time, recalled, "We tried to convince Hubert [Schoemaker] to do a deal with us, and Centoxin turned into a bidding contest between several companies.... I remember a phone call coming in over the weekend saying, "It's going to cost you $100 million in an upfront payment to get Centoxin now." Now it doesn't sound impressive but it was the equivalent of saying a billion today. A $100 million was unheard of. Nobody had ever paid this kind of upfront money." As Garnier explained, "Hubert was a terrific salesman. He whipped up this asset into something that got to be very appealing. He packaged Centoxin very effectively and before you knew it, the bride looked sensational. Everybody was influenced by his sincere belief in the drug and what it could do" [92].

In July 1992, Centocor finalized a licensing agreement with Eli Lilly. Under the agreement Centocor received $100 million upfront from Eli Lilly, an unprecedented large payment for the time. Half of this amount went towards Eli Lilly purchasing 2 million shares in Centocor, thereby giving it a 5 percent stake in the company. The other half went towards providing the much-needed cash to continue developing and seeking clearance for Centoxin. In the event that Centoxin failed, Eli Lilly agreed to pay a further $25 million towards the development of ReoPro®, a cardiovascular drug that Centocor was currently developing clinically [93].

The alliance was strategically useful for Centocor not only because of the capital Eli Lilly was to provide, but because they had a significant presence in the antibiotics field and a strong understanding of the United States infectious disease market crucial for the further development of Centoxin. Eli Lilly was also more receptive to biotechnology than many other pharmaceutical companies, having partnered with Genentech to launch the first genetically engineered insulin and having acquired Hybritech, Centocor's main competitor in mAb diagnostics in 1986 [94]. For Eli Lilly, the alliance gave them a chance to enhance their knowledge in the application of mAbs for infectious disease therapeutics and access to Centocor's European sales team, thereby opening up a new avenue for selling Lilly products [95].

In the following months, Eli Lilly and Centocor worked closely together, overseen by product committees established at both companies, on a new trial for Centoxin, launched in June 1992 [96]. Despite Eli Lilly's support, in January 1993, Centoxin's development was abandoned because interim trial data indicated unexpected high mortality. The poor results were attributed to a flawed trial design. Centoxin proved effective in treating septic shock stemming from gram-negative bacteria, but this accounts for only about a third of patients who present with sepsis. No diagnostic tool existed, however, to detect which of the patients presenting in the trials had gram-negative sepsis. In the absence of a diagnostic tool Centocor's clinical team had insufficient data to convince the FDA of the drug's efficacy [97].

CENTOCOR BECOMES PROFITABLE

Despite the setback with Centoxin, by early 1993, Centocor was financially turning a corner. Its cash burn rate had fallen from $50 million to $30 million between the first and last quarter of 1992. Part of this had been achieved through layoffs, but it had also been helped by the reversion back to collaboration [98]. Good results were also beginning to be reported for other products in Centocor's pipeline.

Some of the most cheering news was the positive data Centocor's clinical team was getting from the cardiovascular drug ReoPro. Licensed from the State University of New York, Stony Brook, in 1986, much of the early development and testing of ReoPro had been undertaken by Centocor with funds raised from a R&D-limited partnership set up in 1987 [99]. By 1992, when Centocor signed its alliance with Eli Lilly, ReoPro was in Phase III clinical trials and Centocor had plans to file for FDA and European regulatory approval the following year [100].

In early 1993 when the first results from the drug's trial emerged positive it was clear Centocor not only possessed a marketable drug, but its future was now secure [101]. Submitted for approval in 1993, ReoPro took just 10 months to be approved by the European regulatory authorities and 12 months by the FDA. These approvals came through in December 1994. ReoPro's approval marked a key milestone for Centocor and placed mAbs firmly on the therapeutic map, showing for the first time they could be used for acute conditions. The drug was the second mAb to win approval as a therapeutic, the first having been approved in 1986 by Johnson & Johnson's Orthoclone® OKT3 (used to prevent kidney transplant rejections) [102]. The first therapeutic product ever to receive simultaneous United States and European approval, ReoPro was the only new biotechnology product sanctioned in 1994. In December 1995, the drug's marketing potential was further boosted when clinical trials showed it was effective for unstable angina, broadening its potential market to more than 1 million patients [103].

Centocor's partnership with Eli Lilly was crucial to the development of ReoPro. While Centocor had undertaken and internally financed much of its early development and clinical trials, the alliance provided the time to do further necessary work [104]. Under the alliance agreement, Eli Lilly exercised its right to market the drug in the United States and most of Western Europe. ReoPro rapidly became a success, with worldwide sales of $23 million in its first year, 1995. By 1999, worldwide sales had increased to $447.3 million. Four years later the drug was being investigated for noncardiac indications, including sickle-cell anemia and cancer [105].

Following ReoPro's success, Centocor's team soon had another major breakthrough with a drug called Remicade®. The drug, based on an antibody called cA2, originated from a collaborative R&D agreement established in January 1984 between Centocor and the laboratory of Jan Vilcek, a scientist based at the New York University School of Medicine [106]. Initially Centocor's researchers investigated cA2 in-house alongside Centoxin to combat sepsis, but clinical studies showed it more promising for treating autoimmune disorders. In 1998, Centocor won FDA approval for Remicade, to treat Crohn's disease. A year later, Remicade was approved for rheumatoid arthritis. By 2007, the drug had received approval in 88 countries for 15 inflammatory disease indications and was being used to treat over 1 million patients worldwide, commanding 23 percent of the arthritis drug market. In 2006, Remicade generated US $3.77 billion in worldwide sales. It would rise to $8 billion in 2010, making it the third medicine in history to top $8 billion in annual sales, and the best-selling biological medicine in the world for that year [107]. The approval of Remicade marked a significant point in the development of mAbs as therapeutics, showing for the first time that mAbs could be deployed for chronic conditions.

The approval of ReoPro and then Remicade signaled how far Centocor had come from its humble beginnings as a company specializing in mAb diagnostics. By 1999, 20 years after its founding, Centocor had raised $1.5 billion and brought to market ten products [108]. Despite this success, Schoemaker and David Holveck, Centocor's chief executive officer from September 1992, realized their company could no longer remain independent if it was to go forward as a serious player. The cash they had secured was insufficient for maintaining and growing the company's R&D program and expanding the company's manufacturing and marketing capabilities. They also recognized that having become so successful, the company could be subject to a take-over bid. In order to prevent a hostile bid, in 1998 they began to assess the company's value and identify possible partners [109]. A year later Holveck and Schoemaker secured a deal for $5.2 billion from Johnson & Johnson. Making Centocor a subsidiary of Johnson & Johnson, the deal allowed Centocor to continue to operate independently while benefiting from the large company's infrastructure, financial resources, and credibility. Within 3 years of the deal, Centocor more than doubled its work force from 1200 people to 2800 worldwide, and more than tripled the number of new drug candidates entering late-stage testing, many in disease areas Centocor had not explored before, including diabetes, organ transplant rejection, and asthma [110].

CONCLUSION

This case study of Centocor is illustrative of the important role collaboration has played in the building up of the biotechnology industry. A key lesson from Centocor is how important R&D partnerships can be to a young company just beginning to create a portfolio and how critical alliances with established companies can be to breaking into a competitive market place. Nearing bankruptcy when straying away from collaboration, the story of Centocor is a salutary reminder of the risks for newly emerging companies of going it alone.

The experiences of Centocor's executives with collaboration and the attempts to go it alone, however, are not universal in the biotechnology industry. Plenty of collaborations between biotechnology companies and large pharmaceutical companies have failed in the past and continue to do so to this day. Amgen, a biotechnology company founded just 1 year after Centocor, landed up in a costly court case over its patents and experienced huge financial losses as a result of the marketing partnership it formed in 1985 with Johnson & Johnson for its first drug erythropoietin, a treatment for anemia [111]. The company had more success when it decided to develop and market its second drug Neupogen, a treatment for neutropenia, independently [112]. The contrast between Centocor and Amgen shows how idiosyncratic the risks and outcomes can be for biotechnology companies when deciding to collaborate or go it alone. This is highly influenced by the personalities involved, market conditions, scientific and technical developments, and the cultural fit between organizations.

ACKNOWLEDGEMENTS

The author would like to thank Anne Faulkner Schoemaker for allowing generous access to Hubert Schoemaker's personal files and reading earlier drafts of this paper. Grateful thanks also go to Stelios Papadopoulos, Alison Kraft, and David Holveck for providing insightful comments on initial drafts of the paper. Much appreciation also goes to all the people who agreed to be interviewed for the research that led to this chapter which was supported by the Chemical Heritage Foundation.

REFERENCES

[1] This figure is based on figures of over 800 deals signed in 2011, each of which was worth approximately $200 million. It is based on data from the EvaluatePharma Deals Database.

[2] Research for this chapter is based on Centocor's company papers and the personal papers of Hubert Schoemaker (hereafter HS-PP) kindly provided by his widow Anne Faulkner Schoemaker and on oral interviews with Centocor's employees undertaken by the author in collaboration with the Chemical Heritage Foundation which houses the interview transcripts. The author conducted all interviews listed below except where specified. Interview transcripts are kept at the Chemical Heritage Foundation.

[3] For Koprowski's biography see Vaughan, R. (2000). Listen to the Music: The Life of Hilary Koprowski. Springer.

[4] HS-PP: Centocor, Centocor Oncogene Research Partners LP, June 9, 1984.

[5] For the early development of monoclonal antibodies see Marks, L. "A Healthtech Revolution: The story of César Milstein and the Making of Monoclonal Antibodies." *www.whatisbiotechnology.org*.

[6] Vaughan, R. Listen to the Music, 174–177.

[7] H. Koprowski and C. Croce, "Method of Producing Tumor Antibodies," U.S. Patent 4,172,124 (filed April 28, 1978, issued October 23, 1979); H. Koprowski, W. Gerhard, and C. Croce, "Method of Producing Antibodies," U.S. Patent 4,196,265 (filed June 15, 1977, issued April 1 1980).

[8] Vaughan, R. Listen to the Music, 179.

[9] Centocor, Centocor Oncogene Research Partners LP, 9 June 1984, HS-PP; Interview with Hilary Koprowski by author and Ted Everson (July 13, 2006), transcript, 16–17; Interview with David Holveck by Lara Marks and Ted Everson (July 14, 2006).

[10] M.A. Wall and E.C. Allen, "Investment Prospectus: Medical Diagnostic Business," date unknown, 34–35, HS-PP.

[11] For a detailed biography of Schoemaker go to his profile on *www.whatisbiotechnology.org/people/Schoemaker*.

[12] Wall and Allen, "Investment Prospectus," 30.

[13] Interview with Tony Evnin, Venrock Associates partner and Centocor director (1981–1999) by author and Ted Everson (September 14, 2006).

[14] Wall and Allen, "Investment Prospectus," 6.

[15] Wall and Allen, "Investment Prospectus," 28, 31. Author unknown, "A Medical Marvel Goes to Market," 56; Author unknown, "Biotechnologists are Ready to Market Another Trick," 87; Author unknown, "Smart Bombs of Biology," 59. For a history of Sera-Labs see Marks, "A healthtech revolution" and L.V. Marks, The "Lock and Key" of Medicine: Monoclonal Antibodies and the Transformation of Healthcare, (forthcoming, Yale University Press), chapter 7.

[16] Author unknown, "A Medical Marvel Goes to Market," 56; M.M. Hamilton, "Competition Feverish in Health Field; Immunodiagnostics in Infancy," The Washington Post, Sunday Final Edition (October 30, 1983) G1.

[17] Vaughan, R. Listen to the Music, 179; interview with Koprowski. See also interview with Michael Dougherty by author and Ted Everson (January 23, 2007), transcript. Dougherty was Centocor's assistant controller, treasurer, chief financial officer and senior vice president (1983–1993).

[18] Interview with Evnin; HS-PP: L.F. Rothschild et al., Centocor Inc: Prospectus for Public Offering (July 22, 1983), 21; R. Teitelman, "Searching for Serendipity: Centocor Combs University Labs for Technology," *Forbes* (May 6, 1985) 80.

[19] R.Teitelman, "Searching for Serendipity: Centocor Combs University Labs for Technology," Forbes (May 6, 1985):80-1.

[20] Interview with former NCI researcher and Centocor collaborator Robert Gallo (July 11, 2006). See also interview with Sarah Cabot, Centocor's technology licensing director (1986–1990), by Jennifer Dionisio (November 7, 2007).

[21] Interviews with Evnin and Anne Faulkner Schoemaker (July 10, 2006). See also HS-PP: Centocor, *Annual Report* (1983), 6. Hereafter all Centocor's *Annual Reports (A/R)*. The *A/Rs* are contained in HS-PP.

[22] Schoemaker cited in Vaughan, R., Listen to the Music, 186 and interview with Faulkner Schoemaker.

[23] HS-PP: L.F. Rothschild et al. Centocor Inc: Prospectus for Public Offering (December 14, 1982), 19 and 25. Stanley Cohen and Herbert Boyer faced similar hostility to the commercialization and patenting of their technology and founding of Genentech (see S. Smith Hughes, "Making Dollars out of DNA: The First Major Patent in Biotechnology and the Commercialization of Molecular Biology, 1974–1980," *ISIS*, 92 (2001) 541–575, 551).

[24] Vaughan, R., Listen to the Music, 182–186.

[25] Interview with Gallo; Schoemaker, cited in Vaughan, R., Listen to the Music, 186.

[26] Before the Bayh-Dole Act, universities wishing to obtain a patent arising from federally funded research required permission from federal authorities to do so. See Smith Hughes, "Making Dollars out of DNA," 551.

[27] Centocor, *A/R* (1985), 5 and Rothschild, *Centocor Inc* (1983), .22; B. Momich, "Building Something Significant at Centocor," *Pennsylvania Technology* (Second Quarter 1990) 25–31.

[28] Interview with Koprowski. Interview with Zurawski by Ted Everson, (January 4, 2007).

[29] Dickinson, S. (May 14, 1990). "Biotech's Centocor Jockeys for Position in Drug Field." The Scientist. 4:1–5.

[30] Wall and Allen, "Investment Prospectus," 6.

[31] Interview with Holveck by author and Ted Everson (July 14, 2006). Holveck was Centocor's head of diagnostics from 1983 and Centocor's chief executive officer from 1992.

[32] Rothschild, Centocor Inc. (1982), 15; Rothschild, *Centocor Inc* (1983), Centocor *A/Rs* (1983), 2 and (1985), 15; Correspondence between author and David Holveck, November 2007; Interview with Holveck.

[33] By 1983 the company had formed a number of marketing and manufacturing partnerships with key companies for distribution of the test in different parts in the world. This included Warner-Lambert to cover the USA, Toray/Fujizoki for Japan, and Byk-Mallinckroft for Europe. Centocor, A/Rs (1983), 2, 14, 18 and (1985), 15.

[34] Interview with Holveck by Sally Smith Hughes (1998, 1999), transcript, 43, Regional Oral History Office, Bancroft Library.

[35] Centocor. A/R 1985:27.

[36] HS-PP: Centocor Press Release, "Centocor Receives FDA Panel Recommendation to Approve Ovarian Cancer Test," November 3, 1986; L. Thompson, "New Test for Ovarian Cancer Detects Residual Cells in the Blood," *The Washington Post* (June 16, 1987).

[37] Interview with Zurawski; Author Unknown, "TWST Names Award Winners Biotechnology," The Wall Street Transcript, 97/11 (December 14, 1987) HS-PP: Centocor, *A/R* (1990), 14.

[38] HS-PP: H. Schoemaker, "Wharton Talk," April 17, 2000 and interview with Holveck.

[39] Bylinsky G. Coming: Star Wars Medicine. Fortune April 27, 1987.

[40] Centocor. A/R 1982.

[41] Rothschild, *Centocor Inc* (1982) and Rothschild, *Centocor Inc* (1983); HS-PP: Paine Webber, Centocor, Common Stock (December 13, 1985), 7; Centocor, *A/R* (1986), (1987), 2 and (1990), 3.

[42] Interviews by author and Ted Everson with PaineWebber investment bankers Stephen Evans-Freke (September 14, 2006) and Stephen Webster (July 13, 2006), and by author with Bruce Peacock, Centocor's chief financial officer 1981–1992 (July 10, 2006). See also Schiff, L. and F. Murray. (2004). "Biotechnology Financing Dilemmas and the Role of Special Purpose Entities." Nature Biotechnology, 22: 271–277.

[43] Interview with Fred A. Middleton, by G.E. Bugos, (2001), transcript, Regional Oral History Office, Bancroft Library.

[44] Interviews with Evans-Freke and Webster. See also HS-PP: Centocor, Centocor Oncogene Research Partners LP; PaineWebber,

Centocor Common Stock, 22; PaineWebber, Tocor II and Centocor Prospectus (January 21, 1992), 5. Centocor, *A/Rs* (1985–1988) and (1989), 31.

[45] Bill Hambrecht, cofounder of Hambrecht and Quist in 1968, an investment bank specializing in emerging high-growth technology companies, was one of Genentech's early investors. See Interview with Middleton, 28. Schoemaker, "Wharton Talk."

[46] For more on the development of recombinant insulin see S. Hall, Invisible Frontiers: The Race to Synthesize a Human Gene, Oxford: Oxford University Press, 1987.

[47] Interview with Centocor's vice president of pharmaceutical development (1988–1993) Renato Fuchs (July 1, 2008). See also Bylinsky, "Coming: Star Wars Medicine."

[48] Bylinsky, "Coming: Star Wars Medicine."

[49] Centocor. A/R 1985:11.

[50] Centocor. Investment Prospectus December 14, 1982. 17; Centocor, *A/R* (1983), 2.

[51] Centocor. A/R 1983:2.

[52] Interview with Fuchs, Interview with Jeffrey Mattis by Lara Marks. Mattis was Centocor's vice president of pharmaceutical development (1979–1998) February 22, 2007. Notes.

[53] BCC Research, "Antibodies for therapeutic and diagnostic imaging applications", Report BIO016D, Feb 2000; BCC Research, "Dynamic Antibody Industry", Report BIO016F, August 2005; R. Wolf, "Centocor makes a deal on product marketing", The Inquirer (December 7, 1987).

[54] PaineWebber, *Centocor Common Stock* (1985), 4, 6, 34; PaineWebber, Tocor II; Centocor, *Annual Report* (1990), 7. Centocor *SEC filing Form 10-K* for the year ending December 31, 1995; Pollack, "The Next Wave of Diagnostics." Interviews with David Holveck by author and Everson, (14 July 2006, and 9 Sept 2009) Harlan Weisman (November 30, 2006) and Mattis. Harlan Weisman was Centocor's president of R&D and team leader for ReoPro development (1990–1999).

[55] Centocor, *A/R* (1988), 4 and (1990), 7; Interview with Mattis; Interviews with Fuchs, notes and with Stelios Papadopolous (October 19, 2006). Papadopolous was an investment banker with Paine Webber (1987–2000). "Centocor's Myoscint Imaging Agent Backed in USA," The Pharmaletter, February 5, 1996. http://www.thepharmaletter.com/file/25880/centocors-myoscint-imaging-agent-backed-in-usa.html.

[56] Centocor. A/R 1983:6.

[57] Centocor, *A/Rs* (1983) 18, 28; (1985) 2; Rothschild, *Centocor Inc* (1983), 47.

[58] Interview with Evans-Freke. Centocor, A/R 1986.

[59] Centocor. A/R 1986:3.

[60] Bylinsky, "Coming: Star Wars Medicine."

[61] Centocor, *A/Rs* (1986), 17 and (1988), 5; Dickinson, "Biotech's Centocor Jockeys for Position," 2.

[62] Interview with Middleton. Interview with Fuchs.

[63] Centocor. A/R 1988;2:12.

[64] Interview with Richard McCloskey (January 19, 2007). McClosky was Centocor's vice president of clinical research and medical research (1990–1997).

[65] Centocor, *A/R* (1985), 29. Interviews with Denise McGinn (September 12, 2006), Zurawski and Fuchs. McGinn was Centocor's development project manager (1983–1999).

[66] Momich, "Building Something Significant at Centocor," 26–28.

[67] Interview with Bernard Schaffer. Schaffer is a Philadelphia-based market analyst; September 11, 2006.

[68] Interview with Evnin.

[69] Interview with Fuchs.

[70] R. Winslow, "Centocor's New Drug Clears FDA Panel;" Dickinson, "Biotech's Centocor Jockeys for Position in Drug Field" and R. Longman, "The Lessons of Centocor, " In Vivo: The Business and Medicine Report (May 1992), 24.

[71] Author unknown, "Centocor Inc. Chief Hubert Schoemaker Adds Chairman's Post."

[72] Interviews with Holveck, Peacock, and Cabot. Joint interview with Sandra Faragalli, Patty Durachko, and Ray Heslip (September 12, 2006). All three were long-time employees of Centocor, working in the administrative, finance, warehouse, and shipping sections. Interview with Centocor's vice president of diagnostics operations (1985–1998), Paul Touhey by author and Ted Everson (September 15, 2006).

[73] Ziegler EJ, Fisher CJ, Sprung CL, et al. Treatment of Gram-Negative Bacteremia and Septic Shock with HA-1A Human Monoclonal Antibody Against Endotoxin. A randomized, double-blind, placebo-controlled trial. The HA-1A Sepsis Study Group. New England J Med February 14, 1991;324/7:429–36.

[74] Author unknown, "Blasting Bacteria," Author unknown, "Centocor, Inc."

[75] S. Usdin, "Wall Street Vents Frustration at Centocor," BioWorld Today (February 20, 1992) 1; D. Shaw, "FDA, Wall Street Bring Bad Tidings to Centocor," The Philadelphia Inquirer (February 20, 1992) B11; Author unknown, "FDA Snag and Loss Hurt Centocor Stock." L.L. Valeriano, "Centocor Stock Slides on News of Drug Snag," The Wall Street Journal (February 20, 1992); A. Newman and D. Pettit, "Biotech Stock Lead Index 0.64% Lower; Centocor Plunges on Worry Over Drug," The Wall Street Journal (February 20, 1992).

[76] Author unknown, "Centocor, Inc."

[77] Patent disputes were common in the industry and could be devastating for the companies concerned. See, for example, the case of CellPro which became bankrupt after failing to win a patent dispute as described in Bar-Shalom, A. and R. Cook-Deegan. (2002). "Patents and Innovation in Cancer: Lessons from CellPro," The Millbank Quarterly, 80/4: 637–676.

[78] Interviews with Centocor's attorney (1987–1999), George Hobbs (September 30, 2006); Papadopoulos; and chief executive officer of Cephalon, Frank Baldino by author and Ted Everson (July 14, 2006). Amgen and Genetics Institute's patent dispute started in 1988 and ended in May 1993 with the Genetics Institute paying Amgen $15.9 million. Amgen SEC filing: Form: 10-Q, 8/10/1994.

[79] Interviews with Faulkner Schoemaker, and Schaffer.

[80] Interviews with Holveck and Papadopoulos. Centocor, *A/R* (1991), 38–39; Valeriano, "Centocor Stock Slides on News of Drug Snag;" L.M. Fisher, "Centocor and Xoma Settle Patent Fight," The New York Times (July 30, 1992).

[81] C.J. Hinds Monoclonal Antibodies in Sepsis and Septic Shock. Br Med J January 18, 1992;304:132–3. Interviews with Peacock, Holveck, and Papadopoulos.

[82] Usdin, "Wall St. Vents Frustration at Centocor"; Shaw, "FDA, Wall Street Bring Bad Tidings to Centocor"; Author unknown, "FDA Snag and Loss Hurt Centocor Stock:" Valeriano, "Centocor Stock Slides on News of Drug Snag:" Newman and Pettit, "Biotech Stock Lead Index 0.64% Lower:" Longman, "The Lessons of Centocor," 25.

[83] Interview with Schaffer.

[84] Interviews with Faulkner Schoemaker, Holveck (by author and Everson), Faragalli, Durachko, and Heslip.

[85] Shaw, "Centocor Absorbs New Blows." See also interview with Papadopoulos.

[86] Author unknown. FDA: Centoxin Data Insufficient. In: 74E, D. Shaw editors. "Centocor Absorbs New Blows", The Philadelphia Inquirer. Interview with Holveck.

[87] Schoemaker, "Wharton Talk"; Longman, "The Lessons of Centocor," 23; interview with Holveck.

[88] Usdin, "Wall Street Vents Frustration at Centocor," 1; Longman, "The Lessons of Centocor," 27.

[89] Interview with Touhey.

[90] HS-PP: Centocor, CenTropics, 1/4, (Fall 1992) 1.

[91] Interview with Papadopoulos.

[92] Interview with J.P Garnier by Ted Everson (July 12, 2006).

[93] Author Unknown, "Lilly to Acquire Marketing Rights to Centocor Drug;" Centocor, Centropics.

[94] Author Unknown, "Lilly to Acquire Marketing Rights to Centocor Drug;" Centocor, Centropics.

[95] Interview with Fuchs; Centocor, CenTropics, 1.

[96] Centocor, CenTropics, 2–4.

[97] Interviews with Holveck. Papadopoulos. Interview with Michael Melore by Ted Everson. Melore was Centocor's head of human resources (1990–1999); May 21, 2007.

[98] Centocor. A/R 1992:7.

[99] Centocor. A/Rs 1987–1988.

[100] Centocor. A/R 1992:4.

[101] Interview with McGinn.

[102] Bylinsky, "Coming: Star Wars Medicine"; Centocor, A/R (1994), 2, 4; B. Cochlovius, M. Braunagel and M. Welschof, "Therapeutic Antibodies," *American Chemical Society: Modern Drug Discovery* (October 2003); C. Farrell, E. Barnathan and H. F. Weisman, "The Evolution of ReoPro Clinical Development," in K. Dembowsky and P. Stadler, eds. Novel Therapeutic Proteins: Selected Case Studies (Weinheim: Wiley-VCH Verlag GmbH, 2003), 323–346.

[103] New York Times December 22, 1995.

[104] Interview with Holveck.

[105] Interview with Holveck.

[106] Interview with Jan Vilcek (July 12, 2006). Vilcek is a microbiology professor at New York University School of Medicine; July 12, 2006.

[107] Wiki analysis, "Arthritis drug market." http://www.wikinvest.com/wiki/Arthritis_Drug_Market#_note-13; PharmaLive, "Top 500 Prescription Medicine," *Special Report* (October 2011).

[108] Schoemaker, "Wharton Talk."

[109] Interview with Holveck; A. Knox, "He is Building on his Success,". *The Philadelphia Inquirer*, May 7, 2000.

[110] J. George, Centocor Now Bigger than Ever. *Philadelphia Business* J, Aug 16, 2002.

[111] A. Moschol and J. Leiter, "Perfect Partnering," *Nature Biotechnology*, Supplement to Vol. 19 (July 2001), BE21±22. For more on Amgen's development and marketing of Epogen see M. Goozner, *The $800 million pill: The Truth Behind the Cost of New Drugs.* (Berkeley: University of California Press 2004), 13–34.

[112] Interview with Papadopoulos.

Chapter 30

Ethical Considerations for Biotechnology Entrepreneurs

Gladys B. White, PhD

Adjunct Professor of Liberal Studies, Georgetown University, Washington, D.C.

It may come as a surprise that the innovation and promise offered by advances in biotechnology raise any ethical issues at all. If biotechnology entrepreneurs are engaged in activities that have as their goal improvements in the health and well-being of humankind, then why is it that these activities warrant ethical scrutiny? If good people with good ideas start, maintain, and operate companies that develop new drugs, devices, and products aimed at the curing of disease and the improvement of human health, what's not to like?

THE NATURE OF ETHICAL REASONING

In order to answer these questions, it is important to first have an understanding of philosophical ethics. In essence, ethics is simply concerned with the examination of important questions related to what it means to be human. Ethical considerations are tools which help us analyze the relevant strengths of arguments about what is right and wrong conduct, or what should be done in important endeavors in life. Because the activities within the biotechnology industry are vital to human health and well-being now and in the future, ethical issues, or arguments, need to be a foundational part of our understanding. What we term ethical "arguments" are simply the reasons and justifications for choosing a particular course of action. Having an understanding of ethics helps one recognize the significance of these arguments and their relative weight when major decisions need to be made. For example, such a decision could be which drug to develop and market for which disease over what period of time with the reason and justification being clearly understood and compelling to others. There is also an ethical aspect to a company's economic decisions. For instance, the strategies that entrepreneurs employ to promote short-term versus long-term profitability should be justifiable and have a rational supporting argument. Cost/benefit analysis and bottom-line viewpoints in the business world are not solely a matter of a computation involving dollars and cents but also judgments about what constitutes the greatest good for

the greatest number of people. The type of ethical analysis and the utilitarian system of justification I describe is not new but dates back to the work of philosophers such as Jeremy Bentham (1748 to 1832) and John Stuart Mill (1806 to 1873) [1]. It is important to recognize that entrepreneurs are faced with significant challenges and alternatives to every rational argument, and in order to support their choices, they must have an understanding of ethical tools and be familiar with ethical principles and theory.

Ethics is simply a "reason-giving" enterprise. This means that ethical arguments leading to good or right actions must be based upon supporting reasons that are both meaningful and understandable to others. Any reason-supporting arguments about what ought to or should be done, in any given circumstance needs to be more than a statement such as "because I said so," or "because it's a rainy day," or "because this is how I feel at the moment." Subjective declarations of how an individual or group feels, or verbalization of the gut reaction of a leader, should not be the primary basis for a sound ethical argument. Poor or weak ethical justifications highlight another important point—often critical decisions are made without ethical reasoning and on a basis that is not rational or objective.

Why should biotechnology entrepreneurs pay attention to the characteristics of sound ethical arguments? There are many reasons why this is relevant and two of the most important reasons are the following:

1. Biotechnology companies are businesses and therefore they must operate using a commonly accepted set of business ethics that include such tenants as fairness, trust, absence of conflict-of-interest, and good business practices.
2. Biotechnology companies face ethical dilemmas as do all companies and the consequences can be devastating for poor decisions. For small biotechnology companies, the cost and stakes are high. There are often competing pressures to achieve goals and accomplish results within

a limited timeframe, and this creates a climate in which ethical dilemmas can arise.

Even in larger organizations, we have seen instances of pharmaceutical product development in human clinical trials revealing adverse conditions which were kept from the U.S. Food and Drug Administration (FDA), and subsequently these products were removed from the market due to deaths during commercialization [2].

A true ethical dilemma is a problem of one of following two types. An ethical dilemma exists when:

1. No matter what action is taken, some harm will occur.
2. There are equally strong-reasoned arguments for taking completely different courses of action.

Accurate facts are crucial to the analysis and resolution of ethical dilemmas, but additional facts alone cannot solve or resolve a true ethical dilemma. A true ethical dilemma requires that the leader make a wise choice. There are key features of reasoned arguments in ethics and the value of each can be assessed based upon the conceptual level or strength of each argument. There are four types of arguments ranging from weak to strong and are found below.

Level 1: Ethical Judgments

Ethical judgment consists of simple pronouncements of right or wrong without stipulating any particular reason. When a particular action is characterized as right or wrong without an identified reason, there is no way another individual can assess its value. Also, no one can associate or compare its reasoning to similar situations because there is no information offered as to why the judgment has been made. This is why ethical judgment alone is relatively weak.

Level 2: Ethical Rules

The second level in the hierarchy of ethical reasoning is ethical rules. Examples of ethical rules are statements such as thou shall not kill, lie, steal, and the like. Ethical rules are found in documents such as the Ten Commandments but also permeate codes of ethics in various professions, codes of good business practices, and corporate policy documents. A rule such as "do not lie" has more power than an ethical judgment because the rule can be used as a guide for ethical action in similar situations. Most of our everyday ethical actions are based upon ethical rules. In this fashion, we readily understand the motivations of our co-workers, business partners, and customers and the use of commonsense ethical rules builds trust.

Level 3: Ethical Principles

The third level of reasoning in ethics takes place at the level of ethical principles. These principles differ from ethical

rules as they are guiding values by which to make decisions rather than hard and fast rules. For ethics in the life sciences, there are already well-defined principles. The Belmont Report published in 1978 was the result of a collaborative effort to determine the characteristics of ethical research when human subjects were involved, and it is generally cited as a key source for ethics in the life sciences [3]. In the Belmont report, these ethical principles are described and explained such as (1) respect for autonomy, (2) beneficence, (3) nonmaleficence, and (4) justice. These are important threads or themes for ethical action. A fifth principle is that of respect for persons as ends unto themselves, rather than merely means to the ends or purposes of others. When individuals are respected as ends unto themselves, their lives, interests, and well-being cannot be compromised in pursuit of the goals of others. Respect for persons carries considerable weight and importance in ethical analysis and is also an important feature of Kantian ethics (see below).

Ethical principles have the advantage of conveying important concepts such as the importance of free and self-directed action (autonomy), being of benefit or good use to others (beneficence), avoiding harm to others (nonmaleficence), and acting in a way such that fair and equal treatment results for individual human beings as well as for groups. Most ethical arguments with sufficient depth and breadth make use of ethical principles as part of their rationale.

Level 4: Ethical Theories

Ethical theories are the most powerful form of reasoning in ethics. Examples of such theories are consequentialism of which utilitarianism is one type and the duty-based theory like that of Immanual Kant which offers a justification for right action. Immanuel Kant (1724 to 1804) developed a theory of ethics based upon duty as perceived by human reason. Ethical analysis serves as a sorting device to unpack complicated ethical dilemmas and simultaneously offer a detailed outline of justification for the right action. Ethical theories are powerful but can also have their weak points. The primary limitation of consequentialist-based ethical reasoning is related to a principle of justice, namely what if by securing the greatest good, or the greatest happiness for the greatest number of individuals, this results in an unacceptable level of harm for a few. For example, what if the risk of death for a few people in the clinical trial of a new drug is high but the eventual research results could benefit many? A utilitarian would regard this as an acceptable risk, whereas a Kantian ethicist would not. That is because Kant believed that the conditions of duty-based ethics should be determined in advance of the actual situation and their consequences. Kant also believed that an argument is very weak if it rests on an assessment of consequences, since we should to be able to discern what our ethical duties are in advance of taking any action.

The basis for determining our duties results from consulting our reason. The result is what Kant identifies as the categorical imperative which has two formulations or forms of expression, namely: (1) always act in such a way that a tenet describing your action can serve as the basis for universal law and (2) always treat human beings as ends in themselves and not merely as means to the ends of others. This theory is in stark contrast to the consequentialist, utilitarian theory of Mill in part because it is prospective and says that we need to decide about right or ethical action in advance of particular circumstances and apart from consequences [4].

In addition to duty-based ethics and consequentialism, there are other ethical theories such as virtue ethics, the ethics of care, casuistry, or case-based analysis and rights-based approaches to ethical problems that offer insights and advantages in understanding important ethical controversies. Due to the limitations of space and time, these possibilities will not be explored in detail here but the reader is referred to other basic survey articles on these topics in the literature of philosophy and ethics. One good online source for more information is the "Stanford Encyclopedia of Philosophy" which can be accessed online at http://plato.stanford.edu/

KEY ISSUES AND PRACTICAL MATTERS FOR BIOTECHNOLOGY ENTREPRENEURS

For biotech entrepreneurs, certain key ethical issues are embedded within their company's everyday practice and product development. Chief among these are informed consent, concepts of ownership of substances ranging from natural resources to human tissues and cells, and justice and intellectual property in the broad sense, to name a few. It is also important that the possible needs and interests of future generations be taken into account by the biotech industry. In ethics, this concept is captured by the term "intergenerational justice" which refers to the obligations and duties we have to ensure that the earth, for example, remains habitable for our future descendants. Even a more futuristic question for biotechnology is how might the creation of synthetic forms of life impact the human race now and in the future?

The responsibilities of an industry, particularly in the for-profit world, are sometimes expressed as corporate social responsibilities. The concept of corporate social responsibility is often a matter of debate and discussion. Some argue that this responsibility is relatively narrow and consists chiefly of staying in business, making a profit, and satisfying customers and shareholders. It is implied that any broader obligations or duties to society are regarded as above and beyond company business, or as something that the government should handle. The "let government do it" notion is generally considered to be a narrow view of corporate social responsibility. This can be contrasted to the broad view of corporate social responsibility which is a more justice-based view for the whole human community in which it is unjust to leave anyone out. This view stands in stark contrast to the utilitarian bottom line calculation of the greatest good for the greatest number irrespective of the consequences for a few. The broad view of corporate social responsibility means that individual companies should look beyond merely making money for themselves. Needless to say, this may be somewhat idealistic or even unreasonable for small biotech start-up companies. Nonetheless, it is important to recognize that all corporations exist within the same global social community and that there is a network of interdependencies, duties, and obligations.

The following themes are pervasive areas of ethical concern that arise in the day-to-day practices and activities of biotechnology and serve as an organizing framework for the case studies that follow.

Informed Consent

Informed consent is required before companies can perform medical research on individuals using their specimens or tissues. Informed consent can be simply defined as autonomous authorization by a competent, comprehending adult who authorizes a professional either to involve the subject in research or to initiate a medical plan for the patient or both [5]. The belief that human beings are entitled to give informed consent arises from the insight and conviction that each individual has the right to say what will, or what will not, be done to their own body. This pertains to all human beings and not just to those who happen to be patients or research subjects. This may appear to be self-evident but in the biotech world, problems can arise for example, when stored biospecimens were collected for purposes other than research and informed consent was never initially sought. Obtaining informed consent is a multifaceted process involving a determination of the consenting individual's competence to decide, the provision of full and objective information, some determination of whether or not the consenting individual has actually comprehended or understood the relevant information, and then the production of a signed written consent form with a copy provided to the consenting individual. No one individual or government official, for example, can give a valid consent to a biotech company or biotech entrepreneur on behalf of an entire community without the knowledge of the consent of the particular individuals who are involved.

Concepts of Ownership

Generally speaking, the concept of ownership implies that an object or entity belongs to a given individual who can control its use and call it theirs. To own something has historically referred to objects or even experiences external to the human person. More recently, the concept of the body as owned property has been highlighted in disputes concerning the status of human tissues and cells, particularly in cases in which something valuable can be created. Biotechnology has had a direct influence on the ability to transform a particular human cell into an immortal cell line which can be patented and then yield profits as royalties that are paid to the patent owner. In cases such as that of John Moore who was diagnosed with hairy cell leukemia in 1976 and the case of Henrietta Lacks who was diagnosed with ovarian cancer in the 1950s, the patients who were the original sources of the cells were not even aware that their biological materials had been developed into something valuable (see Case Study 1 and 2 below).

To what extent is the human body property, and who owns human tissues and cells? Many have argued that, in every case, the body is property and belongs to the human individual. The issue becomes more complicated when particular tissues and cells have been excised as a part of a surgical procedure but were retrieved when they would have otherwise been abandoned.

Justice as Fair and Equal Treatment

Access to medicines domestically and globally is one issue that is of importance to biotech entrepreneurs. Justice, namely, fair and equal treatment globally is one issue that arises again and again with respect to the identification of what is important in pharmaceutical development, namely what drugs to create, which diseases to target, and what population groups to serve. The answers to these questions may pose actual ethical dilemmas; for example, in situations in which the populations who will purchase the individual pharmaceutical downstream are very different from those who participated in the drug development. This is an ethical dilemma that has plagued the HIV/AIDS community for some time [6]. Because the biotechnology industry exists largely in the for-profit world, the presence of consumers who can pay for pharmaceutical products is of practical importance. But if the selection of future research and development (R&D) is shaped solely by the interests and needs of those who can pay, then obviously, important priorities that serve the interests of the developing world will be proportionately overlooked or short-changed. These issues have been deliberated in the fields of philosophy and ethics for a long time even going back to the work of Aristotle in the *Nichomachean Ethics*. Aristotle described the virtue of justice as aimed toward "another's good" [7]. In matters of distribution of resources, he defined justice as a matter of receiving what one deserves. Because of the somewhat imprecise nature of this stipulation, a fuller account of social justice is needed and one can be found in the more recent work

of the philosopher, John Rawls. In his work, *A Theory of Justice,* Rawls identifies two principles of justice which he posits would be selected by a group of rational disinterested human beings who are attempting to establish the structure and shape of a fair or ideal society. These principles are as follows [8]:

> **First principle**—Each person is to have an equal right to the most extensive total system of equal basic liberties compatible with a similar set of liberties for all.
> **Second principle**—Social and economic inequalities are to be arranged so that they are both: (1) to the greatest benefit of the least advantaged and (2) available and accessible to all.

The broad implications of this theory are that everyone in the developed world has obligations to the developing world. Is there a right to essential medicines and correspondingly, does the human right to basic necessities override shareholder rights? Unfortunately, it is often the case that social and economic inequalities come to rest on those who are already least advantaged. From a justice perspective, this is counterintuitive and unfair.

Intellectual Property: How Patenting Raises Ethical Issues

"A patent for an invention is the grant of an exclusive property right to the inventor for a limited amount of time" [9]. The act of patenting serves as a clear incentive for innovation and development as it establishes a structure through which scientists, product developers, and inventors of various types are motivated to engage in competition and can also be rewarded monetarily through the payment of royalties. But this incentive rests on the promise of exclusivity which means that those other than the patent holders may have difficulty accessing the patented product or at least have to pay for the privilege. Because many biotech products are closely aligned with or derived from plant or human substances that exist in nature, restricting access to these products strikes many as unfair. In addition, as the cases that follow indicate, human sources of biological materials and/or their families believe that they are entitled to share in the profits generated from these products.

Traditional knowledge, for example, about the medicinal benefits of plants also seems to be a kind of commodity which has value. This knowledge may be generally available in the developing world but cannot be legitimately borrowed by researchers of the developed world without giving credit and arguably some share of the profits to the sources and points of origin of these materials. Some researchers and policy experts have suggested that what is needed here are "models of cooperation for the benefit of global health" [10] (see Case Studies 3 and 4 which follow).

CASE STUDIES

I. Ownership of Human Tissues and Cells and Patenting Cell Lines

Case 1: John Moore

"In 1976, John Moore was diagnosed as having a rare form of cancer called hairy cell leukemia, a condition that affects an estimated 250 Americans each year. The recommended treatment for Moore's condition was the removal of the spleen and surgery was performed at the University of California, Los Angeles Medical Center. As a patient, Moore had signed a standard surgical consent form (providing for the postoperative disposition of the tissue) to remove his diseased spleen, which had enlarged to approximately 40 times its normal size.

After the surgery, Moore's doctor and his technician developed a cell line (designated "Mo") from a sample of Moore's spleen obtained from the pathologist. (It also appears that some of Moore's blood cells contributed to the development of the cell line. GW.) The scientists found that the cell line developed from the spleen produced high quantities of a variety of interesting and potentially interesting proteins. In 1979, the university applied for a patent on the "Mo" cell line and in 1984 a patent naming the scientists as inventors was obtained and assigned to the university. In 1981, the university, on behalf of the scientists, entered into a 4-year collaborative research program with two biotechnology and pharmaceutical companies for exclusive use of the "Mo" cell line.

In 1984, Moore filed a lawsuit claiming that his blood cells were misappropriated and that he was entitled to share in the profits derived from the commercial uses of these cells and any other products resulting from research on any of his biological materials [2]. John Moore was never successful in convincing the court that he deserved a share of the profits from the patented cell line although it was clear that he had not given informed consent for this particular eventuality.

Discussion This case is one of a number of similar cases in which a patient, through the course of medical treatment and care unwittingly serves as the source of human tissues and cells that are later developed into a valuable product. The unimproved tissues and cells on their own do not have monetary value and also have been excised and discarded in the course of medical care. The development of a cell line which has characteristics of long life or even immortality in a laboratory setting is not something which the patient/research subject or source of the biological material could have accomplished on their own behalf. And yet the product could not have been developed without this source material. Hours of refinement, development, and trial and error research have transformed this biological material into something of

value that can be patented and used for a wide array of useful purposes. It is not surprising that the individual whose cells and tissues have been used in this fashion feels that he has been duped!

Case 2: Henrietta Lacks

Her name was Henrietta Lacks, but scientists know her as HeLa. She was a poor Southern tobacco farmer who worked the same land as her slave ancestors, yet her cells–taken without her knowledge–became one of the most important tools in medicine. The first "immortal" human cells grown in a culture, they are still alive today, though she has been dead for more than 60 years. If you could pile all the HeLa cells ever grown onto a scale, they would weigh more than 50 million metric tons—as much as a hundred Empire State Buildings. HeLa cells were vital for developing the polio vaccine; uncovering secrets of cancer, viruses, and the atom bomb's effects; helping lead to important advances like *in vitro* fertilization, cloning, and gene mapping; and have been bought and sold by the billions. (See Figure 30.1.)

Henrietta Lacks remains virtually unknown and is buried in an unmarked grave. Henrietta's family did not learn of her "immortality" until more than 20 years after her death when scientists investigating HeLa began using her husband and children in research without their informed consent. And though the cells had launched a multimillion-dollar industry that sells human biological materials, her family never saw any of the profits [11]. (See Figure 30.2.)

Discussion In both of the cases of John Moore and Henrietta Lacks, the subjects were not told about the subsequent uses of their biological material even though they each may have signed what was considered to be a standard surgical consent at that particular point in time. They later discovered (the

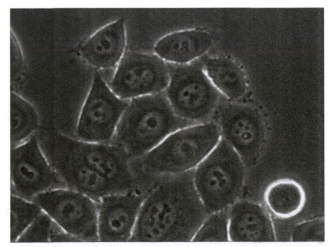

FIGURE 30.1   HeLa Cells: immortal cancer cells of Henrietta Lacks. *(Source: Kristina Yu, © Exploratorium, www.exploratorium.edu)*

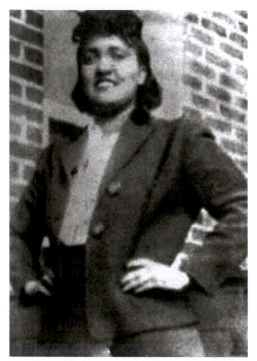

FIGURE 30.2   Henrietta Lacks died of cervical cancer at age 51. *(Source: Wikipedia)*

patient himself in the case of John Moore, and the patient's family in the case of Henrietta Lacks) that profits had accrued from their products and this understandably resulted in their sense of having been seriously wronged. Why couldn't these patients and/or their families have shared in this monetary value? As of this writing, neither the medical research community nor the biotech community at large has been inclined to or figured out a way to share profits with patient sources. In the case of the family of Henrietta Lacks, they have also never shared in the accrued value of the HeLa cell line. They continue to wonder why, given that their mother's body was the source of something so valuable, they cannot even obtain needed health insurance at this point in time. So the ethical question of what is fair in these cases remains to be answered.

II. Biopiracy

The definition of biopiracy is controversial and the legitimacy of the topic as a whole is a matter of debate. But a general definition of biopiracy is "when multinational corporations profit from the medicinal and agricultural uses of plants known to indigenous or native societies and fail to compensate these communities" [12]. One reason why this definition is controversial is that some will argue that plants belong to the global commons, that is, they belong to all of us generally but are not owned by anyone in particular. The same argument might be applied to the knowledge freely shared by indigenous or native societies, namely that if the information is freely given then there is not necessarily a

legitimate expectation for compensation should this knowledge prove to be valuable in the developed world. The two case studies below, one hypothetical and one actual, illustrate what is at stake in this debate.

Case 3: Visplantia

Imagine that a Brazilian scientist visits Wyoming. On his way to the mountains, he encounters a Cheyenne Shaman who joins him. The Shaman is particularly talkative that day so they engage in an entertaining conversation. The Shaman tells the scientist the story of a very important and powerful plant. The Brazilian scientist learns that the Shaman is visiting the mountains to gather this plant that his tribe has nurtured for many generations and that they used to cure a very aggressive disease. The scientist feels curious and decides to visit that site. Once they arrive at the site, the scientist notices that the Shaman is performing a ritual ceremony, after which he picks up some plants. The Shaman explains later that this plant is sacred to the Cheyenne. The scientist takes a sample of the plant back to Brazil and years later patents a medicine based on the plant compounds called Visplantia that cures HIV. Suppose that Visplantia has generated millions of dollars in profit for the Brazilian company and the scientist. The Cheyenne tribal members complain to the United States government arguing that they discovered the plant, they nurtured it for centuries, and they used the plant in important religious ceremonies. The Brazilian pharmaceutical company argues that the plant is a product of nature, that it belongs to humanity, and it is a heritage of "mankind," and that the company spent 10 years and millions of dollars of research to develop the drug [12].

Discussion   In this hypothetical case, it appears that the amount of the plant that was originally taken could not in any way have depleted the source community of this particular vegetation. The traditional community was not deprived of anything that originally existed and in fact, the drug development that took place subsequently was not necessarily anticipated nor did it make use of traditional knowledge. No harm was done initially. The later drug development created an effective therapy for HIV. We do not know if HIV was prevalent in the traditional society, but if it was initially or later when the drug became available, a claim for access to the drug might have some justification. The biotech company could freely provide this drug to the native population or provide it at a discount based upon a broad concept of corporate social responsibility and the ethical principle of beneficence, but they would not necessarily be obliged to do so.

Case 4: Rosy Periwinkle (*Catharanthus Roseus*)

Scientists from developed nations engineered the cancer-fighting medicines vinblastine and vincristine from the rosy periwinkle plant found in Madagascar. Vinblastine has

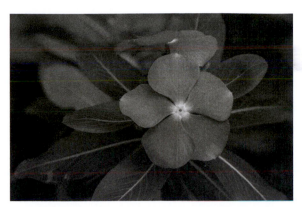

FIGURE 30.3 Rosy periwinkle (*Catharanthus Roseus*).

increased the chance of surviving childhood leukemia and is used to treat Hodgkin's disease. The U.S. pharmaceutical company Eli Lilly has patented and generated huge profits from Vincristine despite the fact that none of the financial benefits have gone to Madagascar or to the indigenous group that first made use of the plant. (See Figure 30.3.)

The difficulty with this situation is that the pharmaceutical industry took the rosy periwinkle out of Madagascar and used it in ways other than what was initially suggested by the indigenous people. This example illustrates the difficulties inherent in the protection of traditional knowledge and biodiversity, especially when the final pharmaceutical use differs from the use suggested by indigenous communities [12].

Discussion Once again, the test that should be applied to this case initially is whether any harm occurred to the indigenous community. Unless the quantity of rosy periwinkle plants was depleted or significantly diminished in Madagascar, it does not appear that any harm was done. In addition, there was no use made of traditional knowledge as the pharmaceutical company discovered uses that were previously unknown and they exploited this discovery. Only a much-expanded notion of corporate social responsibility extending to pure altruism would support the need for any type of in-kind compensation to the traditional community.

SUMMARY

The dynamic world of corporate biotechnology is one of possibility, productivity, and progress. Like other endeavors that exist at the intersections of science, technology, and public policy, there are successes, failures, and hazards along the way. Ethical issues and dilemmas are serious questions about what ought to be done, often in situations of uncertainty. Ethical arguments that make use of judgments, rules, principles, and theories are the rational responses to circumstances in which it is important to decide about the best course of action. Important themes for biotech entrepreneurs are informed consent, ownership of human tissues and cells and derivative products, intellectual property, patenting, and the possibility of biopiracy. The biotechnology industry's response to these issues and others will depend in part on whether the industry as a whole embraces a narrow or a broad concept of corporate social responsibility.

REFERENCES

[1] Mill JS. Utilitarianism. In: Crisp Roger, editor. New York: Oxford University Press; 1998.

[2] U.S. Congress, Office of Technology Assessment. (March 1987). New Developments in Biotechnology: Ownership of Human Tissues and Cells-Special Report, OTA-BA-337, Washington, D.C.: U.S. Government Printing Office.

[3] National Commission for the Protection of Human Subjects of Biomedical and Behavioral Research. The Belmont Report: Ethical Principles and Guidelines for the Protection of Human Subjects of Research. Washington, D.C: DHEW Publication OS; 1978. 78–0012.

[4] Kant I. Foundations of the Metaphysics of Morals. Translation by Lewis White Beck. Indianapolis, Indiana: Bobbs-Merrill; 1959.

[5] Faden R, Beauchamp T. A History and Theory of Informed Consent. Oxford University Press; 1986. pp.276–286.

[6] Treating AIDS, Dilemmas of Unequal Access in Uganda. In: Petrynna AA, Lakaff A, Kleinman, editors. Global Pharmaceuticals, Ethics, Markets, Practices. Durham: Duke University Press; 2006.

[7] Aristotle. The Basic Works of Aristotle. New York: Random House; 1941.

[8] Rawls J. A Theory of Justice. Cambridge, Massachusetts: The Belnap Press of Harvard University Press; 1971.

[9] United States Patent and Trademark Office, *http://www.uspto.gov/web/offices/pac/doc/general/whatis.htm*.

[10] Gupta R, Gabrielsen B, Ferguson SM. Nature's Medicines: Traditional Knowledge and Intellectual Property Management. Case Studies from the National Inst Health, Current Drug Discovery Technol 2005;2:1–17.

[11] Skloot R. The Immortal Life of Henrietta Lacks. New York: Random House; 2010.

[12] Dwyer L. Biopiracy, Trade, and Sustainable Development. Colorado J Int Environ Law and Policy 2008;19:219–56.

Chapter 31

Career Opportunities in the Life Sciences Industry

Toby Freedman, PhD

President, Synapse Search Recruiting, Portola Valley, California

There are many career opportunities in industry, nonprofit organizations, and in government for individuals with science backgrounds. Whether you have an interest in laboratory work, business, sales, marketing, or clinical studies, there are hundreds of different careers in the life sciences industry—and as a consequence, there are numerous opportunities to find that ideal job that matches your unique personality attributes, skills, interests, and long-term goals. A science or medical background is a valuable asset to have. Whether you are writing a patent, marketing a product, conducting a clinical trial, or doing a business deal, having a science background will greatly enhance your career. The chart shown in Figure 31.1 delineates over 100 distinct careers in the life sciences industry where you can apply your scientific or medical educational background.

For those wishing to escape from bench work, the good news is that scientists can transition from bench research to other vocational areas. Most researchers eventually do transition into other careers at some point in time. These additional career areas can provide an opportunity to explore other areas such as general management, team-building, project management, creative writing, and more.

AN OVERVIEW OF THE MANY DIFFERENT VOCATIONAL AREAS IN THE LIFE SCIENCES INDUSTRY

This chapter provides a high-level summary of 24 significant careers in the life sciences industry, as shown in Figure 31.1. If you find a career that interests you, I recommend additional reading in the specific area that piques your interest. At the conclusion of this overview there are two sections to help you move into a particular vocational area, one on steps for making a career transition and the other on job-finding strategies.

1 Entrepreneurship

Do you have a fantastic idea that has the potential of being developed into a successful business? There are few things as exciting as starting a new company and attempting something that no one else has ever done before.

Entrepreneurship can be a stimulating and rewarding career, but it is not for everyone. It helps to be financially secure and to have done it before. However, I have seen postdoctoral fellows, graduate students, professors, and even undergraduates start and manage highly successful ventures without prior business training. If you are considering entrepreneurship, I highly recommend considering a job at one of the growing number of "incubators" or "accelerators" that are cropping up worldwide. An incubator is a supportive place where a cluster of start-up companies thrive. At an incubator, start-ups can share lab equipment, office space, and gain support from fellow entrepreneurs who are working down the hall.

One highly successful example of an incubator is University of California's QB3 (QB3 stands for California Institute for Quantitative Biosciences, which includes three institutions, University of California at San Francisco, Berkeley, and Santa Cruz). QB3's goal is to benefit society by commercializing university research to benefit society. QB3 provides a supportive environment where new companies are being founded on campus in the same buildings where professors, graduate students, and postdocs are conducting research. Venture capital, biopharmaceutical, management consulting, and accounting firms are also actively partnering and assisting these start-up companies. This type of collaborative environment fosters communication, sharing of knowledge, and innovation. To learn more, visit www.qb3.org.

Similar incubators are being created across the United States at top universities such as Harvard University, University of Florida, University of Washington, and SUNY in Brooklyn, for examples. Also consider off-campus

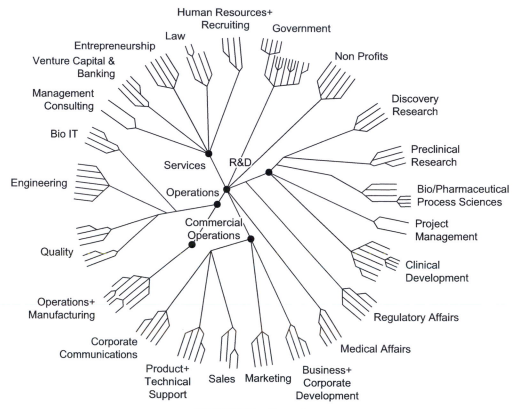

FIGURE 31.1   Career chart.

incubators, such as Phoenix's TGen (Translational Genomics Research Institute), Kendall Square's incubator in Boston, and many others. Working at an incubator will provide you with first-hand experience in a start-up environment where you will be exposed to the challenges of raising capital, building teams, and developing products. Also consider attending "boot camp" programs which can help you develop your business plan, raise venture capital, and be mentored by experienced executives who have built companies before. One to consider is Astia, which is a nonprofit organization dedicated to fostering women-led companies: visit www.astia.org.

2 Venture Capital

A venture capital career is among the most coveted and exciting areas of all the careers in the life sciences industry. This career has real appeal to socially minded and team-oriented scientists because venture capitalists have opportunities to meet and work with successful entrepreneurs that are developing and commercializing ground-breaking technologies.

Most people think of venture capitalists as the people you go to when raising capital to fund their start-ups, but these individuals must first raise money for their own fund which they then use to invest in start-ups. Venture capitalists provide considerably more than just a source of money.

After venture capitalists invest in a start-up company, they may assume positions on the company board of directors to monitor their investment and also to assist the company with the many challenges that are encountered in emerging businesses. Therefore, an operational background and experience in several successful start-ups is considered an optimal background for a venture capitalist.

Corporate venture capitalists work in large pharmaceutical or biotechnology companies and, similar to venture capitalists, they also fund private companies using money from the biopharmaceutical company that they represent. There are institutional investors (also called equity research analysts), who invest in public companies.

If you are interested in seeking a career in venture capital, consider applying for a fellowship with the Kauffman Foundation—a nonprofit organization committed to fostering entrepreneurism. Visit www.kauffman.org for more information. Many venture capital firms also hire associates and advisors (academic scientists or industry experts), consultants, and entrepreneurs-in-residence (EIRs). EIRs are experienced senior-level executives capable of running venture capital portfolio companies and managing their investments.

There are other venture-type careers that involve working with biotech companies. These include angel investors, who are people of high net worth that financially support private companies, usually before venture capitalists invest.

3 Investment Banking

There are three major career areas in investment banking: advisory services, sell-side equity research, and sales trading. Advisory service providers are involved in large financial transactions such as helping their clients raise capital, complete initial public offerings (IPO), or mergers and acquisitions (M&A). This is a highly competitive career and can involve extensive travel, but the payoffs are quite large, as investment bankers are amply compensated for their hard work. If you enjoy transactional work or have an interest in finance, this is a promising career to consider.

Sell-side equity research analysts conduct and publish background research on the particular public companies that they follow. These analysts provide ratings of public companies stock, such as "buy," "sell," or "hold" and they publish informative reports for clients. It is becoming more common for investment banks to hire MDs, Ph.D.s, and MBAs who can analyze and ascertain the chances of success for clinical trials, and by extension, they predict changes in stock value. Sales traders conduct stock sales transactions and promote stock sales.

4 Discovery Research

Discovery research is very similar to academic research and it probably is the most commonly followed path for science graduates wanting to enter into industry. If you enjoy working at the scientific frontier, have an interest in benefiting human health, are an idea generator with a creative mind that can make unique connections; or if you simply enjoy lab work and would like to apply your laboratory skills to industry, this is the career to consider. There are many career levels within discovery research such as a research associate for undergraduates and Master's students as well as a scientist track for Ph.D. graduates.

For creative scientists who do not wish to advance up the administrative path to director and vice president (VP) levels, there are the prestigious "fellow" or "staff scientist" positions which allow scientists to remain close to the research and at the same time minimize their administrative load. There are also nonbench-related positions in discovery research, including project management (see number 10), program management, portfolio management, and more. If your interests evolve over time, discovery research can provide you with an excellent launching pad to other careers in the life sciences industry.

5 Preclinical Research

Preclinical research bridges the gap between discovery research and clinical development and encompasses the areas of pharmacology, toxicology, pharmacokinetics, pathology, and chemical optimization. This is where prospective drug candidates are tested in animals and optimized before entering into human clinical studies. Because research projects are frequently terminated in discovery research, preclinical scientists have an opportunity to work on the "winners"—the most promising drug candidates.

6 Process Sciences

Like discovery research, process sciences offer many great entry-level industry positions for academic scientists, particularly for chemists and biochemists. This is where the steps for chemical synthesis, production of drugs, or products and scale-up processes are developed. A candidate drug might be easy to synthesize in the test tube, but during clinical trials, methods must be developed to scale-up production of the drug for clinical studies and eventually for large-scale manufacturing. This vocational area is a great way to apply your scientific knowledge and laboratory skills to create products and develop synthesis steps that will eventually be used for large-scale manufacturing. Scientists enjoy this field because they can be creatively involved in designing scaled-up reactions and they have the chance to see the end result of their work-products.

If you have a background in process chemistry, formulation, analytical chemistry, or on the biologics side, a background in cell culture, fermentation, purification or biologics scale-up, there are many jobs available in this area.

7 Clinical Development

There are many vocational areas and niches within clinical development—the process of testing drugs in human clinical trials. Clinical development includes areas such as medical monitoring, clinical project management, or working as a clinical research associate (CRA). There are also positions in biometrics (statistics and statistical programming), medical writing, data management, drug safety, and more. People enjoy working in clinical development because of the rapid pace of the work environment and because there is the opportunity to work with the drug candidate "winners" developed in discovery research. Generally, clinical development departments employ people with medical, pharmacological, nursing, or scientific backgrounds.

8 Regulatory Affairs

Regulatory affairs liaisons manage the process of working with project teams and interacting with the regulatory health agencies, such as the Food and Drug Administration (FDA) or the International Conference on Harmonization of Technical Requirements for Registration of Pharmaceuticals for Human Use (ICH). In addition to regulatory affairs liaisons positions, there are a vast array of other career opportunities, such as managing and submitting regulatory information, document management, and publishing.

Positions within regulatory affairs offer excellent job security. The reason is simply supply and demand: not enough people today have experience in regulatory affairs and at the same time, the FDA has increased its standards, requiring more supporting studies and paperwork before products can be approved for human use. To be successful in this position, it helps to be very detail- and process-oriented, and to possess excellent writing, communication, and interpersonal skills.

9 Medical Affairs

After a drug has been approved, medical affairs professionals run additional clinical studies: to test the drug in off-label trials for other disease indications, to study drug-drug interactions, or to test the drug in different patient populations. They are also involved in disseminating this newly discovered information to relevant parties.

There are several departments within medical affairs. Clinical development professionals conduct Phase 4 clinical trials, medical communications executives run medical educational events for practicing physicians, and medical science liaisons (MSLs) provide recently published clinical data to clinicians and doctors of various specialties. Another area of medical affairs is pharmacovigilance and drug safety. This involves monitoring the drug's performance and handling adverse drug events as individual cases after the drug has been approved. If adverse events are associated with the drug, these must be reported to the regulatory authorities. The backgrounds for these positions include medical doctors, nurses, and pharmacists.

10 Project Management

If you are interested in learning about the many nuances of the different steps of drug discovery and development and wish to avoid bench research, consider project management. Project managers don't actually make the critical decisions but facilitate the decision-making process and manage multidisciplinary teams. They spend their time providing vision and leadership, communicating with team members and management, running meetings, allocating resources, doing risk management and problem solving. Each of the areas of drug discovery and development and medical device development require project management. Common areas include discovery research, clinical, and chemistry manufacturing and controls (CMC). Project managers are also needed in many other areas including finance, facility management, portfolio management, and more.

This is a wonderful area to develop your interpersonal, influencing, and leadership abilities, and to gain deeper problem-solving aptitude while moving projects forward.

After working as a project manager you will have developed the ability to enter just about any of the vocational areas in a company. If you are interested in reading more about this career, there is a free chapter on project management careers on my website at www.careersbiotech.com.

11 Business and Corporate Development

Professionals in business and corporate development work with the company's executive team to determine the strategic objectives of the company. For example, they determine which internal products will be funded and which products will be licensed.

Corporate development is the department where strategic decisions are made about securing enough financial resources to ensure continued operations and to reach strategic objectives. Corporate development executives are often involved in the company's fundraising efforts, whether they are raising venture or corporate capital or doing a private investment in a public entity (PIPE) transaction.

Business development is the department that creates and implements the deals which are in alignment with the company's strategic objectives. A deal can be a technology that is in-licensed (acquired) or out-licensed (sold) to another company. Small biotech companies usually don't have the financial resources to bring a drug all the way through clinical trials. Instead, most small biotech companies rely on out-licensing their initial products to larger cash-rich biopharmaceutical companies that are seeking to fill their own drug development pipelines with new products. In exchange, the large biopharmaceutical companies will pay for part, or all, of the remaining clinical development and provide the small biotech company with much-needed milestone-based cash.

There are many steps involved in business development, and each step involves different roles for business and science majors. Examples include commercial strategy consultants and advisors who provide commercial insight into finance and strategic directions; portfolio managers who determine which products have the highest probability of success; technology scouts and analysts who identify and evaluate new business opportunities; licensing officers who are involved in closing deals—they could be involved in negotiations, designing payments, or arranging the final terms of the deal; and finally, alliance managers who implement the deal and manage the partnership. They serve as the main point of contact and ensure that deliverables are met.

If you are currently a student in academia, one of the easiest ways to enter business development is to initially work at the Office of Technology Transfer. There you will learn about patents, technology management, and be exposed to the business of biotech. Alternatively, consider working in sales or patent law—important components to business development. If you are currently working in a company, volunteer to do some business development assessments in your area of expertise. Another great way to gain entry into business development is to work at a trade association.

One final note for job seekers: frequently, a "business development" position really means a "sales" opportunity. In fact, business development is in a way, a sales transaction—it's just that the transaction is longer and more complicated.

12 Marketing

Marketing professionals work with sales executives to determine how products are sold and advertised. They manage brands and determine how the product is perceived by the target consumers. Marketing is about communicating a message to consumers and developing a business strategy. Let's say that you have a great product—how do you tell the world about your wonderful product within the guidelines and purview of the regulatory agencies? There is a psychological component to marketing as well—how do people make purchasing decisions and how do you go about providing the right message to your target market? Marketing is needed throughout a company's life cycle. Even at the early stages of a company, market research analyses might be conducted. Just about every CEO raising money from venture capitalists will discuss the target market in a company's business plan.

Marketing careers provide excellent training in leadership. Many of the large pharmaceutical company CEOs started their careers in marketing. If you have ambitions of eventually becoming a CEO one day, a career in marketing is a great way to acquire some of the strategic leadership training and skills needed to run a company.

Like business development, marketing is an exciting area and a highly coveted career. Once you have gained some marketing experience, it is easier to navigate between the many careers in marketing.

Brand management is being commercially responsible for a specific product. The basic areas of brand management in the life sciences include promotional, medical education, consumer, global, and managed-care marketing. New product-planning professionals help clinical teams strategize on the best market for their drug development plans. In addition, there are other branches of marketing including commercial strategy, data analytics, and forecasting, to name a few.

One of the easiest ways for science graduates to get into marketing is through sales or market research. Market research is a career involved with gathering data about the size of a market, the target customers, and the customer's interest.

13 Sales

Sales executives work directly with customers to develop business and conduct sales transactions. They help customers use products correctly, inform doctors about drugs and products, for example, and ensure that any questions and

concerns that customers have are promptly answered. Sales can be a highly rewarding and lucrative career for those that are highly motivated and energetic. There are many perks to a career in sales, and quite possibly the best, besides the commissions, is that many sales reps work at home. This can provide an opportunity to live in geographically restricted areas where there are limited jobs (like Hawaii, for example). Plus, you can't beat the commute from your kitchen to your home office! However, there can also be extensive travel in sales in order to meet customers and provide sales presentations.

Sales positions provide great entry-level opportunities for new graduates and job changers, and companies generally offer excellent training in sales. Once you have mastered sales basics, you will find a multitude of different positions within sales, including sales management, operations, and account management. There are many types of sales positions such as selling reagents, instruments, microscopes, preclinical and clinical trial services, for example. Specialty and primary drug sales reps visit doctor's offices to promote their products and to establish relations with doctors. For scientists with a driving interest in making science easier to understand for customers, consider technical sales—sales for biological and medical research products such as instruments, biotools, software, services, etc. You might have an opportunity to work with high-level research executives or well-known professors in academia and help them make technical sales decisions. Working closely with the sales reps, Field Application Specialists or Scientists (FAS) provide their technical expertise to help with sales transactions. For recent graduates, this is an exciting entry-level position that will allow you to work with technical leaders in academia and industry, learn business fundamentals, and become an expert in the product that you are promoting.

14 Management Consulting

Management consulting is a great way to apply your analytical skills in a fast-paced, intellectually intense occupation where you can drive change and help companies become more successful. Most management consulting firms offer training and some offer a mini-MBA in which you can learn business fundamentals.

Management consultants serve as high-level strategic advisers to companies. They might conduct strategic analyses on just about any aspect of a company's business, including strategy, portfolio management, pricing, operations, productivity, finance, cost reduction, competition, and more. There are several major global management consulting firms and many small boutiques that specialize in the life sciences. Also consider the many accounting firms which have life science advisory service arms. Management consulting can involve extensive travel, and the position pays well, accordingly.

15 Corporate Communications

If you have a flair for writing, consider corporate communications. Corporate communications is involved in managing the image of the company—how the company is perceived by investors, customers, and the general population.

There are several vocational areas within corporate communications. There are investor relations professionals who interact with the company's investors, public relations professionals who manage the corporate image and news about a company, and government affairs professionals who develop science policies and inform and influence the government. If you are interested in a corporate communications career, consider applying for a policy fellowship with the American Association for the Advancement of Science (AAAS).

Corporate affairs and marketing communications are careers for scientists with an interest in business who possess excellent writing skills. In an entry-level position, you might participate in writing press releases or creating investor packages.

16 Engineering

There are many opportunities for engineers in the life sciences, particularly in the biotools, biofuels, bio-IT, and medical devices industries. Some opportunities include conceiving, developing, and testing human prosthetic devices such as bionic arms, legs, ankles, and hands. There are other opportunities in the development and production of new gene sequencing instruments for researchers in the biotechnology and pharmaceutical industry. In the biofuels sector, chemical and mechanical engineers are needed for developing new methods for renewable fuel sources and the processing machinery that produces them. An engineering, bioengineering, or biochemical engineering background is needed in all sectors of the biotechnology industry including, therapeutics, diagnostics, medical devices, research reagents and tools, bio-agriculture, biofuels, and industrial biotechnology products.

17 Operations

Are you interested in the many operational components of a company and how they work together? A career in operations is focused on manufacturing and distributing products to customers at the highest level of quality for the lowest cost. People in operations enjoy making processes more efficient, and are good at problem-solving and delivering on expectations. This is a fast-paced position, with job variety, where you can apply your science and business acumen and directly affect the company's bottom line.

18 Quality

If one of your strongest attributes is your ability to pay attention to detail, and if you enjoy developing procedures, a quality role might be for you. Quality positions tend to have good job security. Most positions require little if any travel (unless you are an auditor). Quality work ensures that products and procedures are consistent and comply with FDA regulations. For therapeutic companies, quality ensures that products are pure and safe for human or animal consumption.

Quality offers many great entry-level positions for new graduates and career-changers. Quality control specialists test products and make sure that manufactured products meet specifications. Quality assurance provides the documentation that production is being done correctly. Regulatory compliance ensures that systems and procedures in a company have accounted for quality and are compliant with the regulations. Most biotools and medical device companies have a quality systems branch which is involved in validation of computer systems.

19 Bio-IT

A career in bio-IT is for scientists with an interest in information technology, and for computer scientists with an interest in biology—and everything in between. As the biological sciences have evolved over the years, the need to handle large amounts of data has grown tremendously. For example, think of the challenges of handling the tremendous amounts of data generated in genome sequencing. In addition, an IT component is needed in almost every aspect of discovering and developing drugs or products. As such, people with a background in both IT and biological sciences are in high demand.

Career opportunities in bio-IT are diverse. Besides the bioinformatics and "omics" fields, there are also clinical data management, patient registries, IT infrastructure, IT quality, and healthcare IT areas such as electronic health records and mobile health, and much more.

20 Technical and Product Support

If you enjoy working with customers, product and technical support careers are ones to consider. Technical support representatives manage phone calls, answer customer-related questions, and solve technical and product-related problems. They also become experts in each of the specific products that the company develops or in-licenses and, as such, frequently these individuals later move into product development. Technical support can be a collegial and friendly working environment and most positions are 9 to 5 and involve little travel.

If you have a passion for teaching, consider a career as a technical trainer. Technical trainers teach clients how to use new products by developing presentations or setting up workshops. An added perk is that many trainers work from home when they are not offering a workshop.

21 Law

Intellectual property—patents, copyrights, and trademarks are often the most valuable assets held by a biotechnology company, especially at the early stages. Patent attorneys and agents draft and manage the patent applications. But there are other equally interesting areas of law to consider as well, such as transactional, corporate law, and litigation.

Transactional lawyers draft and negotiate business transactions. Corporate lawyers incorporate companies and help structure business deals, such as M&As, IPOs, and venture financings. Litigators are involved in lawsuits, typically patent infringements, which have heated up over the years as large successful biotech companies have more money worth suing for.

There are other law careers, such as regulatory law or working as a general counsel as well as opportunities to work as a patent examiner or attorney at the U.S. Patent and Trademark Office (USPTO) in Alexandria, VA. Law is a highly competitive occupation, but it also is intellectually interesting and financially rewarding.

22 Human Resources and Recruiting

Having the right team in an early-stage start-up is extremely important. It is essential that the company hires people who have the appropriate skill sets and who will also fit in with the team. Your technical knowledge and business acumen can be an asset in human resources and recruiting. The field of human resources, which is managing the corporate culture of a company, employee relations, and governance of employees is generally occupied by people with business backgrounds; however scientists can enter this field as well.

Recruiting can be a gratifying occupation because you are helping companies identify and hire people with the appropriate skill sets and corporate match, and also helping candidates find promising jobs. There are many different types of recruiting companies ranging from the large international executive retained search, to contingency, temp-to-hire, and staffing firms.

23 Careers in Government

Government and nonprofit jobs generally don't pay as well as industry jobs, but they offer much greater job security and pension plans—so in the long term, it can balance out. This is a great way to apply your business and scientific training and contribute to society. There are many jobs in the government sector. At the FDA, there are numerous career fields besides regulatory or medical affairs, such as basic research and pharmacovigilance opportunities. To find out more, and for student internships, visit www.usajobs.com and www.usphs.gov.

In addition to the FDA, there is a plethora of government opportunities, such as working at the Departments of: Agriculture, Energy, Veterans Affairs, and Defense; the CDC, NASA, NIH, Homeland Security, Department of Infectious Diseases, crime labs/forensics, the military, and many more research institutes and government labs.

24 Careers in Nonprofit Organizations

Nonprofit organizations can be a stimulating and altruistic way to apply your scientific and business acumen and work with academics, medical advocacy groups, and philanthropists. In addition to the traditional nonprofit organizations, new business models are cropping up. Many nonprofits are developing their own drug discovery and development or diagnostics efforts in-house, just like a biotech company. For example, the Myelin Repair Foundation, Melanoma Research Alliance, and the Michael J. Fox Foundation are actively involved in advancing treatments through the FDA. As such, the same types of positions discussed in this chapter might also be available in some nonprofit organizations.

There are nonprofit organizations for just about every known disease. Most nonprofits are philanthropic organizations that provide grants for research or patient advocacy for a specific disease, such as the Alzheimer's Association or the American Cancer Society. The Bill and Melinda Gates Foundation's mission is to improve people's health around the world. For example, grants are used for research for cures, for vaccinations, or medical assistance for patients, for epidemiological research or simply for raising awareness for a disease.

There are many different positions for business and science majors in nonprofits, including: project management, social work, development (fundraising), marketing, outreach, operations, scientific affairs, finance, communications, science positions ranging from research associate or scientist to chief scientific officer (CSO), program management, patent and licensing positions, and much more.

There are also a variety of jobs at lobbying and educational nonprofit organizations, such as the Biotechnology Industry Organization (BIO), Pharmaceuticals Research and Manufacturers of America (PhRMA), and the Drug Information Association (DIA). There are many regional nonprofits that serve as lobbying and educational organizations, such as Southern California's BioCom, the American Association for the Advancement of Science (AAAS), and the Massachusetts Biotechnology Council (MassBio). In addition, scientific societies, such as the American Chemical Society provide job opportunities for business and science majors for example. Also consider government-run trade associations and international innovation centers that are located at biotech hubs. These are opportunities to gain exposure to many start-up companies.

MAKING A CAREER TRANSITION

Making a career transition can be quite challenging, depending on the economy. Here are some steps that with proper planning and some good fortune, can help you make the transition smoothly. As shown in Figure 31.2, the first step includes self-assessment. Work with career counselors and take self-assessment tests in order to identify your interests, skills, personality attributes, values, and goals. If you are a student or postdoctoral fellow, most universities provide free career services on campus. If you have already graduated, alumni are frequently provided with free career services on campus. If you are employed in a company, speak to a human resources representative or hire a personal career counselor.

The next step is to identify those vocational areas that best match your self-assessment results to find your "ideal career." After researching the many careers and identifying several possibilities, conduct informational interviews. An informational interview is simply a way to interview professionals currently working in a chosen vocational field that interests you. Note that this is not a job interview—it is a way to learn more about a vocational area or interest. To learn more about informational interviewing, visit your career services department on campus as they generally have an abundance of material on the topic. There is also extensive information available on the Internet.

There may be additional classes, degrees, or certificates that would expedite a career transition. For example, a certificate in project management would provide you with practical experience using the project management tools utilized in companies.

As shown in Figure 31.2, the third step is to prepare a resume specific for the new career and to continue networking by attending local and international conferences and events that are in line with the career area that interests you. For example, if you are interested in a career in business development, you might want to attend the Licensing Executives Society association meeting. If you want to

know how to find the appropriate meetings and societies to attend, simply do a Google search and type in "business development, life science, conference," for example.

For readers who are already working and who wish to make a career transition, try to obtain on-the-job training. For example, if you are interested in a career in project management, become a team member on a project at your existing company and become familiar with the process. If you are interested in business development, ask to help with technical assessments. If you are in academia, consider volunteering at the technology transfer department on campus. Most companies provide employees with degreed training programs at academic institutions, such as MBAs, Master's in Biotechnology degrees, etc.

FINDING A JOB IN THE LIFE SCIENCES INDUSTRY

Most people first look for jobs by applying to the well-established biopharmaceutical companies with name-recognition, such as Amgen, Vertex, Genentech/Roche, Biogen, Gilead, Pfizer, Merck, etc. These companies are also the most competitive to get into. You should also consider the less well known emerging venture-backed companies and start-ups.

Other places to consider are the service companies—such as contract research organizations (CRO) and contract manufacturing organizations (CMO). These companies will provide you with exposure to numerous different processes and products. Because large and small biotech companies tend to outsource many aspects of drug discovery and development, there can be jobs available in the service companies.

Other industries to consider are the many biotech companies that do not develop drugs. For examples, diagnostics, personalized medicine, and next-generation sequencing companies; biotools, which develop products such as microarrays, instruments, reagents, and consulting services; the newly emerging and rapidly growing field of biofuels; industrial biotechnology; systems biology; nanotech; agricultural biotechnology; numerous large and small agencies; and the medical device industry. Apply for jobs in government or in nonprofit organizations. There are many different types of careers in academia in addition to professorships. For example program directorships, working at the office of technology transfer, education-related positions, laboratory management, core facility directorship, working in public relations and development (fundraising), working in an entrepreneurial start-up on campus, working in doctoral career services, and more.

I can't stress enough how important it is to be flexible and open-minded about the types of career opportunities to apply for while looking for a job. Consider job areas that you have not considered before and keep an open mind while exploring your options. Apply for nonglamorous

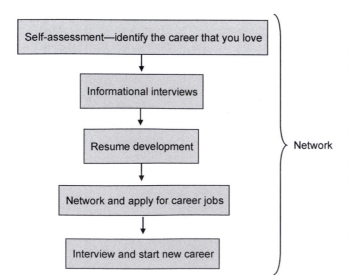

FIGURE 31.2   Basic steps for a career transition.

jobs—they will provide an opportunity to learn new skills, to network, and to gain industry experience. Also consider working as a consultant or on a contract/temporary basis.

NETWORKING

The vast majority of people in industry found their jobs through networking. The reason that networking is so effective is that hiring managers are more likely to consider candidates who came personally vouched for—perhaps a company employee has worked previously with a candidate, or met him or her at a networking event and can forward their resume for consideration to the hiring manager, with an endorsement. Networking is also effective because company employees are frequently financially motivated to bring on hires. The more people that you know, the more likely someone will recommend you for an opportunity.

What does "networking" mean? It means meeting people—whether at local and national meetings, on airplanes, at trade booths at conferences, etc. It means developing personal connections and informing your network about your job status and the types of positions that interest you. It also means being helpful and supportive of your fellow colleagues so that they can contact you for your guidance and support when they are looking for a job.

INTERVIEWING

It is very important to apply for, and interview for, as many positions as possible. The more positions that you interview for, the more likely that you will find the ideal job. Likewise, companies also interview many candidates for each position in order to hire the one with the best technical and corporate match.

CAREERS IN THE LIFE SCIENCES INDUSTRY: JOB SECURITY AND VOLATILITY

Careers in biotechnology can be as volatile as careers in other technology sectors. The reasons for volatility are due to many factors, including the dynamic nature of the life sciences industry, the ever increasing costs of developing drugs, and the increasing difficulty of getting drugs and products approved by regulatory authorities.

If job security is your major concern, some careers offer better job security than others. For example, careers in regulatory affairs or in the government provide significant job security and steady job growth. A particular skill set in a new or uncommon and high-demand area, such as the Clinical Laboratory Improvement Amendment (CLIA) certification, is another way to enhance your job security.

During tough economic times, companies tend to focus on revenues, which translates into a focus on products closest to sales. Therefore, careers in sales, marketing, regulatory affairs, clinical development, and medical affairs tend to be more stable, whereas early drug discovery research jobs may be more volatile. By nature, early-stage biotech start-ups tend to have less job security than the more-established biopharmaceutical companies.

FINAL COMMENTS AND CONCLUSIONS

I hope that I have provided persuasive evidence that there are a myriad of vocational areas in the life sciences industry for you to explore. It is important to find a career that you are passionate about and will enjoy. Make sure that you read about the various career options, and conduct a self-assessment test to determine which career areas best match your skills, interests, and professional and personal goals. Over the years, your interests and personal or professional goals will likely change. You should conduct periodic self-assessments, revisit your "ideal career," or change directions based on the economy.

As opposed to other industries, working in the life sciences provides an unique opportunity to make a real difference in the world—to cure diseases, to improve the quality of people's lives, and much more. This is your chance to make a positive impact on the world and contribute to global health.

In closing, it is my wish that you will be productive in developing drugs or products and services for unmet medical needs, that you will start companies, and be highly successful in your career.

RESOURCES

The data for this chapter was derived from my own insights acquired from many years of working as a recruiter and from my book, *Career Opportunities in Biotechnology and Drug Development,* (published by Cold Spring Harbor Laboratory Press) which was based on interviews with over 200 industry executives. Each chapter describes the aspects of each career area, including descriptions of a typical day; personality attributes to be successful; pros and cons of the job; career potential; experience and educational requirements, and much more. For more information, visit www.amazon.com and www.careersbiotech.com.

Job Posting Websites

Venture Loop—www.ventureloop.com: jobs in venture-backed companies.
Craig's List—www.craigslist.org: postings of entry-level and higher-level jobs; there is a biotech section.
BioSpace—www.biospace.com: perhaps the leading biotech and medical device job posting website and free life sciences news service.
Indeed—www.indeed.com: a good place to source for jobs.

Free Life Science News Services (Many Have Job Postings)

Fierce Biotech—www.fiercebiotech.com: a summary of biotech news.

FierceBiotechResearch—www.fiercebiotechresearch. com: research coverage in the life sciences.

BayBiotechReview—www.baybiotechreview.com: news about the San Francisco Bay Area life sciences.

OnBioVC—www.onbiovc.com: a listing of companies which have received venture capital in the life sciences.

Chapter 32

Summary

Craig Shimasaki, PhD, MBA

President & CEO, Moleculera Labs and BioSource Consulting Group, Oklahoma City, Oklahoma

By now, you may have come to appreciate that the biotechnology industry is tremendously exciting with proven capabilities of delivering innovative and life-saving products previously considered impossible. This industry is immensely diverse and constantly expanding with new scientific discoveries uncovered daily. Biotechnology encompasses a breadth of products such as medical cures and treatments for severe diseases, tests that can predict recurrence of cancer, methods for improving crop yields and unique ways of producing renewable fuels that are environmentally-friendly. Almost all biotechnology products originate from basic research discovered in an academic or research laboratory. However, producing commercial products from this research requires a company and a team of talented individuals to translate these research discoveries into commercial products. A talented entrepreneur is first required to establish and lead these companies down a chosen path that will ultimately deliver these innovative products to the marketplace.

BIOTECHNOLOGY ENTREPRENEURSHIP

For those who are not aware, there are vast differences between the biotechnology industry and most other industries. Some of these differences include the need for tremendous amounts of capital, lengthy product development cycles, and the requirement for extensive field testing, or clinical testing in animals and in humans. Next, there is a need for specialized expertise to overcome stringent regulatory hurdles before any product can reach the market. Once on the market, in order to become successful, these products must be accepted and reimbursed by government agencies and third-party insurers who have stringent criteria of their own. The challenges in this industry are great, but so are the opportunities for success.

A biotechnology entrepreneur is the original company builder, but they are also product developers and risk managers. These individuals are the initial source of the motivation, vision and forward momentum of any new organization. Without them, the company and its products would not exist. Biotechnology entrepreneurship is unique in that it requires individuals who are skilled in both the technology and the business aspects of an enterprise. Biotechnology is the melding of both scientific and business disciplines, and by integrating these activities a company can effectively develop novel products. Success in biotechnology requires individuals who can effectively communicate and understand the language of business and the language of science. A key criteria for any technology leader is the ability to be a multi-disciplined translator. Often this is one of the most challenging aspects of leading and managing a biotechnology business, however, individuals who avail themselves to learning opportunities can become proficient at communicating the central issues in both these disciplines. For those who are interested in reading about additional experiences of early pioneers in the biotechnology industry, there is a wealth of information chronicled at the "Life Sciences Foundation"[a] We can learn valuable lessons from their stories, their successes, as well as their failures.

Biotechnology entrepreneurs are individuals with vision and passion that drives them to pursue their goals with the belief that their product or service will ultimately impact the well-being of multitudes. Much is riding on the shoulders of the biotechnology entrepreneur and, as a result, we have identified some characteristics that will help improve an entrepreneur's success such as:

- A driving passion for their work with an innate ability to inspire others to follow
- The ability to communicate their vision so others can buy into that mission
- Not being afraid to take carefully calculated risks, and accepting responsibility and ownership for problems
- Viewing their environment through optimistic eyes with the desire and humility to learn from others
- Perseverance in the face of adversity, applying creativity and imagination to arrive at resourceful solutions
- An understanding of the real purpose of negotiation

---

a. As of September 9, 2013: http://www.lifesciencesfoundation.org/

- The ability to raise needed capital and manage it well, while simultaneously multitasking critical activities
- Possessing leadership wisdom and an awareness of the Unknown-Unknowns
- Being a multi-disciplined translator with the ability to understand and speak the language of both business and science
- Possessing desirable core values with the ability to identify others who share similar values

The biotechnology entrepreneur cannot accomplish this work alone, but must find and motivate a creative team, and build a culture of innovation in order for their product to be developed and reach commercialization. Without a dedicated and skilled team of individuals it would be impossible for any entrepreneur to accomplish much. Therefore this team of individuals must also be talented, experienced and leaders themselves who can equip and motivate others to contribute in their own unique ways to the enterprise.

BIOTECHNOLOGY SECTORS AND PRODUCT DIVERSITY

As you have already learned, there is a diversity of sectors within the biotechnology industry. On the surface, this industry may appear to be complex because of the vast array of products that biotechnology is capable of producing. When we speak about the "biotechnology industry" it is a general reference to all of the products within each sector which include: therapeutics, biologics, diagnostics, medical devices, clinical laboratory tests, instruments, agricultural, industrial, and biofuel applications.

Each sector focuses on a certain group of products and utilizes many similar tools and methods to create these products. The human health sector creates innovative medical products that decreases human suffering and improves our lives in ways that were not previously possible. New vaccines have been created treat cancer and others have been developed to ward off all types of infectious diseases. More accurate diagnostics have been developed to quickly identify origins of disease and determine treatment options. Many therapies have now been developed to treat orphan diseases, which are debilitating diseases that afflict fewer than 200,000 people, all of whom previously had limited treatments for their conditions. With the aid of biotechnology there are now over 300 FDA-approved treatments for rare diseases with over 450 more in various stages of development.

Advances in personalized medicine are accelerating as practical applications of the human genome research are being developed and used. Breakthroughs in sequencing technology are astounding. To sequence the first human genome it required 13 years and approximately $3 billion dollars, now, within a decade and a half, we have the ability to sequence an entire genome within days for about $1,000. Sequencing technology is advancing so rapidly that it soon will be possible to sequence an individual's entire genome within an hour for about $100. Greater medical advances are realized because of an increased understanding of our genetics and our environment, which will continue to result in novel treatments to enhance our longevity and provide us with a better quality of life. Revolutionary biotechnology research tools continue to be created from innovative discoveries such as polymerase chain reaction (PCR). This technique expanded the field of diagnostic medicine and forensic science by providing us the ability to amplify minuet quantities of genetic material from a human specimen and to determine if a particular individual will respond appropriately to a particular drug.

Major advances are also being made in the food and agriculture biotechnology sector. These include unique ways to more efficiently grow crops, novel ways to increase product yields, and to significantly increase nutritional benefits of the foods we consume. AgBiotechnology has delivered insect resistant crops that greatly reduce the need to use pesticides on our food sources, herbicide tolerance crops that allow farmers to use weed-killers without damaging crops, and to produce crops that have increased resistance to harsh environmental conditions such as drought, floods, extreme cold and heat. Biofuel development and production have significantly advanced because of biotechnology with the use of corn, switchgrass, and cellulostic feedstocks that decrease our dependence on foreign oil and to reduce greenhouse gas emissions. All these advances have been made possible because of the creative ideas of individuals who utilized biotechnology tools and techniques to solve some of the greatest problems of our day.

From the birth of biotechnology in the mid 1970's with the discovery of genetic engineering tools that can transplant a desirable human gene into the genome of bacteria to express this needed protein, the biotechnology industry was begun. Originating from only a handful of start-ups, to now over 10,000 biotechnology companies world-wide, that are creating novel products to solve some of our most challenging problems. These companies forged the way and ushered in the development of additional tools needed to advance research discoveries that, in turn, led to more innovative products. The biotechnology industry is constantly expanding as new scientific and technical discoveries are uncovered and new applications are identified. The overarching goal of this industry is to create unique products and processes that improve life, health and well-being of individuals and society as a whole.

GROWING BIOTECHNOLOGY CLUSTERS

Because of the great value generated by the biotechnology industry, there is wide-spread interest in developing biotechnology clusters in most all countries around the world. Biotechnology companies thrive in an ecosystem with support services, a technically skilled workforce and access to capital. This is evidenced by the many well-established and growing concentrations of biotech activity in United States, United Kingdom, Canada, France, Germany, Netherlands, Switzerland, Europe the Middle East, Japan, Australia with emerging clusters in China, India, Indonesia and Singapore, to name just a few.

Biotechnology clusters provide benefits to the local region and to the community they reside such as creating clean, high-technology, and high-paying jobs. The average wage paid to bioscience industry workers in the US reached $82,697 in 2010, which is more than $36,000 or 79 percent greater than the average paid in the overall national private sector. Of course, these added high-paying jobs generate personal and sales taxes for local government. Biotechnology companies also attract an innovative and skilled workforce, collateral businesses and a host of other support services. Established biotechnology clusters have large talent pools and bring cross-creativity to the local region, and as a result, shorten product development time. As we previously discussed, there are 5 Essential Elements that must be present in any geographical region in order for a biotechnology cluster to develop. These include 1) the abundance of high quality, adequately funded academic research; 2) a ready resource of seasoned and experienced biotechnology entrepreneurs; 3) ready access to sources of at-risk, early and development-stage capital willing to fund startup concepts; 4) an adequate supply of technically-skilled workforce, experienced in the biotechnology industry; and 5) availability of dedicated wet-laboratory and specialized facilities at an affordable rate.

In order to successfully create an environment with these 5 Essential Elements, both industry and government must play a role in the development of biotechnology clusters. Traditionally, the way government has participated is through economic stimulation, financing, and incentives for companies within particular industries. Because funding is always a critical need for biotechnology companies, one of many ways government can help to stimulate private investments in biotechnology companies is by providing investment tax credits for qualified investing in life science companies.

TECHNOLOGY OPPORTUNITIES

Biotechnology companies are birthed from novel product ideas that are conceived to provide value for a specific group of individuals. If you examine the original source of most successful biotechnology products, you will find that the vast majority of them originated from basic research conducted by a scientist, professor, physician or engineer at an academic or research institution. Basic research has a fundamental goal of acquisition and discovery of new knowledge by exploring new ideas, testing new concepts, and better understanding previously unknown processes

in biology, science and engineering. Unfortunately for the commercially-minded, academic research goals rarely include product development or commercialization. Technology transfer offices at universities are increasing efforts to advance basic research ideas further along to early stages of product development. However, academic and research institutions are not typically well-equipped or experienced in assessing the potential (or lack thereof) of technology concepts destined to be blockbuster products, nor do they possess depth of expertise in biotechnology product development. As a result, very few products have been fully-developed within academic and research institutions because this is not one of their major goals. Because the most advanced product development is performed in companies, it is critical for a functional avenue of exchange to be created between research institutions and biotechnology industry enterprises.

For biotechnology entrepreneurs who are considering licensing a basic research technology application from an institution, be sure to first conduct a technology evaluation because that decision has long-term impact on the potential success of your future company. After you select a technology and product application, a team of individuals will be committing an enormous amount of time and resources to the development of this future product. Therefore, technology concepts and product ideas should be selected based upon certain criteria, and some ideas should be avoided because of shortcomings that may limit their likelihood of success. Several criteria have been elaborated upon in this book to assist in evaluating new product technology ideas, and to assess those with the likelihood of future commercial success.

INTELLECTUAL PROPERTY PROTECTION STRATEGIES

Prior to, and during, product development at a biotechnology company, a major asset the company must secure is the intellectual property (IP) rights to the technology. This initially occurs through a negotiated license from the owning institution, but the entrepreneur must pursue additional IP as the product is developed by their company. Much of the early value that investors attribute to a development-stage biotechnology company is the "ownership" of these technological concepts and new product ideas as embodied in the company's IP. In order for a company's product or service to be successful, it must have a technological and beneficial advantage over other products in the market. To gain a competitive advantage, your company must provide something unique. Legal protection of these assets is essential. As improvements, new product concepts and ideas are implemented, it is likely that others will desire to copy them. We previously reviewed a number of legal tools for protecting your assets and for achieving exclusivity or at least a head start over your competition. A good patent counsel is essential in helping you devise a strategy to properly protect these assets through a variety of protective barriers such as: general patents, design patents or industrial designs, utility model patents or petty patents, and plant patents, as well as trademarks, service marks, and layout designs of integrated circuits, commercial names and designations, geographical indications, protection against unfair competition and trade secrets.

COMPANY BUSINESS MODELS

Products are developed and marketed by companies, and every commercial enterprise must operate through an underlying business model. Business models are simply the way in which a company makes money and the manner in which all these functions are interrelated internally and externally. Choosing the right business model is essential to ensure that a company has the best opportunity for success. The selection of a business model should be made during the inception of the company, and chosen to give the future organization a strategic competitive advantage. Selecting the optimal business model is the first step to building business success and reducing the risk of failure. This is because the entrepreneur and leadership team are the "Risk Managers" of the company, and in order to manage risks, they must know what they are. We reviewed business model examples used in the biotechnology industry and described the components that make up a business model. We then discussed five segments of business risk that entrepreneurial leaders must manage in order to optimize success. The purpose was to give the entrepreneur a better understanding of how a business model helps manage and reduce the risks of their company.

THE VIRTUAL COMPANY

Start-up biotechnology companies rarely have enough money to accomplish everything they would like because of limited capital. This is why I am a strong proponent of operating as a "virtual company" during the start-up phase of a company. Operating as a virtual company simply means that the company does not perform all the necessary functions internally but still accomplishes all the necessary activities as if it did. The way this is accomplished is by carefully selecting outsourcing partners. For most early-stage companies, the extent of outsourcing can be significant where almost all development functions are performed under contract through specialty organizations. Sometimes the type of R&D activities required by some early-stage biotechnology companies are so unique and specialized that their only option is to perform these functions in-house; however, the more common functions can still be outsourced to keep overhead costs down. During start-up stages, capital is usually quite limited and a company cannot hire many full-time employees, but substantial progress must still be made in order to gain interest from investors. Operating as a virtual company during the formative stages allows entrepreneurs to extend the time horizon of their operations and it requires much less capital to maintain and sustain the company while their product is initially being developed.

DEVELOPMENT OF A COMPANY CULTURE WITH CORE VALUES

A company's culture is a good predictor of the future success of the organization and their likelihood of achieving their product development and commercialization goals. For a biotech start-up company, developing a corporate culture may not seem like a high priority compared to other pressing needs such as raising capital, hiring a team and quickly making product development progress. One can even temporarily ignore the development of a company culture without much consequence, however, at some point the culture will affect a company's ability to get work done effectively.

Each company should develop a culture suitable for their needs and their particular objectives. It is best to purposefully build a culture that adds strength, rather than a divisive one that occurs by default. At some point the company reaches a critical mass, and the culture of the organization becomes set. Fortunately, most start-up biotechnology companies begin with an entrepreneurial culture. An entrepreneurial culture is one where there is excitement and anticipation about the company's work and mission. Employees have aspirations of contributing to a greater good along with opportunities of professional advancement and expectations about working in an organization with a great future. A one-size-fits-all corporate culture does not work, but there are certain qualities and values that are always advantageous to have.

Just as an organization's strength is the sum total of the strengths of the individuals, the culture of a company is the sum total of the individual core values of the employees. Each one of us possess a set of core values whether we recognize it or not. These are the guiding principles upon which we operate and make decisions. Sometimes these core values are clearly defined, and other times these guiding principles are simply understood. Successful companies have been built upon strong core values. An employee having a core value of "mutual respect for others" will make a different decision about leaving a job unfinished for another employee, and an individual with the core value of "acceptance of responsibility for one's actions" will readily admit a mistake rather than cover it up or blame someone else. These instances may seem inconsequential by themselves, but when you add these up amongst 20, 50, 100 or 1,000 employees this becomes the culture of the company. A fundamental error of business is to focus only on product development and marketing without consideration to the core values of the people that produce these products.

SOURCES OF CAPITAL FOR PRODUCT DEVELOPMENT

A company cannot survive without continued access to capital, no matter how great the technology or product. Fortunately, there are many sources of capital available to biotechnology companies. However, each source has limitations as to the amount of capital they can invest, and the timeframe in which they can invest. The most common sources of capital that are available to biotechnology companies at various stages of development include:

1. Personal Capital
2. Friends and Family
3. Angel Investors
4. Government Grants
5. Local Financing Programs
6. Foundations Focused on your Sector
7. Venture Capital
8. Industry Partnerships
9. Institutional Debt Financing

It is important to remember that each capital source has different investing limitations, different expectations for returns, and different motivations that drive their investing decisions. Most investor groups have well-defined expectations for returns on their investment, and these expectations are commensurate with the level of risk they are taking. Investors typically describe their expectations as a multiple of their investment, a Return on Investment (ROI), and also by the number of years in which to exit. Also, remember that there are "dilution effects" on shareholders, founders and management with each new round of capital raised. Therefore, it is advantageous for the existing shareholders to ensure that the company valuation is constantly increasing as each new round of capital is raised.

We described what we called Funding Alignment Principles. These will improve the likelihood of success in raising the needed amount of capital from the right source at the optimal time of company development. Finding the ideal funding partner is not easy but the likelihood increases by following these Funding Alignment Principles which include:

1. Identify the target capital source that has the greatest interest in the development stage of your company and product.
2. Make sure there is alignment with your company's financial needs and the funding source criteria for investing such as dollar amount, type of equity, length of investment time, etc.
3. Make sure that your opportunity provides the necessary return expected by your target funding source in terms of ROI and multiple-of-investment.
4. Make sure there is alignment in the motivations and core values of your organization with those of the target funding source.

Each of the capital sources we described have a preferred stage at which they like to invest. As companies transition through distinct product development and capital financing stages, these different funding sources become more interested or less interested depending on their investing criteria. Entrepreneurs can save themselves time and energy by focusing only on the funding sources most likely to invest at their particular development stage.

Financing stage terminology may vary but listed below are some of the terms most commonly used. For those that are more familiar with product development stages rather than financing stages, a particular product development stage can be implied by the stage of financing.

1. **Start-up or Pre-seed Capital:** which is also known as Formation Capital and is typically the smallest amount of money the company raises at any one time. These funds are usually used to establish corporate operating and employment agreements, file and prosecute intellectual property and to incrementally advance the technology. Often these are the funds that allow the company to fully develop their business plan and marketing strategy.
2. **Seed Capital:** is sometimes called Proof-of-Concept Capital, and is the next larger round of capital after Start-Up Capital. The money raised in this round can range between $100,000 to over $1,000,000 and is typically used to advance the technology or product to a stage that increases the value of the company by reaching a key development milestone. Other uses of this capital may go towards expanding the target market research, hiring consultants, subcontracting to Contract Research Organizations (CRO) and to hire part-time or temporary employees.
3. **Early-Stage Capital: Series A/B Preferred Rounds:** These are the next significant funding rounds for the organization and may come from a syndicate of Angels or a group of Angels and local funding programs. Early-Stage Capital can also come from institutional investors such as early-stage investing venture capital firms. These rounds can range from a million dollars to multiple millions of dollars.
4. **Mid-stage or Development-stage Capital: Series C/D Preferred Round:** These follow-on rounds usually involve some or all of the investors in the previous preferred rounds plus new investors which typically come from institutions such as venture capital and corporate partners. Greater numbers of VCs invest in Mid-Stage Development companies than in Early-Stage Development companies. The number and size of these subsequent rounds vary and the letter designation increases with each round.
5. **Later-stage and Expansion Capital: Series E/F Preferred Rounds:** Therapeutics and biologics typically

require more funding rounds and larger capital investments as compared to diagnostics, medical devices, and molecular testing products. The good news is that there are greater numbers of VC firms that invest in these later-stage rounds.

6. **Mezzanine Capital:** For companies that need it, this is usually the last round of capital before an exit for investors such as an acquisition or IPO of the company. Venture capital funds are plentiful at this stage when product development risks have been greatly reduced. Investors at this stage enjoy a shorter time from investment to exit than for those who invested at early or development stages.

7. **Acquisition or Initial Public Offering (IPO):** These are exit events where the investors and shareholders can reap a financial reward for their work and perseverance. However, for drug development and biologics companies, the requirement for capital is so high that usually an IPO really becomes another later-stage financing round.

Cash is a precious and limited commodity to a start-up company. The hard fact is that there is just not enough investment capital to fund all the good ideas for every biotechnology company. Securing biotech funding requires perseverance, and the ability to learn from each investor presentation to improve the chances of funding the company at subsequent junctures. The greatest idea imagined, the most powerful drug ever conceived, or the grandest life-saving medical device dreamed, is of no consequence if one cannot finance its development to commercialization. Someone once said "a vision without execution is a hallucination." To have a vision without funds to execute it is an exercise in frustration and futility. Perseverance, flexibility, creativity, and finding a team of exceptional people are key ingredients to successful fundraising.

COMPANY GROWTH STAGES

All companies transition through growth stages along their pathway to commercialization and maturity. This transition is a real process that occurs subtly over time. As this transition takes place, there is a corporate culture that becomes established and it originates from the core values of the leaders, to the sum total of the core values of the majority of the new hires. There are distinct growth stages of every company, and during these stages there are transition phases in which a company moves to another growth stage successfully or unsuccessfully. The ability of the organization to make this transition is dependent upon the leadership and their ability to make management style changes as the company grows. For individuals who work daily within an organization, these transition stages and changes are not obvious, whereas for those coming into the organization from the outside, it is very obvious.

As a company works to accomplish its objective of creating a valuable product or service, it adds staff, expands activities, and establishes corporate relationships and its business practices evolve. Changes will also occur in the process of how a company makes decisions. A company that is comprised of 10,000 employees, and manufactures and markets products world-wide, typically makes decisions differently than a start-up organization with a handful of employees and one product in development. The optimal methods and processes of decision-making for an early-stage company does not necessarily work well for a mature company and vice versa, however, even though the methods and processes may change, the culture should not, nor does it need to change with growth.

BIOLOGICS MANUFACTURING

Once a biotechnology product has been fully-developed it must be manufactured in large enough quantities to meet the demand for the product. In the case of biologics manufacturing (or biomanufacturing, for short), it is quite different from traditional small molecule pharmaceutical manufacturing. Biomanufacturing is a complex process using recombinant DNA technology to develop procedures and analytics to manufacture these biologic products. These biologic product processes are developed using several platforms such as, whole *multi-cellular* systems encompassing transgenic plants, animals and *unicellular* microbial (bacteria and yeast), insect and mammalian cell culture. The discovery and "proof of concept" from the research bench is transferred to a process and analytical group that will use science and engineering as well as regulatory experience to scale-up the product efficiently. The process for different biologics platforms are complex and unlike traditional chemical synthesis the biologic product resulting from a living system is not as an exact science as chemistry. Because of this complexity it is important to remember that "the process is *the* product" and any variation in the process could impart a change in the products safety and efficacy, and ultimately regulatory approval.

REGULATORY APPROVAL FOR BIOTECHNOLOGY PRODUCTS

The entrepreneurial team must develop a clear regulatory strategy during the early stages of product development which can later be presented to national regulatory authorities (NRAs) such as the FDA. NRAs regulate products developed for treating and diagnosing patients to facilitate access to high quality, safe and effective products, and restrict access to those products that are unsafe or have limited clinical use. Regulatory procedures will have an impact on all stages of biomedical product development. Biotechnology companies must have well thought-out plans for safety review during research and development stages, regulatory approval, and legal registration which are all required before product commercialization. When appropriately implemented, this type of regulation and oversight ensures public health benefits and safety for patients, healthcare workers and the broader medical community. Therefore, it is essential that developers of biomedical products (drugs, biologics, devices, *in vitro* diagnostics or some combination) possess the knowledge and awareness of the regulatory challenges and opportunities to expedite the development of safe and effective products in a cost-effective manner.

BIOTECHNOLOGY PRODUCTS HAVE THREE CUSTOMERS

Compounding these challenges that have been described, the biotechnology entrepreneur and management team must be sure that their product meets the needs of three different "customers" rather than just one. Each of these three: the Patient, the Physician (or provider), and the Payer, all need to recognize value in your product in order for it to be successful. In the biotechnology industry, one customer is the decision-maker who decides *which* product should be used, another customer makes an independent decision whether or not to *pay* for the product (and how *much* to pay for the product) and a totally different customer *uses* the product. In other industries, the customer is the same individual who makes the decision to purchase, and he or she is the same one who uses the product. This is *not* how product decisions, purchasing and utilization occurs for biomedical products. This partitioning of customer decisions is an aspect that can hamper the success of many biotechnology companies. It is vital to have a clear understanding of the three independent customers of biotechnology products and to provide a compelling value proposition to each. This can be accomplished if you understand each of their motivations and responsibilities which will then improve your product marketing success.

BUSINESS DEVELOPMENT AND PARTNERING

For biotechnology companies it seems like the need for cash is constant. Very few, if any, biotech companies have been able to raise enough capital to cover all their research, development, clinical, regulatory and manufacturing costs through to commercialization. Venture capital has provided a significant portion of the later-stage funding for many companies, but there are still requirements for larger amounts of capital at final stages of human clinical trials, and a need for a commercialization partner. For therapeutic, biologic and many medical devices, forming partnerships with large pharmaceutical companies or medical device companies can provide the needed capital and a valuable marketing partner. Therefore, it is important for the entrepreneurial team to assess who these likely future partners

may be, and to keep them apprised of your product development progress along the way. The benefits of having a strategic partner are many. In a typical partnership, the biotech company may receive up-front payments, milestone payments, fee-for-service payments and, eventually, royalties on sales. In exchange, the partner receives ownership or exclusive license and marketing rights to the biotechnology company's product. Also, this partnership event may also be, or precede, the exit event for your investors. Having a strategic commercial partner is almost essential, but keep in mind that successful deals can take at least 12 months to bring about so be sure to plan and prepare early.

PUBLIC RELATIONS FOR BIOTECHNOLOGY COMPANIES

Finding the right partner can be difficult especially when the management team usually has more priorities than it has resources. One great tool to help potential partners to find you is through Public Relations (PR), which is the art of creating, broadcasting and maintaining your message and company image with your targeted audiences.

Public relations is often overlooked by many early-stage biotechnology companies but it is a excellent tool for supporting your company objectives such as finding funding, partnerships, customers or employees, or just carrying out various business activities. One critical step in reaching a particular audience is to determine the story you want to tell about your company and products, in terms of your target audience's needs and interests. Once you have defined your positioning and key messages, these can then be tailored to specific objectives for specific audiences, and used as part of a strategic communications program that supports your corporate goals. Entrepreneurs should consider the various PR methods, including building a steady stream of news and media coverage, contributed articles, speaking platforms, and strategic use of social media. Strategically incorporating these tools will help you reach your desired audience and will help potential partners find you, along with providing visibility and credibility for your company over time.

ETHICS IN BIOTECHNOLOGY

All companies are faced with challenges, and some challenges are greater than others. Biotechnology companies may also face ethical dilemmas at some time, even in an industry where life-saving products are developed for the good of others. For small biotechnology companies, consequences can be devastating for poor decisions, and the cost and stakes are high. Challenges can arise because of competing pressures to achieve goals and accomplish results within a limited timeframe, and this could set up a climate in which a bad choice could be made and, as a consequence, ethical dilemmas can arise. We have seen the set-backs of

ImClone, the developers of the chemotherapeutic Erbitux, in 2002 when Sam Waksal their CEO was convicted of securities fraud, bank fraud, obstruction of justice, and perjury. Even in larger organizations, we have also seen instances of pharmaceutical products such as Vioxx, where the product was subsequently removed from the market due to heart attack deaths during commercialization. There were indications in human studies supporting the drug's association with increased incidents of heart attack much earlier, but they were not made public. All companies must strive to operate in a manner that would not provide reason for the public to be skeptical about its motives or its mission and purpose. Biotechnology companies will also need to operate using a commonly accepted set of business ethics that include such tenets as fairness, trust, absence of conflict-of-interest and good business practices.

In rare cases, companies may find themselves in a dilemma when no matter what action is taken, some harm will occur and there are equally strong reasons for taking either course of action. In these cases, accurate facts are vital to resolving ethical dilemmas but facts alone will not solve the problem. Ethical dilemmas require that the leader make wise choices. The choices individuals make are based upon core values. Fortunately, these instances described are rare, and the examples of dilemmas will most likely arise because of a series of, unethical or at best, poor decisions made over time, rather than one solitary decision. For a biotechnology company to have success it is vital that the leader and the entrepreneurial team possess similar core values, and that they lead and manage using these values to inspire their team to follow. By doing this, your company will improve its decision-making skills and this will exceedingly reduce the number of ethical issues that might be faced in the future.

CAREER OPPORTUNITIES IN THE LIFE SCIENCES INDUSTRY

Individuals with a life science education and background are essential to the biotechnology industry and a company's success. You should realize that having this background does not limit your career to just laboratory research and bench work. We have described a number of sectors within the biotechnology industry and within each of these sectors there are diverse career opportunities. Life science careers are not limited to biotechnology sectors either, as there are a multitude of opportunities in other industries such as those that support the biotechnology industry. A sample of career opportunities for individuals with life science backgrounds include: discovery and preclinical research, process sciences, clinical development, regulatory or medical affairs, project management, business and corporate development, marketing, sales, technical and product support, management consulting, corporate communications, operations, manufacturing, quality control, bio-IT, law, human resources and recruiting, venture capital and investment banking and careers in nonprofit organizations and in government. Whether or not you have an interest in laboratory work, business, sales, marketing or clinical studies, there are hundreds of different career options. Some of the different career paths can lead you to writing a patent, marketing a product, conducting a clinical trial or doing a business deal. It is important to realize that there are numerous opportunities to find that ideal job that matches your unique personality attributes, skills, interests and long-term goals.

For individuals with a scientific or technology background who are conducting laboratory bench work and want to transition from bench research to other vocational areas, the good news is that many scientists do transition to other careers and bring with them the depth of experience and knowledge within the science field. Be sure to pursue your interests and explore the various opportunities available. As I tell students, be sure to find the career opportunity that inspires you and the one that you would do even if you did not get paid, for that is the place where you will excel and fulfill your vocational destiny.

CONCLUSIONS

The information and examples in this book are intended to supply you the concepts and background needed to start, manage and lead a life science company or to give you a background and understanding to operate as an "intrepreneur" or team member within this amazing industry. The first goal of this book has been to equip and train future biotechnology leaders and managers to become more successful by learning from previous generations of entrepreneurs and companies who are sharing their experiences, knowledge and life lessons. Another key purpose is to educate and expand the workings within this industry to the vital service providers and partners that are essential to the success of biotechnology companies.

It would be impossible to cover in enough detail all the topics and information that are relevant to this growing biotechnology industry. However, it is our desire to provide enough information to help you become better equipped to operate, manage, lead within, or support, companies in the biotechnology industry. I hope that the material presented, along with the experiences and teachings, have given you knowledge and inspiration to pioneer new product opportunities, to lead and manage more effectively, to overcome technical, financing and regulatory challenges as you journey alongside the multitudes of individuals within this vast and growing industry. A familiar saying to some is "There is no trying, only doing". All biotechnology entrepreneurs must start with a foundational belief that their technology and product possesses great value to those in need of their treatment, test, or service. And it is through the continual "doing" rather than "trying" you will have an opportunity to make a difference in this world. Keep "doing" and don't quit.

Best wishes for your future and for your success!

Index

Note: Page numbers followed by "f," "t," and "b" denote figures, tables, and boxes, respectively.

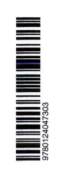